# Practical Neuropathology

# Practical Neuropathology

Editor: Josh Vaughan

AMERICAN
MEDICAL PUBLISHERS
www.americanmedicalpublishers.com

AMERICAN
MEDICAL PUBLISHERS
www.americanmedicalpublishers.com

**Cataloging-in-Publication Data**

Practical neuropathology / edited by Josh Vaughan.
p. cm.
Includes bibliographical references and index.
ISBN 978-1-63927-328-7
1. Nervous system--Diseases. 2. Nervous system--Diseases--Pathophysiology.
3. Neurology. I. Vaughan, Josh.
RC347 .P73 2022
616.8--dc23



American Medical Publishers,
41 Flatbush Avenue,
1st Floor, New York,
NY 11217, USA

ISBN 978-1-63927-328-7 (Hardback)

# Contents

# Preface

The understanding of the diseases affecting the nervous system tissue particularly the brain, viz. brain tumors, degenerative diseases, neuromuscular diseases, brain trauma, multiple sclerosis and stroke can be approached through neuropathological studies. Neuropathology is aided in this direction with small surgical biopsies and in some cases, whole-body autopsies. Another aspect of neuropathology is the analysis and examination of muscle and peripheral nerve biopsies. Muscle biopsies are performed to diagnose muscle diseases such as mitochondrial myopathy, polymyositis, etc. while peripheral nerve biopsies assess suspected cases of peripheral neuropathies that are secondary to amyloidosis and vasculitis. Epidermal nerve fiber density testing is a modern neuropathology test which is often seen as a minimally invasive replacement of the traditional sural nerve biopsy. This book discusses the fundamentals as well as modern approaches of neuropathology. It will also provide interesting topics for research which interested readers can take up. Coherent flow of topics, student-friendly language and extensive use of examples make this book an invaluable source of knowledge.

This book has been the outcome of endless efforts put in by authors and researchers on various issues and topics within the field. The book is a comprehensive collection of significant researches that are addressed in a variety of chapters. It will surely enhance the knowledge of the field among readers across the globe.

It gives us an immense pleasure to thank our researchers and authors for their efforts to submit their piece of writing before the deadlines. Finally in the end, I would like to thank my family and colleagues who have been a great source of inspiration and support.

**Editor**

# 1

# Exceptional in vivo catabolism of neurodegeneration-related aggregates

Zsolt Datki[1*], Zita Olah[1], Tibor Hortobagyi[2,3], Lilla Macsai[1], Katalin Zsuga[4], Livia Fulop[5], Zsolt Bozso[5], Bence Galik[6], Eva Acs[7,8], Angela Foldi[8], Amanda Szarvas[1] and Janos Kalman[1]

**Abstract:** Neurodegenerative diseases are linked to a systemic enzyme resistance of toxic aggregated molecules and their pathological consequences. This paper presents a unique phenomenon that *Philodina acuticornis*, a bdelloid rotifer, is able to catabolize different types of neurotoxic peptide and protein aggregates (such as beta-amyloids /Aβ/, alpha-synuclein, and prion) without suffering any damage. *P. acuticornis* is capable of using these aggregates as an exclusive energy source (i.e., as 'food', identified in the digestive system and body) in a hermetically isolated microdrop environment, increasing their survival. As regards Aβ1–42, five other bdelloid rotifer species were also found to be able to perform this phenomenon. Based on our experiments, the Aβ1–42-treated bdelloid rotifers demonstrate significantly increased survival (e.g. mean lifespan = 51 ± 2.71 days) compared to their untreated controls (e.g. mean lifespan = 14 ± 2.29 days), with similar improvements in a variety of phenotypic characteristics. To our knowledge, no other animal species have so far been reported to have a similar capability. For all other microscopic species tested, including monogonant rotifers and non-rotifers, the treatment with Aβ1–42 aggregates proved to be either toxic or simply ineffective. This paper describes and proves the existence of an unprecedented in vivo catabolic capability of neurotoxic aggregates by bdelloid rotifers, with special focus on *P. acuticornis*. Our results may provide the basis for a new preclinical perspective on therapeutic research in human neurodegenerative diseases.

**Keywords:** Alpha-synuclein, Bdelloid rotifer, Beta-amyloid, Catabolism, Lifespan, Prion

## Introduction

Neurodegenerative disorders, such as Alzheimer's disease (AD), Parkinson's disease (PD), and prion disease, could be regarded as phenotypes secondary to the progressive functional impairment of proteomes. [29, 52, 53]. The molecular basis of aging in the brain may be described as an accelerated accumulation accompanied by a decreased clearance and degradation of misfolded proteins [46]. There is a clear correlation between protein aggregation and aged-related pathologies. The intramolecular regions arranged in β-sheet conformation are highly resistant to enzymatic degradation. [32, 51] The various neurotoxic aggregates, such as those composed of beta-amyloid (Aβ), alpha-synuclein (α-Syn), and prion (normal cellular prion protein /PrPC/ and pathogenic prion protein 'scrapie' /PrPSc/), share common features, with their accumulation and aggregation facilitating neurodegeneration. The peptide and protein aggregates in neurodegenerative diseases have several characteristics in common; however, their different molecular structures and pathomechanism may lead to differences in their toxicity [38]. Therefore, investigation of aggregate degradation has emerged from a marginal area of protein chemistry to become a highly relevant field in neuropharmacological science [25]. Although the pathological role of these aggregates has been well established, at present, no universal and satisfactory method exists for their in vivo degradation as a potential therapeutic tool. Misfolded peptide and protein aggregates can be partially digested by several endogenous enzymes, such as insulin-degrading enzyme (IDE) [23], neprilysin (NEP) [16], endothelin-converting enzyme [12], angiotensin-converting enzyme [14], plasmin [47] and matrix metalloproteinases [1]; however, their presence and function is apparently insufficient in a scenario that leads to neurodegenerative disorders.

Amyloids, such as Aβs, are key molecules in aging-associated diseases, representing a starting point in the

* Correspondence: datki.zsolt@med.u-szeged.hu; datkizsolt@gmail.com
[1]Department of Psychiatry, Faculty of Medicine, University of Szeged, Kalvaria sgt. 57, Szeged H-6725, Hungary
Full list of author information is available at the end of the article

development of dementias. Therefore, their accumulation is one of the most important toxic processes during the course of cerebral Aβ-related pathologies, which is potentiated by a reduced clearance and insufficient degradation [30]. The understanding and modulation of Aβ toxicity and its metabolism might provide novel approaches in the treatment of Aβ-related dementias, including AD and cerebral amyloid angiopathy.

Physiologically, two major enzymes are predominantly implicated in the partial degradation of Aβs: NEP and IDE [6, 16]. NEP is a membrane-anchored zinc-dependent endopeptidase, being able to cleave both Aβ monomers and oligomers. The role of NEP in the pathogenesis of AD is indicated by its decreased expression in the AD brain, particularly in vulnerable regions such as the hippocampus and the midtemporal gyrus, a phenomenon associated with increased Aβ-deposition [54]. IDE, a thiol- and zinc-dependent metallopeptidase, appears to participate in the catabolism of insulin and Aβ as well, and its decreased expression was reported in the hippocampus of AD patients [55]. Although IDE mediates these processes in vivo, it still remains a question how this cytoplasmic protein can degrade extracellular Aβ aggregates in the brain. Further relevant membrane proteases involved in Aβ degradation include plasmin, cathepsin B, endothelin-converting enzyme, and certain members of matrix metalloproteinase family, which are highly tissue- and brain region-specific [2]. Potential therapeutic approaches to reduce the accumulation of harmful neurotoxic proteins include the facilitation of anti-aggregation processes or the enhancement of their clearance. As an example, β-sheet breakers bind to the central hydrophobic core of Aβ1–42 and attenuate the formation of the β-sheet structures. These molecules could destabilize the senile plaques; however, they do not provide adequate solution to the degradation and catabolism of overexpressed toxic aggregates. [40] Therefore, an ideal protective strategy against aggregate-induced neuronal damage requires more complex and practical solutions, with dual mechanisms of action targeting both the destabilization and degradation of toxic aggregates.

Treatments with different exogenous Aβ isoforms are widely used models of AD and earlier studies used various in vitro and in vivo systems to reveal their exact effects. Several studies were performed on human neuroblastoma cells [7, 36], invertebrates, rodents, and primates [13, 20, 42]; however, only a single publication aimed at describing the effects of Aβ on bdelloid rotifers, e.g. *Philodina* species [36]. This unique study by Poeggeler et al. [36] reported the treatment of rotifers with Aβ1–42 in order to test the efficacy of an antioxidant molecule (LPBNAH) against the supposed neurotoxicity of the peptide aggregates. In their in vivo studies with rotifers, the authors applied doxorubicin instead of Aβ1–42, because this toxin gave more consistent results in rotifers. In fact, the neurotoxic effect of Aβ1–42 in this model could not be proven. Our aim was to investigate this intriguing phenomenon that was only slightly touched upon in the paper of Poeggeler.

Bdelloid rotifers, as microinvertebrates, are one of the most commonly used animal models in toxicity-, aging-, and longevity-related research. These organisms are multicellular animals with well-defined anatomical characteristics, possessing a ciliated head structure, bilateral ovaries, mastax, ganglia, muscles, digestive, nervous, and secretory systems, and photosensitive, and tactile organs. [5, 15]. Due to their peculiar anatomy and physiology, these animals have outstanding advantages in terms of culturing and are rather easy to work with [44]. Rotifers are extremely resistant to environmental alterations and successfully adapt to the different types and amounts of nutrients present in their natural habitat. The natural decomposition of organic materials is a process that results in the formation of precipitates and aggregates, which represent potential nutrients for rotifers [50]. The metabolic utilization of all these available organic material resources is their special property [4].

In a prior publication, we reported the development of a unique and straightforward method [34], which enables the investigation of the effect of several different agents or impacts on various phenotypic parameters of microinvertebrates. The oil-covered microdrop technology, adopted from human in vitro fertilization, is a well-controllable construction to assess the lifespan and other features of a single isolated animal (one-housed rotifer).

In our present study, we examined the effect of various neurodegeneration-related peptide and protein aggregates under complete dietary restriction, ensuring that the individual rotifers had no other organic source to be used for gluconeogenesis. Observing an intriguing increase in survival upon treatment with aggregates, as a next step, we investigated different types of micro-entities in neurotoxic aggregate-supplemented environment. To our knowledge, this study is the first to address the in vivo catabolism of these molecules as dietary sources in microscopic animals such as rotifers. Our findings may provide a starting point to understand the possible ways of degradation of abnormally folded neurotoxins despite their aggregated state and consequent protease resistance, a subject with high potential relevance in the treatment of neurodegenerative proteinopathies.

## Materials and methods

### Materials

The Aβ1–42, Aβ1–42 [Gln22], Aβ1–40, Aβ25–35, two scrambled isoforms (Aβ1–42 S1: LKAFDIGVEYNKVGEG-FAISHGVAHLDVSMFGEIGRVDVHQA and Aβ1–42 S2:

KVKGLIDGAHIGDLVYEFMDSNSAIFREGVGAGHVHV AQVEF) were prepared in the Department of Medical Chemistry, University of Szeged, Szeged, Hungary. The peptides were synthesized on an Fmoc-Ala-Wang resin using Nα-Fmoc-protected amino acids with a CEM Liberty microwave peptide synthesizer (Matthews, NC, USA). The peptide Aβ11–42 (H-7668.1000) was purchased from Bachem (Torrance, CA, USA), whereas Aβ1–28 (A0184) and α-Syn (type E46K human; S4447) were purchased from Sigma-Aldrich (St. Louis, MO, USA). The mature part (25–244) of recombinant bovine prion protein (PrPC, AG210) was obtained from Merck Millipore (Darmstadt, Germany). EZ4U (BI-5000; Biomedica Medizinprodukte, Wien, Austria) and Calcein-AM (17,783; Sigma-Aldrich) cell viability assays were used to measure the toxicity of the aggregates. For in vivo and in vitro investigations of the different aggregates, we applied Bis-ANS (4,4′-dianilino-1,1′-binaphthyl-5,5′-disulfonic acid dipotassium salt; D4162) and Congo red (CR; C6277) dyes obtained from Sigma-Aldrich. To detect gold-tagged beta-amyloid (Au-Aβ1–42) in *P. acuticornis* with scanning electron microscopy (SEM), we used Gold(III) chloride (AuCl3 x $2H_2O$; 01216, Reanal, Budapest, Hungary) and Aβ1–42 aggregates. Distilled water (DW) was prepared in our laboratory (Millipore-type, ultrapure, demineralized DW).

### Preparation of aggregating peptides and proteins

The synthesis and characterization of the Aβ peptides were conducted as previously described by Bozso et al. [3] with minor modifications: the concentrations of the stock solutions were 1 mg/mL (DW); the aggregation time was 3 h or 3 days (25 °C, pH 3.5); the neutralization (to pH 7.5) was performed with NaOH (1 N) [17]; after 10-fold dilution with standard medium, the final (working) concentrations were 100 μg/mL. The amount of diluted cations and anions in standard medium (mg/L): $Ca^{2+}$ 31.05; $Mg^{2+}$ 17.6; $Na^+$ 0.9; $K^+$ 0.25; $Fe^{2+}$ 0.001; $HCO_3^-$ 153.097; $SO_4^-$ 3; $Cl^-$ 0.8; $F^-$ 0.02; $H_2SiO_3$ 3.3 (pH = 7.5) [41]. To prepare the PrPSc form of PrPC, the stock solution of PrPC was aggregated for 24 h at pH 2 [49, 57]. The pH of the prepared prion was also adjusted to pH 7.5 before being used to treat the rotifers.

### Collection, isolation, identification and harvesting of different animal species

To collect and isolate different microscopic species, we used the method described by Debortoli et al. [9] with minor modifications. The sampling sites were distributed within two areas of about 500 $m^2$ near Szeged (Southern Great Plain, Hungary) and Saint-George (Transylvania, Romania). Fifty patches of highly hydrated moss (with minimal soil) were collected from the northern side of trees (of the genera Acer and Platanus) and from their close environment. Briefly, the collected samples were hydrated with the standard medium in separate flasks. After identifying the species by using methods described in the literature [18, 21, 24, 33, 48] we applied species-specific information (e.g., body size in relation to age) to collect relatively young (approximately 3–5 days old) and individuals of the same size. The isolation protocol from the samples was in line with the method of Debortoli et al. [9]. However, instead of culturing; we collected and isolated these animals (using micropipette) to create monoclonal populations. After washing these groups with standard medium, we harvested as many individuals as needed ($n = 30$) for the experiments. The species collected in Hungary comprised *Philodina vorax Janson, 1893; Philodina megalotrocha Ehrenberg, 1832; Lepadella patella Müller, 1773; Lecane arcula Harring, 1914; Lecane agilis Bryce, 1892; Lecane hamata Stokes, 1896; Lecane closterocerca Schmarda, 1859; Brachionus diversicornis Daday, 1883; Brachionus calyciflorus calyciflorus Pallas, 1766; Brachionus forficula Wierzejski, 1891; Caenorhabditis elegans Maupas, 1900; Typhloplana viridata Abildgaard, 1789; Vorticella convallaria Linnaeus, 1758; Stylonychia mytilus Müller, 1773*. The species collected in Romania comprised *Mniobia russeola Zelinka, 1891; Adineta steineri Bartoŝ, 1951; Habrotrocha elusa Milne, 1916; Filinia terminalis Plate, 1886; Lindia torulosa Dujardin, 1841; Hypsibius dujardini Doyère, 1840; Centropyxis aculeata Ehrenberg, 1832*. Processes related to culturing and harvesting *Philodina acuticornis Murray, 1906* were performed (in artificial environment) as previously described by our group [34]. The animals were photographed (Nikon D5500, Nikon Corp., Kanagawa, Japan) under the light microscope (at 200× magnification; Leitz Labovert FS, Wetzlar, Germany) by taking serial images at every 5-μm intervals, yielding a total of 20–30 photographic layers per animal, which were subsequently merged into one superimposed picture (by using Photoshop CC software, Adobe Systems Inc., San Jose, CA, USA) to achieve better resolution.

### In vitro and in vivo treatment and monitoring

To test the previously described neurotoxic effects of the examined aggregates in vitro, we used a differentiated SH-SY5Y human neuroblastoma cell line (Sigma-Aldrich), with the related culturing and differentiating methods based completely on our previous works [7, 26]. Five-day-old animals (as determined by BSI) were chosen for the experiments, an age that precedes the beginning of the reproductive stage (i.e., egg production) by 2 days. Before treatment (using micropipette) of individual rotifers with aggregated molecules (0.1, 10 and 100 μg/mL), the stock solutions (1 mg/mL) were ultrasonicated (Emmi-40 HC, EMAG AG, Mörfelden-Walldorf, Germany) for 10 min at 45 kHz to achieve sterilization and homogenization.

During the in vivo experiments, the viability assay, the assessments of descriptive characteristics (such as normalized mean lifespan /NML/, body size index /BSI/, bright light disturbance /BLD/, mastax contraction frequency /MCF/, and cellular reduction capacity /CRC/), and the assembly of the experimental setup (with the oil-covered microdrop) were carried out as presented in detail previously [34].

### Detections of exo- and endogenic Aβ1–42 in *P. acuticornis*

*Optical analysis in live rotifers* (Fig. 1a-d): The juvenile (5 days old) animals were identified on the basis of their body size as read from a calibration curve previously described [34]. For the treatment (in 96-well plate; 3695, Costar, Corning Inc., USA) of preselected and 1-day starved rotifers, we used unlabelled Aβ1–42 (3 h and 3 days aggregated) as 'food' source. After 12 days the content of the wells were changed to labelled Aβ1–42, aggregated for 3 h (in vitro marked with 10 μM Bis-ANS fluorescent dye for 30 min) or 3 days (in vitro marked with 50 μM CR dye for 1 h). Applying 5 h treatment ('feeding'), we detected the optical signals (at 200× magnification) in the digestive system (stomach and intestine) of individual rotifers by an optical/fluorescence microscope (Olympus IX71, OLYMPUS, Budapest, Hungary). The representative images demonstrate the localization of Aβ1–42 in the body of rotifers compared to untreated, normally fed (600 μg/mL yeast suspension) and unfed (starved) controls (Fig. 1a-d). Unfed individuals labelled with these two dyes (control background without Aβ1–42 treatment) have no signal (photo not shown).

*Searching for endogenous Aβ1–42 in rotifers*: The immunological detection of the presence or absence of natural Aβ1–42 in *P. acuticornis* species has a central role in interpreting the relations of Aβ1–42 and rotifers. After harvesting, the animals were put into − 75 °C for 30 min in standard medium. The number of rotifers were $10^4$ per sample. The thawed animals were ultrasonicated (at 45 kHz at room temperature for 10 min). The rotifer homogenate was centrifuged (300 x g for 5 min at 24 °C) to eliminate the exoskeletons of the dead animals. The protein concentration of the supernatant was determined by the Qubit Protein Assay Kit (Q33212; Thermo Fisher Scientific, Wilmington, DE, USA) following the manufacturer's protocol. The concentration of the stock suspension was 340.54 μg/mL, which was diluted to the final protein concentrations (μg/mL) of 20, 15, 10, 5 and 1 in standard medium. Commercially available Aβ1–42-specific sandwich ELISA kits (Innotest Aβ1–42, 81,576, Fujirebio, Gent, Belgium) were used according to the manufacturer's protocol for the quantitative detection of Aβ1–42 in the diluted rotifer homogenate.

*The Au-Aβ1–42 complex detection with SEM* (Fig. 1f, g): The stock solutions of Aβ1–42 (1 mg/mL) and $AuCl_3$ (2.8 mg/mL) were prepared with DW. The 3-day-aggregated Aβ1–42 solution was mixed for 2 h with the $AuCl_3$ solution in a 1:4 M ratio, according to the number of Au-binding sites of monomeric Aβ1–42 (one methionine and three histidine residues). To remove excess Au ions, two rounds of centrifugation (25,000 x g for 10 min at 24 °C) with supernatant replacement were used. NaOH (1 N) was applied to adjust the pH to 7.5. Peptide content of the final pellet was determined by the Qubit™ Protein Assay Kit (Thermo Fisher Scientific). The middle-aged (15 days old) harvested rotifers were starved (i.e., complete food deprivation) for 2 days. After washing the rotifers in 6-well plates (containing $10^4$ adherent animals per well), each well was treated with Au-Aβ1–42 complex in a dose of 100 μg/mL for 1 day. The wells were decanted and washed twice with standard medium and after an incubation period of 6 h (the time to empty the digestive tract of the animals), the wells were washed again and the populations were fixed and dehydrated with 96% EtOH at − 75 °C for 5 min, followed by a partial rehydration with 30% EtOH at room temperature for 30 min. After fixation with 1% paraformaldehyde (for 30 min), the wells were washed twice with DW. The collected animals were transferred with pipette to the centre of a round glass coverslip (diameter: 12 mm, thickness: 0.15 mm; 89,167–106, VWR International, Houston, TX, USA), and were allowed to dry. The samples were not coated with gold. The structural integrity of the rotifer bodies was controlled with digitally recorded photographs (Nikon D5500). The selected bodies (based on their quality) were subjected to SEM (Zeiss EVO MA 10, Carl Zeiss, Oberkochen, Germany) [2]. The sample-carrier coverslip was fixed onto a stub using a double-sided carbon tape. The fine structure of the rotifers was observed and photo-documented with the SEM (Fig. 1f, g), operating at 10 kV with an 8-mm working distance, using a backscattered electron detector in variable pressure mode at 30 Pa. The white balance of SEM photographs was normalized.

### Congo red aggregation assay

The methods described by Klunk et al. [19] and Datki et al. [8] were used for these experiments. The preparation and aggregation of the peptides and proteins for the CR assay was the same as described in the in vitro and in vivo treatment protocols. A volume of 10 μL CR stock solution (0.5 mM) was added to each aggregate-containing tube (490 μL; 100 μg/mL) and these mixtures were incubated for

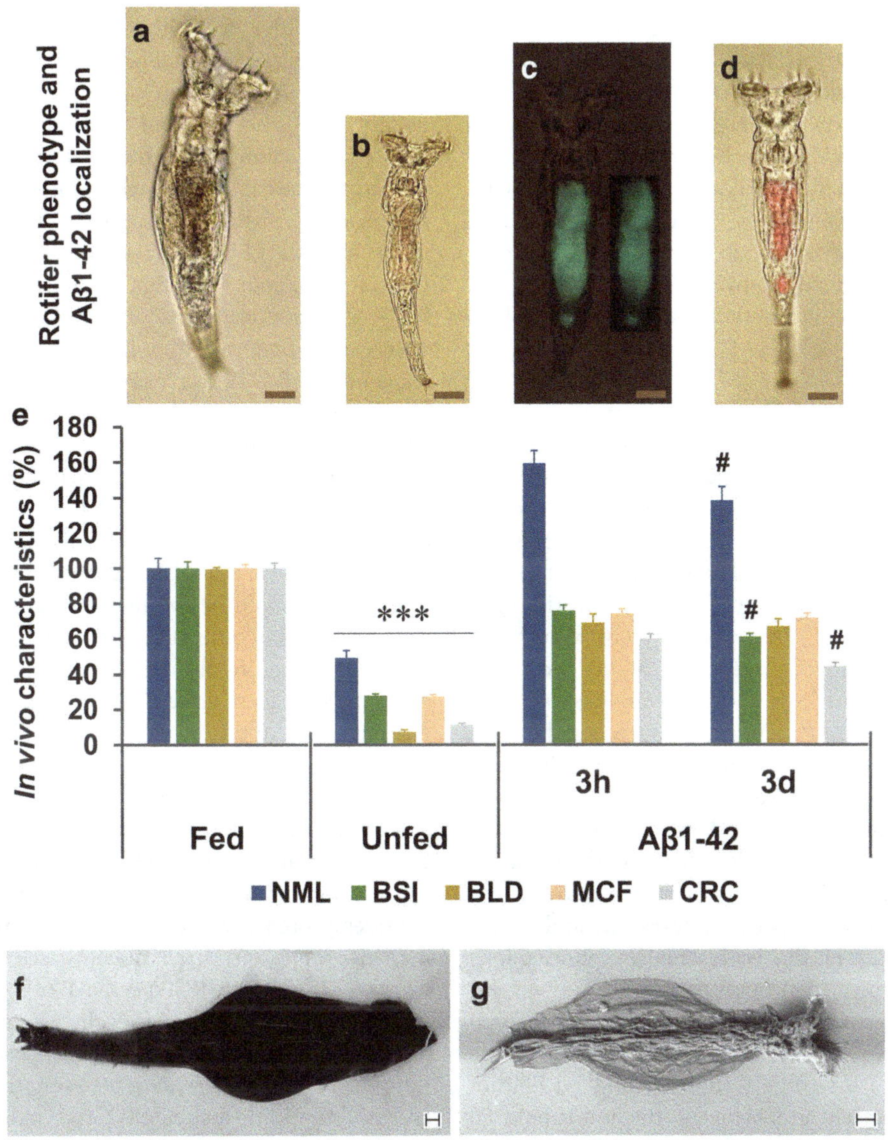


**Fig. 1** Localization and demonstration of the beneficial effects of aggregated Aβ1–42 on *P. acuticornis*. Juvenile rotifers were selected in different groups after 1-day starvation: fed (**a**; 12 days normal feeding), unfed (**b**; 12 days starvation) and Aβ1–42 treated (for 12 days). The Aβ1–42 in the digestive system (stomach and intestine) of live rotifers were visualized by fluorescent Bis-ANS (**c**; green colour in the representative photograph; 3 h = aggregated for 3 h) and absorbent Congo red (**d**; red colour in the representative photograph; 3d = aggregated for 3 days). Untreated individuals labelled with these two dyes showed no signal (not shown). **e** The normalized mean lifespan (NML) of the Aβ1–42-treated animals was significantly longer than that of their normally fed and unfed untreated controls, with a significant difference between the 3 h- and 3d–aggregated forms. Besides NML, four viability markers were measured, including body size index (BSI), bright light disturbance (BLD), mastax contraction frequency (MCF), and cellular reduction capacity (CRC). The Aβ1–42-treated rotifers performed significantly better than their unfed untreated controls and there were significant differences between the subgroups treated with two the differently aggregated forms in BSI and CRC. The concentration of Aβ1–42 was 100 μg/mL; $n = 30$ (NML), 50 (BSI), 20 (BLD), and 24 (MCF) one-housed individual rotifers per group; $n = 24$, well with normalized absorbance to rotifer number (CRC). The scale bars in the proportional representative photographs represent 20 μm (*, significant difference from the fed and Aβ1–42-treated groups; #, significant difference from the group treated with the 3 h aggregated form). The possible distribution of the exogenous Au-Aβ1–42 complex was studied in vivo with SEM in the body of *P. acuticornis*: **f** rotifer without treatment (background); **g** Au-Aβ1–42-treated rotifer. Homogenously signals of gold can be detected in Au-Aβ1–42-treated entities. Scale bar represents 10 μm

20 min at room temperature and shaken every 5 min (at 50 rpm for 10 s), followed by centrifugation at 25,000 x g for 15 min. The supernatant was carefully removed with a pipette and the sediment (pellet) was resuspended in standard medium (0.5 mL). The aggregate-bound CR content of the suspensions was measured spectrophotometrically at 540 nm with a BMG NOVOStar plate reader (BMG Labtech, Ortenberg, Germany), using a 96-well plate (Costar).

### Statistics

The error bars represent the standard error of the mean (S.E.M.). For comparative statistical analysis, the one-way ANOVA was used followed by the Bonferroni post hoc test with SPSS 23.0 software for Windows. A $p \leq 0.05$ was regarded as statistically significant, with the different levels of significance indicated as follows: $p^{\#} \leq 0.05$, $p^{**} \leq 0.01$ and $p^{***} \leq 0.001$. Kaplan-Meier curves were applied to present the survival of the groups. The GraphPad Prism 7.0b software (GraphPad Software Inc., La Jolla, CA, USA) was used for the illustration and statistical analysis (log-rank; Mantel-Cox) of survival.

## Results

To investigate the background of less 'consistent results' with Aβ1–42 toxicity in bdelloid rotifers reported by Poeggeler et al. [36], we investigated the effect of different neurodegeneration-related protein aggregates on one-housed *P. acuticornis* in an experimental setup [34] inspired by that applied human in vitro fertilization (i.e., oil-covered microdrop). This assay system allows the observation of our model organisms at an individual level. First, we examined the effect of Aβ1–42, which we predicted to be toxic to *P. acuticornis*. Surprisingly; however, treatment of the animals with Aβ1–42 resulted in a significantly longer mean lifespan (51 ± 2.71 days) than in the case of unfed (14 ± 2.29 days) and normally fed (32 ± 2.72 days) controls. To localize and demonstrate the presence of Aβ1–42 aggregates in the body of the rotifers, we used β-sheet-specific fluorescent and absorbent dyes. Animals in the representative photographs (Fig. 1a-d) are shown in proportional sizes and display the strong differences between the groups. The Fig. 1c, d show the presence of the exogenous Aβ1–42 in the digestive system of the rotifers after 'feeding' ad libitum (above is the stomach and below is the intestine). To characterize the Aβ1–42-treated *P. acuticornis* animals, we applied some previously published [34] experimental monitoring assays. The results (Fig. 1e) are evidences to the fact that this bdelloid rotifer can use the Aβ1–42 as food in isolated environment without the presence of any other organic material. The NML of groups treated with either 3 h or 3 days aggregated Aβ1–42 significantly increased compared to unfed (starved) controls. The BSI and the BLD indicated phenotypical and physiological changes of the treated animals. These characteristics were increased by 40% and 60% compared to untreated starved controls, respectively. The MCF and the CRC suggested intensified energy level as represented by neuromuscular and cellular-redox activities. These two markers were increased by 46% and 42% compared to unfed entities, correspondingly. The Aβ1–42-treated one-housed rotifer individuals performed much better in the measured parameters than their unfed controls, and they do not drastically differ from the normally fed counterparts. These results suggest that Aβ1–42 is not toxic to *P. acuticornis* and it could be used by them as an exclusive dietary source to live and develop in an hermetically-isolated environment. As the next step, we aimed at detecting the possible presence of endogenous Aβ1–42 in *P. acuticornis* species. We applied ELISA for the quantitative analysis of Aβ1–42 in the rotifer homogenates. Interestingly, our findings indicate that endogenous Aβ1–42 is practically absent in *P. acuticornis* species, an observation first reported in the literature. To localize exogenous Aβ1–42 aggregates in the live (Fig. 1a) rotifers (beyond the digestive system) we applied Au-tagged Aβ1–42 aggregates, detected with SEM (Fig. 1f, g). After fixating and drying the Au-Aβ1–42-treated and untreated animals, we monitored the possible distribution of the remnants of the potentially catabolized peptide. We found that in Au-Aβ1–42-treated animals, the signal of gold-ions could be found homogeneously everywhere in their body in contrast to the untreated ones. The only possible source of gold in the samples was the Au-Aβ1–42 complex taken up during life, as no aspecific gold coating was applied. These SEM photos are only representative.

In our study, we used eleven different peptides and proteins, with some of them being accepted as neurotoxic aggregates in neurodegenerative diseases (Fig. 2). To test and confirm the toxic effect of these aggregated peptides/proteins, we used a differentiated SH-SY5Y human neuroblastoma cell model, based on our previous works [7, 8]. The CRC-specific EZ4U and cytoplasmic enzyme activity-sensitive Calcein-AM assays were used to test the potential effect of the various aggregates. The time-dependent differences between the respective aggregate solutions incubated for 3 h and 3 days were measured with CR spectrophotometric assay [8, 19]. The data demonstrated an inverse correlation between CR-binding property and cellular toxicity of aggregates. The Aβ1–28, the scrambled isoforms Aβ1–42 S1 and S2, and PrPC demonstrated low affinity to CR and were not toxic to SH-SY5Y cells, accordingly.

In our next experiment, we examined whether the *P. acuticornis* is capable of catabolizing other neurotoxic aggregates as well (Fig. 3). To investigate the dose-dependency of the effect of Aβ1–42 on rotifers, we used three different treatment concentrations (0.1, 10, and 100 μg/mL), comparing the results with those of groups treated with equivalent concentrations of bovine serum albumin (BSA). Interestingly, we observed the highest median survival in the case of 100 μg/mL Aβ1–42 treatment (Fig. 3a). We found that almost all Aβ peptide forms tested (Aβ1–42, Aβ1–42 [Gln22], Aβ1–40, Aβ11–42, Aβ1–28, Aβ1–42 S1; Aβ1–42 S2) were favourable

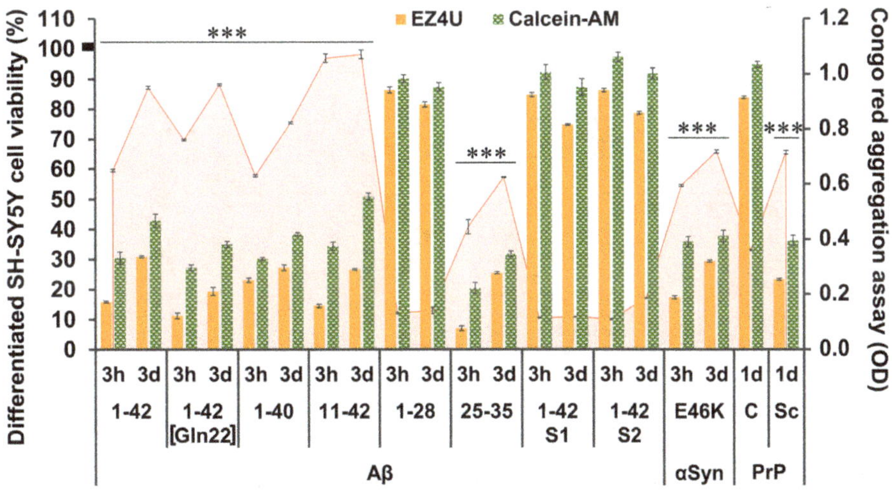


**Fig. 2** Aggregation-dependent neurotoxicity of different neurodegeneration-related peptides and proteins in cell culture. To test the previously described [10, 11] toxic effect of neurodegeneration-related aggregates, we used a differentiated SH-SY5Y human neuroblastoma cell model. The EZ4U and Calcein-AM cell viability assays were used to detect the NADH- and esterase-activity-dependent cell viability of the cultures (presented in orange and green columns of the chart, respectively). The mean viability of the untreated control wells was regarded as 100% (the S.E.M. of the mean was ±2.8%). The aggregation level of the proteins was measured with Congo red spectrophotometric assay (red line in the background of the chart). The length of incubation and aggregation time (3 h = 3 h and 3d = 3 days) influenced the toxicity of the treatment in most of the peptides and proteins tested. Significant differences ($p \leq 0.01$) were detected between the 3 h- and 3d-groups (no markers on columns) in both viability assays. Significant differences could be detected between the 3 h- and 3d-aggregated forms in the Congo red assay for all Aβs, except for Aβ11–42, Aβ1–28, Aβ1–42 S1, and Aβ1–42 S2. Alpha-synuclein (α-Syn, type E46K) and prepared 'scrapie' (PrPSc) form of prion protein also showed significant in vitro toxicity, contrasting with the ineffective normal cellular prion (PrPC). The aggregation time of the prions was 1 day (1d). Each molecule was used in 100 μg/mL concentration; $n = 8$ (for EZ4U and Calcein-AM) and 20 (for Congo red) wells per group. The error bars present the S.E.M. For statistical analysis, one-way ANOVA was used followed by the Bonferroni post hoc test, and the level of significance were $p^{***} \leq 0.001$ (*- the significant rate of deviation from the non-toxic and non-aggregated forms /Aβ 1–28, 1–42 S1, 1–42 S2, PrPC/ in both viability and Congo red assays)

nutrient sources, contrasting with Aβ25–35, which proved to be toxic to the rotifers (Fig. 3 b-c). This 'short' type of Aβ has a relatively low molecular weight (1060.27 g/mol) compared to the longer Aβ peptides (e.g., Aβ1–42), resulting in higher molar concentration (94.3 μM) in a 100-μg/mL dose. We tested this artificial Aβ aggregate in a dose of 10 μg/mL as well, and we found it also significantly toxic (NML 58 ± 5.8%; $p \leq 0.01$) when analysing the survival of the treated group compared to that of unfed controls. In addition to various Aβ isoforms, *P. acuticornis* was also able to catabolize one of the most aggregation-prone forms of α-Syn (type E46K) as well as the physiological (PrPC) and pathological forms (PrPSc) of prion protein (Fig. 3d). The Kaplan-Meier survival curves demonstrate significant differences in all treatment groups compared to the respective untreated control curve (Fig. 3a).

To investigate the universal capability of one-housed microscopic entities to catabolise Aβ1–42 (aggregated for 3 h before treatment; Fig. 4), we examined 22 species with different phylogenetic backgrounds. These species included bdelloid rotifers: *P. acuticornis, P. vorax, P. megalotrocha, M. russeola, A. steineri, H. elusa*; monogonant rotifers: *L. patella, L. arcula, L. agilis, L. hamate, L. closterocerca, B. diversicornis, B. calyciflorus calyciflorus, B. forficula, F. terminalis, L. torulosa*; non-Rotifers: *C. elegans, H. dujardini, T. viridata, V. convallaria, C. aculeate, S. mytilus.* In order to provide adequate basis for comparison, we used an NML where the mean lifespan of the unfed (starved) control group within the respective species were regarded as 100% (contrasting with the comparisons in Fig. 1 where 100% was the mean lifespan of the normally-fed group). From the all examined species, bdelloids (Fig. 4a-f) were the only ones that demonstrated significantly longer NMLs (240–290%) compared to their unfed (starved) controls (100%). As regards other species, Aβ1–42 was either toxic (Fig. 4g-o of monogonants and Fig. 4s-v of non-rotifers) or had no effect (Fig. 4p-r of both groups).

The results strongly suggest that *P. acuticornis* can catabolize various form of toxic and non-toxic Aβs, α-Syn, and prion aggregates and that the investigated bdelloid rotifer species are also able to use the neurotoxic Aβ1–42 aggregates as nutrients (ad libitum). This agent is either toxic or has no effect on the lifespan of other microinvertebrates examined, suggesting that the catabolism of aggregates with proteinopathy is an exceptional property of bdelloid rotifers (Fig. 5).

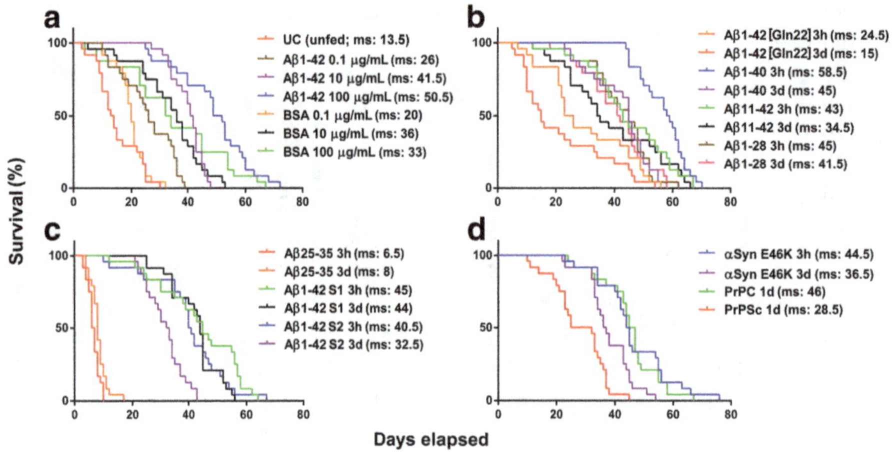


**Fig. 3** The effect of different neurodegeneration-related aggregates on the survival of *P. acuticornis*. The Kaplan-Meier curves demonstrate the survival of rotifers (n = 24 one-housed individuals per sample type; aggregation time: 3 h = 3 h and 3d = 3 days). **a** *Dose dependency*: the effect of 3 h–aggregated Aβ1–42 and BSA were tested in three different concentrations. This neurotoxic peptide as well as the non-toxic protein served as nutriments to rotifers. The survival was dose-dependent (0.1, 10, and 100 μg/mL) and was significantly higher in both type of treatments compared to the untreated control group (UC; $p < 0.001$; log-rank test). **b** *Natural Aβ isoforms:* we tested four natural variants of the Aβ peptide (1–42 [Gln22], 1–40, 11–42 and 1–28) on rotifers in two different aggregated forms (3 h and 3d). All types of natural Aβs had a positive effect on the survival of the treated rotifers compared to the UC (**a**). **c** *Artificial Aβ isoforms:* the rotifers were able to use both scrambled forms of Aβ1–42 (S1 and S2) as nutrients. As a unique exception in the series, Aβ25–35 was toxic to the rotifers, decreasing their survival as compared to the UC (**a**). All three types of artificial Aβs were measured in 3 h- and 3d–aggregated forms. **d** *Non-Aβ proteins:* the animals treated with alpha-synuclein (α-Syn, type E46K; in 3 h- and 3d–aggregated forms) and the cellular (PrPC) or 'scrapie' (PrPSc) forms of prion protein (1d = aggregated for 1 day) also showed a significantly longer lifespan compared to the UC (**a**). Each protein was used in 100 μg/mL concentration. The significance of log-rank (Mantel-Cox) test was $p < 0.0001$ in the statistical analyses in panels **b-d**. Median survival (ms) values in days are presented in the graphs. The statistical analysis of survival was performed by GraphPad Prism 7.0b

## Discussion

The formation and accumulation of aggregated proteins is a central feature of several neurodegenerative diseases. The age-related dyshomeostasis promotes the aggregation of misfolded proteins. Neurodegeneration is associated with the resistance of various aggregated peptides and proteins to enzymatic degradation [39]. In transmissible spongiform encephalopathies, the endogenous PrPC, composed of the pure protein without any presence of nucleic acid components, is converted to the pathogenic and infectious form (PrPSc) [37]. The α-Syn is a presynaptic neuronal protein, which contributes to the pathogenesis of PD via its toxic aggregation [35]. Aβ peptides can accumulate as senile plaques, which are regarded as one of the hallmark alterations in AD [2, 43].

Although the degradation of these amino acid-containing organic macromolecules has been in the focus of neuropharmaceutical science for decades, there have been no proper treatments developed or methods identified for the elimination of these toxic aggregates from living systems to date. Moreover, only a fraction of these peptides and proteins can be efficiently digested by proteolytic enzymes either in vitro or in vivo. [22]

In our study, we are the first to describe the existence of the in vivo catabolism of neurotoxic aggregates by bdelloid rotifers (e.g., *Philodina acuticornis*), as these microinvertebrates are capable of using even neurotoxic aggregates as exclusive energy and organic material sources, prolonging their lifespan. The one-housed and aggregated Aβ1–42-treated [3] *P. acuticornis* individuals have significantly longer lifespan and better viability compared to their untreated controls under complete dietary restriction in a fully isolated environment. This capability to improve (NML) or maintain (BSI, BLD, MCF and CRC) viability showed a correlation with the aggregation state (i.e., CR affinity) of Aβ1–42. The administered exogenous peptide aggregates were first localized and distributed within the digestive system of the rotifers, providing evidence of being consumed (Fig. 1). First in the literature, we demonstrated that this species have no detectable endogenous Aβ1–42 production. Since the treated *P. acuticornis* maintained its well-being, function, and redox capacity, we presume that these aggregates may serve as an obligatory energy source for gluconeogenesis in these experimental conditions. Prolonged starvation of animals causes significant physiological changes supplying glucose from amino

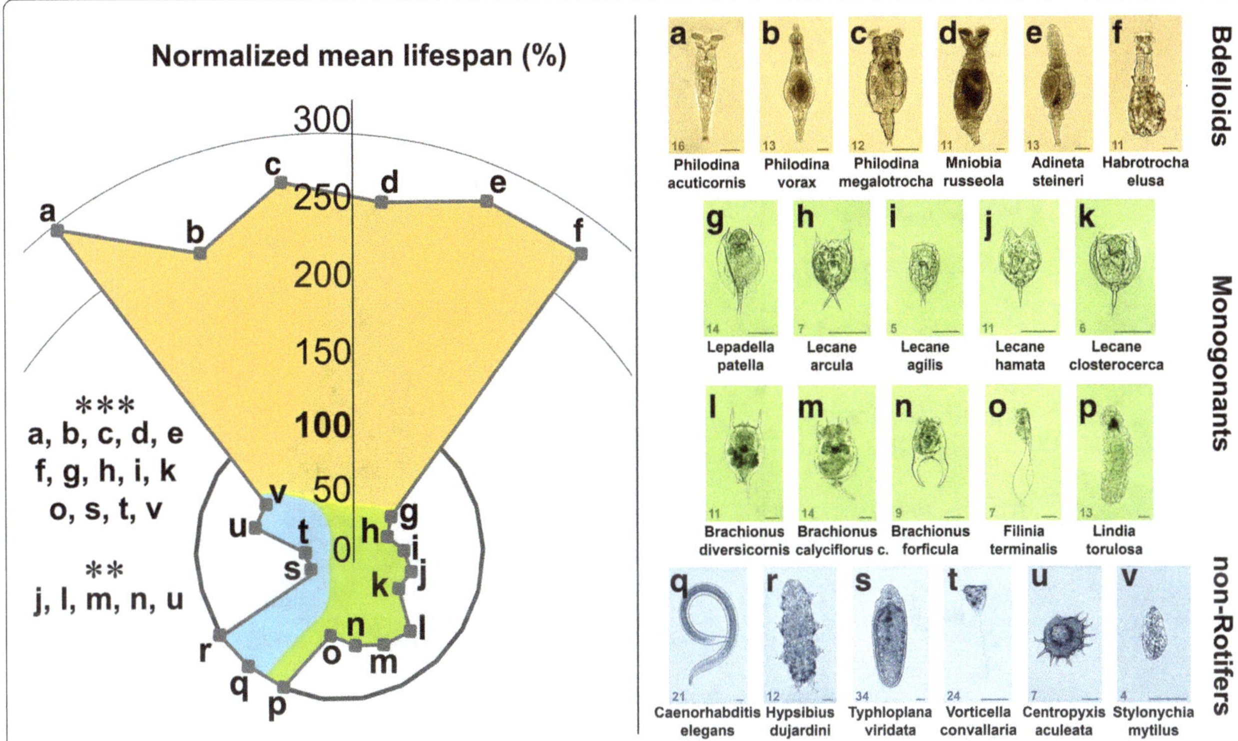


**Fig. 4** The effect of Aβ1–42 on the normalized mean lifespan of different microscopic species. To investigate the universality of the ability to catabolise 3 h-aggregated Aβ1–42 in one-housed entities, we tested 6 Bdelloids (**a-f**), 10 Monogonants (**g-p**), and 6 non-Rotifers (**q-v**). The data were normalized in percent, where the mean survival of the untreated starved group of the respective species were regarded as 100%. Only bdelloids demonstrated significantly longer lifespan compared to their starved controls after Aβ1–42 treatment. For monogonant rotifers, Aβ1–42 was either toxic (**g-o**) or ineffective (**p**) compared to their untreated controls. A similar effect was detected in non-rotifer species, where the aggregated peptide likewise either had no effect (**q** and **r**) or was toxic (**s-v**). The number in the bottom left corner of the images represents the measured real mean survival lifespan (in days) of the untreated starved control individuals. The concentration of Aβ1–42 was 100 μg/mL n = 30 one-housed individuals per group. For statistical analysis, one-way ANOVA was used followed by the Bonferroni post hoc test, and the levels of significance were $p^{**} \leq 0.01$ and $p^{***} \leq 0.001$ (*- significant difference from the untreated starved control). Scale bars represent 50 μm

acids by metabolism, including ketogenesis and gluconeogenesis. The main function of gluconeogenesis is to maintain the glucose level via its endogenous de novo production from non-carbohydrate substrates, such as glycerol, lactate, or glycogenic amino acids [28]. In rotifers, the resting eggs contain large amounts of non-carbohydrate substrates as obligatory sources for vital anabolic processes during dormancy and hatching via glyoxylate cycle and gluconeogenesis [10]. The bdelloids are extremely resistant to starvation, which has been shown to extend their lifespan [31], suggesting that the enzymatic machinery required for endogenous de novo glucose production may play a crucial role in their metabolism. On this basis, their observed survival in the presence of an aggregated peptide suggests its partial catabolism.

In order to assess the toxicity of the examined aggregated molecules, the same treatment agents were tested on differentiated SH-SY5Y neuroblastoma cell cultures [7, 26]. The α-Syn and PrPSc, similar to the known toxic Aβs, caused significant reduction of viability, in correlation with their aggregation state (CR affinity). Our in vitro results (Fig. 2) were in line with our a priori expectations and the academic literature [45, 56].

The catabolic capability of *P. acuticornis* was not limited to Aβ1–42 (Fig. 3). In the absence of any other potential dietary source, the presence of other neurodegeneration-related aggregates, such as natural (Fig. 3b) or artificial (Fig. 3c) Aβs; α-Syn, PrPC, or PrPSc (Fig. 3d) likewise prolonged the survival of the treated animals compared to the untreated (unfed) controls, except for Aβ25–35, which resulted in reduced survival. The median survival showed association with the aggregation state. These results together led us to the conclusion that this extraordinary catabolic activity is universal as regards almost any type of peptide and protein aggregates. In their natural habitat, bdelloids constantly have to cope with extreme fluctuations in nutrient availability [4]. Furthermore, their native food source includes particulate organic detritus, dead bacteria, algae, and protozoa, which offer a large variety of natural

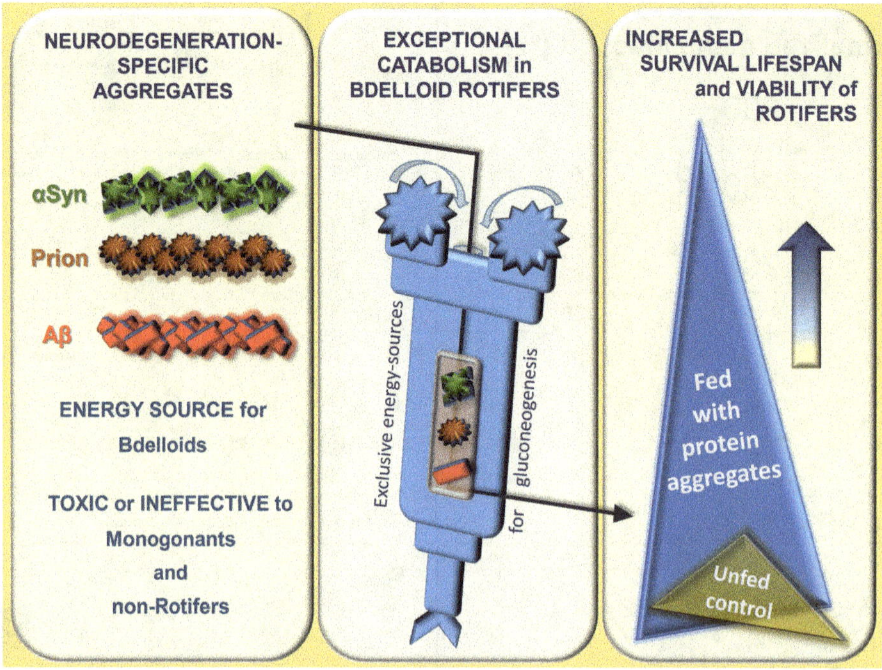


**Fig. 5** The general capability of bdelloid rotifers to catabolise neurotoxic aggregates. Neurodegeneration-related peptide and protein aggregates can be utilized as nutrients when given as the only potential energy source for starved bdelloid rotifer species. These agents proved to be either toxic or ineffective for monogonant and non-rotifer species. A currently unidentified mechanism in bdelloid rotifers is hypothesized to enable the utilization of amino acids derived from the degraded aggregates for gluconeogenesis. Compared to the unfed (starved) controls, the bdelloid rotifers treated with aggregates ('fed') demonstrate increased survival and viability

aggregates [50]. Therefore, the capability of these animals to metabolize almost every type of aggregated peptides and proteins might be an evolutionary strategy for adaption and survival.

Our aim was to describe the existence of the in vivo catabolism of neurodegeneration-related aggregates by bdelloid rotifers. The results strongly indicate that these animals can use these toxic agents as an exclusive dietary source to live and grown in an hermetically isolated environment. The available literature does not describe any other metazoan species with a similar capability. In species widely applied in the animal modelling of AD, such as *Caenorhabditis elegans, Drosophila melanogaster, Danio rerio,* or rodents, the Aβ1–42 are toxic [11, 20, 27, 41]. Based on our experiments (Fig. 4), the Aβ1–42 aggregates were also toxic or ineffective to the other microscopic entities tested (monogonant rotifers and non-rotifers). The universal capability of bdelloid rotifers to catabolise peptide and protein aggregates (including such that are known to be neurotoxic) implied that the hypothetic catabolic pathway might consist of degrading enzyme(s), their possible cofactors, and/or anti-aggregation compounds. The comprehensive identification of the molecular background of this unique phenomenon requires further analyses.

## Conclusion

In summary (Fig. 5), we present findings indicating the exceptional capability of the investigated bdelloids to catabolise neurotoxic aggregates in vivo, which is to our knowledge unprecedented in the literature regarding any multicellular animals. In our experimental system, only amino acids could be used for gluconeogenesis by the rotifers; therefore, the aggregates applied represented the only material to be catabolised in the absence of any other food source in this isolated environment. The one-housed *P. acuticornis* individuals maintain their normal phenotypic characteristics and demonstrate significant activity during their life, which require constant energy production. The prolonged lifetime in the presence of (almost all types of) Aβs, α-Syn, PrPC or PrPSc suggests the universal catabolic capability of our model species as regards a wide range of peptide or protein aggregates.

The understanding of the unique catabolic capability of bdelloid rotifers, including *P. acuticornis,* on neurotoxic aggregates in an isolated environment without any other energy source available may provide the basis of a novel therapeutic approach (identification of key molecules and metabolic pathways) in neurodegenerative proteinopathies.

### Abbreviations

α-Syn: Alpha-synuclein; AD: Alzheimer's disease; Au-Aβ: Gold-tagged beta-amyloid; Aβ: Beta-amyloid; BLD: Bright light disturbance; BSA: Bovine serum albumin; BSI: Body size index; CR: Congo red; CRC: Cellular reduction capacity; CSF: Cerebrospinal fluid; DW: Distilled water; EtOH: Ethanol; IDE: Insulin-degrading enzyme; MCF: Mastax contraction frequency; NEP: Neprilysin; NML: Normalized mean lifespan; PD: Parkinson's disease; PrPC: Normal cellular prion protein; PrPSc: Pathogenic prion protein 'scrapie'; SEM: Scanning electron microscope; UC: Untreated control

### Acknowledgements

The authors wish to thank for the contribution of Anna Szentgyorgyi MA (Institute of English and American Studies, University of Szeged, Szeged, Hungary), Ilona Hatvani, and Prof. Botond Penke. We are grateful to Levente Szalardy MD, PhD (Department of Neurology, University of Szeged) for his valuable contribution in proofreading the manuscript.

### Funding

This research was supported by the GINOP-2.3.2–15–2016-00019 grant to EA and AF.

### Authors' contributions

ZsD was the scientific advisor and together with ZO and LM designed and performed the experiments and wrote the manuscript. TH was the medical advisor and contributed with his expertise in neurodegenerative proteinopathies to our experiments. KZs identified the microscopic species. LF and ZsB synthesized and prepared the Aβ peptides. BG and ASz helped to analyze the data and carried out the statistical analysis. EA and AF took the SEM photographs. JK coordinated and obtained the resources. All authors approved the final manuscript.

### Competing interests

The authors declare that they have no competing interests.

### Author details

[1]Department of Psychiatry, Faculty of Medicine, University of Szeged, Kalvaria sgt. 57, Szeged H-6725, Hungary. [2]MTA-DE Cerebrovascular and Neurodegenerative Research Group, Department of Neuropathology, Institute of Pathology, University of Debrecen, P.O. Box 24, Debrecen H-4012, Hungary. [3]Department of Old Age Psychiatry, Institute of Psychiatry Psychology & Neuroscience, King's College London, Box PO70, De Crespigny Park, Denmark Hill, London SE5 8AF, UK. [4]Agrint Kft., Facan sor 56, Godollo H-2100, Hungary. [5]Department of Medical Chemistry, Faculty of Medicine, University of Szeged, Semmelweis u. 6, Szeged H-6725, Hungary. [6]Bioinformatics & Scientific Computing, Vienna Biocentre Core Facilities, Dr. Bohr-Gasse 3, 1030 Vienna, Austria. [7]Danube Research Institute, MTA Centre for Ecological Research, Karolina ut 29-31, Budapest H-1113, Hungary. [8]Sustainable Ecosystems Group, MTA Centre for Ecological Research, Klebelsberg Kuno u. 3, Tihany H-8237, Hungary.

### References

1. Backstrom JR, Lim GP, Cullen MJ, Tökés ZA (1996) Matrix metalloproteinase-9 (MMP-9) is synthesized in neurons of the human hippocampus and is capable of degrading the amyloid-beta peptide (1-40). J Neurosci 16:7910–7919
2. Baranello RJ, Bharani KL, Padmaraju V, Chopra N, Lahiri DK, Greig NH et al (2015) Amyloid-beta protein clearance and degradation (ABCD) pathways and their role in Alzheimer's disease. Curr Alzheimer Res 12:32–46
3. Bozso Z, Penke B, Simon D, Laczkó I, Juhász G, Szegedi V et al (2010) Controlled in situ preparation of a beta(1-42) oligomers from the isopeptide "iso-a beta(1-42)", physicochemical and biological characterization. Peptides 31:248–256. https://doi.org/10.1016/j.peptides.2009.12.001
4. Castro BB, Antunes SC, Pereira R, Soares AMVM, Gonçalves F (2005) Rotifer community structure in three shallow lakes: seasonal fluctuations and explanatory factors. Hydrobiologia 543:221–232. https://doi.org/10.1007/s10750-004-7453-8
5. Clément P, Amsellem J, Cornillac AM, Luciani A, Ricci C (1980) An ultrastructural approach to feeding behaviour in Philodina Roseola and Brachionus calycyflorus (rotifers). Hydrobiologia 73:137–141. https://doi.org/10.1007/BF00019437
6. Cook DG, Leverenz JB, McMillan PJ, Kulstad JJ, Ericksen S, Roth RA, Schellenberg GD et al (2003) Reduced hippocampal insulin-degrading enzyme in late-onset Alzheimer's disease is associated with the apolipoprotein E-epsilon4 allele. Am J Pathol 162:313–319
7. Datki Z, Juhász A, Gálfi M, Soós K, Papp R, Zádori D et al (2003) Method for measuring neurotoxicity of aggregating polypeptides with the MTT assay on differentiated neuroblastoma cells. Brain Res Bull 62:223–229
8. Datki Z, Papp R, Zádori D, Soós K, Fülöp L, Juhász A et al (2004) In vitro model of neurotoxicity of Abeta 1-42 and neuroprotection by a pentapeptide: irreversible events during the first hour. Neurobiol Dis 17:507–515. https://doi.org/10.1016/j.nbd.2004.08.007
9. Debortoli N, Li X, Eyres I, Fontaneto D, Hespeels B, Tang CQ et al (2016) Genetic exchange among Bdelloid rotifers is more likely due to horizontal gene transfer than to meiotic sex. Curr Biol 26:723–732. https://doi.org/10.1016/j.cub.2016.01.031
10. Denekamp NY, Thorne MA, Clark MS, Kube M, Reinhardt R, Lubzens E (2009) Discovering genes associated with dormancy in the monogonant rotifer Brachionus Plicatilis. BMC Genomics 10:108. https://doi.org/10.1186/1471-2164-10-108
11. Donnini S, Solito R, Cetti E, Corti F, Giachetti A, Carra S et al (2010) Abeta peptides accelerate the senescence of endothelial cells in vitro and in vivo, impairing angiogenesis. FASEB J 24:2385–2395. https://doi.org/10.1096/fj.09-146456
12. Eckman EA, Reed DK, Eckman CB (2001) Degradation of the Alzheimer's amyloid beta peptide by endothelin-converting enzyme. J Biol Chem 276:24540–24548. https://doi.org/10.1074/jbc.M007579200
13. Harkany T, Abrahám I, Timmerman W, Laskay G, Tóth B, Sasvári M et al (2000) Beta-amyloid neurotoxicity is mediated by a glutamate-triggered excitotoxic cascade in rat nucleus basalis. Eur J Neurosci 12:2735–2745
14. Hemming ML, Selkoe DJ, Farris W (2007) Effects of prolonged angiotensin-converting enzyme inhibitor treatment on amyloid beta-protein metabolism in mouse models of Alzheimer disease. Neurobiol Dis 26:273–281. https://doi.org/10.1016/j.nbd.2007.01.004
15. Hochberg R, Litvaitis MK (2000) Functional morphology of the muscles in Philodina sp. (Rotifera: Bdelloidea). Hydrobiologia 432:57–64. https://doi.org/10.1023/A:1004003509017
16. Iwata N, Tsubuki S, Takaki Y, Watanabe K, Sekiguchi M, Hosoki E et al (2000) Identification of the major Abeta1-42-degrading catabolic pathway in brain parenchyma: suppression leads to biochemical and pathological deposition. Nat Med 6:143–150. https://doi.org/10.1038/72237
17. Kalweit AN, Yang H, Colitti-Klausnitzer J, Fülöp L, Bozsó Z, Penke B et al (2015) Acute intracerebral treatment with amyloid-beta (1-42) alters the profile of neuronal oscillations that accompany LTP induction and results in impaired LTP in freely behaving rats. Front Behav Neurosci 9:103. https://doi.org/10.3389/fnbeh.2015.00103
18. Kertész K (1894) Budapest és környékének Rotatoria-Faunája. Rózsa Kálmán és Neje Print, Budapest
19. Klunk WE, Jacob RF, Mason RP (1999) Quantifying amyloid beta-peptide (Abeta) aggregation using the Congo red-Abeta (CR-abeta) spectrophotometric assay. Anal Biochem 266:66–76. https://doi.org/10.1006/abio.1998.2933
20. Kong Y, Li K, Fu T, Wan C, Zhang D, Song H et al (2016) Quercetin ameliorates Aβ toxicity in drosophila AD model by modulating cell cycle-related protein expression. Oncotarget 7:67716–67731. https://doi.org/10.18632/oncotarget.11963

21. Koste W (1978) Rotatoria - Die Radertiere Mitteleuropas. Ein Bestimmunsgwerk, begründet von Max Voigt. Überornung Monogononta. Berlin - Stuttgart. p. 285-289. doi:https://doi.org/10.1002/iroh.19800650226
22. Kuo YM, Webster S, Emmerling MR, De Lima N, Roher AE (1998) Irreversible dimerization/tetramerization and post-translational modifications inhibit proteolytic degradation of a beta peptides of Alzheimer's disease. Biochim Biophys Acta 1406:291–298
23. Kurochkin IV, Goto S (1994) Alzheimer's beta-amyloid peptide specifically interacts with and is degraded by insulin degrading enzyme. FEBS Lett 345:33–37
24. Kutikova LA (1970) Kolovratki fauna SSSR. Fauna SSSR, vol. 4. Akademia Nauk Leningrad, pp. 362-367
25. Langer F, Eisele YS, Fritschi SK, Staufenbiel M, Walker LC, Jucker M (2011) Soluble Aβ seeds are potent inducers of cerebral β-amyloid deposition. J Neurosci 31:14488–14495. https://doi.org/10.1523/JNEUROSCI.3088-11.2011
26. Li J, Liu CN, Wei N, Li XD, Liu YY, Yang R et al (2016) Protective effects of BAY 73-6691, a selective inhibitor of phosphodiesterase 9, on amyloid-β peptides-induced oxidative stress in in-vivo and in-vitro models of Alzheimer's disease. Brain Res 1642:327–335. https://doi.org/10.1016/j.brainres.2016.04.011
27. Link CD (2006) C. Elegans models of age-associated neurodegenerative diseases: lessons from transgenic worm models of Alzheimer's disease. Exp Gerontol 41:1007–1013. https://doi.org/10.1016/j.exger.2006.06.059
28. Liu P, Wang Y, Du X, Yao L, Li F, Meng Z (2015) Transcriptome analysis of thermal parthenogenesis of the domesticated silkworm. PLoS One 10: e0135215. https://doi.org/10.1371/journal.pone.0135215
29. Makin S (2016) Pathology: the prion principle. Nature 538:S13–S16. https://doi.org/10.1038/538S13a
30. Mawuenyega KG, Sigurdson W, Ovod V, Munsell L, Kasten T, Morris JC, Yarasheski KE, Bateman RJ (2010) Decreased clearance of CNS beta-amyloid in Alzheimer's disease. Science 330:1774. https://doi.org/10.1126/science.1197623
31. Marotta R, Uggetti A, Ricci C, Leasi F, Melone G (2012) Surviving starvation: changes accompanying starvation tolerance in a bdelloid rotifer. J Morphol 273:1–7. https://doi.org/10.1002/jmor.11000
32. Morell M, Bravo R, Espargaró A, Sisquella X, Avilés FX, Fernàndez-Busquets X et al (2008) Inclusion bodies: specificity in their aggregation process and amyloid-like structure. Biochim Biophys Acta 1783:1815–1825. https://doi.org/10.1016/j.bbamcr.2008.06.007
33. Nogrady T, Segers H (2002) Rotifera Vol. 6: Asplanchnidae, Gastropodidae, Lindiidae, Microcodidae, Synchaetidae, Trocoshphaeridae and Filinia. In: H.J. Dumont ed.: guides to the identification of the microinvertebrates of the continental waters of the world. Leiden. p. 59-79
34. Olah Z, Bush AI, Aleksza D, Galik B, Ivitz E, Macsai L et al (2017) Novel in vivo experimental viability assays with high sensitivity and throughput capacity using a bdelloid rotifer. Ecotoxicol Environ Saf 144:115–122. https://doi.org/10.1016/j.ecoenv.2017.06.005
35. Peelaerts W, Bousset L, Van der Perren A, Moskalyuk A, Pulizzi R, Giugliano M et al (2015) α-Synuclein strains cause distinct synucleinopathies after local and systemic administration. Nature 522:340–344. https://doi.org/10.1038/nature14547
36. Poeggeler B, Durand G, Polidori A, Pappolla MA, Vega-Naredo I, Coto-Montes A et al (2005) Mitochondrial medicine: neuroprotection and life extension by the new amphiphilic nitrone LPBNAH acting as a highly potent antioxidant agent. J Neurochem 95:962–973. https://doi.org/10.1111/j.1471-4159.2005.03425.x
37. Prusiner SB (1991) Molecular biology of prion diseases. Science 252:1515–1522
38. Riek R, Eisenberg DS (2016) The activities of amyloids from a structural perspective. Nature 539:227–235. https://doi.org/10.1038/nature20416
39. Saido T, Leissring MA (2012) Proteolytic degradation of amyloid β-protein. Cold Spring Harb Perspect Med 2:a006379. https://doi.org/10.1101/cshperspect.a006379
40. Salahuddin P, Fatima MT, Abdelhameed AS, Nusrat S, Khan RH (2016) Structure of amyloid oligomers and their mechanisms of toxicities: targeting amyloid oligomers using novel therapeutic approaches. Eur J Med Chem 114:41–58. https://doi.org/10.1016/j.ejmech.2016.02.065
41. Sasaguri H, Nilsson P, Hashimoto S, Nagata K, Saito T, De Strooper B et al (2017) APP mouse models for Alzheimer's disease preclinical studies. EMBO J 36:2473–2487. https://doi.org/10.15252/embj.201797397
42. Sharma N, Khurana N, Muthuraman A (2017) Lower vertebrate and invertebrate models of Alzheimer's disease - a review. Eur J Pharmacol S0014-2999:30603-9. https://doi.org/10.1016/j.ejphar.2017.09.017
43. Selkoe DJ, Abraham CR (1986) Isolation of paired helical filaments and amyloid fibers from human brain. Methods Enzymol 134:388–404
44. Snell TW (2014) Rotifers as models for the biology of aging. Int Rev Hydrobiol 99:84–95. https://doi.org/10.1080/07924259.2014.925516
45. Song J, Kim BC, Nguyen DT, Samidurai M, Choi SM (2017) Levodopa (L-DOPA) attenuates endoplasmic reticulum stress response and cell death signaling through DRD2 in SH-SY5Y neuronal cells under α-synuclein-induced toxicity. Neuroscience 358:336–348. https://doi.org/10.1016/j.neuroscience.2017.06.060
46. Tomita T (2017) Aberrant proteolytic processing and therapeutic strategies in Alzheimer disease. Adv Biol Regul 64:33–38. https://doi.org/10.1016/j.jbior.2017.01.001
47. Tucker HM, Kihiko M, Caldwell JN, Wright S, Kawarabayashi T, Price D et al (2000) The plasmin system is induced by and degrades amyloid-beta aggregates. J Neurosci 20:3937–3946
48. Varga L (1966) Rotifers I. Hungarian Academy of Sciences, Budapest
49. Vila-Viçosa D, Campos SR, Baptista AM, Machuqueiro M (2012) Reversibility of prion misfolding: insights from constant-pH molecular dynamics simulations. J Phys Chem B 116:8812–8821. https://doi.org/10.1021/jp3034837
50. Wallace RL, Snell TW (2010) Rotifera, Chapter 8 In: Thorp JH and Covich AP (Eds), Ecology and classification of North American freshwater invertebrates Oxford: Elsevier, p 173–235
51. Wang L, Maji SK, Sawaya MR, Eisenberg D, Riek R (2008) Bacterial inclusion bodies contain amyloid-like structure. PLoS Biol 6:e195. https://doi.org/10.1371/journal.pbio.0060195
52. Wildburger NC, Esparza TJ, LeDuc RD, Fellers RT, Thomas PM, Cairns NJ et al (2017) Diversity of amyloid-beta Proteoforms in the Alzheimer's disease brain. Sci Rep 7:9520. https://doi.org/10.1038/s41598-017-10422-x
53. Wyss-Coray T (2016) Ageing, neurodegeneration and brain rejuvenation. Nature 539:180–186. https://doi.org/10.1038/nature20411
54. Yasojima K, Akiyama H, McGeer EG, McGeer PL (2001) Reduced neprilysin in high plaque areas of Alzheimer brain: a possible relationship to deficient degradation of beta-amyloid peptide. Neurosci Lett 297:97–100
55. Zhao Z, Xiang Z, Haroutunian V, Buxbaum JD, Stetka B, Pasinetti GM (2007) Insulin degrading enzyme activity selectively decreases in the hippocampal formation of cases at high risk to develop Alzheimer's disease. Neurobiol Aging 28:824–830. https://doi.org/10.1016/j.neurobiolaging.2006.05.001
56. Zhao C, Wang X, He L, Zhu D, Wang B, Du W (2014) Influence of gold-bipyridyl derivants on aggregation and disaggregation of the prion neuropeptide PrP106-126. Metallomics 6:2117–2125. https://doi.org/10.1039/c4mt00219a
57. Zhou GP, Huang RB (2013) The pH-triggered conversion of the PrP(c) to PrP(sc.) Curr Top Med Chem 13:1152–1163

2

# Different tau species lead to heterogeneous tau pathology propagation and misfolding

Simon Dujardin[1,2,3], Séverine Bégard[1†], Raphaëlle Caillierez[1†], Cédrick Lachaud[1†], Sébastien Carrier[1], Sarah Lieger[1], Jose A. Gonzalez[2,3], Vincent Deramecourt[1], Nicole Déglon[4], Claude-Alain Maurage[1], Matthew P. Frosch[2,3], Bradley T. Hyman[2,3], Morvane Colin[1*†] and Luc Buée[1*†]

**Abstract**

Tauopathies are a heterogeneous group of pathologies characterized by tau aggregation inside neurons. Most of them are sporadic but certain tauopathies rely on tau gene (MAPT) mutations. They particularly differ from one to another by their different neuropathological signatures e.g. lesion shapes, regions affected and molecular composition of aggregates. Six isoforms of tau exist, but they do not all co-aggregate in each tauopathy but rather have a unique signature for each one. In some tauopathies such as Alzheimer's disease (AD), tau protein aggregation follows stereotypical anatomical stages. Recent data suggest that this progression is due to an active process of tau protein propagation from neuron-to-neuron. We wondered how tau isoforms or mutations could influence the process of tau aggregation and tau propagation. In human neuropathological material, we found that MAPT mutations induce a faster misfolding compared to tau found in sporadic AD patients. In the rat brain, we observed cell-to-cell transfer of non-pathological tau species irrespective of the tested isoform or presence of a mutation. By contrast, we found that the species of tau impact the propagation of tau pathology markers such as hyperphosphorylation and misfolding. Indeed, misfolding and hyperphosphorylated tau proteins do not spread at the same rate when tau is mutated, or the isoform composition is modified. These results clearly argue for the existence of specific folding properties of tau depending on isoforms or mutations impacting the behavior of pathological tau species.

**Keywords:** Tau, Propagation, Isoforms, Misfolding, Alzheimer's disease, Heterogeneity

## Introduction

Tau is a microtubule-associated protein mainly found in the axonal part of neurons. Resulting from an alternative splicing mechanism, six major isoforms of tau coexist in the human brain with the presence of either 3 or 4 repeated sequences (named below as 3R-tau or 4R-tau) known as the microtubule-binding regions [8, 28]. The hyperphosphorylation and deposition of tau proteins in insoluble aggregates inside neurons are a hallmark of around 20 pathologies called tauopathies including the well-known Alzheimer's disease (AD) [8, 25]. These aggregates progressively invade the whole neuron and form specific intraneuronal lesions named neurofibrillary degeneration (NFD) ultimately leading to cell death. However, the kinetics of this pathological cascade as well as the exact factors leading to cell death are still poorly understood [61]. Furthermore, even if tauopathies share common features, this group of pathologies is very heterogeneous with a vast variety of clinical presentations including fronto-temporal dementias (e.g. Pick's disease (PiD)), movement disorders/parkinsonism (e.g. progressive supranuclear palsy (PSP)) or Alzheimer's type dementia such as AD or argyrophilic grain disease (AGD) [39]. This heterogeneity may be explained by strong histopathologic differences and differential laminar and regional brain distribution but also by molecular variations such as isoform composition and posttranslational modifications. For example, in AD, the six isoforms of tau co-aggregate, in contrast to pathologies like PSP or AGD, in which only the 4R-tau isoforms aggregate, and

* Correspondence: morvane.colin@inserm.fr; luc.buee@inserm.fr
†Séverine Bégard, Raphaëlle Caillierez and Cédrick Lachaud contributed equally to this work.
†Morvane Colin and Luc Buée contributed equally to this work.
[1]Univ. Lille, Inserm, CHU-Lille, UMR-S 1172, Alzheimer & Tauopathies, School of Medicine, 1 rue Polonovski, 59045 Lille, France
Full list of author information is available at the end of the article

Pick's disease, where the aggregates are only comprised of 3R-tau [39]. Adding additional complexity, around 50 autosomal dominant mutations in the tau gene (MAPT) have been reported to promote strong tau aggregation and clinically lead to dramatic fronto-temporal lobar degeneration (formerly FTDP-17 now referred to as genetic FTLD-Tau) [21, 23].

Likely due to the molecular heterogeneity of tauopathies, different morphologies of lesions can be observed, with mainly flame-shaped neurofibrillary tangles in AD, argyrophilic grains and/or glial lesions in AGD or PSP and Pick bodies in Pick's disease [39]. These lesions affect different part of the brain and the pathology evolves differently. Thus, histopathological studies in some sporadic tauopathies such as AD [6, 15, 24], PSP [66, 69] and AGD [55] show that, specifically for each disease, tau lesions appear progressively and hierarchically in the brain along anatomical connections. The mechanisms underlying such evolution had remained unexplained for many years and are still poorly understood [60]. Increasing evidence both in vitro and in vivo, support the ideas that the evolution across brain areas is the result of the active propagation of NFD within the brain. Indeed, our group and others recently showed that tau assemblies are transferred from cell-to-cell and, by being taken up by a second cell, seed the aggregation of endogenous tau leading to the propagation of tau lesions in the brain [13, 14, 19, 57, 65] reviewed in [48].

Interestingly, in these studies, 4R-tau human constructs were always used to observe tau propagation/seeding. In human tauopathies, the spatio-temporal evolution of NFD was also only reported in three sporadic tauopathies in which the 4R-tau isoforms aggregate (AD, AGD and PSP). Conversely, it is still controversial whether 3R-tau can propagate in genetic FTLD-Tau (mutant tau) or Pick's disease (3R-tau) [33].

Phosphorylation plays essential roles in tau physiology particularly by controlling its binding with microtubules [5, 49]. In AD, tau hyperphosphorylation leads to the misfolding of tau protein and its oligomerization in highly structured, insoluble aggregates [3]. Nowadays, this hypothesis has been widened to all human tauopathies. Tau misfolding is thought to be responsible for the seeding propensity of tau that ultimately becomes aggregated and insoluble [45]. This sequence of event is however not yet completely clear and some intriguing data obtained with a transgenic mouse model overexpressing mutant tau strongly suggest that the appearance of the epitopes of misfolding (particularly with the antibodies Alz50/MC1) precede hyperphosphorylation (particularly with the antibody AT8) [29]. Interestingly, in genetic FTLD-Tau (mutant tau), tau proteins show conformational changes even without hyperphosphorylation [35, 46, 67, 68]. In the present study, we re-explore these issues in human neuropathological samples and experimentally in a rat model, to understand how isoforms and mutations influence tau propensity to misfold and propagate from neuron-to-neuron.

We analyzed NFD by immunohistochemistry in different brains areas from genetic FTLD-Tau (3 different mutations) and AD patients (at different Braak stages) using either conformation-dependent or phospho-dependent antibodies. Conformational changes might occur before hyperphosphorylation only in genetic FTLD-Tau patients and not in AD. To further explore these observations, we used a rat model of tauopathies [10, 19], to examine the pathophysiological propagation of tau using different species, 3R or 4R, mutant or wild-type (WT). As previously described, 4R-tau propagates physiologically and pathologically from neuron-to-neuron to distant brain areas [19]. Interestingly, when mutant or 3R-tau constructs are used, the transfer of non-pathological species of tau remains functional but tau pathology does not spread and stays in the vicinity of the initiation site. Early conformational changes as indicated by the MC-1 immunoreactivity might facilitate aggregation and neurodegeneration rather than propagation. Therefore, our results suggest that different tau species may encounter different misfolding processes that could explain such differences.

## Materials & methods

### Viral vectors

The procedures to produce the lentiviral vectors (LVs) batches have been previously described [10, 16, 31]. Briefly, the packaging construct pCMVΔR8.92, the pRSV-Rev, pMD.2G and the human Tau cDNA (htau1N4R, htau1N4R-P301L, htau1N4R-P332S, htau1N3R or htau1N3R-P332S) were co-transfected in human 293T cells and lentiviral vectors particles were concentrated from successive ultracentrifugation of the culture medium 48 h later.

### Animals

Wistar male rats were purchased from Janvier Laboratories and housed in a temperature-controlled room maintained on a 12 h day/night cycle with food and water provided ad libitum. Animal experiments were performed in compliance with and with the approval of the local ethics committee (agreement 2015101320441671, 2016–2021), standards for the care and use of laboratory animals, and the French and European Community guidelines as well as the Massachusetts General Hospital's Institutional Animal Care and Use Committee.

### Stereotaxic injections, cerebro-spinal (CSF) and interstitial fluids (ISF) sampling and sacrifice procedures

Rats were housed and stereotactically injected with PBS or lentiviral vectors (LVs) (Coordinates from bregma:

Anteroposterior − 5.3 mm, Mediolateral +/− 6.2 mm, Dorsoventral − 7 and -6 mm; for detailed procedures see [19]) encoding either htau1N4R (*n* = 9 for histology, *n* = 3 for RNA extraction), htau1N4R-P301L (*n* = 5 for histology, n = 3 for RNA extraction), htau1N4R-P332S (*n* = 6 for histology, *n* = 3 for RNA extraction), htau1N3R (*n* = 8 for histology, n = 3 for RNA extraction) or htau1N3R-P332S (n = 5 for histology, n = 3 for RNA extraction). The negative control consists in injection of the vehicle (PBS, 1% *v*/*w* BSA; n = 3 for histology, n = 3 for RNA extraction). For histology analysis, eight months post-injection, animals were deeply anesthetized (pentobarbital 50 mg/kg) and transcardially perfused first with cold 0.9% NaCl followed by cold 4% PFA for 20 min. The brains were immediately removed, fixed overnight in 4% PFA, placed in 20% sucrose for 24 h and frozen until further use. Free-floating coronal cryostat sections (40 μm thickness) were used for immunohistochemical analysis. For RNA extraction, 2 weeks post-injection, were deeply anesthetised (pentobarbital 50 mg/kg). Brains were dissected, and 1-mm-thick coronal sections were generated using an acrylic rat brain matrix (Electron Microscopy Sciences). The sections were immediately frozen on dry ice and stored at − 80 °C until further use.

### Immunohistochemistry

For rats, immunohistochemistry procedures were previously described [19]. Briefly, sections from the entire brain were washed in PBS-0.2% Triton X-100 and treated for 30 min with $H_2O_2$ (0.3%). Non-specific binding was blocked using goat serum (1:100 in PBS, Vector) for 60 min. Sections were incubated overnight at 4 °C with the monoclonal antibodies AT8 (Thermo Scientific; MN1020–1:400; phosphorylated residues 202, 205 and 208 of tau) [42], ADx-215 [10, 54] (1:10,000; human specific total tau) or MC1/Alz50 (kind gifts from Dr. Peter Davies – 1:10,000; misfolded tau) in PBS-0.2% Triton X-100. After several washes, labelling was amplified by incubation with an anti-mouse biotinylated IgG (1:400 in PBS-0.2% Triton X-100, Vector) for 60 min followed by the application of the ABC kit (1:400 in PBS, Vector) prior to visualization with 0.5 mg/ml DAB (Vector) in Tris-HCl 50 mmol/L, pH 7.6, containing 0.075% $H_2O_2$. Brain sections were counter-stained in a cresyl violet solution (0.5%) and mounted with Vectamount (Vector) for microscopic analysis.

For human sections, 9 μm thick paraffin-embedded sections of hippocampus, temporal cortex and visual cortex of 10 human cases (Table 1) were cut using a microtome and placed on glass slides. Slides were incubated at 55 °C for 4 h before being immerged in successive 8 min baths of xylene twice, EtOH 100% twice, EtOH 95%, EtOH 70%, EtOH 50% and PBS three times. Slides were then incubated in boiling citrate buffer (citric acid anhydrous 10 mM, Tween20 0.05%, pH = 6) in a microwave at low power for 20 min. Slides were immerged in Tris-Buffered Saline (TBS) with 0.5% triton X-100 for 30 min followed by blocking with TBS, 10% Normal Goat Serum for 1 h. Slides were incubated overnight at 4 °C with primary antibodies (Alz50, kind gift of Dr. Peter Davis: 1/50 and AT8 1/400) in TBS, 5% NGS, 0.05% Triton X-100. Slides were washed 4 times with TBS and then incubated with secondary antibodies (anti-mouse IgM 568 and anti-mouse IgG 488 1/400, Invitrogen) diluted in TBS, 5% NGS. Slides were washed 4 times with TBS and counterstained with Sudan black (0.1% in 70% EtOH, filtered) for 20 min. Slides were washed 4 times with TBS and coversliped with Fluoromount G with Dapi (Thermo Fisher Scientific). Slides were scanned using an Olympus VS-120 slide scanner and then 100% of neurons were counted using the cellSens software. All human tissues come from the Lille Neurobank and the Massachusetts Alzheimer's Disease Research center and written consent forms have been

**Table 1** Human case demographics

| Case | Age at death | Sex (M/F) | PMI (hours) | Neuropathology diagnosis | Braak stage (if applicable) | MAPT mutation (if applicable) | Neurobank |
|---|---|---|---|---|---|---|---|
| 1 | 70 | M | 12 | genetic FTLD-Tau | N/A | P301L | Massachusetts ADRC |
| 2 | 56 | M | 6 | genetic FTLD-Tau | N/A | P301L | Massachusetts ADRC |
| 3 | 85 | F | 20 | genetic FTLD-Tau | N/A | P332S | Lille Neurobank |
| 4 | 33 | M | 33 | genetic FTLD-Tau | N/A | G389R | Massachusetts ADRC |
| 5 | > 90 | F | 8 | Control | I | N/A | Massachusetts ADRC |
| 6 | 68 | M | 27 | Control | I | N/A | Massachusetts ADRC |
| 7 | 63 | M | 16 | AD | IV | N/A | Massachusetts ADRC |
| 8 | 69 | M | 6 | AD | IV | N/A | Massachusetts ADRC |
| 9 | 68 | M | 14 | AD | VI | N/A | Massachusetts ADRC |
| 10 | 69 | F | 4 | AD | VI | N/A | Massachusetts ADRC |

*M* Male, *F* Female, *PMI* Post Mortem interval, *genetic FTLD-Tau* genetic FrontoTemporal Lobar Dementia-Tau, *AD* Alzheimer's Disease, *N/A* Non-Applicable obtained accordingly to the local legislations and ethical committees. Human brains extracts were obtained from the Massachusetts Alzheimer's Disease Research Center (grant number P50 AG005134, under IRB protocol 1999P003693) and the Lille Neurobank (CRB/CIC1403 Biobank, BB-0033-00030, agreement DC-2008-642) fulfilling criteria of the local laws and regulations on biological resources with donor consent, data protection and ethical committee review.

### RNA extraction from brain sections and RT-PCR/PCR

The brain slices were lysed, and total RNA was extracted using the RNeasy Lipid Tissue kit (Qiagen) according to the manufacturer's instructions and adjusted to 1 µg/mL. RNA were retro-transcripted using the 'High-capacity' cDNA reverse transcription kit (Applied Biosystems); cDNA was generated after reverse transcription of 1 µg of RNA with 4 mM of dNTPs, 10X random primers, 1 units/ µl of RNAse inhibitor, 1.25 ng/µl of oligo dT, 2.5 units/µl of MultiScribe reverse transcriptase. Real time PCR was then performed using the 'Taqman gene expression Master Mix' (Thermofisher) containing probe against MAPT (ref probe: Hs00902194_m1). Results were normalized to 18S transcripts (ref probe: 4308329). Reactions and data analysis were carried out with a StepOnePlus thermocycler (Applied Biosystems).

### Statistical assays

The *P* values have been determined using one-way ANOVA tests and a Tukey post-hoc test or a Pearson's Chi-squared test with Yates' continuity correction as indicated in the figure legend. Differences were considered to be statistically significant if $p < 0.05$.

## Results

### Differential misfolding/hyperphosphorylation profile in human MAPT mutant carriers compared to sporadic AD

We hypothesized that the mechanisms of tau deposition are different in sporadic tauopathies than when a mutation of MAPT gene is present. Therefore, we investigated the presence of tau misfolding and hyperphosphorylation epitopes in human brain samples. We selected six Alzheimer's disease patients (two Braak I, two Braak IV, two Braak VI) and 4 patients with Fronto-temporal dementia associated with a mutation of MAPT gene (two P301L, one P332S and one G389R). We stained brain sections from three different regions following the Braak stages: hippocampus, temporal cortex and visual cortex with AT8 antibody for tau hyperphosphorylation and Alz50 for tau misfolding. Three different phenotypes can be observed: neurons positive for both Alz50 and AT8 (Fig. 1a-c, arrows), neurons positive only for AT8 (Fig. 1a-c, arrowheads) and, more rarely, neurons positive only for Alz50 (Fig. 1a, star). We quantified in each case the number of neurons in each category. We counted a total number of 27,214 neurons for the AD cases and 15,460 for the mutant cases. Most of the neurons were positive both for tau misfolding and hyperphosphorylation in all cases (AD: $n = 17,588$, mutants $n = 12,516$ Fig. 1d, Additional file 1: Figure S1 and Additional file 2: Table S1). The number of neurons with only tau hyperphosphorylation was also prominent most of the time (AD: n = 17,588, mutants $n = 2731$ Fig. 1d, Additional file 1: Figure S1 and Additional file 2: Table S1). More interestingly, we found significantly more Alz50 positive-only neurons (213) in mutants compared to only 4 in AD cases (only in the visual cortex of Braak VI cases, Fig. 1d, Additional file 1: Figure S1 and Additional file 2: Table S1). Distributions of frequencies of both Alz50-only or AT8-only neurons were compared in mutant versus AD using a Pearson's Chi-squared test with Yates' continuity correction both globally (all regions pooled) and in the hippocampus. Interestingly, and taking into account the limitations of statistical analysis on such heterogenous cohort with a small number of cases, there is a significant link between having a mutation and having Alz50-only positive neurons both overall ($p < .001$; $chi^2 = 391$) and in the hippocampus ($p < .001$; $chi^2 = 656$). There is also a significant link between having a mutation and having AT8-only positive neurons overall ($p < .001$; $chi^2 = 171$) but not in the hippocampus ($p = 0.43$; $chi^2 = .64$). These results suggest that in AD, hyperphosphorylation precedes or accompanies misfolding in a large majority of neurons. By contrast, when the MAPT gene is mutated, misfolding seems to precede hyperphosphorylation in a small portion of neurons arguing for folding differences of mutant tau proteins.

### Cell-to-cell transfer of all tau species

We observe in human brains that hyperphosphorylation seems to appear first in sporadic cases such as AD patients but appears after misfolding in genetic FTLD-Tau. We next tested this hypothesis in an animal model. We described, in a previous study, the transfer of human tau proteins from the rat hippocampus to different distant secondary regions including limbic or olfactive regions following the injection of LVs encoding human wild-type 4R-tau [19]. Using this model of tau propagation, we wanted to assess whether different tau species (mutant tau and 3R-tau) act in a similar manner and also propagates from neuron-to-neuron. Different cohorts of Wistar male rats were bilaterally injected into the CA1 layer of the hippocampus with LVs encoding the human 3R-tau or 4R-tau either mutant or WT. We selected two different mutations: the widely used P301L only present on 4R-tau isoforms and the mutation P332S present on all isoforms [16] resulting in 5 different groups of animals referred above as 3R-tau, P332S-3R-tau, 4R-tau,

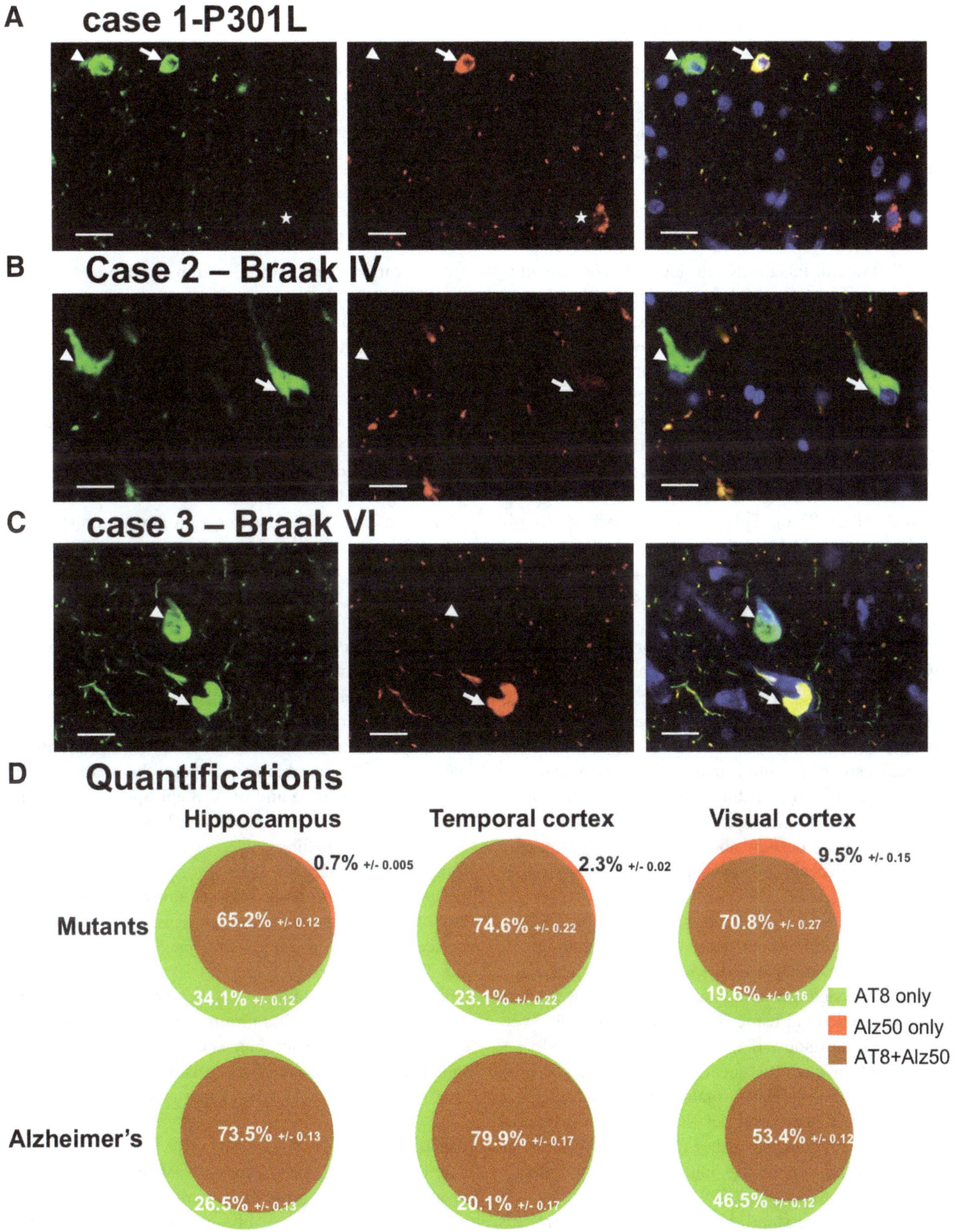


**Fig. 1** (See legend on next page.)

(See figure on previous page.)

**Fig. 1** Tau misfolding and hyperphosphorylation in human brains with AD and genetic FTLD-Tau. (**a, b** and **c**) human brain sections from a genetic FTLD-Tau case (**a**), a Braak IV AD case (**b**) and a Braak VI AD case (**c**) stained with AT8 (green), Alz50 (red) and Dapi (blue) showing neurons Alz50 and AT8 positive (arrows), neurons only AT8 positive (arrowhead) and neurons only Alz50 positive (star). Scale bars represent 20 μm (**d**) Quantification of the percentage of neurons single or double positive for Alz50 and AT8 in MAPT mutants ($n = 4$, top panels) or AD cases ($n = 6$, low panels) in hippocampus (left), temporal cortex (middle) and visual cortex (right). The percentages for each category: double positive (brown), AT8 only (green) and Alz50 only (red) are indicated along with standard deviations. Statistical test used: Pearson's Chi-squared test with Yates' continuity correction was used to assess the distribution of Alz50-only neurons and AT8-only neurons in mutant versus AD cases. The presence of Alz50-only positive neurons was significantly linked to the presence of a MAPT mutation both taking into account all regions ($p < .001$; $chi^2 = 391$) and in the hippocampus ($p < .001$; $chi^2 = 656$). The presence of AT8-only positive neurons could only be linked with the presence of a mutation taking into account all regions ($p < .001$; $chi^2 = 171$)

P301L-4R-tau and P332S-4R-tau (Fig. 2a). We stained by immunohistochemistry the brain sections with a human specific N-terminal tau antibody (ADx215) in order to properly discriminate the exogenous over-expressed tau from the endogenous tau. With similar level of expression (Additional file 3: Figure S2) and no observable retrograde transfer of the viral vectors [19], 8 months post-injection, tau proteins can be detected in cell bodies in various long-distance regions such as limbic areas, cortical areas or olfactory area for all the tested groups of animals (Figs. 2b-c). This transfer is particularly observable in the granular cell layer of the olfactory bulb more than 10 mm away from the injection site (Fig. 2c) and in cortical caudal regions situated 3 mm behind the injection (Fig. 2d). These data clearly indicate that all species of tau, regardless of being 3R or 4R-tau, mutants or WT, transfer from neuron-to-neuron.

### Tau species-dependent differential propagation of tau pathology

We previously highlighted major differences between WT 4R-tau and P301L-4R-tau regarding hyperphosphorylation, misfolding and aggregation in this rat model [19]. The data we present above on human brains also argue for a difference between WT and mutant tau in the folding properties.

Based on these data, we investigated the impact of tau isoforms and mutations on tau pathology spreading. We stained the brain sections with epitopes of tau pathology: hyperphosphoryled tau using the antibody AT8 [42, 44, 53] and misfolded tau using the antibody MC1 (IgG version of Alz50 antibody, [34, 36]). We first verified that, at the injection site, the focal overexpression of both constructs resulted in the formation of tau pathology in the CA1 of rats. 8 months post-injection, the neuronal expression of all isoforms, either mutant or WT, results in the formation of strong tau hyperphosphorylation (Fig. 3a) and misfolding (Fig. 3b).

In order to understand how tau pathology spreads through the brain, we analyzed the presence of tau lesions in the whole rat brain, from the olfactory bulb (rostro-caudal coordinates + 6 mm from bregma in coronal sections) to the end of the cortical areas (rostro-caudal coordinates − 9 mm from bregma in coronal sections). As a sensor for tau pathology spreading from the initiation site to secondary regions, we determined for each animal the rostral-most and caudal-most coordinates where we could see tau pathology, either in neurites or in cell bodies. We confirmed our previous data showing that in rats injected with LVs encoding 4R-tau the AT8 immunoreactivity was found in the cell body of second order neurons in several connected regions (e.g. the granular layer of the olfactory bulb) as far as 11 mm away from the injection site. Interestingly, in rats injected with LVs encoding P332S-4R-tau, P301L-4R-tau, 3R-tau or P332S-3R-tau, AT8 immunoreactivity was significantly restricted to the vicinity of the initiation site both for neurites or cell bodies (Fig. 3c).

In order to compare the appearance of tau hyperphosphorylation and tau misfolding in our model, we also stained by immunohistochemistry the epitope of misfolding MC1 in the different cohorts of rats. We determined the rostral-most and caudal-most coordinates for each animal to be able to compare the spatial appearance of MC1 epitope and of AT8 epitope. In the animals overexpressing the WT proteins 3R-tau and 4R-tau, the MC1 immunolabelling stayed significantly closer to the initiation site than the AT8 immunolabelling (Fig. 3d). Indeed, numerous brain regions show hyperphosphorylated tau without misfolding tau. It is really intriguing to notice that when a mutant tau species is overexpressed, the MC1 immunolabelling is retrieved in regions significantly more (or equally for P301L) distant from the initiation site than the AT8 immunolabelling (Fig. 3d) clearly suggesting a difference between WT proteins and mutant proteins in terms of tau misfolding and hyperphosphorylation in the context of spatial spreading.

## Discussion

The data in the present study reveal new aspects of the propagation of tau proteins by demonstrating that different species of tau have different behaviors in terms of pathological spreading and folding properties. Since the discovery of tau protein as the principal component of NFD [7, 26], around 20 pathologies involving aggregated tau were described with various time-courses, lesions

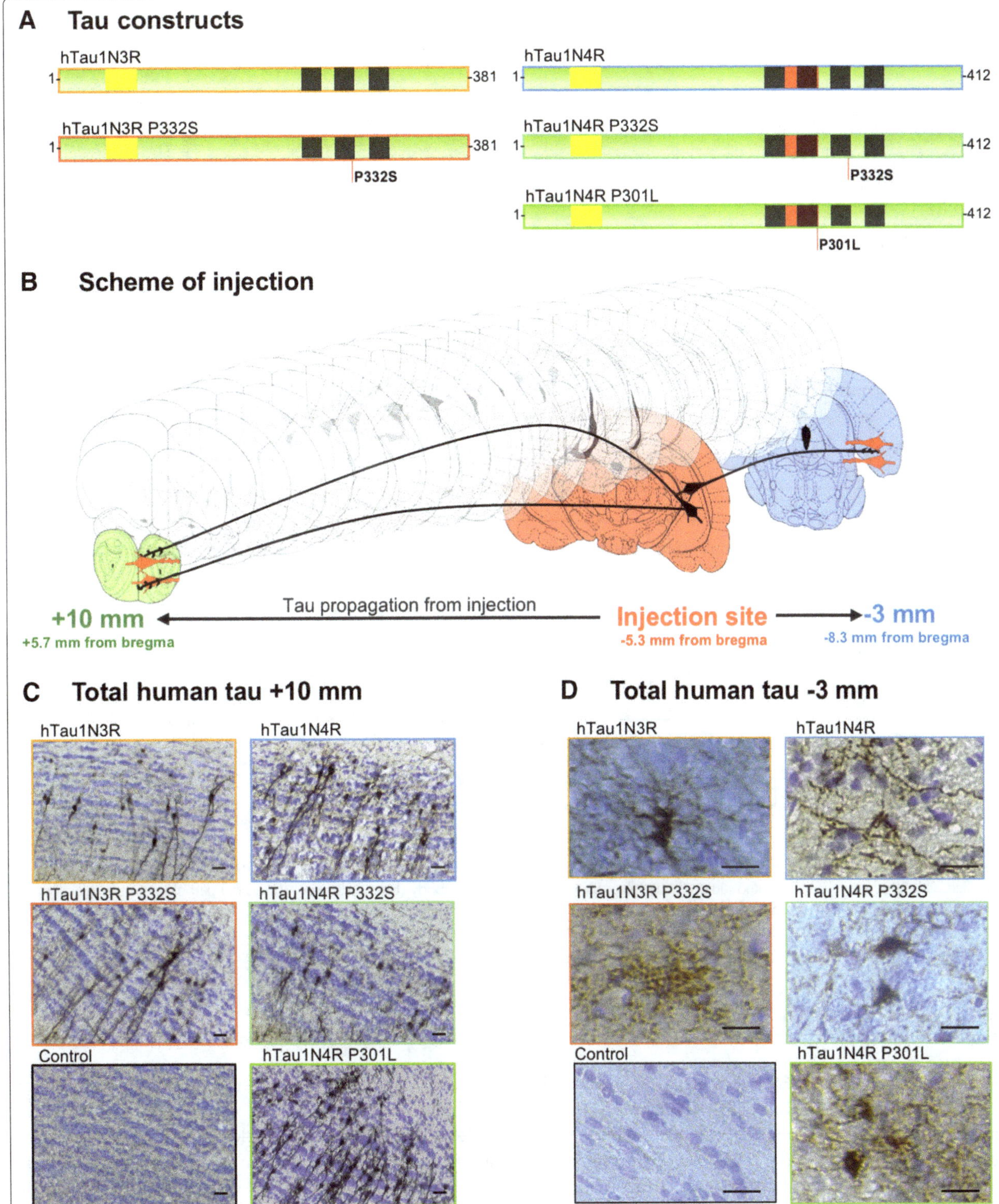


**Fig. 2** All tau species are transferred from neuron-to-neuron. **(a)** Schematic representations of tau construct used in this study. **(b)** Schematic representation of rat brain showing the injection coordinates in red and some of the rostral-most and caudal-most regions where we can find tau propagation. **(c** and **d)** Rat brains sections at coordinates + 5.7 mm **(c)** -8.3 mm **(d)** from bregma stained with a total human tau antibody (Adx215) showing transfer of tau for every species. htau1N4R ($n = 9$), htau1N4R-P301L ($n = 5$), htau1N4R-P332S (n = 6), htau1N3R ($n = 8$) or htau1N3R-P332S ($n = 5$). Scale bars represent 20 µm

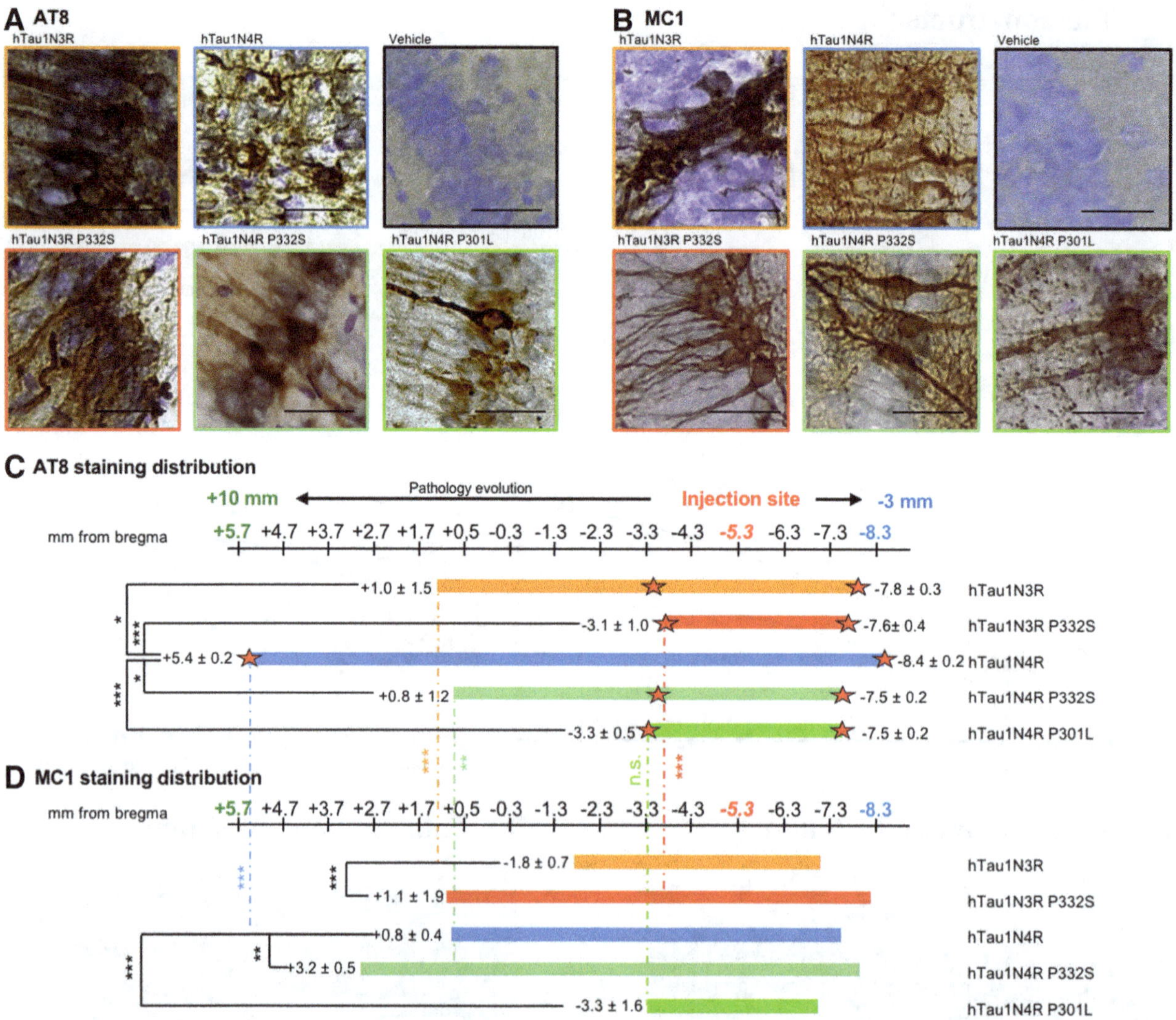


**Fig. 3** Differential of spreading of tau pathology between tau species. **(a** and **b)** Rat brains sections at − 5.3 mm from bregma for each group labelled with AT8-hyperphosphorylated tau antibody **(a)** or MC1-misfolded tau antibody **(b)** and showing strong tau pathology at the injection site. Scale bars represent 40 μm **(c** and **d)** Distribution of the AT8 **(c)** or MC1 **(d)** staining in coronal sections throughout the brains for each group is represented with bars along the scale of antero-posterior coordinates from Bregma. Bars represents the average of rostral-most to caudal-most staining (cell body or neurite) observed for each cohort. Red stars represent the coordinate of the last cell body observed. htau1N4R ($n = 9$), htau1N4R-P301L ($n = 5$), htau1N4R-P332S ($n = 6$), htau1N3R ($n = 8$) or htau1N3R-P332S ($n = 5$). The mean and standard deviations are indicated at the end of each bars. Statistical test used: One-way ANOVA test followed by a Tuckey post-hoc test was used to assess statistical differences between each group

and involved tau species [39]. This group includes pathologies with aggregated 3R-tau, 4R-tau, or both isoforms. Rare fronto-temporal dementia cases also involve mutation in the tau gene [23]. These latter proteins are pro-aggregative [4, 12] often showing strong tau pathology when overexpressed and therefore are widely used in the modelling of tau pathologies [18]. The in vivo studies dealing with tau propagation are also mainly based on the overexpression or injection of mutant 4R-tau proteins [1, 13, 14, 32, 41, 63]. However, in view of the neuroanatomical and biochemical differences among human tauopathies [2, 4, 22], one may ask if the different tau species trigger the same pathological mechanisms.

Here, we studied the misfolding and hyperphosphorylation status of tau proteins in human brains with AD or with MAPT mutations. In all groups, we found a majority of tangles showing both misfolding and hyperphosphorylation and also a high number of neurons showing only hyperphosphorylation. More interestingly though, the misfolding-only neurons were most prevalent in mutant tau brains (Fig. 1). This result doesn't show per se that tau misfolding precedes hyperphosphorylation in MAPT-mutant patients and the contrary in AD patients but seems to indicate that the mutant-tau may have different folding properties compared to WT tau.

To model such differences, we took advantage of lentiviral technology to induce the accumulation of 3R or 4R WT or mutant tau, and to investigate the propagation of both the protein and the pathology. We show that regardless of the isoform or mutation, all tau proteins are capable of long-distance propagation through the brain (Fig. 2) consistent with the existence of a cell-to-cell transfer mechanism as previously suggested [14, 19, 41]. Our study indicates that most of the tau species, travel in a non-pathological, non-phosphorylated, non-misfolded state. Indeed, we clearly see transfer for every species studied (Fig. 2) but only some of them show long distance pathological epitopes presence (Fig. 3). It is clear in this model that at least part of tau cell-to-cell transfer is physiological, as tau does not seem to be either misfolded or hyperphosphorylated. This finding is in line with numerous studies showing that secreted tau is mostly monomeric and non-phosphorylated [11, 17, 37, 38, 47, 50–52, 56, 58, 62, 64, 70].

We also show differences in tau pathology between species of tau in the human brains (Fig. 1). Therefore, we wondered if, in the rat model, the propagation of pathological epitopes is impacted by the species. Indeed, all constructs trigger the development of tau pathology in the hippocampus of rats, but these pathologies evolve in a different manner in the whole brain. 4R-tau leads to a strong long-distance spreading of tau pathology when 3R-tau or mutant-tau mediated-pathologies stay in the vicinity of the pathology initiation site and don't spread in long-distant brain areas (Fig. 3). These observations using mutant tau confirm our previous data obtained with the P301L mutation [19], located in the 2nd tau repeat, and extend our conclusions to another genetic FTLD-Tau mutation located in the 3rd tau repeat [16]. Given the reproducibility of our results among several cohorts of animals, as well as our observations in human brains, such differences between WT-4R-tau and 3R-tau or mutant-tau are likely to be due to intrinsic properties of mutant tau proteins. First, both mutant-tau and 3R-tau are known to induce better fibrillogenesis than WT-4R-tau [12, 59] probably due to conformational changes in the protein when tau protein is mutated [2, 20, 22]. For 3R-tau, the presence of a single cysteine in its sequence allows for the formation of intermolecular bridges initiating tau conversion/aggregation. Conversely, the two cysteines (C291, C322) present in 4R tau mostly drive the formation of intramolecular bridges, potentially slowing-down the process of oligomerization and subsequent aggregation [59].

Indeed, in this study, we suggest that 3R-, 4R- or mutant-tau support different types of pathological conversion. The classical view regarding the pathological conversion of tau proteins from a disordered state to insoluble, ordered and hyperphosphorylated aggregates suggests that tau becomes hyperphosphorylated inducing first the misfolding of the protein, and then its oligomerization. This hypothesis is further supported by the early appearance during the pathology of certain epitopes of phosphorylation [3, 43]. However, recently, Diamond's team showed in a transgenic mouse model overexpressing the mutant P301S-tau that the seeding propensity of tau proteins is the first detectable indicator of tau pathology, before misfolding (MC1 antibody) and then hyperphosphorylation (AT8) [29]. We also previously reported the precocious appearance of tau misfolding epitopes and not hyperphosphorylation when mutant tau was overexpressed (As early as 2 months post lentiviral vectors injection, see [10]). By contrast, it is obvious that when overexpressing WT tau, hyperphosphorylation occurs first at the initiation site [10] but also in distant regions ([19], Fig. 3). Here, we confirm that when mutant-tau proteins accumulate, tau may first acquire misfolding properties (Figs. 1 and 3). This supports the existence of an intrinsic misfolding in mutant-tau proteins leading to the early appearance of a misfolding epitope and to the formation of fibrils with different structures [2, 20, 22]. Interestingly, the structure of these fibrils is transmissible to other tau species [20, 22]. This prominent misfolding might be the cause of the higher toxicity and neurodegeneration reported when mutant tau is expressed compared to WT [10, 30].

The phosphorylation state of tau may be a key player in the propagation processes. We know that tau is retained within axons due to its binding with microtubules which is highly dependent on phosphorylation [40]. Given that 3R-tau and mutant-tau show weaker binding to microtubules compared to 4R-WT-tau [9, 16, 27], it is very unlikely for 3R-phospho-tau and mutant-phospho-tau to stay in the axons. We hypothesize that they relocalize to the soma and therefore be less available for trans-synaptic transfer than 4R-tau. These results also suggest the presence of different tau species within the same individual (e.g. non-phosphorylated tau, phosphorylated tau, misfolded tau, truncated tau, dimers, oligomers, polymers, seeding-competent tau) that act differentially for tau transfer and pathological propagation. Most of them can be called "tau pathological species" but it is rather difficult to clearly identify the role of each in the pathology. In further studies, these different tau species should be analyzed independently to understand the part of each in the pathophysiological processes such as tau pathology spreading, misfolding or aggregation.

To conclude, the mechanisms of tau propagation and cell-to-cell transfer are highly dependent on tau species and our study is the first to identify this differential propensity of tau isoforms/mutations to mediate tau pathology spreading. This observation probably relies on intrinsic differences between tau species such as folding. These characteristics are consistent with what is observed in the human tauopathies and could explain their phenotypic specificities. This study also highlights the fundamental difference between tau physiological cell-to-cell transfer and tau pathological propagation. Those two mechanisms probably involve different species of tau that behave differently in the brain. This concept must be carefully taken into account and addressed in further studies dealing with tau propagation.

## Additional files

**Additional file 1: Figure S1.** Tau misfolding and hyperphosphorylation in human brains with AD and genetic FTLD-Tau-detailed figure. Details of each individual is indicated to show the patient-to-patient variability. Rows represent patients (numbered from 1 to 10), columns represent the regions studied. In each Venn diagram are indicated the percentage of neurons counted for each patient in each region. AT8 only neurons are indicated in green, Alz50-only in red and double-positive neurons in brown. MAPT mutants ($n = 4$), AD cases ($n = 6$). (TIFF 6255 kb)

**Additional file 2: Table S1.** Detailed neuronal counts for each patient are indicated here. MAPT mutants ($n = 4$), AD cases ($n = 6$). (DOCX 16 kb)

**Additional file 3: Figure S2.** No difference in transgene expression. Expression of MAPT gene in the different cohorts show no statistical difference between the expression of the different constructs. htau1N4R ($n = 3$), htau1N4R-P301L ($n = 3$), htau1N4R-P332S ($n = 3$), htau1N3R ($n = 3$) or htau1N3R-P332S ($n = 3$). Statistical test used: One-way ANOVA test followed by a Tuckey post-hoc test was used to assess statistical differences. (TIFF 5 mb)

**Acknowledgements**
We are grateful from LabEx DISTALZ, Association France Alzheimer, Fondation Plan Alzheimer, ANR Spreadtau, CNRS, DN2M VicTaur for funding this work. We also wanted to thank Lille NeuroBank and the Massachusetts Alzheimer's Disease Research Center for providing human tissues and Dr. Peter Davis for the gift of Alz50 and MC1 antibodies. Simon Dujardin is supported by a grant from the Alzheimer's Association (2018-AARF-591935). Massachusetts Alzheimer's Disease Research Center is supported by a grant from National Institute of Health grant number P50 AG005134.

**Funding**
This work has been funded by LabEx DISTALZ, Association France Alzheimer, Fondation Plan Alzheimer, ANR Spreadtau, CNRS, DN2M VicTaur. Simon Dujardin is supported by a grant from the Alzheimer's Association (2018-AARF-591935). Massachusetts Alzheimer's Disease Research Center is supported by a grant from National Institute of Health grant number P50 AG005134.

**Authors' contributions**
SD, MC and LB Conceived and designed the experiments and analysis. SD, SB, RC, SL, CL, and SC performed the experiment and collected the data. SD and MC analyzed the data. SD, MC and LB wrote the paper. ND and BTH gave critical opinion and revised the manuscript. JAG, VD, CAM and MPF performed the human tissue selection and distribution. All authors read and approved the final manuscript.

**Ethics approval**
Animal experiments were performed in compliance with and with the approval of the local ethics committee (agreement 2,015,101,320,441,671, 2016–2021), standards for the care and use of laboratory animals, and the French and European Community guidelines as well as the Massachusetts General Hospital's Institutional Animal Care and Use Committee.
All human tissues come from the Lille Neurobank and the Massachusetts Alzheimer's Disease Research center and written consent forms have been obtained accordingly to the local legislations and ethical committees. Human brains extracts were obtained from the Massachusetts Alzheimer's Disease Research Center (grant number P50 AG005134, under IRB protocol 1999P003693) and the Lille Neurobank (CRB/CIC1403 Biobank, BB-0033-00030, agreement DC-2008-642) fulfilling criteria of the local laws and r egulations on biological resources with donor consent, data protection and ethical committee review.

**Competing interests**
The authors declare no conflicts of interest.

**Author details**
[1]Univ. Lille, Inserm, CHU-Lille, UMR-S 1172, Alzheimer & Tauopathies, School of Medicine, 1 rue Polonovski, 59045 Lille, France. [2]Department of Neurology, Massachusetts General Hospital, MassGeneral Institute of Neurodegenerative Diseases (MIND), Charlestown, MA, USA. [3]Department of Neurology, Harvard Medical School, Boston, MA, USA. [4]Lausanne University Hospital (CHUV), Neuroscience Research Center (CRN), Laboratory of Neurotherapies and Neuromodulation (LNTM), CH-1011 Lausanne, Switzerland.

**References**
1. Ahmed Z, Cooper J, Murray TK, Garn K, McNaughton E, Clarke H, Parhizkar S, Ward MA, Cavallini A, Jackson S, Bose sS, Clavaguera F, Tolnay M, Lavenir I, Goedert M, Hutton ML, O'Neill MJ (2014) A novel in vivo model of tau propagation with rapid and progressive neurofibrillary tangle pathology: the pattern of spread is determined by connectivity, not proximity. Acta Neuropathol 127:667–683. https://doi.org/10.1007/s00401-014-1254-6
2. Aoyagi H, Hasegawa M, Tamaoka A (2007) Fibrillogenic nuclei composed of P301L mutant tau induce elongation of P301L tau but not wild-type tau. J Biol Chem 282:20309–20318. https://doi.org/10.1074/jbc.M611876200
3. Augustinack JC, Schneider A, Mandelkow EM, Hyman BT (2002) Specific tau phosphorylation sites correlate with severity of neuronal cytopathology in Alzheimer's disease. Acta Neuropathol 103:26–35
4. Barghorn S, Zheng-Fischhofer Q, Ackmann M, Biernat J, von Bergen M, Mandelkow EM, Mandelkow E (2000) Structure, microtubule interactions, and paired helical filament aggregation by tau mutants of frontotemporal dementias. Biochemistry 39:11714–11721
5. Biernat J, Gustke N, Drewes G, Mandelkow EM, Mandelkow E (1993) Phosphorylation of Ser262 strongly reduces binding of tau to microtubules: distinction between PHF-like immunoreactivity and microtubule binding. Neuron 11:153–163
6. Braak H, Braak E (1991) Neuropathological stageing of Alzheimer-related changes. Acta Neuropathol 82:239–259
7. Brion J, Passareiro H, Nunez J, Flament-Durand J (1985) Mise en évidence immunologique de la protéine tau au niveau des lésions de dégénérescence neurofibrillaires de la maladie d'Alzheimer. Arch Biol (Brux): 229–235
8. Buee L, Bussiere T, Buee-Scherrer V, Delacourte A, Hof PR (2000) Tau protein isoforms, phosphorylation and role in neurodegenerative disorders. Brain Res Brain Res Rev 33:95–130
9. Butner KA, Kirschner MW (1991) Tau protein binds to microtubules through a flexible array of distributed weak sites. J Cell Biol 115:717–730

10. Caillierez R, Begard S, Lecolle K, Deramecourt V, Zommer N, Dujardin S, Loyens A, Dufour N, Auregan G, Winderickx J, Hantraye P, Deglon N, Buee L, Colin M (2013) Lentiviral delivery of the human wild-type tau protein mediates a slow and progressive neurodegenerative tau pathology in the rat brain. Mol Ther 21:1358–1368. https://doi.org/10.1038/mt.2013.66
11. Chai X, Dage JL, Citron M (2012) Constitutive secretion of tau protein by an unconventional mechanism. Neurobiol Dis 48:356–366. https://doi.org/10.1016/j.nbd.2012.05.021
12. Chang E, Kim S, Yin H, Nagaraja HN, Kuret J (2008) Pathogenic missense MAPT mutations differentially modulate tau aggregation propensity at nucleation and extension steps. J Neurochem 107:1113–1123. https://doi.org/10.1111/j.1471-4159.2008.05692.x
13. Clavaguera F, Bolmont T, Crowther RA, Abramowski D, Frank S, Probst A, Fraser G, Stalder AK, Beibel M, Staufenbiel M, Jucker M, Goedert M, Tolnay M (2009) Transmission and spreading of tauopathy in transgenic mouse brain. Nat Cell Biol 11:909–913. https://doi.org/10.1038/ncb1901
14. de Calignon A, Polydoro M, Suarez-Calvet M, William C, Adamowicz DH, Kopeikina KJ, Pitstick R, Sahara N, Ashe KH, Carlson GA, Spires-Jones TL, Hyman BT (2012) Propagation of tau pathology in a model of early Alzheimer's disease. Neuron 73:685–697. https://doi.org/10.1016/j.neuron.2011.11.033
15. Delacourte A, David JP, Sergeant N, Buee L, Wattez A, Vermersch P, Ghozali F, Fallet-Bianco C, Pasquier F, Lebert F, Petit H, Di Menza C (1999) The biochemical pathway of neurofibrillary degeneration in aging and Alzheimer's disease. Neurology 52:1158–1165
16. Deramecourt V, Lebert F, Maurage CA, Fernandez-Gomez FJ, Dujardin S, Colin M, Sergeant N, Buee-Scherrer V, Clot F, Ber IL, Brice A, Pasquier F, Buee L (2012) Clinical, neuropathological, and biochemical characterization of the novel tau mutation P332S. J Alzheimers Dis 31:741–749. https://doi.org/10.3233/JAD-2012-120160
17. Dujardin S, Begard S, Caillierez R, Lachaud C, Delattre L, Carrier S, Loyens A, Galas MC, Bousset L, Melki R, Auregan G, Hantraye P, Brouillet E, Buee L, Colin M (2014) Ectosomes: a new mechanism for non-exosomal secretion of tau protein. PLoS One 9:e100760. https://doi.org/10.1371/journal.pone.0100760
18. Dujardin S, Colin M, Buee L (2015) Invited review: animal models of tauopathies and their implications for research/translation into the clinic. Neuropathol Appl Neurobiol 41:59–80. https://doi.org/10.1111/nan.12200
19. Dujardin S, Lecolle K, Caillierez R, Begard S, Zommer N, Lachaud C, Carrier S, Dufour N, Auregan G, Winderickx J, Hantraye P, Deglon N, Colin M, Buee L (2014) Neuron-to-neuron wild-type tau protein transfer through a trans-synaptic mechanism: relevance to sporadic tauopathies. Acta Neuropathol Commun 2:14. https://doi.org/10.1186/2051-5960-2-14
20. Falcon B, Cavallini A, Angers R, Glover S, Murray TK, Barnham L, Jackson S, O'Neill MJ, Isaacs AM, Hutton ML, Szekeres PG, Goedert M, Bose S (2015) Conformation determines the seeding potencies of native and recombinant tau aggregates. J Biol Chem 290:1049–1065. https://doi.org/10.1074/jbc.M114.589309
21. Forrest SL, Kril JJ, Halliday GM (2018) Reply: will FTLD-tau work for all when FTDP-17 retires? Brain. https://doi.org/10.1093/brain/awy179
22. Frost B, Ollesch J, Wille H, Diamond MI (2009) Conformational diversity of wild-type tau fibrils specified by templated conformation change. J Biol Chem 284:3546–3551. https://doi.org/10.1074/jbc.M805627200
23. Ghetti B, Oblak AL, Boeve BF, Johnson KA, Dickerson BC, Goedert M (2015) Invited review: frontotemporal dementia caused by microtubule-associated protein tau gene (MAPT) mutations: a chameleon for neuropathology and neuroimaging. Neuropathol Appl Neurobiol 41:24–46. https://doi.org/10.1111/nan.12213
24. Giannakopoulos P, Herrmann FR, Bussiere T, Bouras C, Kovari E, Perl DP, Morrison JH, Gold G, Hof PR (2003) Tangle and neuron numbers, but not amyloid load, predict cognitive status in Alzheimer's disease. Neurology 60:1495–1500
25. Goedert M (2016) The ordered assembly of tau is the gain-of-toxic function that causes human tauopathies. Alzheimers Dement 12:1040–1050. https://doi.org/10.1016/j.jalz.2016.09.001
26. Grundke-Iqbal I, Iqbal K, Quinlan M, Tung YC, Zaidi MS, Wisniewski HM (1986) Microtubule-associated protein tau. A component of Alzheimer paired helical filaments. J Biol Chem 261:6084–6089
27. Hasegawa M, Smith MJ, Goedert M (1998) Tau proteins with FTDP-17 mutations have a reduced ability to promote microtubule assembly. FEBS Lett 437:207–210
28. Himmler A, Drechsel D, Kirschner MW, Martin DWJ (1989) Tau consists of a set of proteins with repeated C-terminal microtubule-binding domains and variable N-terminal domains. Mol Cell Biol 9:1381–1388
29. Holmes BB, Furman JL, Mahan TE, Yamasaki TR, Mirbaha H, Eades WC, Belaygorod L, Cairns NJ, Holtzman DM, Diamond MI (2014) Proteopathic tau seeding predicts tauopathy in vivo. Proc Natl Acad Sci U S A 111:E4376–E4385. https://doi.org/10.1073/pnas.1411649111
30. Hoover BR, Reed MN, Su J, Penrod RD, Kotilinek LA, Grant MK, Pitstick R, Carlson GA, Lanier LM, Yuan LL, Ashe KH, Liao D (2010) Tau mislocalization to dendritic spines mediates synaptic dysfunction independently of neurodegeneration. Neuron 68:1067–1081. https://doi.org/10.1016/j.neuron.2010.11.030
31. Hottinger AF, Azzouz M, Deglon N, Aebischer P, Zurn AD (2000) Complete and long-term rescue of lesioned adult motoneurons by lentiviral-mediated expression of glial cell line-derived neurotrophic factor in the facial nucleus. J Neurosci 20:5587–5593
32. Iba M, McBride JD, Guo JL, Zhang B, Trojanowski JQ, Lee VM (2015) Tau pathology spread in PS19 tau transgenic mice following locus coeruleus (LC) injections of synthetic tau fibrils is determined by the LC's afferent and efferent connections. Acta Neuropathol 130:349–362. https://doi.org/10.1007/s00401-015-1458-4
33. Irwin DJ, Brettschneider J, McMillan CT, Cooper F, Olm C, Arnold SE, Van Deerlin VM, Seeley WW, Miller BL, Lee EB, Lee VM, Grossman M, Trojanowski JQ (2016) Deep clinical and neuropathological phenotyping of pick disease. Ann Neurol 79:272–287. https://doi.org/10.1002/ana.24559
34. Jeganathan S, Hascher A, Chinnathambi S, Biernat J, Mandelkow EM, Mandelkow E (2008) Proline-directed pseudo-phosphorylation at AT8 and PHF1 epitopes induces a compaction of the paperclip folding of tau and generates a pathological (MC-1) conformation. J Biol Chem 283:32066–32076. https://doi.org/10.1074/jbc.M805300200
35. Jicha GA, Berenfeld B, Davies P (1999) Sequence requirements for formation of conformational variants of tau similar to those found in Alzheimer's disease. J Neurosci Res 55:713–723. https://doi.org/10.1002/(SICI)1097-4547(19990315)55:6<713::AID-JNR6>3.0.CO;2-G
36. Jicha GA, Bowser R, Kazam IG, Davies P (1997) Alz-50 and MC-1, a new monoclonal antibody raised to paired helical filaments, recognize conformational epitopes on recombinant tau. J Neurosci Res 48:128–132
37. Karch CM, Jeng AT, Goate AM (2012) Extracellular tau levels are influenced by variability in tau that is associated with tauopathies. J Biol Chem 287:42751–42762. https://doi.org/10.1074/jbc.M112.380642
38. Katsinelos T, Zeitler M, Dimou E, Karakatsani A, Muller HM, Nachman E, Steringer JP, Ruiz de Almodovar C, Nickel W, Jahn TR (2018) Unconventional secretion mediates the trans-cellular spreading of tau. Cell Rep 23:2039–2055. https://doi.org/10.1016/j.celrep.2018.04.056
39. Kovacs GG (2015) Invited review: neuropathology of tauopathies: principles and practice. Neuropathol Appl Neurobiol 41:3–23. https://doi.org/10.1111/nan.12208
40. Li X, Kumar Y, Zempel H, Mandelkow EM, Biernat J, Mandelkow E (2011) Novel diffusion barrier for axonal retention of tau in neurons and its failure in neurodegeneration. EMBO J 30:4825–4837. https://doi.org/10.1038/emboj.2011.376
41. Liu L, Drouet V, Wu JW, Witter MP, Small SA, Clelland C, Duff K (2012) Trans-synaptic spread of tau pathology in vivo. PLoS One 7:e31302. https://doi.org/10.1371/journal.pone.0031302
42. Malia TJ, Teplyakov A, Ernst R, Wu SJ, Lacy ER, Liu X, Vandermeeren M, Mercken M, Luo J, Sweet RW, Gilliland GL (2016) Epitope mapping and structural basis for the recognition of phosphorylated tau by the anti-tau antibody AT8. Proteins 84:427–434. https://doi.org/10.1002/prot.24988
43. Maurage CA, Sergeant N, Ruchoux MM, Hauw JJ, Delacourte A (2003) Phosphorylated serine 199 of microtubule-associated protein tau is a neuronal epitope abundantly expressed in youth and an early marker of tau pathology. Acta Neuropathol 105:89–97. https://doi.org/10.1007/s00401-002-0608-7
44. Mercken M, Vandermeeren M, Lubke U, Six J, Boons J, Van de Voorde A, Martin JJ, Gheuens J (1992) Monoclonal antibodies with selective specificity for Alzheimer tau are directed against phosphatase-sensitive epitopes. Acta Neuropathol 84:265–272
45. Mirbaha H, Chen D, Morazova OA, Ruff KM, Sharma AM, Liu X, Goodarzi M, Pappu RV, Colby DW, Mirzaei H, Joachimiak LA, Diamond MI (2018) Inert and seed-competent tau monomers suggest structural origins of aggregation. Elife 7. https://doi.org/10.7554/eLife.36584

46. Mocanu MM, Nissen A, Eckermann K, Khlistunova I, Biernat J, Drexler D, Petrova O, Schonig K, Bujard H, Mandelkow E, Zhou L, Rune G, Mandelkow EM (2008) The potential for beta-structure in the repeat domain of tau protein determines aggregation, synaptic decay, neuronal loss, and coassembly with endogenous tau in inducible mouse models of tauopathy. J Neurosci 28:737–748. https://doi.org/10.1523/JNEUROSCI.2824-07.2008
47. Mohamed NV, Plouffe V, Remillard-Labrosse G, Planel E, Leclerc N (2014) Starvation and inhibition of lysosomal function increased tau secretion by primary cortical neurons. Sci Rep 4:5715. https://doi.org/10.1038/srep05715
48. Mudher A, Colin M, Dujardin S, Medina M, Dewachter I, Alavi Naini SM, Mandelkow EM, Mandelkow E, Buee L, Goedert M, Brion JP (2017) What is the evidence that tau pathology spreads through prion-like propagation? Acta Neuropathol Commun 5:99. https://doi.org/10.1186/s40478-017-0488-7
49. Noble W, Hanger DP, Miller CC, Lovestone S (2013) The importance of tau phosphorylation for neurodegenerative diseases. Front Neurol 4:83. https://doi.org/10.3389/fneur.2013.00083
50. Plouffe V, Mohamed NV, Rivest-McGraw J, Bertrand J, Lauzon M, Leclerc N (2012) Hyperphosphorylation and cleavage at D421 enhance tau secretion. PLoS One 7:e36873. https://doi.org/10.1371/journal.pone.0036873
51. Polydoro M, Dzhala VI, Pooler AM, Nicholls SB, McKinney AP, Sanchez L, Pitstick R, Carlson GA, Staley KJ, Spires-Jones TL, Hyman BT (2014) Soluble pathological tau in the entorhinal cortex leads to presynaptic deficits in an early Alzheimer's disease model. Acta Neuropathol 127:257–270. https://doi.org/10.1007/s00401-013-1215-5
52. Pooler AM, Phillips EC, Lau DH, Noble W, Hanger DP (2013) Physiological release of endogenous tau is stimulated by neuronal activity. EMBO Rep 14: 389–394. https://doi.org/10.1038/embor.2013.15
53. Porzig R, Singer D, Hoffmann R (2007) Epitope mapping of mAbs AT8 and Tau5 directed against hyperphosphorylated regions of the human tau protein. Biochem Biophys Res Commun 358:644–649. https://doi.org/10.1016/j.bbrc.2007.04.187
54. Rosseels J, Van den Brande J, Violet M, Jacobs D, Grognet P, Lopez J, Huvent I, Caldara M, Swinnen E, Papegaey A, Caillierez R, Buee-Scherrer V, Engelborghs S, Lippens G, Colin M, Buee L, Galas MC, Vanmechelen E, Winderickx J (2015) Tau monoclonal antibody generation based on humanized yeast models: impact on tau oligomerization and diagnostics. J Biol Chem 290:4059–4074. https://doi.org/10.1074/jbc.M114.627919
55. Saito Y, Ruberu NN, Sawabe M, Arai T, Tanaka N, Kakuta Y, Yamanouchi H, Murayama S (2004) Staging of argyrophilic grains: an age-associated tauopathy. J Neuropathol Exp Neurol 63:911–918
56. Saman S, Kim W, Raya M, Visnick Y, Miro S, Saman S, Jackson B, McKee AC, Alvarez VE, Lee NC, Hall GF (2012) Exosome-associated tau is secreted in tauopathy models and is selectively phosphorylated in cerebrospinal fluid in early Alzheimer disease. J Biol Chem 287:3842–3849. https://doi.org/10.1074/jbc.M111.277061
57. Sanders DW, Kaufman SK, DeVos SL, Sharma AM, Mirbaha H, Li A, Barker SJ, Foley AC, Thorpe JR, Serpell LC, Miller TM, Grinberg LT, Seeley WW, Diamond MI (2014) Distinct tau prion strains propagate in cells and mice and define different tauopathies. Neuron 82:1271–1288. https://doi.org/10.1016/j.neuron.2014.04.047
58. Santa-Maria I, Varghese M, Ksiezak-Reding H, Dzhun A, Wang J, Pasinetti GM (2012) Paired helical filaments from Alzheimer disease brain induce intracellular accumulation of tau protein in aggresomes. J Biol Chem 287: 20522–20533. https://doi.org/10.1074/jbc.M111.323279
59. Schweers O, Mandelkow EM, Biernat J, Mandelkow E (1995) Oxidation of cysteine-322 in the repeat domain of microtubule-associated protein tau controls the in vitro assembly of paired helical filaments. Proc Natl Acad Sci U S A 92:8463–8467
60. Selkoe DJ, Hardy J (2016) The amyloid hypothesis of Alzheimer's disease at 25 years. EMBO Mol Med 8:595–608. https://doi.org/10.15252/emmm.201606210
61. Simic G, Babic Leko M, Wray S, Harrington C, Delalle I, Jovanov-Milosevic N, Bazadona D, Buee L, de Silva R, Di Giovanni G, Wischik C, Hof PR (2016) Tau protein hyperphosphorylation and aggregation in Alzheimer's disease and other Tauopathies, and possible neuroprotective strategies. Biomolecules 6: 6. https://doi.org/10.3390/biom6010006
62. Simon D, Garcia-Garcia E, Royo F, Falcon-Perez JM, Avila J (2012) Proteostasis of tau. Tau overexpression results in its secretion via membrane vesicles. FEBS Lett 586:47–54. https://doi.org/10.1016/j.febslet.2011.11.022
63. Stancu IC, Vasconcelos B, Ris L, Wang P, Villers A, Peeraer E, Buist A, Terwel D, Baatsen P, Oyelami T, Pierrot N, Casteels C, Bormans G, Kienlen-Campard P, Octave JN, Moechars D, Dewachter I (2015) Templated misfolding of tau by prion-like seeding along neuronal connections impairs neuronal network function and associated behavioral outcomes in tau transgenic mice. Acta Neuropathol 129:875–894. https://doi.org/10.1007/s00401-015-1413-4
64. Tang Z, Ioja E, Bereczki E, Hultenby K, Li C, Guan Z, Winblad B, Pei JJ (2015) mTor mediates tau localization and secretion: implication for Alzheimer's disease. Biochim Biophys Acta 1853:1646–1657. https://doi.org/10.1016/j.bbamcr.2015.03.003
65. Tardivel M, Begard S, Bousset L, Dujardin S, Coens A, Melki R, Buee L, Colin M (2016) Tunneling nanotube (TNT)-mediated neuron-to neuron transfer of pathological tau protein assemblies. Acta Neuropathol Commun 4:117. https://doi.org/10.1186/s40478-016-0386-4
66. Verny M, Jellinger KA, Hauw JJ, Bancher C, Litvan I, Agid Y (1996) Progressive supranuclear palsy: a clinicopathological study of 21 cases. Acta Neuropathol 91:427–431
67. von Bergen M, Barghorn S, Biernat J, Mandelkow EM, Mandelkow E (2005) Tau aggregation is driven by a transition from random coil to beta sheet structure. Biochim Biophys Acta 1739:158–166. https://doi.org/10.1016/j.bbadis.2004.09.010
68. von Bergen M, Barghorn S, Li L, Marx A, Biernat J, Mandelkow EM, Mandelkow E (2001) Mutations of tau protein in frontotemporal dementia promote aggregation of paired helical filaments by enhancing local beta-structure. J Biol Chem 276:48165–48174. https://doi.org/10.1074/jbc.M105196200
69. Williams DR, Holton JL, Strand C, Pittman A, de Silva R, Lees AJ, Revesz T (2007) Pathological tau burden and distribution distinguishes progressive supranuclear palsy-parkinsonism from Richardson's syndrome. Brain 130: 1566–1576. https://doi.org/10.1093/brain/awm104
70. Yamada K, Holth JK, Liao F, Stewart FR, Mahan TE, Jiang H, Cirrito JR, Patel TK, Hochgrafe K, Mandelkow EM, Holtzman DM (2014) Neuronal activity regulates extracellular tau in vivo. J Exp Med 211:387–393. https://doi.org/10.1084/jem.20131685

3

# 5-HIAA induces neprilysin to ameliorate pathophysiology and symptoms in a mouse model for Alzheimer's disease

Christian Klein, Guy Roussel, Susana Brun, Cristina Rusu, Christine Patte-Mensah[†], Michel Maitre[*†] and Ayikoe-Guy Mensah-Nyagan[*†]

**Abstract**

Serotoninergic activation which decreases brain Aβ peptides is considered beneficial in mouse models for Alzheimer's disease (AD), but the mechanisms involved remain unclear. Because growing evidence suggested that the stimulation of proteases digesting Aβ, especially the endopeptidase neprilysin (NEP) may be effective for AD therapy/prevention, we explored the involvement of serotonin precursors and derivatives in NEP regulation. We found that 5-hydroxyindolacetic acid (5-HIAA), the final metabolite of serotonin, considered until now as a dead-end and inactive product of serotonin catabolism, significantly reduces brain Aβ in the transgenic APPSWE mouse model for AD-related Aβ pathology and in the phosphoramidon-induced cerebral NEP inhibition mouse model. 5-HIAA treatment improves memory performance in APPSWE mice. Furthermore, 5-HIAA and its precursors increase NEP level in vivo and in neuroblastoma cells. Inhibition of ERK 1/2 cascade by 5-HIAA or SCH772984 enhanced NEP levels, suggesting MAP-kinase pathway involvement in 5-HIAA-induced regulation of NEP expression. Our results provide the first demonstration that 5-HIAA is an active serotonin metabolite that increases brain Aβ degradation/clearance and improves symptoms in the APPSWE mouse model for AD.

**Keywords:** Alzheimer's disease, Neprilysin, Aβ peptides, 5-HIAA, Serotonergic transmission, ERK and GSK-3 pathways

## Introduction

Alzheimer's disease (AD) is a multifactorial neurodegenerative disorder resulting from proteinopathies characterized by the accumulation/ aggregation of β amyloid peptides (Aβ) and hyperphosphorylation followed by aggregation of microtubule-associated protein Tau [48, 52]. Before the symptomatic expression of the disease, a long incubation time over decades is characterized by micro-inflammation, vasculopathy, metabolic disturbances that favorize the appearance of neurodegenerative processes in aged population. Alterations of the genes encoding amyloid precursor protein (APP), presenilin-1 or 2 (PS1 or PS2), Adamalysin 10 or Apolipoprotein E4 (APOE4) are frequent in familial AD [12], but the large majority of AD patients show increased brain levels of neurotoxic Aβ without changes of the gene aforementioned. In aged patients, it is postulated that various accumulated mutations determine or favor deleterious proteinopathies, the most frequent being an anomaly in the synthesis or elimination of amyloid peptides [41]. This in turn initiates a cascade of post-translational disturbances, including mainly the hyperphosphorylation and accumulation of Tau. These events produce an early symptomatology made of significant memory and cognitive impairment, generally accompanied by measurable brain atrophy due to neurodegeneration [49].

Several approaches have been proposed to limit Aβ synthesis or to increase their elimination [2]. To reach this goal, the potentiation of some protease activities able to disaggregate pathologic Aβ substrates has been studied since several years. Among possible proteolytic enzymes, the most promising seems to be neprilysin (NEP) [39]. This enzyme belongs to the family of human M13 zinc-dependent endopeptidases which cleave a wide spectrum of brain regulatory peptides, including Aβ peptides [36]. Hyper-expression of NEP gene in the

* Correspondence: maitre@unistra.fr; gmensah@unistra.fr
[†]Christine Patte-Mensah, Michel Maitre and Ayikoe-Guy Mensah-Nyagan contributed equally to this work.
Biopathologie de la Myéline, Neuroprotection et Stratégies Thérapeutiques, INSERM U1119, Fédération de Médecine Translationnelle de Strasbourg (FMTS), Université de Strasbourg, Bâtiment 3 de la Faculté de Médecine, Strasbourg, France

brain of transgenic mouse models for AD decreases the incidence of amyloid pathology, and NEP activity is age dependently reduced in the rodent and human brain [2].

Besides the genetic manipulation of NEP expression, pharmacological approaches used to modulate NEP activity revealed that somatostatin and various polyphenols up-regulate NEP activity in the brain [44]. Epigenetic mechanisms via HDAC inhibition also seem to be a strategy to potentiate brain NEP expression and to protect against AD progression [35]. Valproic acid and gamma-hydroxybutyrate for example have been reported to decrease brain Aβ concentration, ameliorating in parallel memory performance in mouse models for AD [28, 51].

In this context, it is known that several metabolites of tryptophan pathways through kynurenine or serotonin metabolism are implicated in neuroprotection, regulation of brain Aβ levels, excitotoxicity, cognitive and synaptic maintenance [30]. Thus, several metabolites of kynurenine and serotonin pathways are suspected to be involved in AD-related neurodegenerative processes. However, the balance between these two pathways seems to be regulated by numerous factors among which neuroinflammation may promote the kynurenine pathway and in parallel impact serotonin synthesis. Because several indications favor a role of SSRI and serotonin receptors in AD pathophysiology and progression in human and animal models [24], we examined the possible interference of serotonin intermediates on brain Aβ clearance and evidenced a specific role for 5-HIAA which is generally thought to be a dead-end and inactive product of serotonin catabolism. To strengthen our investigations and consolidate our findings, we have used two different experimental models, namely the transgenic APPSWE mouse model for AD-related Aβ pathology (Tg2576) and the mouse model of phosphoramidon-evoked brain NEP inhibition [17, 20–22, 54].

## Materials and methods

### In vitro experiments

#### *Cell culture*

Human neuroblastoma SH-SY5Y cells and human neuroblastoma SH-SY5Y-APPwt cells stably transfected with DNA constructs harboring human wild-type APP695 (APPwt) were maintained in a humidified atmosphere of 95% air and 5% $CO_2$ at 37 °C [28]. Cells were seeded into plates or 100 mm dishes in Dulbecco modified Eagle medium, supplemented with 10% (vol/vol) fetal bovine serum, 100 U/mL penicillin, 100 µg/mL streptomycin (Fisher Scientific, France) and for the transfected cells with 300 µmg/mL hygromycin (Sigma-Aldrich, France), a selective antibiotic. Between 70 and 90% confluency, cells were incubated during various time periods and/or with various concentrations of compounds to be tested.

#### *RNA isolation and quantitative PCR*

Total RNA was extracted from SH-SY5Y cells after 0, 30, 60 and 90 min of treatment with 30 µM 5-HIAA, using the Nucleospin RNA L protocol (Macherey-Nagel, Düren, Germany). This protocol included a treatment of isolated RNA by DNase I. Integrity and purity of RNA was checked by spectrophotometry.

Reverse transcription was performed with 1 µg RNA using Biorad iScript® cDNA synthesis kit. q-PCR was performed in an iCycler thermal cycler (Biorad, Hercules, CA, USA) using SYBR Green dye (iQ SYBR green Supermix, Biorad). For each sample, the reaction mix was a make-up of 320 nM forward primer (F), 320 nM reverse primer (R), 200 nM probe, and 4 µL cDNA template in a total reaction volume of 20 µl [3]. Using the iCycler iQ optical system software (version 3.1, Bio-Rad), a standard curve based on successive cDNA dilutions was performed and was used to calculate starting quantities. To ensure a thorough calculation, starting quantities of genes of interest were reported to those of a housekeeping gene (U6 or Actin) in the same plate.

All samples were analyzed in triplicates, and the mean and standard deviation were calculated. After each q-PCR, specificity of the amplification was controlled by a melting curve ranging from 55 to 95 °C whereby a single peak corresponding to the amplicon was present.

The following primer pairs were used to amplify cDNAs after reverse transcription experiments [26]:

| Gene | Primer |
|---|---|
| Neprilysin | F 5′-CCTGGAGATTCATAATGGATCTTGT-3′ |
| | R 5′-AAAGGGCCTTGCGGAAAG-3′ |
| U6 | F 5′-CTCGCTTCGGCAGCACA-3′ |
| | R 5′-AACGCTTCACGAATTTGCGT-3′ |
| Actin | F 5′-CGCAGCAGTCAGGGACATTT-3′ |
| | R 5′-TTCACATACAGCTTGGGAAGC-3′ |

#### *Measurement of neprilysin protein level*

SH-SY5Y cells were washed with PBS and homogenized with lysis buffer containing a protease inhibitor cocktail (Sigma-Aldrich). The proteins in whole cell lysates were quantified using the BCA protein assay kit with BSA as a standard (Pierce, Rockford, IL, USA).

NEP protein levels were measured by using a DuoSet ELISA kit (R&D Systems Europe, Oxford, UK) according to the manufacturer's guidelines with minor modifications. Goat anti-human NEP (1.6 mg/mL) diluted in PBS (pH 7.4) was coated overnight on a high-binding 96 well plate (R&D Systems Europe) at room temperature (RT). The plates were washed 3 times in PBS containing 0.5%

Tween-20 (Sigma-Aldrich) (PBS-T). Non-specific binding of antibody was blocked by addition of PBS completed with 1% Bovine serum albumin (Sigma-Aldrich) (1% PBS-BSA) for 3 h at RT, then the plates were washed a further 3 times. Serial dilutions of recombinant human NEP or crude homogenates diluted in 1% PBS-BSA or 1% PBS-BSA alone as a control were incubated for 2 h with continuous shaking at RT. After a further 3 washes, biotinylated anti-NEP (1.6 mg/mL) was added for 2 h before another wash and incubation with streptavidin-peroxidase (1200) for 20 min in the dark. Substrate solution (tetramethyl benzidine; R&D Systems, Europe) was added for 30 min, and the optical density for each well was read at 450 nm and 540 nm or 570 nm in a plate reader (Elisa reader model Sigma 960, Metertech, Taipei, Taiwan).

The NEP protein levels were interpolated from the standard curve generated from serial dilutions of recombinant human NEP (R&D Systems Europe). Each measurement was repeated on 3 occasions, and the average value was calculated.

#### *Cell treatment with precursors or inhibitors of the serotonin pathway*

Different concentrations (0 to 100 µM) of 5-HIAA, 5-HTP, Serotonin hydrochloride (5-HT, Sigma-Aldrich) and Tryptophan (Trp, Sigma-Aldrich), were used. Pharmacological treatments were performed with specific inhibitors ((S)-(−)-carbidopa monohydrate (Abcam, Cambridge, UK), tranylcypromine hydrochloride (2-PCPA, Abcam), clorgyline hydrochloride (Abcam) were added to the SH-SY5Y cells 90 min or 24 h before harvest.

ERK inhibitor SCH772984 (Carbosynth, Compton Berkshire, UK), MEK ½ inhibitor GSK 1120212 (Targetmol, USA) or GSK-3 inhibitor CHIR99021 (Sigma-Aldrich, France) was added 30 min before the measurement of NEP protein.

#### *SH-SY5Y-APP cell treatment and Western blot analysis*

According to experimental design [26], the SH-SY5Y cells were incubated either with 10 mM ammonium chloride ($NH_4Cl$, Sigma-Aldrich) or 30 µM 5-HIAA (Sigma-Aldrich) for 24 h. Non-treated cells were used as control. After 24 h of treatment, the cells were rinsed twice with cold PBS pH 7.4, harvested and pelleted by centrifugation. The cell's pellets were lysed in RIPA buffer (10 mM Tris/HCl pH 8.0, 150 mM NaCl, 1% (vol/vol) Nonidet P-40, 0.5% (wt/vol) sodium deoxycholate, 5 mM EDTA) with complete inhibitor mix from Roche diagnostics (Basel, Switzerland) at 0 °C for 20 min. The lysates were homogenized through 21-G needles 10 times, and then clarified by centrifugation at 2800 x g for 10 min. Protein concentration of lysates was determined using a BCA protein assay kit.

A total of 50 µg proteins were fractionated by 4–20% TGX SDS polyacrylamide gels (BioRad, Hercules, CA, USA). After electrotransfer to polyvinylidene fluoride membranes (BioRad), these membranes were blocked overnight at 4 °C in Tris-buffered saline (TBS: 50 mM Tris, 150 mM NaCl) containing 0.1% (vol/vol) Tween-20 (Sigma-Aldrich) (TBS-T) and 5% (wt/vol) skimmed milk powder. Membranes were incubated 2 h at RT with primary antibodies, Rabbit antibody against anti-APP C-terminal fragment (APP intracellular domain, AICD, Sigma-Aldrich) and Mouse monoclonal anti-β-actin antibody (Sigma-Aldrich) (1: 1000 and 1: 5000, respectively). After washing 3 times with TBS-T, the membranes were probed with corresponding peroxidase conjugated secondary antibodies rabbit anti-mouse or goat anti-rabbit (Abliance former Paris, France) (1: 4000) at RT for 1 h. Detection was carried out by using a chemiluminescence detection kit (Clarity Western ECL substrate, Biorad). After washing steps, signals were detected with ChemiDoc MP (Biorad).

The relative intensity of bands was densitometrically determined by Image J software 1.46r (NIH, USA). For statistical analysis, all data from 3 independent experiments were expressed as the ratio to optical density values of the corresponding β-actin control [53]. The values were expressed as a percentage of the control group arbitrarily set at 100%. The statistical analysis was done with a Student t-test.

#### *Fluorescence-activated cell sorting (FACS) by flow cytometry*

After 24 h of treatment with 100 µM 5-HIAA, SH-SY5Y cells were harvested, centrifuged for 10 min at 1000 x g at RT and re-suspended with 0.5% PBS-BSA before being gently fixed in 4% paraformaldehyde (PFA, Sigma-Aldrich) in PBS for 1 h. Thereafter, the cells were submitted to two centrifugation steps (10 min at 1000 x g) separated by a washing step using 0.5% PBS-BSA. Cells were then incubated in permeabilization buffer (0.1% Triton X-100 in 0.1% sodium citrate) for 2 min on ice. An additional round of washing and centrifugation was performed before incubating the cells with anti-NEP antibody (Merck-Millipore; 1:200) in PBS for 25 min at 4 °C. At the end of the incubation, the cells were washed and centrifuged again for 10 min at 1000 x g. Supernatants were removed and the pellets were suspended and incubated with a secondary antibody for 25 min at 4 °C. The cells were washed and centrifuged a last time, the supernatants were removed, and the pellets were suspended in PBS before being analyzed.

#### *Proteome profiler Phospho-MAPK array*

After ½ hour of treatment with 100 µM 5-HIAA or without treatment, SH-SY5Y cells were harvested, centrifuged for 5 min at 300 x g at RT, and then solubilized at $1 \times 10^7$ cells/ml in the Lysis Buffer provided with the kit for ½ hour. The level of phosphorylation was determined by using a Proteome Profiler Antibody Kit (Human Phospho-MAPK Array Kit, R&D Systems Europe, Oxford, UK). Briefly, two nitrocellulose membranes, containing 26 different capture antibodies printed in duplicate, were blocked for 1 h under agitation at RT. During the same time, the protein extracts were incubated with a detection antibody cocktail. After one hour, the blocking buffer was replaced by the mix protein extract - antibody cocktail and incubated overnight at 2–8 °C under agitation. Then the membranes were washed 3 times in wash buffer, and were put in a solution of Streptavidin-HRP for ½ hour under agitation at RT. After a further 3 washes, the membranes were covered with a Chemi-reagent mix for 1 min before detection of the signal with ChemiDoc MP (Biorad). The relative intensity of bands was densitometrically determined by Image J software 1.46r (NIH, USA).

#### *Neprilysin activity assay*

SH-SY5Y cells were harvested and washed with PBS after 0, 30, 60 and 90 min of treatment with 30 µM 5-HIAA (Sigma-Aldrich). The cells were then sonicated in iced Tris buffer (50 mM Tris-HCl, pH 7.4) and store at – 80 °C.

Measurement of neprilysin activity was performed according to the technical details given by the manufacturer for the fluorescent SensoLyte 520 kit (AnaSpec Inc., Fremont, CA, US). Briefly, 100 µg of total protein were placed in the wells of a non-binding 96-well plate (Corning) before adding the substrate working solution. The reagents were mixed by shaking the plate gently for 30 s and the fluorescence signal was immediately measured at Ex/Em = 490 nm/520 nm continuously and the data were recorded every 5 min for 1 h.

The initial reaction velocity was determined by the slope of the linear portion of the data plot and the results were expressed in percentage by reference to control condition.

#### *Immunocytochemistry*

Coverslips were prepared with SH-SY5Y cells treated or not by 5-HIAA at a concentration of 100 µM. The cells were fixed in 4% PFA for 15 min and then permeabilized with 100% ethanol for 5 min and incubated in PBS with 5% fetal bovine serum overnight at 4 °C. A rabbit polyclonal anti-neprilysin antibody (Merck; 1:200) was applied for 2 h at RT then a pre-adsorbed Goat polyclonal anti-Mouse IgG - H&L (Alexa Fluor® 647) antibody (Abcam; 1:500) was used as secondary antibody. Coverslips were mounted in glycerol mounting medium with DAPI and DABCO™ (Abcam) before microscopic analysis using a Zeiss microscope equipped for fluorescence.

### In vivo experiments

#### *Animals and treatments*

Procedures involving animals and their care were conducted in compliance with a European Communities Council Directive (86/609/EEC) and under the supervision of authorized investigators. In addition, all the protocols were reviewed and approved by the Alsace Head Office of the French Department of Veterinary and Public Health Guide for the Care and Use of Laboratory Animals. Mice were individually housed per cage in a room with 12/12-h light-dark cycle. The room was maintained under constant temperature and humidity conditions. Water and food were available ad libitum.

#### *Mice models*

Two mice models were used:

- Female Swiss albino mice, 3-month-old, outbreeded, about 20 g (Janvier Labs, France),
- Male APPSWE hemizygote mice (B6, SJL-Tg (APPSWE) 2576 Kha, tested for heterozygous RD1, Taconic Europe, Denmark) carrying a transgene coding for the 695-amino acid isoform of human Alzheimer APP (Tg 2576) and the corresponding wild type (WT), 13-month-old. All animals were 30-35 g body weight.

#### *Phosphoramidon model of NEP inhibition and Aβ 1–40 or Aβ 1–42 quantification*

Four groups of 5 Swiss Albino mice were treated for 5 consecutive days. Group 1 received the NEP inhibitor Phosphoramidon (Peptide Institute, Osaka, Japan) each day via intranasal route. Phosphoramidon was dissolved in PBS (with 1 mM ascorbic acid) at a concentration of 30 mM and was administered intranasally as previously described [28]. Group 2 was treated with 5-HIAA via intranasal route (24 µL of a 30 mM solution). Group 3 received PBS alone. Group 4 received both phosphoramidon and 5-HIAA.

#### Aβ 1–40 and Aβ 1–42 quantification

After 5 days of treatment, the mice were euthanized for tissue collection 2 h after the last administration. The brains were removed, the two hemispheres separated and immediately frozen in liquid nitrogen and stored at – 80 °C.

The tissues of one hemisphere were homogenized in 8 volumes of ice-cold guanidine buffer (5.0 M guanidine-HCl/50 mM Tris-HCl, pH 8.0). Homogenates were mixed for 3–4 h at RT. The quantification of total proteins was done with a BCA protein assay kit (Pierce, Rockford, IL, USA). The lysates were then aliquoted and stored at – 80 °C until quantification of Aβ 1–40 and 1–42 peptides, according to the technical details given by the manufacturer (Fisher former Invitrogen, Carlsbad, CA, USA).

Samples were briefly diluted with cold Reaction buffer and centrifuged at 16,000 g for 20 min at 4 C. Supernatant was decanted and sample was stored on ice until use. Hundred μL of the diluted homogenates or of the Aβ peptide standards were incubated on the pre-coated 96-well plate for 2 h at RT. The plate was washed 4 times and 100 μL of the primary antibody was added for 1 h at RT. After 4 further washes, 100 μL of the secondary antibody was added for 30 min at RT. After 4 new washes, 100 μl of Stabilized Chromogen was added to each well for 30 min at RT in the dark. Finally, the reaction was stopped by 100 μL of Stop Solution to each well and the optical density was read at 450 nm in a plate reader (Elisa reader model Sigma 960, Metertech, Taipei, Taiwan).

The β peptides levels were interpolated from the standard curve generated from serial dilutions of synthetic peptide. Each measurement was repeated on 3 occasions, and the average value was calculated.

The results were analyzed with an analysis of variance (ANOVA $p < 0.0001$) to evaluate the effects of genotype and treatment factors. Post hoc analyses were performed with the Bonferroni test.

#### *Tg 2576 and WT mice treatment*

Two groups of mice (12 Tg 2576 and 12 WT) were administered daily via intra-nasal route with 4 μL of a 30 mM solution of 5-HIAA (Sigma-Aldrich, France) in PBS [20, 21]. In parallel, 24 other animals (12 Tg 2576 and 12 WT) were treated for 5 consecutive days with 48 mg/kg 5-Hydroxy-L-tryptophan (5-HTP, Sigma-Aldrich) administrated IP. Control groups were obtained by administration of PBS (12 Tg 2576 and 12 WT). These mice were the used for the neprilysin activity assay or for the spatial novelty task.

#### *Neprilysin activity assay*

To measure NEP activity in the mouse brain, the animals were treated daily for 5 consecutive days and euthanized for tissue collection 2 h after the last administration for the Tg 2576 mouse (sub-chronical treatment) and at various times (0 to 120 min) for the Swiss mice (acute treatment). The brains were removed, the two hemispheres separated and immediately frozen in liquid nitrogen and stored at − 80 °C. The tissues of one hemisphere were homogenized in 5 volumes of ice-cold PBS, centrifuged at 15000 x g for 5 min at 4 °C and the supernatant was decanted and stored at − 80 °C. The quantification of total proteins was done by a BCA protein assay kit).

Measurement of neprilysin activity was performed according to the technical details given by the manufacturer for the fluorescent SensoLyte 520 kit (AnaSpec Inc., Fremont, CA, US). Briefly, 100 μg of total protein were placed in the wells of a non-binding 96-well plate (Corning) before adding the substrate working solution. The reagents were mixed by shaking the plate gently for 30 s and the fluorescence signal was immediately measured at Ex/Em = 490 nm/520 nm continuously and the data were recorded every 5 min for 1 h.

The initial reaction velocity was determined by the slope of the linear portion of the data plot and the results were expressed in percentage by reference to control condition.

#### *Spatial novelty task*

This task is based on the spontaneous tendency of mice to preferentially explore objects which have been displaced within a familiar arrangement of objects. Tg 2576 mice are deeply impaired in this task as early as 7 to 8 months of age, independently of the rd mutation [38, 57].

The spatial novelty task was performed in a square Plexiglas open field (52 × 52 × 40 cm). For each testing period, a specific set of 7 different objects (4 for the habituation phases and 3 for the spatial recognition task), which differed in shape, color, and materials, were used. Each object was available in duplicate (one for each trial when required) and was wiped with 70% ethanol as the whole open field between each trial. On days 1 and 2, the mice received a habituation trial of 10 min with 2 different objects each day.

On day 3 (5th day of treatment), the mice explored the spatial configuration of 3 new objects during a 10-min acquisition trial, returned in their home cage for 3 min, and then received a 10-min retention trial with a new spatial configuration resulting from the shifting of one of the 3 objects to a new location. Recognition performances were calculated as the additional time spent exploring the displaced object during the retention trial when mice are the most involved in exploring the objects. This value was compared with the 0 value (no detection of the spatial change) with a Student t-test to measure whether spatial novelty detection occurred and was also compared among groups with an analysis of variance (ANOVA $p < 0.0001$) to evaluate the effects of genotype and treatment factors. Post-hoc analyses were performed with the Newman-Keuls test.

#### *Immunocytochemistry on brain tissue slices*

Tg 2576/APPSWE mice chronically treated with 5-HIAA were perfused through the heart with cold 4% PFA. The brains were fixed in a 4% PFA solution for 72 h at 4 °C and afterwards were immersed in PBS containing 20% sucrose for 48 h. The brains were cut in a vibratome Leica VT1000M (80 μm thick) and the slices were collected in a Watson medium.

Floating sections were immunostained as follows: Tissue slides were rehydrated with PBS for 1 h at RT then blocked overnight at 4 °C with 5% (*v*/*v*) fetal bovine serum in PBS. Sections were stirred overnight at 4 C with the primary antibodies (mouse monoclonal Anti-β Amyloid 1–40 antibody (Abcam) and rabbit polyclonal anti-Neprilysin antibody (Merck Millipore) at a dilution of 1:200. Sections were then washed 10 to 12 times for 1 h in PBS pH 7.4. Then the sections were stirred with species-specific secondary antibodies (pre-adsorbed Goat polyclonal anti-Mouse IgG - H&L (Alexa Fluor® 647) antibody (Abcam) and pre-adsorbed Goat polyclonal anti-Rabbit IgG - H&L (Alexa Fluor® 488) antibody (Abcam), at a dilution of 1:500, overnight at 4 C in the dark. Sections were washed again (10 to 12 times for 1 h) with PBS pH 7.4. After this second period of washing, the sections were mounted in glycerol mounting medium with DAPI and DABCO™ (Abcam) before microscopic analysis using a microscope (Zeiss AxioImager Z2).

### Statistical analysis

GraphPad Prism was used for all statistical analysis. For ANOVA multiple statistical comparisons, Newman-Keuls or Bonferroni tests were used and two-sided unpaired Student's *t*-test for single statistical comparison. Statistical distribution for the Post-hoc analyses was: * $p < 0.05$, ** $p < 0.005$ and *** $p < 0.0001$. Errors are standard error of mean (SEM).

## Results

### The synthesis and activity of NEP in SH-SY5Y neuronal cells increase time-dependently in the presence of graded concentrations of 5-HIAA

The serotonin catabolite 5-HIAA at a dose of 100 µM increases NEP activity in SH-SY5Y cells with time. The maximum activity culminates at 90–120 min after addition of the compound and decrease to basal level 3 h later (Fig. 1a). Under the same conditions, the corresponding NEP mRNA messenger was measured in cell cultures until 90 min of incubation. An increase was noticed starting at 30 min and was elevated by about 30 times after 90 min, which corresponds to the maximum of NEP activity (Fig. 1b). The neo-synthesis of NEP protein, measured in cells cultured in the presence of increased amounts of 5-HIAA by an ELISA method, showed an $EC_{50}$ of 8 ± 3 µM (Fig. 1c). This concentration is within the range of 5-HIAA concentration found in brain tissue [50].

### 5-HIAA or 5-HTP administration in vivo increases NEP activity in the mouse brain

Tg 2576 mice were intranasally administered either 24 µL of a 30 mM solution of 5-HIAA or with 48 mg/kg I.P of 5-HTP consecutively for 5 days. At the end of treatment, NEP activities were measured. Both 5-HTP and 5-HIAA treatments increase the level of NEP activity in brain, the treatment with 5-HIAA being the more active (Fig. 1f). In a second series of experiments, Swiss albino mice were treated with 5-HIAA at time zero (24 µL of a 30 mM solution) and the NEP activity was determined in brain every 30 min until 120 min. A rapid increase in this activity was shown with a maximum at 90 min, confirming in vivo the result obtained in cell cultures (Fig. 1g).

### Cell analysis by flow cytometry confirms the stimulatory effect of 5-HIAA on NEP expression

The induction of NEP expression by 5-HIAA is rapid when measured in a cell's homogenate. However, NEP protein targeting the cell membrane is a prolonged process [25]. For this reason, we confirmed the induction of NEP protein in SH-SY5Y neuronal cells using flow cytometry analysis after incubation for 24 h with 100 µM 5-HIAA. The cells were labeled with a NEP specific antibody. Figure 1d represents a qualitative analysis of the intensity of NEP antibody-induced immunolabeling in 5-HIAA-treated and control SH-SY5Y cells. A quantitative approach has been used to count cells by flow cytometry. Figure 1e shows the percentage of NEP positive cells under control conditions (46%) and in the presence of 100 µM 5-HIAA (89%).

### Effect of 5-HIAA in a pharmacological model of brain Aβ accumulation

Adult Swiss albino mice treated for 5 days by intranasal administrations of the NEP inhibitor phosphoramidon ($K_i$ of about 2 nM) showed increased brain concentrations of both 1–40 Aβ (+ 39%) and 1–42 Aβ (+ 144%) compared to control mice treated with saline. Administration of 5-HIAA alone to healthy mice reduced brain basal levels of 1–40 and 1–42 Aβ about 14 and 32%, respectively. The co-treatment of phosphoramidon-receiving mice with 5-HIAA decreased the brain 1–40 Aβ (–15%) and 1–42 Aβ (– 45%) concentrations. These results reveal that 5-HIAA is capable of counteracting Aβ accumulation in the brain under physiological or pharmacologically-evoked (phosphoramidon-induced NEP inhibition) conditions (Fig. 2a and b and Table 1).

### 5-HIAA treatment reduces brain Aβ concentration in APPSWE mice

Tg 2576 APPSWE mice are well characterized as a model for AD-related Aβ pathology expressing brain 1–40 and 1–42 Aβ accumulations [17, 22, 54]. We measured the concentration of 1–40 and 1–42 Aβ peptides in cerebral hemispheres of 14 months aged APPSWE mice treated (5 consecutive days) or not by intranasal

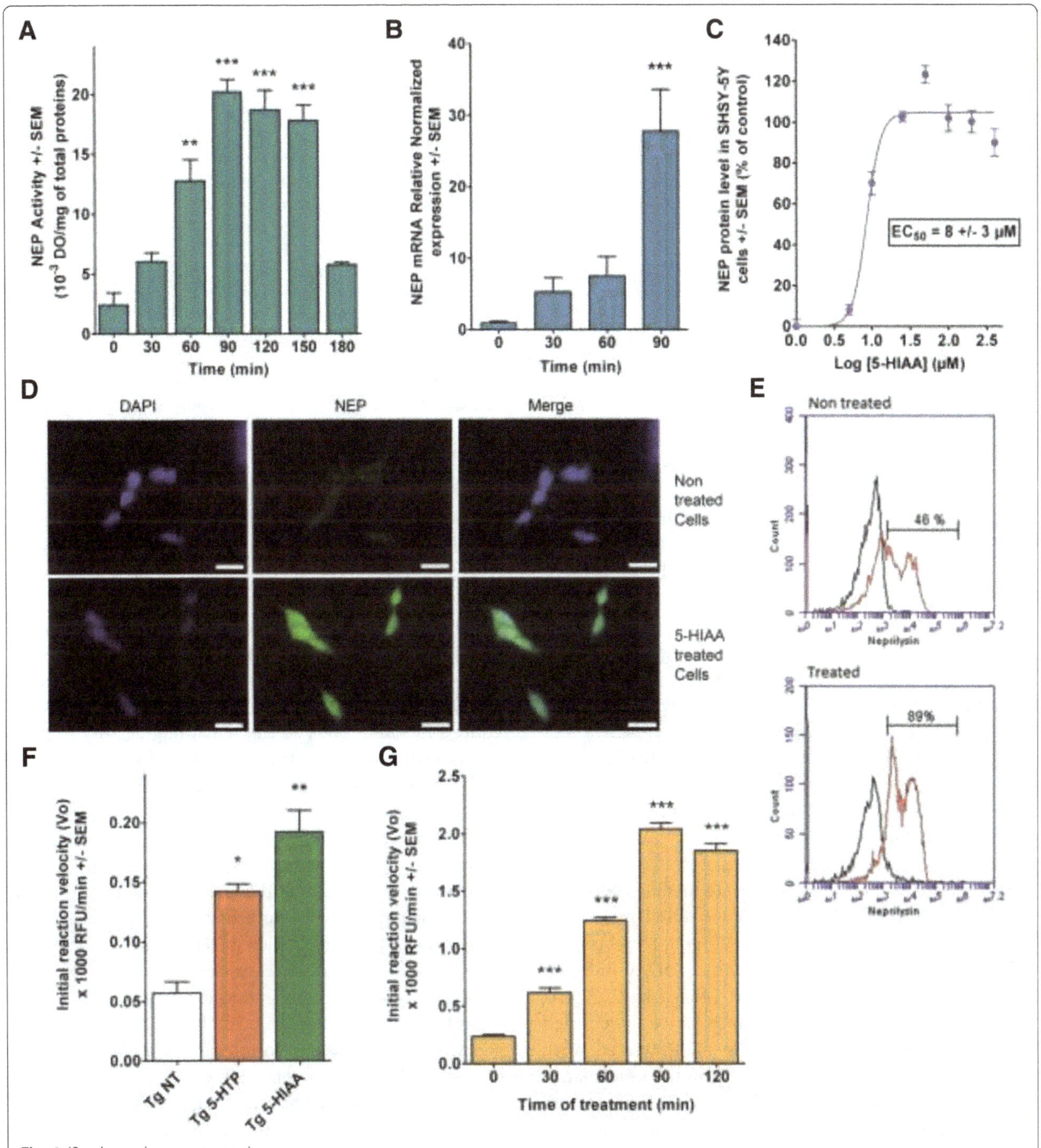

**Fig. 1** (See legend on next page.)

(See figure on previous page.)
**Fig. 1** Effects of 5-HIAA on NEP expression and activity in SH-SY5Y neuronal cells and mouse brain. **a**, **b**, **c**: Experiments in SH-SY5Y neuroblastoma cells. **a** Kinetic of NEP activity as a function of incubation time (0 to 180 min) in cells treated by 100 μM 5-HIAA. NEP activity was determined with a fluorescent SensoLyte 520 kit (AnaSpec Inc., Fremont, CA, US). NEP activity culminates at 90–120 min after addition of the compound, with quantitative values corresponding to 20 +/− 1 and 19 +/ 2 $10^3$ DO/mg of total proteins, respectively. These maximal values decrease to basal level after 3 h. **b** q-PCR assessment of NEP mRNA increase as a function of incubation time (0 to 90 min) in SH-SY5Y cells treated by 100 μM 5-HIAA. The increase of NEP mRNA level already detectable at 30 min, reached a value 30 times higher at 90 min which represents the time point corresponding to NEP maximal activity. **c** ELISA test determination of the dose-response effect of 24 h 5-HIAA treatment on NEP activity. Evaluation of the effects of increasing doses of 5-HIAA showed an $EC_{50}$ of 8 ± 3 μM, a concentration within the range of 5-HIAA concentration found in brain tissue. The statistical analysis of triplicate samples was done by an ANOVA completed with a Bonferroni's Multiple Comparison Test. ** $p < 0.005$, *** $p < 0.0001$. **d** Immunocytochemistry with anti-NEP antibody of SH-SY5Y cells treated with 100 μM 5-HIAA for 24 h versus non-treated controls. Scale bars: 20 μm. **e** Fluorescence-activated cell sorting (FACS) by flow cytometry on SHSY-5Y cells treated with 5-HIAA (100 μM) for 24 h versus controls. 46% of cells were neprilysin-positive in control cells while 89% were positively labeled in treated cells. Black curve: no secondary antibody; Red curve: cells treated with NEP secondary antibody. **f**, **g**: Experiments on mouse brain in vivo. **f** Effects of 5-HTP (48 mg/kg, I.P.) or 5-HIAA (24 μL of a 30 mM solution, intra-nasal) on NEP activity in 14 months APPSWE mice brain ($n = 5$ for each treatment). Drugs were administered each day during five consecutive days. Both 5-HTP and 5-HIAA treatments increase the level of NEP activity in brain (142 +/− 7 and 192 +/− 18 Relative Fluorescence Units (RFU)/min, respectively). However, 5-HIAA treatment was the most effective. **g** Kinetics of NEP enzymatic activity in 3 months Swiss Albinos mice ($n = 5$ at each time point) treated by an intra-nasal administration of 24 μL of a 30 mM solution of 5-HIAA at time zero. The brain NEP activity was determined every 30 min until 120 min. A rapid increase of NEP activity was detected at 90 min with a maximum value of 2040 +/− 50 RFU/min. The statistical analysis was done by an ANOVA completed with a Bonferroni's Multiple Comparison Test. * $p < 0.05$; ** $p < 0.005$; *** $p < 0.0001$ by reference to NT or time zero

5-HIAA or by 5-HTP (48 mg/kg) injected IP. This last compound is a precursor of 5-HIAA in the brain, but also of serotonin (Fig. 3a). Six hours after the last administration of each compound, the animals were killed and brain Aβ concentrations were determined.

In the wild type counterparts of Tg 2576 mice, 5-HIAA treatment reduces brain 1–40 and 1–42 Aβ concentrations by 19 and 39%, respectively. In APPSWE mice, the decrease of brain 1–40 Aβ level was − 39% and − 69% after 5-HIAA or 5-HTP administration while the reduction of cerebral 1–42 Aβ level was − 14% and − 45% after 5-HIAA or 5-HTP treatment, respectively (Fig. 2c and Table 2).

### 5-HIAA or 5-HTP treatments ameliorate memory task performance in both WT and Tg 2576 APPSWE mice

Tg 2576 APPSWE mice and their WT counterparts were treated for five consecutive days with 5-HIAA (intranasal administration) or by 5-HTP (48 mg/kg I.P). Six hours after the last administration, the mice were tested for spatial recognition test. WT mice treated with 5-HTP or 5-HIAA exhibited an improved performance than control animals treated with saline; 5-HIAA-treated animals showed the best performance. Non-treated Tg 2576 APPSWE mice performed very poorly compared to transgenic animals treated with 5-HTP or 5-HIAA under the same conditions. Retention performances of the non-treated APPSWE groups were lower than those of treated APPSWE, treated WT and non-treated WT groups respectively (Newman-Keuls: $p < 0.001$, APPSWE control groups compared to each other group) (Fig. 2e).

### A role for 5-HIAA precursors in NEP induction?

Tryptophan, 5-HTP and serotonin (5-HT) are the main precursors of 5-HIAA in the brain. We examined in a series of experiments the potential role of these compounds to induce NEP via the production of 5-HIAA. Tryptophan is both the precursor of kynurenic acid through the kynurenic pathway and of 5-HIAA through serotonin catabolism (Fig. 3a). Kynurenic acid has been found to be a NEP inducer and its neuroprotective properties are well documented [29]. In the presence of IMAO (A + B), the induction of NEP by tryptophan is reduced by about 50%, so the remaining activity of tryptophan could be due to the formation of kynurenic acid. In the absence of inhibitor, L-tryptophan possesses an $EC_{50}$ of 19 ± 2 μM for the induction of NEP in SH-SY5Y cell cultures (Fig. 3b and c).

5-HTP is a well-known precursor of serotonin and of 5-HIAA in the brain. In the presence of either carbidopa, which inhibits its decarboxylation into serotonin or of tranylcypromine which blocks its transformation into 5-HIAA, the inductive capacity of 5-HTP on NEP expression is significantly reduced compared to 5-HTP tested without inhibitors (Fig. 3c). In the presence of carbidopa, 5-HTP possesses an intrinsic activity on NEP induction with an $EC_{50}$ of 5 ± 1 μM (Fig. 3b), but the maximum activity reaches a plateau at 20%.

Finally, increasing doses of serotonin incubated in the presence of tranylcypromine showed no effect on NEP induction (Fig. 3b, green). Also, serotonin at 100 μM exerted no significant effect on NEP expression in the presence of IMAO (Fig. 3c). Serotonin incubated alone exhibited some effect, probably because of its role as a precursor of 5-HIAA.

### 5-HIAA induces NEP neo-expression via a MAP-kinase driven mechanism

The level of phosphorylation of the principal intermediates of MAP-kinase pathway was determined by using

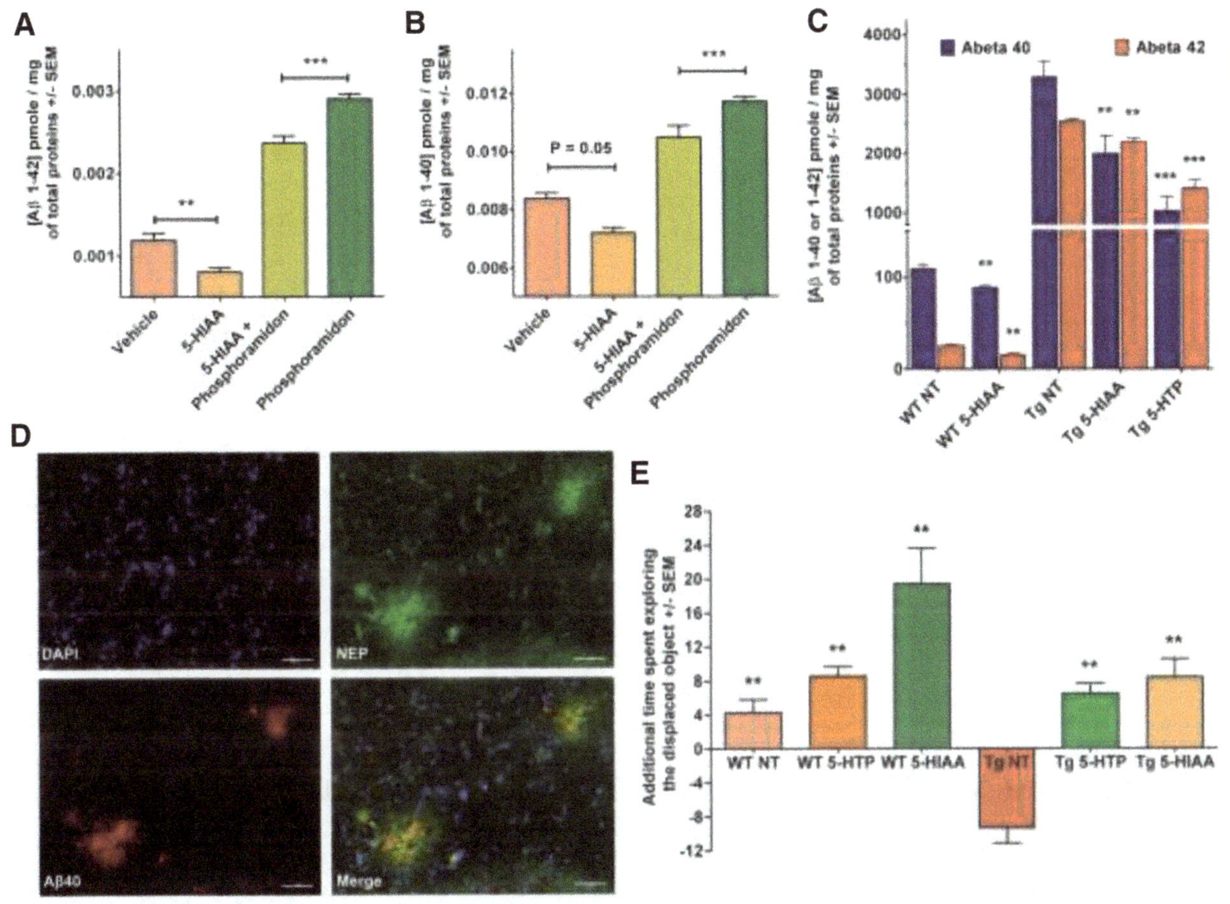


**Fig. 2** Effects of 5-HIAA on brain amyloid peptide accumulation and memory performance. **a**, **b**: Inhibitory action of 5-HIAA against phosphoramidon-induced brain Aβ accumulation in 3-month-old Swiss albino mice ($n = 7$ for each group). **a** Phosphoramidon induces an increase in Aβ 1–42 peptide which is counteracted by 5-HIAA treatment. The effect of 5-HIAA can be seen also in control mice non-treated with Phosphoramidon (see also Table 1). Statistical analysis by an ANOVA completed with a Bonferroni's Multiple Comparison Test. * $p < 0.05$, ** $p < 0.005$, *** $p < 0.0001$. **b**: Same results than in A with the Aβ 1–40 peptide. **c** 5-HIAA- or 5-HTP-induced decrease of brain Aβ peptide level in 14-month-old Tg 2576/APPSWE mice (Tg). The mice ($n = 7$ for each group) were treated daily during 5 consecutive days with 5-HTP (48 mg/kg, I.P.) or 5-HIAA (24 μL of a 30 mM, intra-nasal). 5-HIAA treatment reduces brain 1–40 and 1–42 Aβ concentrations in wild type (WT) and APPSWE mice. 5-HTP treatment is also active in APPSWE mice (see also Table 2). The statistical analysis was done by an ANOVA completed with a Bonferroni's Multiple Comparison Test of NT (non-treated) WT (wild-type) or Tg (Tg 2576/APPSWE) mice. **d** Photomicrographs showing the co-localization of NEP and 1–40 Aβ peptide in the cortex of Tg 2576/APPSWE mice brain. Scale bars: 50 μm. This image is an illustration of the distribution of NEP and amyloid deposits co-localization. **e** Effects of 5 consecutive days intra-nasal 5-HIAA (24 μl of a 30 mM solution) or I.P. 5-HTP (48 mg/kg) treatments on the spatial novelty performances of 14-month-old wild-type (WT) and Tg 2576/APPSWE (Tg) mice ($n = 7$ for each group). Results are shown as the mean additional time (SEM) spent in exploring the displaced object versus the non-displaced objects during the retention trial. This value was compared to the 0 value (no detection of the spatial change) with a Student t-test (** $p < 0.01$) to determine whether spatial novelty detection occurred. Treated WT mice exhibited an improved performance compared to control animals; 5-HIAA-treated mice showed the best performance. Non-treated (NT) Tg 2576/APPSWE mice performed very poorly compared to treated transgenic animals. The various groups were compared with an ANOVA ($P < 0.0001$) completed with a Newman-Keuls Multiple Comparison Test to evaluate the effects of treatments. Retention performances of the non-treated (NT) APPSWE groups were lower than those of treated APPSWE, treated WT and non-treated WT groups, respectively

the Proteome Profiler Antibody Kit (R&D Systems). This system detects the phosphorylation of 26 human kinases simultaneously. SH-SY5Y cells were treated during 30 min with 100 μM 5-HIAA and then were analyzed according to the recommended protocol. Figure 4a represents the integrated spots that were significantly different from the non-treated cells. From these results, we decided to explore particularly the ERK pathway, which appears to be down-regulated by 5-HIAA. The modification of GSK-3 α/β, a strategic factor for tau phosphorylation, was also significantly affected by the treatment, together with the transcription factor CREB. The phosphorylation of all these intermediates and transcription factor are decreased by the cell's treatment with 5-HIAA.

SCH772984 is a specific inhibitor of ERK1/2 with $IC_{50}$ values of 4 nM and 1 nM in cell-free assays [8]. We incubated this compound alone or in combination with

**Table 1** Variations of brain amyloid peptide level in phosphoramidon-treated and control mice after 5-HIAA or vehicle treatment

| | Vehicle | 5-HIAA | Phosphoramidon | 5-HIAA + Phosphoramidon | |
|---|---|---|---|---|---|
| Aβ42 | 1.2 | 0.8 | 2.9 | 2.4 | Mean (pg/total proteins) |
| | 100 | 68 | 244 | 199 | Mean compared with vehicle (%) |
| | 0 | −32 | 144 | 99 | % of variation compared to Vehicle |
| | −144 | − 176 | 0 | −45 | % of variation compared to Phosphoramidon |
| Aβ40 | 8.4 | 7.2 | 11.7 | 10.5 | Mean (pg/total proteins) |
| | 100 | 86 | 140 | 125 | Mean compared with vehicle (%) |
| | 0 | −14 | 40 | 25 | % of variation compared to Vehicle |
| | −39 | −54 | 0 | −15 | % of variation compared to phosphoramidon |

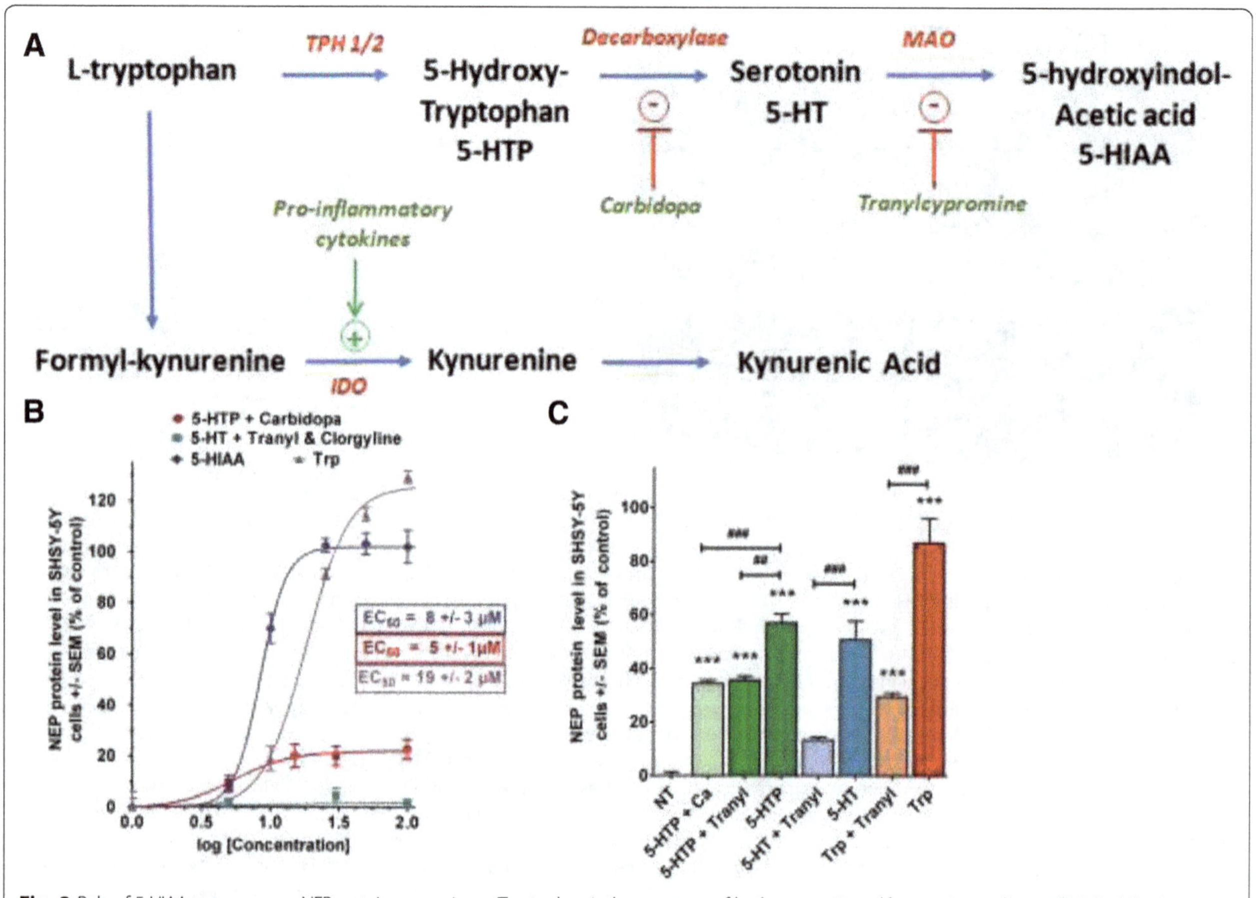


**Fig. 3** Role of 5-HIAA precursors on NEP protein expression. **a** Tryptophan is the precursor of both serotonin and kynurenine pathways. IDO (indolamine dioxygenase 2,3 dioxygenase) induction by inflammatory cytokines favorizes the production of kynurenine pathway intermediates, including kynurenic acid. Tryptophan, 5-hydroxytryptophan (5-HTP) and serotonin (5-HT) are precursors of 5-HIAA. 5-HTP degradation is prevented by carbidopa while serotonin catabolism is blocked by IMAO (tranylcypromine + clorgyline). **b** Dose-response curves for the induction of NEP protein in SH-SY5Y cells. Effect of tryptophan, 5-HIAA, 5HTP + carbidopa (100 μM), Serotonin + tranylcypromine (30 μM) and clorgyline (20 μM) on NEP protein level in SH-SY5Y cells after 30-min treatment. In the absence of inhibitor, 5-HIAA and L-tryptophan exhibit an $EC_{50}$ of 8 ± 3 μM and 19 ± 2 μM for NEP induction, respectively. In the presence of carbidopa, 5-HTP shows an intrinsic activity on NEP induction with an $EC_{50}$ of 5 ± 1 μM but the maximum activity is 20%. Incubation of SH-SY5Y cells with increasing doses of serotonin in the presence of tranylcypromine showed no effect on NEP induction. **c** Effects of 24-h pharmacological inhibition of 5-HIAA synthesis from precursors (Tryptophan, 5-HTP, or 5-HT) on NEP protein expression in SH-SY5Y cells. In the presence of Tranylcypromine, NEP induction by tryptophan is reduced from 87 +/− 9 to 30 +/− 1%. In the presence of either carbidopa (inhibitor of 5-HTP decarboxylation into 5-HT), or tranylcypromine (blocker of 5-HTP conversion into 5-HIAA), NEP induction by 5-HTP was significantly reduced compared to 5-HTP tested without inhibitors (respectively 35 +/− 1 and 36 +/− 1% vs 57 +/− 3%). 5-HT at 100 μM exhibited some effect on NEP (51 +/− 7%) because of its role as a precursor of 5-HIAA. Consistently, the effect of 5-HT was inhibited by tranylcypromine (13 +/− 1%). The statistical analysis of triplicatesamples was done by an ANOVA completed with a Bonferroni's Multiple Comparison Test. ## $p < 0.005$, ### or *** $p < 0.0001$. * by reference to non-treated (NT) cells, or # by reference to treatments with specific enzyme's inhibitor

**Table 2** Variations of brain amyloid peptide level in APPSWE and WT mice after 5-HIAA or 5-HTP treatment

| | WT NT | WT 5HIAA | Tg NT | Tg 5HIAA | Tg 5HTP | |
|---|---|---|---|---|---|---|
| Aβ40 | 109.2 | 88.6 | 3285 | 1996 | 1031 | Mean (pg/total proteins) |
| | 100 | 81 | 100 | 61 | 31 | Mean compared with NT (%) |
| | 0 | −19 | 0 | −39 | −69 | % of variation compared to corresponding NT |
| Aβ42 | 25.2 | 15.3 | 2544 | 2192 | 1408 | Mean (pg/total proteins) |
| | 100 | 61 | 100 | 86 | 55 | Mean compared with NT (%) |
| | 0 | −39 | 0 | −14 | −45 | % of variation compared to corresponding NT |

5-HIAA in SH-SY5Y incubation medium to confirm the role of ERK pathway inhibition in the neo-expression of NEP. As shown in Fig. 4b, NEP protein expression is strongly stimulated by the presence of SCH772984 after 90 min of incubation and the addition of 100 μM 5-HIAA increases this stimulation significantly. Similarly, the MEK inhibitor (GSK 1120212, Trametinib) which plays a role as a MEK/MAPK/ERK kinase inhibitor, induces NEP with an $EC_{50}$ in the nanomolar range. These results constitute additional evidence for a role of MAP-kinase cascade in NEP expression mediated by 5-HIAA. However, as several reports described a role for AICD peptide (intra-cellular domain of APP) in the control of NEP expression [18], this possibility was tested in the same experimental model. While $NH_4Cl$ strongly induced AICD, this peptide was down-regulated by 5-HIAA, suggesting that the mechanism activated by 5-HIAA to induce NEP expression does not involve or depend on AICD stimulation (Fig. 4c).

## Discussion and conclusions

In its early stage of clinical expression, sporadic AD is heterogeneous with cognitive, behavioral or psychological symptoms of many kinds, including alterations of mood, emotive disorders, confusion, agitation and anxiety or modifications in the sleep-wake cycle [46]. Serotonin and its brain innervations are known to modulate these alterations and pharmacological manipulations of the serotonergic system have long been used as therapeutic approach for these symptoms [11]. This therapeutic strategy includes the potentiation of serotonin synthesis by tryptophan or 5-HTP administration, the inhibition of serotonin transport by SSRI's or degradation by IMAO. Among the large family of serotonergic receptors (5-HT1 to 5-HT7, each of them containing several isoforms), several classes appear to be implicated in AD related mechanisms. 5-HT2 receptors (2A, 2B, 2C) which activate phospholipase C pathway and 5-HT4, 5-HT6 that are coupled to Gs, have been reported to regulate the proteolytic cleavage of APP, neuroinflammation and cognitive deficits. The mechanisms involved in these processes are unknown, and serotonin is supposed to activate the complete set of its receptors with a global effect to be defined regarding AD [24]. This disease is characterized by diffuse brain atrophy due to neuronal degeneration and synaptic loss affecting multiple regions in the brain. The neurodegeneration results from Aβ accumulation and hyperphosphorylation of Tau which affect neuron survival [9]. Interestingly, it has been shown that the dorsal raphe nucleus exhibits cytoskeletal lesions at early stages of the disease, suggesting a possible role for the ascending serotonergic pathway in early manifestations of AD [5, 19, 43]. Amyloid protein accumulation in the brain is a prolonged process induced by chronic inflammation, reduction of energy metabolism and promotion of apoptotic mechanisms which precede the development of microtubule-associated protein Tau hyperphosphorylation and loss of functions [13]. Several mutations and gene variants are in favor of a closed link between Aβ proteinopathy and progressive occurrence of dementia in AD [1, 42]. The accumulation of amyloid oligomers is tightly regulated in the normal brain, in part by a fine control of their clearance. The cellular proteolysis of many brain proteins involves the proteasome and the lysosome, but also many proteolytic activities including Insulin-degrading enzyme, Endothelin or angiotensin converting enzyme and matrix metalloproteinases among others [33, 56]. However, a pivotal role is assigned to NEP, a cell-surface ectoenzyme degrading several key neuropeptides (enkephalins, substance P), which has been identified as a major Aβ degrading enzyme in the brain. Over-expression of NEP in Drosophila or in transgenic mice could suppress amyloid plaques formation or reduce brain Aβ levels. By contrast, a reduction of NEP expression has been evidenced in the brain of aged or AD patients [23, 33]. However, NEP activity seems to be stimulated in brain cells in contact with amyloid deposits in human brain. It appears that NEP up-regulation could be an adaptive mechanism counteracting brain Aβ accumulation and protecting thus neuron survival during the disease incubation [40]. Since several years, a pharmacological approach has been suggested to increase NEP activity in the brain and several compounds were identified as NEP expression modulators, some of them being potential actors regulating NEP homeostasis in vivo [28,

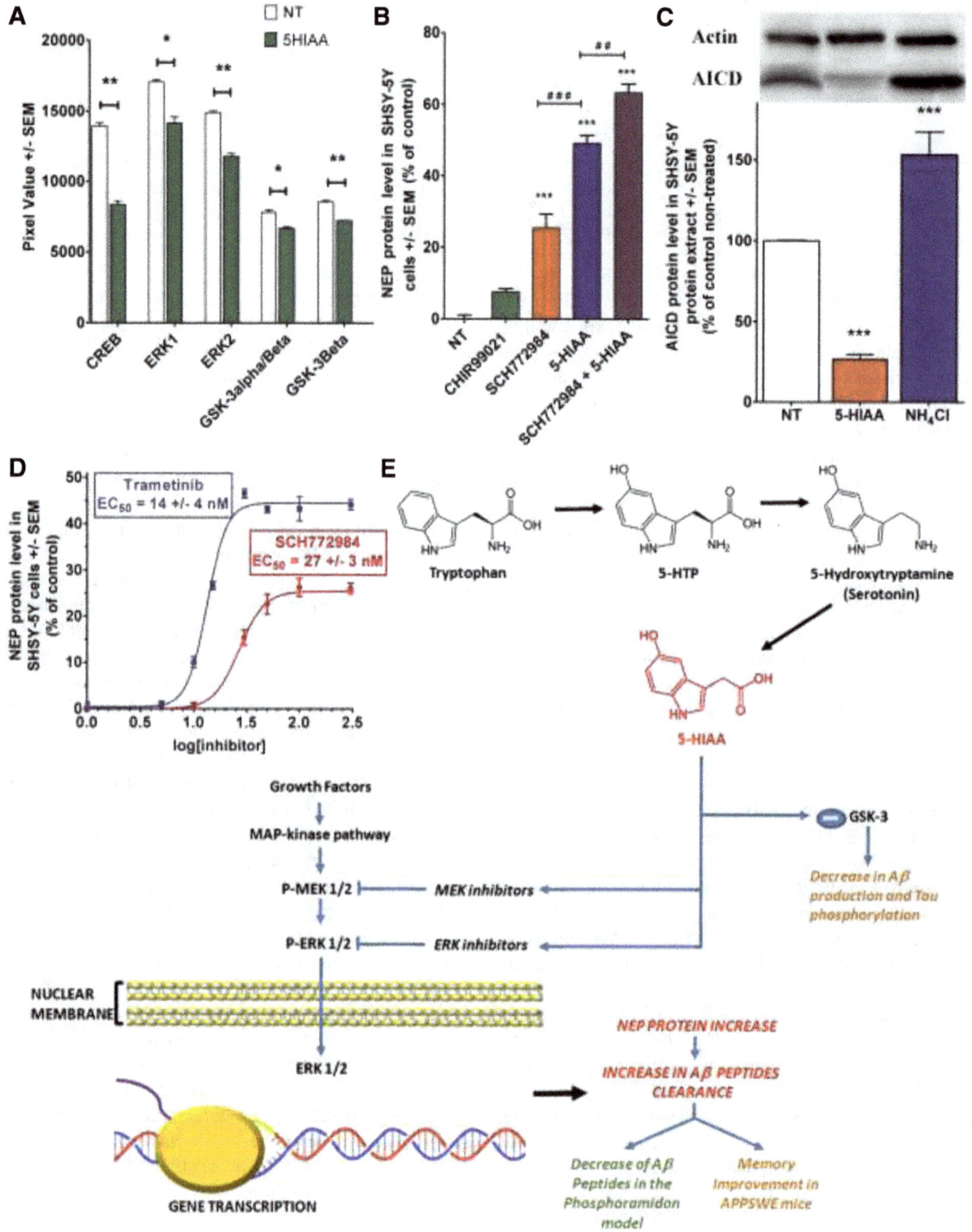


**Fig. 4** (See legend on next page.)

(See figure on previous page.)
**Fig. 4** 5-HIAA induces NEP expression via the MAP-kinase/ERK ½ pathway. **a** Down-regulatory effect of 5-HIAA on ERK ½, MEK ½ and GSK-3 expression in SH-SY5Y cells after 30 min treatment. The ERK pathway was down-regulated by 5-HIAA (mean decrease of ERK1–17% and ERK2–21%). GSK-3 α/β, a strategic factor for tau phosphorylation, was also significantly affected by the treatment (mean decrease of GSK-3α/β and GSK-3β – 15%), together with the transcription factor CREB (mean decrease – 40%). The statistical analysis of triplicate samples was done with a Student t-test. * $p < 0.05$, ** $p < 0.005$ by reference to non-treated cells (NT). **b** Effects of separated or combined treatments with the ERK ½ inhibitor SCH772984 and/or 5-HIAA on NEP expression in SH-SY5Y cells after 90 min treatment. NEP protein expression was stimulated by SCH772984 (26 +/– 4%) or 100 μM 5-HIAA (49 +/– 2%) tested separately. The combined treatment containing 100 μM 5-HIAA and SCH772984 showed a higher increase percentage of NEP expression (63 +/– 2%) compared to the separate treatments. The statistical analysis of triplicate samples was done by an ANOVA completed with a Bonferroni's Multiple Comparison Test. ## $p < 0.005$, ### or *** $p < 0.0001$. * by reference to non-treated cells (NT), or # by reference to treatments with 5-HIAA. **c** Inhibitory action of 5-HIAA on AICD expression in SH-SY5Y cells. $NH_4Cl$ as positive control. The statistical analysis ($n = 5$ in each group) was performed by an ANOVA completed with a Bonferroni's Multiple Comparison Test. *** $p < 0.0001$ by reference to non-treated cells (NT). **d** Dose-response effect and $EC_{50}$ of SCH772984 and Trametinib on NEP expression in SH-SY5Y cells. Both MEK inhibitor (GSK 1120212, Trametinib) and ERK kinase inhibitor (SCH772984) induce NEP with an $EC_{50}$ of 14 +/– 4 and 27 +/– 3 nM, respectively. **e** Graphical summary of potential mechanisms involved in 5-HIAA-induced NEP expression. The MAP-kinase pathway is involved in NEP expression in SH-SY5Y cells: inhibition of MEK/ERK ½ phosphorylation increased NEP protein levels. Phosphorylation of GSK-3 is also down-regulated by 5-HIAA treatment. These effects may explain 5-HIAA-induced increase in Aβ peptide clearance

29, 34, 51]. The fundamental interest of these studies is to try to slow-down the occurrence of AD clinical symptoms and beneficial effects against memory deficits have been reported in animal models following NEP up-regulation.

The present work describes the role of 5-HIAA, the final product of serotonin metabolism, as an inducer of NEP expression in the brain. This compound is not a ligand for serotonin receptors and was until now considered only as a dead-end product, with no functional role. However, 5-HIAA was implicated recently in the negative control of RAS/MAPK signaling pathway in *C. elegans* [45]. Interestingly, NT-3 treatment significantly increased Aβ in primary neuron cultures, an effect which was abolished by the MEK 1/2 inhibitor UO126 [25]. The Ras/MAP-kinases pathway was reported to be elevated in initial stages of AD, before the accumulation and pathology driven by Aβ [15, 16]. A pathological link between Aβ generation and altered MAP/phospho-ERK signaling seems to exist. Phospho-ERK contributes to tau phosphorylation but GSK-3 is also involved in this process, together with several other kinases [27]. GSK-3 promotes every major pathological process in AD, including apoptosis and GSK-3 inhibitors improve several cognitive functions in transgenic mice models for AD [4]. We demonstrate that in SH-SY5Y cell cultures, 5-HIAA-induced neo-expression of NEP protein and this effect is partially reproduced by the inhibition of ERK 1/2 pathway. 5-HIAA reduces also the expression of GSK-3 and this action may additionally ameliorate AD symptoms in APPSWE transgenic mice. Moreover, P-CREB decrease observed after 5-HIAA administration may probably result from the down-regulation of MAP-kinase/GSK-3 pathways but it is difficult to estimate the direct impact of this effect on the behavior of APPSWE mice owing to the involvement of P-CREB in various events related to brain plasticity [7].

Independently from the effect of 5-HIAA on NEP gene expression, its possible inhibitory action at the hamster prion promoter controlling the mutated human APP isoform expression in APPSWE mice is worthy of attention. 5-HIAA may act via this mechanism to reduce mutated APP expression and decrease Aβ accumulation in APPSWE mice. However, the probability of such action appears extremely low since the removal of $PrP^c$ prion from human APP-transgenic mice did not modify APP proteolysis, Aβ levels or pathologic phenotype [55].

Consistently, we observed that 5-HIAA increased NEP expression and decreased brain Aβ in the mouse model of intranasal phosphoramidon-induced NEP inhibition and cerebral accumulation of amyloid oligomers [21]. However, besides NEP inhibition, phosphoramidon may also reduce the activity of other Aβ degrading enzymes including the endothelin-converting enzyme [14]. Therefore, the possibility that in addition to NEP induction, 5-HIAA may also promote the activity of other Aβ degrading enzymes cannot be ruled out. Moreover, it has been reported that intracerebroventricular injection of the protease inhibitor phosphoramidon into wild type mice increased brain Aβ deposits and concomitantly induced neurodegeneration of hippocampal neurons and neuroinflammation [37]. Interestingly, we found that in the transgenic mouse model of AD expressing a human-mutated APP (APP Swedish) and accumulating brain Aβ, in vivo administration of 5-HIAA treatment during 5 consecutive days significantly reduced brain Aβ concentration and counteracted memory deficits in a spatial recognition task. The possibility exists that a longer period of treatment could induce a deeper elimination of Aβ, since there is no obvious toxicity of 5-HIAA. However, as the intra-nasal route was used to circumvent the blood brain barrier, this mode of administration may have some limitations for very long-term therapies. Therefore, a possibility could be the use of precursors of 5-HIAA such as tryptophan or 5-HTP that can be absorbed per os. Serotonin is also degraded into 5-HIAA in vitro and the global activity of the serotonergic system influences 5-HIAA levels in vivo. Thus, we explored a possible effect of these three substances using pharmacological treatment of SH-SY5Y neuronal cultures. We found that tryptophan, 5-HTP and serotonin induce NEP and these effects were strongly reduced by the presence of carbidopa or pargyline which inhibits dopa-decarboxylase or MAO, respectively. Thus, these three substances appear to act on NEP protein levels via the synthesis of 5-HIAA. For tryptophan, whose dietary increase reduces intraneuronal Aβ density in transgenic animals [32], the blockade of its degradation into 5-HIAA by MAO inhibition strongly reduced its ability to induce NEP synthesis. But tryptophan is the precursor of both kynurenine and serotonin pathways, and chronic inflammation is thought to drive tryptophan metabolism into the kynurenine pathway after induction of indolamine 2,3-dioxygenase, in detriment of serotonin metabolism [30]. A role of some intermediates of kynurenine pathway has been described in the pathophysiology of neurodegenerative diseases, including AD [6, 31]. Concerning 5-HTP, a direct precursor of both serotonin and 5-HIAA, the inhibition of dopa-decarboxylase decreases its effect on NEP induction, but this compound has also a direct role on NEP protein levels in cell cultures with an $EC_{50}$ of about 5 μM.

The role of serotonin appears more complex. The synthesis of serotonin is associated with lower Aβ levels in animals and humans [10]. In the presence of a MAO inhibitor, the stimulatory effect of serotonin on NEP protein in cell cultures disappeared, indicating that the reported beneficial effect of serotonin on Aβ levels is partly due to its catabolism into 5-HIAA. Serotonin itself has no effect on NEP but this neurotransmitter has been reported to exert several beneficial effects on AD via other mechanisms, as demonstrated by the pharmacological action of some SSRI and agonists/antagonists at 5-HT receptors [47]. Moreover, it is well demonstrated that the raphe nuclei are affected by neurofibrillary tangles very early in AD pathogenesis, suggesting the occurrence of early serotoninergic alterations that may facilitate AD progression [5, 19, 43]. Therefore, our results showing a beneficial role and mechanisms of action of serotonin metabolite 5-HIAA (until now considered only as a dead-end inactive product) in a mouse model of AD, may contribute to improve the efficacy of serotoninergic derivatives-based strategies against AD.

In conclusion, the present report, which provides the first demonstration that 5-HIAA sub-chronic therapy actively increases brain Aβ degradation/clearance and ameliorates symptoms in the APPSWE mouse model for AD, also contributes to elucidate the role of tryptophan/kynurenine/serotonin interrelated pathways in AD pathophysiology and progression.

**Abbreviations**

5-HIAA: 5-hydroxyindolacetic acid; APPSWE: Transgenic mice, B6; ERK ½: Extracellular signal-regulated kinases; GSK-3: Glycogen synthase kinase-3; MEK ½: Mitogen extracellular signal-regulated kinases; NEP: Neprilysin; SJL-Tg: (APPSWE) 2576Kha

**Acknowledgements**

This work was supported by grants from Institut National de la Santé et de la Recherche Médicale (INSERM, France) and Université de Strasbourg (France). Additional support was provided by the NeuroRhine Consortium coordinated by AGMN and funded by INTERREG IV Program (European Fund for Regional Development) in the Upper Rhine Region and the Offensive Science Call 2012. Authors would like to thank Dr. Martine Schmitt for the chemical advices.

**Authors' contributions**

CK performed biochemical, cell cultures and behavioral studies and analyzed the data. GR performed immunocytochemical studies and microscope analysis. SB performed flow cytometry analysis. CR participated to cell culture studies. CPM contributed to the design of the research project, supervised biochemical, cell culture studies and analyzed the data. MM and AGMN designed the whole research project, supervised all the studies, analyzed the data and wrote the manuscript. All authors read and approved the final manuscript.

**Competing interests**

The authors declare that they have no competing interests.

**References**

1. Bagyinszky E, Youn YC, An SS, Kim S (2014) The genetics of Alzheimer's disease. Clin Interv Aging 9:535–551
2. Baranello RJ, Bharani KL, al PV (2015) Amyloid-beta protein clearance and degradation (ABCD) pathways and their role in Alzheimer's disease. Curr Alzheimer Res 12:32–46
3. Benosman S, Gross I, N C et al (2007) Multiple neurotoxic stresses converge on MDMX proteolysis to cause neuronal apoptosis. Cell Death Differ 14: 2047–2057
4. Beurel E, Grieco SF, Jope RS (2015) Glycogen synthase kinase-3 (GSK3): regulation, actions, and diseases. Pharmacol Ther 148:114–131
5. Braak H, Thal DR, Ghebremedhin E, Del Tredici K (2011) Stages of the pathologic process in Alzheimer disease: age categories from 1 to 100 years. J Neuropathol Exp Neurol 70:960–969
6. Breda C, Sathyasaikumar KV, Sograte Idrissi S et al (2016) Tryptophan-2,3-dioxygenase (TDO) inhibition ameliorates neurodegeneration by modulation of kynurenine pathway metabolites. Proc Natl Acad Sci U S A 113:5435–5440
7. Carlezon WA Jr, Duman RS, Nestler EJ (2005) The many faces of CREB. Trends Neurosci 28:436–445
8. Chaikuad A, Tacconi EM, Zimmer J et al (2014) A unique inhibitor binding site in ERK1/2 is associated with slow binding kinetics. Nat Chem Biol 10: 853–860
9. Chiti F, Dobson CM (2017) Protein Misfolding, amyloid formation, and human disease: a summary of Progress over the last decade. Annu Rev Biochem 86:27–68
10. Cirrito JR, Disabato BM, Restivo JL et al (2011) Serotonin signaling is associated with lower amyloid-beta levels and plaques in transgenic mice and humans. Proc Natl Acad Sci U S A 108:14968–14973
11. Claeysen S, Bockaert J, Giannoni P (2015) Serotonin: a new Hope in Alzheimer's disease? ACS Chem Neurosci 6:940–943
12. Cooper-Knock J, Kirby J, Ferraiuolo L, Heath PR, Rattray M, Shaw PJ (2012) Gene expression profiling in human neurodegenerative disease. Nat Rev Neurol 8:518–530
13. Doyle KM, Kennedy D, Gorman AM, Gupta S, Healy SJ, Samali A (2011) Unfolded proteins and endoplasmic reticulum stress in neurodegenerative disorders. J Cell Mol Med 15:2025–2039
14. Eckman EA, Reed DK, Eckman CB (2001) Degradation of the Alzheimer's amyloid beta peptide by endothelin-converting enzyme. J Biol Chem 276: 24540–24548

15. Gartner U, Holzer M, Arendt T (1999) Elevated expression of p21ras is an early event in Alzheimer's disease and precedes neurofibrillary degeneration. Neuroscience 91:1–5
16. Gartner U, Holzer M, Heumann R, Arendt T (1995) Induction of p21ras in Alzheimer pathology. Neuroreport 6:1441–1444
17. Good MA, Hale G (2007) The "Swedish" mutation of the amyloid precursor protein (APPswe) dissociates components of object-location memory in aged Tg2576 mice. Behav Neurosci 121:1180–1191
18. Grimm MO, Mett J, Stahlmann CP et al (2015) APP intracellular domain derived from amyloidogenic beta- and gamma-secretase cleavage regulates neprilysin expression. Front Aging Neurosci 7:77
19. Grinberg LT, Rub U, Ferretti RE et al (2009) The dorsal raphe nucleus shows phospho-tau neurofibrillary changes before the transentorhinal region in Alzheimer's disease. A precocious onset? Neuropathol Appl Neurobiol 35:406–416
20. Hanson LR, Fine JM, Svitak AL, Faltesek KA (2013) Intranasal administration of CNS therapeutics to awake mice. J Vis Exp. https://doi.org/10.3791/4440
21. Hanson LR, Hafez D, Svitak AL et al (2011) Intranasal phosphoramidon increases beta-amyloid levels in wild-type and NEP/NEP2-deficient mice. J Mol Neurosci 43:424–427
22. Hsiao K, Chapman P, Nilsen S et al (1996) Correlative memory deficits, Abeta elevation, and amyloid plaques in transgenic mice. Science 274:99–102
23. Iijima-Ando K, Iijima K (2010) Transgenic Drosophila models of Alzheimer's disease and tauopathies. Brain Struct Funct 214:245–262
24. Jankowska A, Wesolowska A, Pawlowski M, Chlon-Rzepa G (2017) Multi-target-directed ligands affecting serotonergic neurotransmission for Alzheimer's disease therapy: advances in chemical and biological research. Curr Med Chem 25:2045–2067
25. Kakiya N, Saito T, Nilsson P et al (2012) Cell surface expression of the major amyloid-beta peptide (Abeta)-degrading enzyme, neprilysin, depends on phosphorylation by mitogen-activated protein kinase/extracellular signal-regulated kinase kinase (MEK) and dephosphorylation by protein phosphatase 1a. J Biol Chem 287:29362–29372
26. Kerridge C, Belyaev ND, Nalivaeva NN, Turner AJ (2014) The Abeta-clearance protein transthyretin, like neprilysin, is epigenetically regulated by the amyloid precursor protein intracellular domain. J Neurochem 130:419–431
27. Kirouac L, Rajic AJ, Cribbs DH, Padmanabhan J (2017) Activation of Ras-ERK signaling and GSK-3 by amyloid precursor protein and amyloid Beta facilitates neurodegeneration in Alzheimer's disease. eNeuro 4. https://doi.org/10.1523/ENEURO.0149-16.2017
28. Klein C, Mathis C, Leva G et al. (2015) Gamma-Hydroxybutyrate (Xyrem) ameliorates clinical symptoms and neuropathology in a mouse model of Alzheimer's disease. Neurobiol Aging 36: 832–844
29. Klein C, Patte-Mensah C, Taleb O et al (2013) The neuroprotector kynurenic acid increases neuronal cell survival through neprilysin induction. Neuropharmacology 70:254–260
30. Lovelace MD, Varney B, Sundaram G et al (2017) Recent evidence for an expanded role of the kynurenine pathway of tryptophan metabolism in neurological diseases. Neuropharmacology 112:373–388
31. Maddison DC, Giorgini F (2015) The kynurenine pathway and neurodegenerative disease. Semin Cell Dev Biol 40:134–141
32. Musumeci G, Castrogiovanni P, Szychlinska MA et al (2017) Protective effects of high tryptophan diet on aging-induced passive avoidance impairment and hippocampal apoptosis. Brain Res Bull 128:76–82
33. Nalivaeva NN, Beckett C, Belyaev ND, Turner AJ (2012) Are amyloid-degrading enzymes viable therapeutic targets in Alzheimer's disease? J Neurochem 120(Suppl 1):167–185
34. Nalivaeva NN, Belyaev ND, Lewis DI et al (2012) Effect of sodium valproate administration on brain neprilysin expression and memory in rats. J Mol Neurosci 46:569–577
35. Nalivaeva NN, Belyaev ND, Turner AJ (2016) New insights into epigenetic and pharmacological regulation of amyloid-degrading enzymes. Neurochem Res 41:620–630
36. Nilsson P, Loganathan K, Sekiguchi M et al (2015) Loss of neprilysin alters protein expression in the brain of Alzheimer's disease model mice. Proteomics 15:3349–3355
37. Nisemblat Y, Belinson H, Dolev I, Michaelson DM (2008) Activation of the amyloid cascade by intracerebroventricular injection of the protease inhibitor phosphoramidon. Neurodegener Dis 5:166–169
38. Ognibene E, Middei S, Daniele S et al (2005) Aspects of spatial memory and behavioral disinhibition in Tg2576 transgenic mice as a model of Alzheimer's disease. Behav Brain Res 156:225–232
39. Pacheco-Quinto J, Eckman CB, Eckman EA (2016) Major amyloid-beta-degrading enzymes, endothelin-converting enzyme-2 and neprilysin, are expressed by distinct populations of GABAergic interneurons in hippocampus and neocortex. Neurobiol Aging 48:83–92
40. Park MH, Lee JK, Choi S et al (2013) Recombinant soluble neprilysin reduces amyloid-beta accumulation and improves memory impairment in Alzheimer's disease mice. Brain Res 1529:113–124
41. Piaceri I, Nacmias B, Sorbi S (2013) Genetics of familial and sporadic Alzheimer's disease. Front Biosci (Elite Ed) 5:167–177
42. Rosenberg RN, Lambracht-Washington D, Yu G, Xia W (2016) Genomics of Alzheimer disease: a review. JAMA Neurol 73:867–874
43. Rub U, Del Tredici K, Schultz C, Thal DR, Braak E, Braak H (2000) The evolution of Alzheimer's disease-related cytoskeletal pathology in the human raphe nuclei. Neuropathol Appl Neurobiol 26:553–567
44. Saito T, Iwata N, Tsubuki S et al (2005) Somatostatin regulates brain amyloid beta peptide Abeta42 through modulation of proteolytic degradation. Nat Med 11:434–439
45. Schmid T, Snoek LB, Frohli E, van der Bent ML, Kammenga J, Hajnal A (2015) Systemic regulation of RAS/MAPK signaling by the serotonin metabolite 5-HIAA. PLoS Genet 11:e1005236
46. Simic G, Babic Leko M, Wray S et al (2017) Monoaminergic neuropathology in Alzheimer's disease. Prog Neurobiol 151:101–138
47. Smith GS, Barrett FS, Joo JH et al (2017) Molecular imaging of serotonin degeneration in mild cognitive impairment. Neurobiol Dis 105:33–41
48. Stroo E, Koopman M, Nollen EA, Mata-Cabana A (2017) Cellular regulation of amyloid formation in aging and disease. Front Neurosci 11:64
49. Tentolouris-Piperas V, Ryan NS, Thomas DL, Kinnunen KM (2017) Brain imaging evidence of early involvement of subcortical regions in familial and sporadic Alzheimer's disease. Brain Res 1655:23–32
50. Vermeiren Y, Van Dam D, Aerts T, Engelborghs S, De Deyn PP (2014) Monoaminergic neurotransmitter alterations in postmortem brain regions of depressed and aggressive patients with Alzheimer's disease. Neurobiol Aging 35:2691–2700
51. Wang Z, Zhang XJ, Li T, Li J, Tang Y, Le W (2014) Valproic acid reduces neuritic plaque formation and improves learning deficits in APP(Swe) /PS1(A246E) transgenic mice via preventing the prenatal hypoxia-induced down-regulation of neprilysin. CNS Neurosci Ther 20:209–217
52. Weiner MW, Veitch DP, al APS (2017) Recent publications from the Alzheimer's disease neuroimaging initiative: reviewing progress toward improved AD clinical trials. Alzheimer's Dement 13:e1–e85
53. Wendt G, Kemmel V, Patte-Mensah C et al (2014) Gamma-hydroxybutyrate, acting through an anti-apoptotic mechanism, protects native and amyloid-precursor-protein-transfected neuroblastoma cells against oxidative stress-induced death. Neuroscience 263:203–215
54. Westerman MA, Cooper-Blacketer D, Mariash A et al (2002) The relationship between Abeta and memory in the Tg2576 mouse model of Alzheimer's disease. J Neurosci 22:1858–1867
55. Whitehouse IJ, Brown D, Baybutt H et al (2016) Ablation of prion protein in wild type human amyloid precursor protein (APP) transgenic mice does not Alter the proteolysis of APP, levels of amyloid-beta or pathologic phenotype. PLoS One 11:e0159119
56. Whyte LS, Lau AA, Hemsley KM, Hopwood JJ, Sargeant TJ (2017) Endo-lysosomal and autophagic dysfunction: a driving factor in Alzheimer's disease? J Neurochem 140:703–717
57. Yassine N, Lazaris A, Dorner-Ciossek C et al (2013) Detecting spatial memory deficits beyond blindness in tg2576 Alzheimer mice. Neurobiol Aging 34: 716–730

# 4

# Dichotomous scoring of TDP-43 proteinopathy from specific brain regions in 27 academic research centers: associations with Alzheimer's disease and cerebrovascular disease pathologies

Yuriko Katsumata[1,2*], David W. Fardo[1,2], Walter A. Kukull[3] and Peter T. Nelson[2,4]

**Abstract**

TAR-DNA binding protein 43 (TDP-43) proteinopathy is a common brain pathology in elderly persons, but much remains to be learned about this high-morbidity condition. Published stage-based systems for operationalizing disease severity rely on the involvement (presence/absence) of pathology in specific anatomic regions. To examine the comorbidities associated with TDP-43 pathology in aged individuals, we studied data from the National Alzheimer's Coordinating Center (NACC) Neuropathology Data Set. Data were analyzed from 929 included subjects with available TDP-43 pathology information, sourced from 27 different American Alzheimer's Disease Centers (ADCs). Cases with relatively unusual diseases including autopsy-proven frontotemporal lobar degeneration (FTLD-TDP or FTLD-tau) were excluded from the study. Our data provide new information about pathologic features that are and are not associated with TDP-43 pathologies in different brain areas—spinal cord, amygdala, hippocampus, entorhinal cortex/inferior temporal cortex, and frontal neocortex. Different research centers used cite-specific methods including different TDP-43 antibodies. TDP-43 pathology in at least one brain region was common (31.4%) but the pathology was rarely observed in spinal cord (1.8%) and also unusual in frontal cortex (5.3%). As expected, TDP-43 pathology was positively associated with comorbid hippocampal sclerosis pathology and with severe AD pathology. TDP-43 pathology was also associated with comorbid moderate-to-severe brain arteriolosclerosis. The association between TDP-43 pathology and brain arteriolosclerosis appears relatively specific since there was no detected association between TDP-43 pathology and microinfarcts, lacunar infarcts, large infarcts, cerebral amyloid angiopathy (CAA), or circle of Willis atherosclerosis. Together, these observations provide support for the hypothesis that many aged brains are affected by a TDP-43 proteinopathy that is more likely to be seen in brains with AD pathology, arteriolosclerosis pathology, or both.

**Keywords:** FTD, VCID, Arteriosclerosis, Apolipoprotein E

* Correspondence: katsumata.yuriko@uky.edu
[1]Department of Biostatistics, University of Kentucky, 725 Rose Street, Lexington, KY 40536, USA
[2]Sanders-Brown Center on Aging, University of Kentucky, Lexington, KY 40536, USA
Full list of author information is available at the end of the article

## Introduction

There is an evolving appreciation of a common brain disease with TAR-DNA binding protein 43 (TDP-43) proteinopathy that mimics Alzheimer's disease (AD) clinically [5, 25, 26, 34, 39, 50] and affects 10–25% of persons aged 85 or older [5, 19, 21, 33, 50]. The defining characteristics of this disease are recognized by neuropathologic observations: TDP-43 pathology, often with comorbid neuronal loss and astrocytosis pathology in the hippocampus [1, 33], the latter two features collectively termed hippocampal sclerosis (HS). The literature that pertains to this disease was initially focused on HS pathology (TDP-43 pathology was discovered as a disease marker in 2006 [38]), but it is now recognized that TDP-43 pathology is the most sensitive and specific marker of the disease. For example, cases with HS pathology due to acute anoxia is immunonegative for TDP-43 and is considered a fundamentally different disease [2, 20, 33]. Importantly, the presence of TDP-43 proteinopathy, with or without comorbid HS pathology, is independently associated with cognitive impairment [5, 26, 29, 31].

"TDP-43 pathology" lacks a universally applied specific connotation, but refers to phosphorylated TDP-43 deposits in cytoplasmic (where it may appear like speckles, skeins, or tangles), intranuclear, perivascular, and/or neurite-like structures. TDP-43 pathology may also manifest as a decrease in the normal (non-phosphorylated) TDP-43 in the nucleus [4], or within twig-like deposits of phosphorylated TDP-43 detected immunohistochemically in the subpial or subependymal regions [11, 18, 30]. In prior published papers that have studied the spectrum of TDP-43 pathologies in aged brains (often with comorbid AD pathology), the severity of TDP-43 proteinopathy has been mostly graded according to stage-based classification systems where the presence of any TDP-43 pathology in a given region defines a particular stage [15, 17, 27, 29, 44]. For example, the amygdala seems to be affected very early so this is the first stage. By contrast, in cases with extensive pathology, the frontal neocortex may be affected and if this region has any detectable TDP-43 pathology, that is indicative of a late disease stage. Unfortunately, there currently is no consensus as to a specific antibody or combination of antibodies recommended for detecting TDP-43 proteinopathy. Further, the stage-based classification systems for common age-related disease differ from TDP-43 pathologic staging systems that were developed for amyotrophic lateral sclerosis (ALS) and/or frontotemporal lobar degeneration (FTLD)-TDP [6, 10, 45].

Prior published findings suggest that vascular factors may cause or exacerbate the disease process that manifests neuropathologically as TDP-43 (with or without HS pathology) in the aged brain [8, 41, 47, 49]. In prior work, arteriolosclerosis – dysmorphic changes in small arterioles – was preferentially associated with this disease [36]. Further, arteriolosclerosis was observed in regions outside of the hippocampal formation in cases with comorbid HS pathology, indicating a "whole-brain disease" rather than a disease process isolated to the medial temporal lobe [37]. However, the precise underlying mechanisms are not understood, and more work is required to determine how the clinical and pathologic endpoints are associated with each other.

The AD Centers (ADCs) program has constituted a critical resource for research on AD and related dementias in the U.S. This network derived from a National Institutes of Health (NIH)-funded initiative that started in 1984 and has included more than 30 different ADCs geographically dispersed across the U.S. Each ADC follows a longitudinal cohort of generally elderly individuals reflecting a broad spectrum of clinical diseases and pathologic manifestations. The National Alzheimer's Coordinating Center (NACC) oversees data collection by the ADCs. For research subjects that died and came to autopsy, a standardized form was created by NACC to describe the neuropathology in a systematic manner, and for correlation with clinical, radiographic, genetic, and biochemical parameters in the same persons. The latest Neuropathology (NP) Form was updated in 2014, and is referred to as version 10 (v10). The NACC NP Form v10 incorporated detailed neuropathological data including Thal phase for Aβ plaques [43], relatively newly categorized FTLD neuropathologic changes [23], ALS/motor neuron disease (MND), HS of the CA1 and/or subiculum, and distributions of TDP-43 immunoreactive inclusions in five brain regions. The summary data for the updated v10 form was recently described [3]. Here we focused on the clinical and pathologic correlates of TDP-43 pathology in the NACC NP v10 data set among individuals lacking unusual conditions such as FTLD.

## Materials and methods

### Participants

For the current study, data (before exclusion criteria were applied) derived from 30 different ADCs with autopsies reported using the NACC NP v10 form, which started in 2014, through the data freeze of July 11th 2018. Autopsies were performed within each of the contributory ADCs. The database comprises a standardized set of data collected based on the NACC NP v10 data collection form (https://www.alz.washington.edu/NONMEMBER/NP/rdd_np.pdf). Inclusion criteria for this study were neuropathology data available through the NACC NP Form v10, age at death ≥65 years, and non-missing data on TDP-43 referent to at least one of the five brain regions of interest (see below). Exclusion criteria were the presence of at least one of 19 rare neurological diseases (see Additional file 1: Table S1). Research using the NACC database was approved by the University of Washington Institutional Review Board. Informed consent was obtained from all participants at the individual ADCs. The NACC data were de-identified.

### Measurements

#### *Neuropathology data*

TDP-43-immunoreactive inclusions were evaluated in five brain regions: spinal cord, amygdala, hippocampus, entorhinal cortex/inferior temporal cortex (EC/inferior TCTX), and frontal neocortex, with the response categories "no", "yes", "not assessed", and "missing/unknown". Because data on TDP-43 pathology in spinal cord contained more "not assessed"' or "missing/unknown" values (Additional file 1: Table S2), we considered TDP-43 inclusions in four brain regions (all except spinal cord) in the subsequent multivariable regression analyses. HS was determined by the variable of "hippocampal sclerosis of CA1 and/or subiculum" ("unilateral", "bilateral", or "present but laterality not assessed"). Data was obtained from all 30 contributory ADCs on whether the antibody used was phospho-specific or non-phospho-specific. A survey was sent to all the ADC Neuropathology Core leaders as to what specific antibodies were used. The phospho-specific antibodies were mostly 1D3 (EMD Millipore), followed by 11–9 (Cosmo Bio) and the polyclonal Cosmo Bio antibody (TIP-PTD-P02). The non-phospho-specific antibodies were almost all Proteintech 10,782–2-AP (rabbit polyclonal), with one center reporting to use Sigma C-term (T1580). Examples of results from the two most frequently used antibodies are shown in Fig. 1. For AD-related pathology, data were included on density of diffuse plaques ("none", "sparse", "moderate", or "frequent"), density of neocortical neuritic plaques ("none", "sparse", "moderate", or "frequent"), Thal phase for Aβ distribution (Thal Aβ phases 0 to 5), Braak stage for neurofibrillary degeneration (Braak NFT stages 0 to VI). For cerebrovascular pathology, data were available on atherosclerosis severity in the circle of Willis ("none", "mild", "moderate", or severe), cerebral amyloid angiopathy ("none", "mild", "moderate", or "severe"), infarct and lacunes (no or yes), microinfarcts (no or yes), hemorrhages and microbleeds (no or yes), and arteriolosclerosis ("none", "mild", "moderate", or "severe"; see Fig. 2). The detailed response categories of these variables and the dichotomized scoring are shown in Additional file 1: Table S3.

### Statistical analysis

Descriptive statistical analyses were performed for sex, age at death (both available in the NACC NP Form v10), and years of education, apolipoprotein E (*APOE*) genotype (no ε4 alleles = 0, one ε4 allele = 1, or pair of ε4 alleles = 2), and other health conditions at the last clinical visit (via self-report) including diabetes, hypertension, hypercholesterolemia, and thyroid disease (all from the NACC Uniform Data Set (UDS)).

Comparisons of characteristics of individuals with and without the TDP-43 pathology were performed using t-tests for continuous variables and Pearson's chi-square test for categorical variables. Multivariable logistic regression was used to examine the associations of TDP-43 pathology with AD and cerebrovascular disease pathologies. We controlled for sex, age at death, *APOE* genotype, and the type of TDP-43 antibody in the analyses for AD pathologies, and additionally for Braak NFT stage and Thal Aβ phase in the analyses for cerebrovascular disease pathologies. All statistical analyses were carried out with R version 3.4.4 [40]. Statistical significance was set at 0.05.

## Results

Subjects who were assessed by ADC neuropathologists using the NACC NP Form v10 and died at age 65 years or older ($n = 1968$) were extracted from the NACC NP dataset. We excluded 476 subjects who had at least one rare neurological disease listed in Additional file 1: Table S1, and we also excluded 562 subjects who had no TDP-43 pathology (i.e., missing) data reported in all five brain regions and 1 subject with "other" reported as the TDP-43 antibody used (Fig. 3). Following exclusions, a total of 929 subjects were included in this study. For these subjects, TDP-43 pathology data were sourced from 27 different ADCs (range of the number of subjects with any TDP-43 pathology in this study: 1–123 cases per center), including ADCs that only recently began to perform autopsies for inclusion in this dataset. The mean number of the subjects analyzed per ADC was 34 (median 33). Overall, 67.3% of the subjects were stained with phospho-specific antibodies; the rest with non-phospho-specfic antibodies. Among the 20 different ADCs that submitted 10 or more subjects with relevant TDP-43 immunohistochemistry (IHC) data to NACC, 13 ADCs used all or mostly phospho-specific antibodies for TDP-43 IHC, whereas 7 ADCs used all or mostly non-phospho-specific TDP-43 antibodies (Additional file 1: Table S4).

Table 1 shows the characteristics of the study subjects in total and stratified by TDP-43 pathology absent or present in at least one brain region. In all included subjects, the mean (standard deviation (SD)) age at death was 83.1 (8.7), 51.8% were males, and the mean of years of education was 15.5 (3.1). The subjects with TDP-43 pathology in at least one region died older ($p$-value < 0.001). There were no statistically significant differences

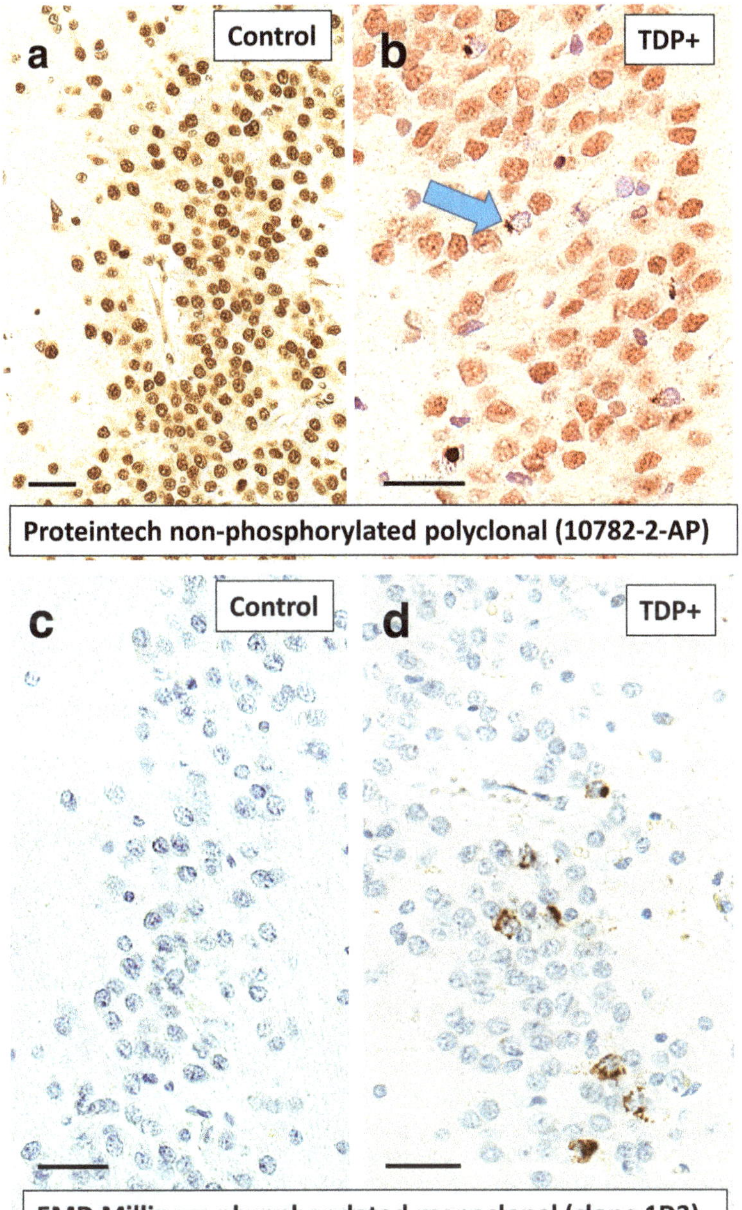


**Fig. 1** Examples of TDP-43 immunohistochemistry performed with the most commonly used antibodies against non-phosphorylated TDP-43 (**a**,**b**: Proteintech 10,782–2-AP), and phosphorylated TDP-43 (**c**,**d**: EMD Millipore clone 1D3) in the Alzheimer's Disease Centers (ADCs) that contribute to the NACC neuropathology dataset. These sections are counterstained with hematoxylin (blue-stained nuclei). Shown are portions of dentate granule cells from the hippocampi of cases without TDP-43 pathology (**a**,**c**) which are contrasted against cases with detectable TDP-43 pathology (**b**,**d**). In normal brains, non-phosphorylated TDP-43 protein is seen in cell nuclei (**a**). In cases with TDP-43 pathology, the non-phosphorylated TDP-43 protein can be seen in some cells' cytoplasm instead of the cell nucleus (**b**). The antibody against phosphorylated TDP-43 protein shows no brown reaction product in normal brain (**c**), with only the hematoxylin (blue) counterstain evident. By contrast, there are clearly intracellular aggregates (brown-colored chromagen) of phosphorylated TDP-43 protein in panel (**d**). Scale bars = 30 μm

in sex, *APOE* genotype, educational attainment, and other health conditions between subjects with and without TDP-43 pathology.

We compared TDP-43 pathology frequencies between HS present and absent in each brain region (Fig. 4). HS pathology was strongly associated with TDP-43 pathology in each brain region except spinal cord. Table 2 shows the associations between TDP-43 and AD-related pathologies in each brain region. AD pathologies were strongly and positively associated with TDP-43 pathology in amygdala, hippocampus, and EC/inferior TCTX, although the association between

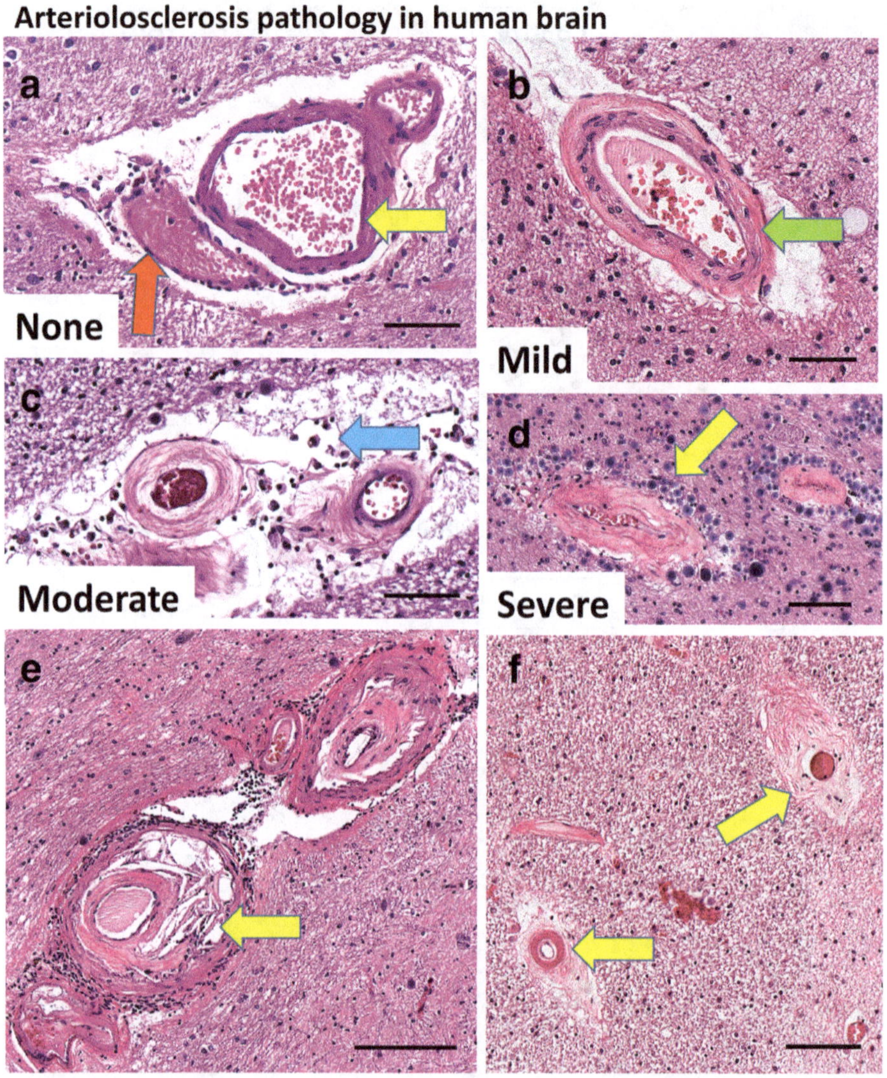


**Fig. 2** Arteriolosclerosis pathology in the aged human brain. The present study used a 0–3 scale of severity for arteriolosclerosis pathology, which is illustrated in panels (**a-d**). These photomicrographs depict vascular profiles in sections of amygdala or peri-amygdaloid regions from aged individuals at various stages of arteriolosclerosis pathology. Panel (**a**) shows an arteriole (yellow arrow) next to a presumed venule (red arrow), which have histopathologic features within normal limits in aging, including some eosinophilic material in the vessel wall and Virchow-Robin space [*] that may be partly an artifact of fixation and embedding. Panel (**b**) shows an arteriole with thicker vessel wall and intact cellular constituents, but with eosinophilic material (green arrow) in the adventitia. Panel (**c**) depicts arteriolosclerosis of moderate severity with some "onion-skinning" of the vessel wall and extravasation of macrophages (blue arrow) in the Virchow-Robin space. Panel (**d**) shows severe arteriolosclerosis in two vessels that have extensive proliferation of eosinophilic material in the vessel wall, attenuation of normal arteriolar cellular contents, apparent partial occlusion of the vessel itself, and the vessels are surrounded by corpora amylacea (yellow arrow) indicating localized brain injury. The pathologic appearance of brain arteriolosclerosis is heterogeneous, particularly in the area of the brain (amygdala; panels **e**,**f**) that is at high risk for incipient TDP-43 pathology. In panel (**e**), one can see pathologically affected blood vessel(s) with surrounding leukocytes and eosinophilic and small slit-like profiles that appear to be cholesterol clefts in the vessel wall. In panel (**f**), two vessels are seen (arrows) with largely attenuated cellular contents in the vessel walls. Scale bars = 150 um (**a**,**d**); 100 um (**b**,**c**), 300 um (**e**), 250 um (**f**)

dichotomized diffuse plaques (moderate/frequent vs. no/sparse) and TDP-43 pathology in hippocampus was not statistically significant. Among cerebrovascular disease pathologies, there were no significant associations (or even consistent trends) between TDP-43 pathology in any brain regions with atherosclerosis of the circle of Willis, cerebral amyloid angiopathy, infarct and lacunes, microinfarcts, hemorrhages or microbleeds.

By contrast, arteriolosclerosis pathology was associated with TDP-43 pathology in amygdala and EC/inferior TCTX when adjusted for sex, age at death, *APOE* genotype, and the type of TDP-43 antibody. The significant

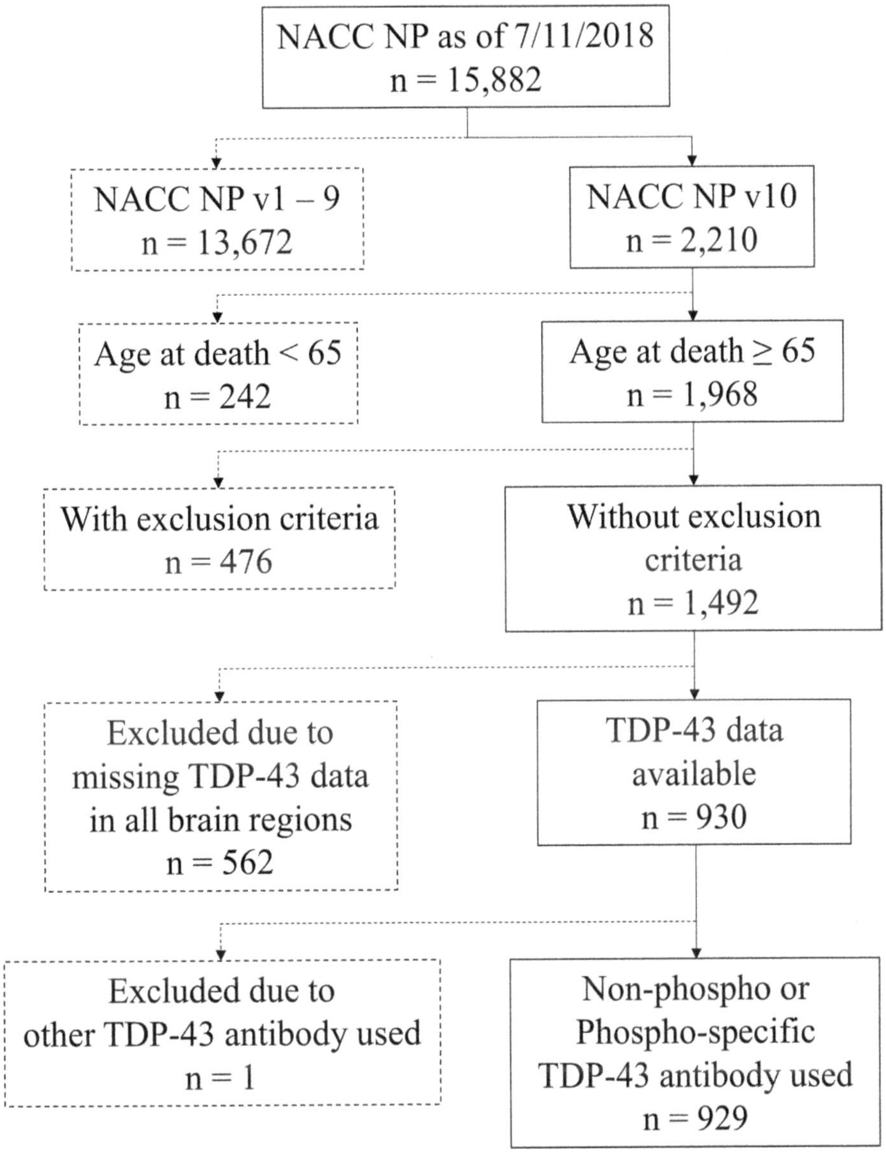


**Fig. 3** Included study subjects for the present study. NACC = National Alzheimer's Coordinating Center; NP = Neuropathology

association in EC/inferior TCTX remained after AD-pathologies were added as covariates in the model (Table 3). To examine whether *APOE* genotype difference affects the association between TDP-43 pathology and arteriolosclerosis pathology, we further performed logistic regression analyses stratified by *APOE* genotype. As shown in Table 4, the associations of TDP-43 pathology in amygdala and EC/inferior TCTX with arteriolosclerosis pathology were observed in the subjects with *APOE* −/− or −/ε4 genotype. The significant association of TDP-43 in EC/inferior TCTX remained after including Thal Aβ phase and Braak NFT stage as additional covariates in the model. However, in persons with *APOE* ε4/ε4 ($n = 77$), TDP-43 pathologies in amygdala, hippocampus, and frontal neocortex were not associated with arteriolosclerosis pathology.

## Discussion

Here we present data focusing on TDP-43 pathology in the aged human brain, using a large sample with autopsy confirmation, sourced from multiple high-quality research centers. Our data provide new information about comorbidities that are and are not apparently associated with TDP-43 pathologies in different brain regions. TDP-43 pathology is strongly associated with advanced AD and brain arteriolosclerosis pathologies.

There are some potential pitfalls in our study sample, as we have discussed previously [3]. Contributory ADC

**Table 1** Characteristics of included study subjects

| Characteristic | All included subjects ($n = 929$) | No TDP-43 pathology ($n = 637$) | TDP-43 pathology at least one region[a] ($n = 292$) | *P*-value[b] | Excluded subjects[c] ($n = 563$) | *P*-value[d] |
|---|---|---|---|---|---|---|
| Age at death, mean ± SD | 83.1 ± 8.7 | 82.4 ± 8.8 | 84.8 ± 8.5 | **< 0.001** | 84.4 ± 9.0 | **0.012** |
| Gender, n (%) | | | | | | |
| Male | 481 (51.8) | 341 (53.5) | 140 (47.9) | 0.13 | 287 (51.0) | 0.81 |
| Female | 448 (48.2) | 296 (46.5) | 152 (52.1) | | 276 (49.0) | |
| Education (years), mean ± SD | 15.5 ± 3.1 | 15.5 ± 3.1 | 15.5 ± 3.2 | 0.95 | 15.2 ± 3.3 | 0.10 |
| *APOE*, n (%) | | | | | | |
| −/− | 370 (49.0) | 275 (51.6) | 95 (42.8) | 0.063 | 229 (52.8) | 0.43 |
| −/ε4 | 309 (40.9) | 210 (39.4) | 99 (44.6) | | 162 (37.3) | |
| ε4/ε4 | 76 (10.1) | 48 (9.0) | 28 (12.6) | | 43 (9.9) | |
| Diabetes, n (%) | | | | | | |
| Recent/remote | 91 (15.5) | 66 (15.6) | 25 (15.2) | 1 | 56 (13.2) | 0.35 |
| Absent | 495 (84.5) | 356 (84.4) | 139 (84.8) | | 368 (86.8) | |
| Hypertension, n (%) | | | | | | |
| Recent/remote | 375 (64.3) | 270 (64.1) | 151 (64.8) | 0.95 | 281 (67.9) | 0.27 |
| Absent | 208 (35.7) | 105 (35.9) | 57 (35.2) | | 133 (32.1) | |
| Hypercholesterolemia, n (%) | | | | | | |
| Recent/remote | 411 (63.7) | 300 (63.6) | 111 (64.2) | 0.96 | 297 (66.4) | 0.39 |
| Absent | 234 (36.3) | 172 (36.4) | 62 (35.8) | | 150 (33.6) | |
| Thyroid disease present, n (%) | | | | | | |
| Yes | 70 (24.4) | 48 (24.5) | 22 (24.2) | 1 | 31 (22.5) | 0.75 |
| No | 217 (75.6) | 148 (75.5) | 69 (75.8) | | 107 (77.5) | |

[a]TDP-43 pathology at least one of the five regions: spinal cord, amygdala, hippocampus, EC/inferior TCTX, and frontal neocortex
[b]The p-values were computed for the associations with TDP-43 inclusions statuses
[c]Subjects excluded due to missing TDP-43 data in all regions or other TDP-43 antibody used
[d]The *p*-values were computed for the associations between all included subjects and the subjects with no data on TDP-43 inclusions
*SD* standard deviation
Bold *p*-value represents the statistical significance

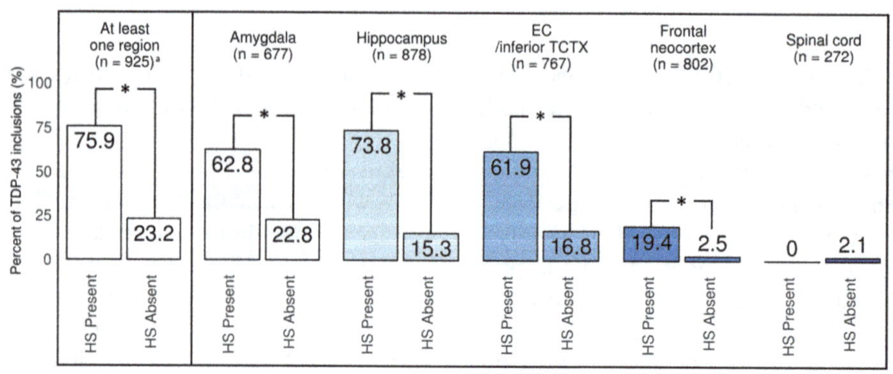


**Fig. 4** Comparisons in percent of TDP-43 pathology in each brain region between hippocampal sclerosis present and absent. Note that there is a strong association between hippocampal sclerosis (HS) pathology and TDP-43 pathology. However, only a minority of cases, with or without comorbid HS pathology, have TDP-43 pathology detected in frontal cortex or spinal cord. [a] $n = 4$ had missing data on hippocampal sclerosis (HS) pathology. * $p < 0.001$. EC = entorhinal cortex; TCTX = temporal cortex

**Table 2** Associations between TDP-43 and Alzheimer's disease pathologies using binary logistic regression ($n = 929$)

| Region | OR (95% CI)[a] | *P*-value |
|---|---|---|
| Diffuse plaques (moderate + frequent vs. no + sparse) | | |
| Amygdala | 3.34 (1.47–8.99) | **0.0079** |
| Hippocampus | 1.45 (0.81–2.71) | 0.23 |
| EC/inferior TCTX | 2.61 (1.20–6.53) | **0.025** |
| Frontal neocortex | 2.30 (0.63–14.93) | 0.28 |
| Neuritic plaques (moderate + frequent vs. no + sparse) | | |
| Amygdala | 2.84 (1.57–5.44) | $\mathbf{9.1 \times 10^{-4}}$ |
| Hippocampus | 2.56 (1.58–4.29) | $\mathbf{2.2 \times 10^{-4}}$ |
| EC/inferior TCTX | 4.04 (2.11–8.43) | $\mathbf{6.6 \times 10^{-5}}$ |
| Frontal neocortex | 1.88 (0.71–5.92) | 0.23 |
| Thal Aβ phase (phase 4 + 5 vs. phase 0 to 3) | | |
| Amygdala | 2.78 (1.56–5.21) | $\mathbf{8.5 \times 10^{-4}}$ |
| Hippocampus | 2.34 (1.44–3.93) | $\mathbf{8.5 \times 10^{-4}}$ |
| EC/inferior TCTX | 2.52 (1.41–4.77) | **0.0029** |
| Frontal neocortex | 1.42 (0.53–4.50) | 0.51 |
| Braak NFT stage (stage V + VI vs. stage 0 to IV) | | |
| Amygdala | 3.38 (1.99–5.95) | $\mathbf{1.3 \times 10^{-5}}$ |
| Hippocampus | 2.90 (1.86–4.63) | $\mathbf{4.2 \times 10^{-6}}$ |
| EC/inferior TCTX | 3.15 (1.86–5.53) | $\mathbf{3.4 \times 10^{-5}}$ |
| Frontal neocortex | 1.22 (0.52–3.06) | 0.66 |

[a]Odds ratios were adjusted for sex, age at death, *APOE* genotype, and the type of TDP-43 antibody
*OR* odds ratio, *CI* confidence interval, *EC* entorhinal cortex, *TCTX* temporal cortex, *NFT* neurofibrillary tangle
Bold *p*-value represents the statistical significance

**Table 3** Associations between TDP-43 and cerebrovascular disease pathologies using binary logistic regression ($n = 929$)

| Region | Model 1[a] | | Model 2[b] | |
|---|---|---|---|---|
| | OR (95% CI) | *P*-value | OR (95% CI) | *P*-value |
| Atherosclerosis of the circle of Willis (moderate + severe vs. none + mild) | | | | |
| Amygdala | 0.96 (0.63–1.47) | 0.87 | 0.90 (0.58–1.39) | 0.63 |
| Hippocampus | 1.07 (0.74–1.55) | 0.70 | 0.98 (0.67–1.43) | 0.93 |
| EC/inferior TCTX | 1.16 (0.77–1.75) | 0.48 | 1.07 (0.70–1.62) | 0.77 |
| Frontal neocortex | 1.03 (0.47–2.27) | 0.93 | 1.00 (0.45–2.21) | 0.99 |
| Cerebral amyloid angiopathy (moderate + severe vs. none + mild) | | | | |
| Amygdala | 0.82 (0.52–1.28) | 0.38 | 0.66 (0.41–1.04) | 0.077 |
| Hippocampus | 0.89 (0.59–1.32) | 0.57 | 0.71 (0.47–1.07) | 0.10 |
| EC/inferior TCTX | 0.99 (0.64–1.52) | 0.97 | 0.79 (0.50–1.22) | 0.29 |
| Frontal neocortex | 1.16 (0.49–2.60) | 0.73 | 1.11 (0.46–2.56) | 0.81 |
| Infarct and lacunes (yes vs. no) | | | | |
| Amygdala | 0.77 (0.43–1.32) | 0.35 | 0.84 (0.47–1.45) | 0.54 |
| Hippocampus | 0.76 (0.45–1.23) | 0.28 | 0.81 (0.48–1.33) | 0.42 |
| EC/inferior TCTX | 0.79 (0.45–1.32) | 0.38 | 0.87 (0.49–1.48) | 0.61 |
| Frontal neocortex | 1.64 (0.63–3.82) | 0.27 | 1.66 (0.63–3.89) | 0.26 |
| Microinfarcts (yes vs. no) | | | | |
| Amygdala | 1.15 (0.73–1.79) | 0.55 | 1.08 (0.68–1.70) | 0.74 |
| Hippocampus | 1.14 (0.76–1.70) | 0.51 | 1.14 (0.75–1.70) | 0.54 |
| EC/inferior TCTX | 1.25 (0.80–1.94) | 0.31 | 1.21 (0.77–1.88) | 0.41 |
| Frontal neocortex | 1.76 (0.78–3.84) | 0.16 | 1.77 (0.78–3.86) | 0.16 |
| Hemorrhages and microbleeds (yes vs. no) | | | | |
| Amygdala | 0.65 (0.26–1.44) | 0.32 | 0.65 (0.25–1.47) | 0.33 |
| Hippocampus | 0.71 (0.30–1.50) | 0.40 | 0.69 (0.29–1.46) | 0.36 |
| EC/inferior TCTX | 0.57 (0.21–1.29) | 0.21 | 0.55 (0.20–1.26) | 0.19 |
| Frontal neocortex | 0.45 (0.02–2.34) | 0.45 | 0.44 (0.02–2.32) | 0.44 |
| Arteriolosclerosis (moderate + severe vs. none + mild) | | | | |
| Amygdala | 1.56 (1.03–2.37) | **0.038** | 1.38 (0.90–2.13) | 0.14 |
| Hippocampus | 1.31 (0.92–1.89) | 0.14 | 1.16 (0.80–1.69) | 0.42 |
| EC/inferior TCTX | 1.77 (1.17–2.72) | **0.0078** | 1.61 (1.05–2.49) | **0.029** |
| Frontal neocortex | 0.97 (0.45–2.13) | 0.95 | 0.93 (0.43–2.06) | 0.86 |

[a]Odds ratios were adjusted for sex, age at death, *APOE* genotype, and the type of TDP-43 antibody used
[b]Thal Aβ phase and Braak NFT stage were included as additional covariates in model 2
*OR* odds ratio, *CI* confidence interval, *EC* entorhinal cortex, *TCTX* temporal cortex
Bold *p*-value represents the statistical significance

cohorts tend to be enriched for rare, genetic, early-onset, and "pure" subtypes of diseases, including AD and many other degenerative conditions. In particular, this sample may be biased toward individuals with a clinical syndrome that mimics AD. The NACC-contributory ADCs also tend to recruit (and achieve autopsy consent for) Caucasian/white individuals of relatively high socioeconomic status; thus, there are relatively few non-Caucasian individuals or those lacking formal education. Further, ADCs apply exclusion criteria that can limit the number of autopsied participants with mental illness, substance abuse, physical disability, or other prevalent conditions. There also are challenges in data interpretation related to the lack of methodologic standardization between the ADCs in terms of TDP-43 IHC methods. This problem will probably plague multi-center studies for some time since our study confirms that different state-of-the-art research centers use different reagents to operationalize TDP-43 proteinopathy (~ 2/3rd of ADCs use phospho-specific TDP-43 antibodies, whereas the remaining ADCs use antibodies that recognize non-phosphorylated epitopes). We also recognize the current lack of knowledge about underlying mechanisms is a limitation, and our study does not describe how the brain arteriolosclerosis pathology spatially relates to the TDP-43 proteinopathy.

Despite the challenges and potential pitfalls, there also are considerable strengths related to this use of the NACC NP data set. We note that despite the abovementioned sources of data variability, our study found

**Table 4** Associations between TDP-43 and arteriolosclerosis (moderate/severe vs. none/mild) pathologies among included subjects stratified by *APOE* genotype

| Region | *APOE* −/− or −/ε4 ($n = 679$)[a] | | *APOE* ε4/ε4 ($n = 76$)[a] | |
|---|---|---|---|---|
| | OR (95% CI) | *P*-value | OR (95% CI) | *P*-value |
| Model 1[b] | | | | |
| Amygdala | 1.66 (1.07–2.59) | **0.023** | 0.71 (0.16–3.19) | 0.65 |
| Hippocampus | 1.40 (0.96–2.05) | 0.083 | 0.89 (0.29–2.79) | 0.84 |
| EC/inferior TCTX | 1.82 (1.18–2.86) | **0.0080** | 1.43 (0.35–6.55) | 0.62 |
| Frontal neocortex | 1.13 (0.50–2.61) | 0.76 | 0.26 (0.01–3.04) | 0.30 |
| Model 2[c] | | | | |
| Amygdala | 1.43 (0.91–2.26) | 0.12 | 0.57 (0.12–2.67) | 0.47 |
| Hippocampus | 1.19 (0.80–1.77) | 0.39 | 0.80 (0.25–2.56) | 0.70 |
| EC/inferior TCTX | 1.60 (1.02–2.54) | **0.041** | 1.13 (0.27–5.26) | 0.87 |
| Frontal neocortex | 1.08 (0.47–2.52) | 0.86 | 0.21 (0.01–2.47) | 0.23 |

[a]A total of 755 subjects had data on *APOE* genotype (those data were missing in 174 subjects)
[b]Odds ratios were adjusted for sex, age at death, and the type of TDP-43 antibody used
[c]Thal Aβ phase and Braak NFT stage were included as additional covariates in model 2
*OR* odds ratio, *CI* confidence interval, *EC* entorhinal cortex, *TCTX* temporal cortex
Bold *p*-value represents the statistical significance

evidence of strong associations between TDP-43 proteinopathy and other factors (age, HS pathology, AD pathology, and arteriolosclerosis pathology). These data were collected from individuals who died and came to autopsy over the past 4 years (NACC NP Form v10), providing both fresh data and relatively up-to-date clinical and pathological testing modalities. The study of nearly 1000 brains with *APOE* genotype and TDP-43 pathology status in multiple brain regions is unusual, and the statistical power it provides is important. Further, the derivation of data from 27 different research centers with expertise in research in AD and related dementias is a strength because the autopsy data may be considered more generalizable than the results from a single neuropathologist or small group of pathologists. For the foreseeable future, it seems unlikely that all research centers will agree on a single protocol for TDP-43 IHC, and we consider it a strength that the current study incorporates results from multiple research centers using site-specific protocols.

There are three main findings that we describe: TDP-43 pathology is strongly associated with advanced AD pathology; TDP-43 pathology is associated with increasingly severe arteriolosclerosis pathology (particularly in non *APOE* ε4/ε4 carriers); and age-related TDP-43 pathology is predominantly seen in the medial temporal cortex, uncommon in frontal neocortex, and very rare in spinal cord.

There is a relatively large extant literature on the relatively common comorbidity of TDP-43 pathology with AD, providing a compelling evidence that the pathologies co-occur whether or not they directly interact mechanistically [14, 16, 27, 30, 48]. Staging schema have been proposed to describe how TDP-43 pathology is distributed in brains with comorbid AD pathology [15, 17, 27]. Notably, in multiple cohorts of aged persons, TDP-43 pathology is more strongly linked to HS than *early* AD pathology [5, 7, 26, 28, 33]. However, within the amygdala of subjects with *advanced* AD, protein misfolding (tau, Aβ, α-synuclein, and TDP-43 pathologies alike) tends to occur [14, 16].

Compared with AD, the literature on the association between TDP-43 pathology and cerebrovascular is smaller, and overlaps with the paradigm of hypoxia/ischemia. As stated by Zarow et al. [49], "HS has long been hypothesized to result from ischemic-hypoxic insult to the brain. The CA1 sector is fed by small end-arterioles from the anterior choroidal and posterior cerebral arteries and is known to be susceptible to hypoxic injury" (with citation to Ref [9]). Others have also published data compatible with a link between HS pathology and cerebrovascular disease [22, 41, 46, 47, 49]. However, we have found in various data sets previous evidence of a relatively specific association between the type of HS that frequently is comborbid with TDP-43 pathology, and brain arteriolosclerosis [12, 35–37]. In the present study, the specificity of that association was underscored since no other subtype of cerebrovascular pathology was linked to TDP-43 pathology. There currently is no proven mechanistic explanation for this association. We note that factors that are conventionally associated with arteriolosclerosis, such as diabetes or hypertension, do not appear to be specifically associated with TDP-43 pathology. Intriguingly, Montagne and colleagues recently showed that subtle blood-brain barrier dysfunction and "leaky vessels" in the human hippocampus precede cognitive impairment in advanced aging [24]. Winkler et al. [42] reported that pericyte damage could contribute to cognitive impairment through disruption of the neurovascular unit, which may relate to TDP-43 proteinopathy, rather than AD. There also have been described some genetic risk factors that may help explain the link between brain arteriolosclerosis and TDP-43 pathology [32], but more work is required in this area. We speculate that there may be some reason that the TDP-43 pathology is usually confined to the medial temporal lobe of aged individuals, perhaps analogous to how primary age-related tauopathy [13], in the absence of comorbid Aβ plaques, tends not to progress beyond Braak NFT stage IV. Considering this analogy, there may be, in some of the brains, a disease-accelerating factor, analogous to Aβ, which promotes TDP-43 pathology outside of the medial temporal lobe.

**Acknowledgments**

We are extremely grateful to the many patients, clinicians, and other colleagues, who have worked so hard to provide and organize these data. The NACC database is funded by NIA/NIH Grant U01 AG016976. NACC data are contributed by the NIA-funded ADCs: P30 AG019610 (PI Eric Reiman, MD), P30 AG013846 (PI Neil Kowall, MD), P50 AG008702 (PI Scott Small, MD), P50 AG025688 (PI Allan Levey, MD, PhD), P50 AG047266 (PI Todd Golde, MD, PhD), P30 AG010133 (PI Andrew Saykin, PsyD), P50 AG005146 (PI Marilyn Albert, PhD), P50 AG005134 (PI Bradley Hyman, MD, PhD), P50 AG016574 (PI Ronald Petersen, MD, PhD), P50 AG005138 (PI Mary Sano, PhD), P30 AG008051 (PI Thomas Wisniewski, MD), P30 AG013854 (PI M. Marsel Mesulam, MD), P30 AG008017 (PI Jeffrey Kaye, MD), P30 AG010161 (PI David Bennett, MD), P50 AG047366 (PI Victor Henderson, MD, MS), P30 AG010129 (PI Charles DeCarli, MD), P50 AG016573 (PI Frank LaFerla, PhD), P50 AG005131 (PI James Brewer, MD, PhD), P50 AG023501 (PI Bruce Miller, MD), P30 AG035982 (PI Russell Swerdlow, MD), P30 AG028383 (PI Linda Van Eldik, PhD), P30 AG053760 (PI Henry Paulson, MD, PhD), P30 AG010124 (PI John Trojanowski, MD, PhD), P50 AG005133 (PI Oscar Lopez, MD), P50 AG005142 (PI Helena Chui, MD), P30 AG012300 (PI Roger Rosenberg, MD), P30 AG049638 (PI Suzanne Craft, PhD), P50 AG005136 (PI Thomas Grabowski, MD), P50 AG033514 (PI Sanjay Asthana, MD, FRCP), P50 AG005681 (PI John Morris, MD), P50 AG047270 (PI Stephen Strittmatter, MD, PhD).

**Funding**

Funding included NIH grants P30 AG028383, R01 AG057187, R01 AG042475, R01 AG054060, and U01 AG016976 from the National Institute on Aging (NIA)/National Institutes of Health (NIH). For more on NACC-related funding, please see Acknowledgment section.

**Authors' contributions**

Acquisition, analysis and interpretation of the data: YK, PTN. Manuscript preparation and conceptualization: YK, PTN. Critical revision of the manuscript for intellectual content: PTN, DWF, WAK. All authors read and approved the final manuscript.

**Competing interests**

The authors declare that they have no competing interests.

**Author details**

[1]Department of Biostatistics, University of Kentucky, 725 Rose Street, Lexington, KY 40536, USA. [2]Sanders-Brown Center on Aging, University of Kentucky, Lexington, KY 40536, USA. [3]National Alzheimer's Coordinating Center, Department of Epidemiology, University of Washington, Seattle, WA 98105, USA. [4]Department of Pathology, Division of Neuropathology, University of Kentucky, Lexington, KY 40536, USA.

**References**

1. Amador-Ortiz C, Dickson DW (2008) Neuropathology of hippocampal sclerosis. Handb Clin Neurol 89:569–572. https://doi.org/10.1016/S0072-9752(07)01253-5
2. Amador-Ortiz C, Lin WL, Ahmed Z, Personett D, Davies P, Duara R, Graff-Radford NR, Hutton ML, Dickson DW (2007) TDP-43 immunoreactivity in hippocampal sclerosis and Alzheimer's disease. Ann Neurol 61:435–445. https://doi.org/10.1002/ana.21154
3. Besser LM, Kukull WA, Teylan MA, Bigio EH, Cairns NJ, Kofler JK, Montine TJ, Schneider JA, Nelson PT (2018) The revised National Alzheimer's coordinating Center's neuropathology form-available data and new analyses. J Neuropathol Exp Neurol 77:717–726. https://doi.org/10.1093/jnen/nly049
4. Braak H, Ludolph AC, Neumann M, Ravits J, Del Tredici K (2017) Pathological TDP-43 changes in Betz cells differ from those in bulbar and spinal alpha-motoneurons in sporadic amyotrophic lateral sclerosis. Acta Neuropathol 133:79–90. https://doi.org/10.1007/s00401-016-1633-2
5. Brenowitz WD, Monsell SE, Schmitt FA, Kukull WA, Nelson PT (2014) Hippocampal sclerosis of aging is a key Alzheimer's disease mimic: clinical-pathologic correlations and comparisons with both alzheimer's disease and non-tauopathic frontotemporal lobar degeneration. J Alzheimers Dis 39: 691–702. https://doi.org/10.3233/JAD-131880
6. Brettschneider J, Del Tredici K, Toledo JB, Robinson JL, Irwin DJ, Grossman M, Suh E, Van Deerlin VM, Wood EM, Baek Y et al (2013) Stages of pTDP-43 pathology in amyotrophic lateral sclerosis. Ann Neurol 74:20–38. https://doi.org/10.1002/ana.23937
7. Cykowski MD, Takei H, Van Eldik LJ, Schmitt FA, Jicha GA, Powell SZ, Nelson PT (In Press) Hippocampal sclerosis, but not normal aging or Alzheimer's disease, is associated iwth TDP-43 pathology in aged persons' basal forebrain. J Neuropathol Exp Neurol
8. Dickson DW, Davies P, Bevona C, Van Hoeven KH, Factor SM, Grober E, Aronson MK, Crystal HA (1994) Hippocampal sclerosis: a common pathological feature of dementia in very old (> or = 80 years of age) humans. Acta Neuropathol 88:212–221
9. Duvernoy HM (2005) The human Hippocampus: functional anatomy, vascularization and serial sections with MRI. Srpinger-Verlag, City
10. Fatima M, Tan R, Halliday GM, Kril JJ (2015) Spread of pathology in amyotrophic lateral sclerosis: assessment of phosphorylated TDP-43 along axonal pathways. Acta Neuropathol Commun 3:47. https://doi.org/10.1186/s40478-015-0226-y
11. Geser F, Robinson JL, Malunda JA, Xie SX, Clark CM, Kwong LK, Moberg PJ, Moore EM, Van Deerlin VM, Lee VM et al (2010) Pathological 43-kDa transactivation response DNA-binding protein in older adults with and without severe mental illness. Arch Neurol 67:1238–1250. https://doi.org/10.1001/archneurol.2010.254
12. Ighodaro ET, Abner EL, Fardo DW, Lin AL, Katsumata Y, Schmitt FA, Kryscio RJ, Jicha GA, Neltner JH, Monsell SE et al (2017) Risk factors and global cognitive status related to brain arteriolosclerosis in elderly individuals. J Cereb Blood Flow Metab 37:201–216. https://doi.org/10.1177/0271678X15621574
13. Jellinger KA, Alafuzoff I, Attems J, Beach TG, Cairns NJ, Crary JF, Dickson DW, Hof PR, Hyman BT, Jack CR Jr et al (2015) PART, a distinct tauopathy, different from classical sporadic Alzheimer disease. Acta Neuropathol 129: 757–762. https://doi.org/10.1007/s00401-015-1407-2
14. Josephs KA, Dickson DW, Tosakulwong N, Weigand SD, Murray ME, Petrucelli L, Liesinger AM, Senjem ML, Spychalla AJ, Knopman DS et al (2017) Rates of hippocampal atrophy and presence of post-mortem TDP-43 in patients with Alzheimer's disease: a longitudinal retrospective study. Lancet Neurol 16:917–924. https://doi.org/10.1016/S1474-4422(17)30284-3
15. Josephs KA, Murray ME, Whitwell JL, Parisi JE, Petrucelli L, Jack CR, Petersen RC, Dickson DW (2014) Staging TDP-43 pathology in Alzheimer's disease. Acta Neuropathol 127:441–450. https://doi.org/10.1007/s00401-013-1211-9
16. Josephs KA, Murray ME, Whitwell JL, Tosakulwong N, Weigand SD, Petrucelli L, Liesinger AM, Petersen RC, Parisi JE, Dickson DW (2016) Updated TDP-43 in Alzheimer's disease staging scheme. Acta Neuropathol 131:571–585. https://doi.org/10.1007/s00401-016-1537-1
17. Josephs KA, Murray ME, Whitwell JL, Tosakulwong N, Weigand SD, Petrucelli L, Liesinger AM, Petersen RC, Parisi JE, Dickson DW (2016) Updated TDP-43 in Alzheimer's disease staging scheme. Acta Neuropathol. https://doi.org/10.1007/s00401-016-1537-1
18. Josephs KA, Whitwell JL, Knopman DS, Hu WT, Stroh DA, Baker M, Rademakers R, Boeve BF, Parisi JE, Smith GE et al (2008, 1850) Abnormal TDP-43 immunoreactivity in AD modifies clinicopathologic and radiologic phenotype. Neurology 70:–1857. https://doi.org/10.1212/01.wnl.0000304041.09418.b1
19. Kero M, Raunio A, Polvikoski T, Tienari PJ, Paetau A, Myllykangas L (2018) Hippocampal sclerosis in the oldest old: a Finnish population-based study. J Alzheimers Dis 63:263–272. https://doi.org/10.3233/JAD-171068
20. Lee EB, Lee VM, Trojanowski JQ, Neumann M (2008) TDP-43 immunoreactivity in anoxic, ischemic and neoplastic lesions of the central nervous system. Acta Neuropathol 115:305–311. https://doi.org/10.1007/s00401-007-0331-5

21. Leverenz JB, Agustin CM, Tsuang D, Peskind ER, Edland SD, Nochlin D, DiGiacomo L, Bowen JD, McCormick WC, Teri L et al (2002) Clinical and neuropathological characteristics of hippocampal sclerosis: a community-based study. Arch Neurol 59:1099–1106
22. Leverenz JB, Lipton AM (2008) Clinical aspects of hippocampal sclerosis. Handb Clin Neurol 89:565–567. https://doi.org/10.1016/S0072-9752(07)01252-3
23. Mackenzie IR, Neumann M, Bigio EH, Cairns NJ, Alafuzoff I, Kril J, Kovacs GG, Ghetti B, Halliday G, Holm IE et al (2010) Nomenclature and nosology for neuropathologic subtypes of frontotemporal lobar degeneration: an update. Acta Neuropathol 119:1–4. https://doi.org/10.1007/s00401-009-0612-2
24. Montagne A, Barnes SR, Sweeney MD, Halliday MR, Sagare AP, Zhao Z, Toga AW, Jacobs RE, Liu CY, Amezcua L et al (2015) Blood-brain barrier breakdown in the aging human hippocampus. Neuron 85:296–302. https://doi.org/10.1016/j.neuron.2014.12.032
25. Montine TJ, Phelps CH, Beach TG, Bigio EH, Cairns NJ, Dickson DW, Duyckaerts C, Frosch MP, Masliah E, Mirra SS et al (2012) National Institute on Aging-Alzheimer's Association guidelines for the neuropathologic assessment of Alzheimer's disease: a practical approach. Acta Neuropathol 123:1–11. https://doi.org/10.1007/s00401-011-0910-3
26. Murray ME, Cannon A, Graff-Radford NR, Liesinger AM, Rutherford NJ, Ross OA, Duara R, Carrasquillo MM, Rademakers R, Dickson DW (2014) Differential clinicopathologic and genetic features of late-onset amnestic dementias. Acta Neuropathol 128:411–421. https://doi.org/10.1007/s00401-014-1302-2
27. Nag S, Yu L, Boyle PA, Leurgans SE, Bennett DA, Schneider JA (2018) TDP-43 pathology in anterior temporal pole cortex in aging and Alzheimer's disease. Acta Neuropathol Commun 6:33. https://doi.org/10.1186/s40478-018-0531-3
28. Nag S, Yu L, Capuano AW, Wilson RS, Leurgans SE, Bennett DA, Schneider JA (2015) Hippocampal sclerosis and TDP-43 pathology in aging and Alzheimer disease. Ann Neurol 77:942–952. https://doi.org/10.1002/ana.24388
29. Nag S, Yu L, Wilson RS, Chen EY, Bennett DA, Schneider JA (2017) TDP-43 pathology and memory impairment in elders without pathologic diagnoses of AD or FTLD. Neurology 88:653–660. https://doi.org/10.1212/WNL.0000000000003610
30. Nelson PT, Abner EL, Patel E, Anderson S, Wilcock DM, Kryscio RJ, Van Eldik LJ, Jicha GA, Gal Z, Nelson RS et al (2018) The amygdala as a locus of pathologic Misfolding in neurodegenerative diseases. J Neuropathol Exp Neurol 77:2–20. https://doi.org/10.1093/jnen/nlx099
31. Nelson PT, Abner EL, Schmitt FA, Kryscio RJ, Jicha GA, Smith CD, Davis DG, Poduska JW, Patel E, Mendiondo MS et al (2010) Modeling the association between 43 different clinical and pathological variables and the severity of cognitive impairment in a large autopsy cohort of elderly persons. Brain Pathol 20:66–79. https://doi.org/10.1111/j.1750-3639.2008.00244.x
32. Nelson PT, Jicha GA, Wang WX, Ighodaro E, Artiushin S, Nichols CG, Fardo DW (2015) ABCC9/SUR2 in the brain: implications for hippocampal sclerosis of aging and a potential therapeutic target. Ageing Res Rev 24:111–125. https://doi.org/10.1016/j.arr.2015.07.007
33. Nelson PT, Schmitt FA, Lin Y, Abner EL, Jicha GA, Patel E, Thomason PC, Neltner JH, Smith CD, Santacruz KS et al (2011) Hippocampal sclerosis in advanced age: clinical and pathological features. Brain 134:1506–1518. https://doi.org/10.1093/brain/awr053
34. Nelson PT, Smith CD, Abner EL, Wilfred BJ, Wang WX, Neltner JH, Baker M, Fardo DW, Kryscio RJ, Scheff SW et al (2013) Hippocampal sclerosis of aging, a prevalent and high-morbidity brain disease. Acta Neuropathol 126: 161–177 https://doi.org/10.1007/s00401-013-1154-1
35. Nelson PT, Trojanowski JQ, Abner EL, Al-Janabi OM, Jicha GA, Schmitt FA, Smith CD, Fardo DW, Wang WX, Kryscio RJ et al (2016) "new old pathologies": AD, PART, and cerebral age-related TDP-43 with sclerosis (CARTS). J Neuropathol Exp Neurol 75:482–498. https://doi.org/10.1093/jnen/nlw033
36. Neltner JH, Abner EL, Baker S, Schmitt FA, Kryscio RJ, Jicha GA, Smith CD, Hammack E, Kukull WA, Brenowitz WD et al (2014) Arteriolosclerosis that affects multiple brain regions is linked to hippocampal sclerosis of ageing. Brain 137:255–267. https://doi.org/10.1093/brain/awt318
37. Neltner JH, Abner EL, Jicha GA, Schmitt FA, Patel E, Poon LW, Marla G, Green RC, Davey A, Johnson MA et al (2016) Brain pathologies in extreme old age. Neurobiol Aging 37:1–11. https://doi.org/10.1016/j.neurobiolaging.2015.10.009
38. Neumann M, Sampathu DM, Kwong LK, Truax AC, Micsenyi MC, Chou TT, Bruce J, Schuck T, Grossman M, Clark CM et al (2006) Ubiquitinated TDP-43 in frontotemporal lobar degeneration and amyotrophic lateral sclerosis. Science 314:130–133. https://doi.org/10.1126/science.1134108
39. Pao WC, Dickson DW, Crook JE, Finch NA, Rademakers R, Graff-Radford NR (2011) Hippocampal sclerosis in the elderly: genetic and pathologic findings, some mimicking Alzheimer disease clinically. Alzheimer Dis Assoc Disord 25:364–368. https://doi.org/10.1097/WAD.0b013e31820f8f50
40. R Development Core Team (2013) R: a language and environment for statistical computing. 3.0.2 edn. R. Foundation for Statistical Computing, City
41. Reed BR, Mungas DM, Kramer JH, Ellis W, Vinters HV, Zarow C, Jagust WJ, Chui HC (2007) Profiles of neuropsychological impairment in autopsy-defined Alzheimer's disease and cerebrovascular disease. Brain 130:731–739. https://doi.org/10.1093/brain/awl385
42. Sagare AP, Bell RD, Zhao Z, Ma Q, Winkler EA, Ramanathan A, Zlokovic BV (2013) Pericyte loss influences Alzheimer-like neurodegeneration in mice. Nat Commun 4:2932. https://doi.org/10.1038/ncomms3932
43. Thal DR, Attems J, Ewers M (2014) Spreading of amyloid, tau, and microvascular pathology in Alzheimer's disease: findings from neuropathological and neuroimaging studies. J Alzheimers Dis 42(Suppl 4): S421–S429. https://doi.org/10.3233/JAD-141461
44. Uchino A, Takao M, Hatsuta H, Sumikura H, Nakano Y, Nogami A, Saito Y, Arai T, Nishiyama K, Murayama S (2015) Incidence and extent of TDP-43 accumulation in aging human brain. Acta Neuropathol Commun 3:35. https://doi.org/10.1186/s40478-015-0215-1
45. Verde F, Del Tredici K, Braak H, Ludolph A (2017) The multisystem degeneration amyotrophic lateral sclerosis - neuropathological staging and clinical translation. Arch Ital Biol 155:118–130. https://doi.org/10.12871/00039829201746
46. White L (2009) Brain lesions at autopsy in older Japanese-American men as related to cognitive impairment and dementia in the final years of life: a summary report from the Honolulu-Asia aging study. J Alzheimers Dis 18: 713–725. https://doi.org/10.3233/JAD-2009-1178
47. White L, Petrovitch H, Hardman J, Nelson J, Davis DG, Ross GW, Masaki K, Launer L, Markesbery WR (2002) Cerebrovascular pathology and dementia in autopsied Honolulu-Asia aging study participants. Ann N Y Acad Sci 977: 9–23
48. Yang HS, Yu L, White CC, Chibnik LB, Chhatwal JP, Sperling RA, Bennett DA, Schneider JA, De Jager PL (2018) Evaluation of TDP-43 proteinopathy and hippocampal sclerosis in relation to APOE epsilon4 haplotype status: a community-based cohort study. Lancet Neurol 17:773–781. https://doi.org/10.1016/S1474-4422(18)30251-5
49. Zarow C, Sitzer TE, Chui HC (2008) Understanding hippocampal sclerosis in the elderly: epidemiology, characterization, and diagnostic issues. Curr Neurol Neurosci Rep 8:363–370
50. Zarow C, Weiner MW, Ellis WG, Chui HC (2012) Prevalence, laterality, and comorbidity of hippocampal sclerosis in an autopsy sample. Brain Behavior 2:435–442. https://doi.org/10.1002/brb3.66

# 5

# Homozygous TBC1 domain-containing kinase (TBCK) mutation causes a novel lysosomal storage disease – a new type of neuronal ceroid lipofuscinosis (CLN15)?

Stefanie Beck-Wödl[1†], Klaus Harzer[2†], Marc Sturm[1], Rebecca Buchert[1], Olaf Rieß[1], Hans-Dieter Mennel[4], Elisabeth Latta[3^], Axel Pagenstecher[4] and Ursula Keber[4*]

**Abstract**

Homozygous mutation of TBC1 domain-containing kinase (*TBCK*) is the cause of a very recently defined severe childhood disorder, which is characterized by severe hypotonia, global developmental delay, intellectual disability, epilepsy, characteristic facies and premature death. The link between TBCK loss of function and symptoms in patients with TBCK deficiency disorder (TBCK-DD) remains elusive. Here we demonstrate for the first time the histopathological characteristics of TBCK deficiency consisting of 1) a widespread and massive accumulation of lipofuscin storage material in neurons of the central nervous system without notable neuronal degeneration, 2) storage deposits in few astrocytes, 3) carbohydrate-rich deposits in brain, spleen and liver and 4) vacuolated lymphocytes. Biochemical examinations ruled out more than 20 known lysosomal storage diseases. These investigations strikingly uncover TBCK-DD as a novel type of lysosomal storage disease which is characterized by different storage products rather than one specific type of accumulated material. Due to the clear predominance of intraneuronal lipofuscin storage material and the characteristic clinical presentation we propose to classify this disease as a new subtype of neuronal ceroid lipofuscinosis (CLN15). Our results and previous reports suggest an autophagosomal-lysosomal dysfunction caused by enhanced mTORC1-mediated autophagosome formation and reduced Rab-mediated autophagosome-lysosome fusion, thus disclosing potential novel targets for therapeutic approaches in TBCK-DD.

**Keywords:** Infantile muscular hypotonia with psychomotor retardation and characteristic facies 3 (IHPRF3), Central nervous system (CNS), Vacuolated lymphocytes, Autophagy, Mammalian target of rapamycin (mTOR), Rab

## Introduction

Homozygous mutation of TBC1 domain-containing kinase (*TBCK*) leads to a very recently defined severe disorder in childhood, which is characterized by infantile muscular hypotonia, psychomotor retardation and characteristic facies (IHPRF3; OMIM: 616900). To date, more than 30 patients with various homozygous *TBCK* mutations have been reported [1, 4, 9, 17, 20, 31, 35, 51]. The disease is often accompanied by global developmental delay, distinctive facial features like deeply set eyes and tented upper lip vermilion, medication refractory epilepsy and chronic respiratory failure [51]. Typical brain imaging signs are brain atrophy and progressive leukoencephalopathy with a thinned corpus callosum. The disease has a generally short survival and only exceptional clinical courses up to two decades have been described [17, 35].

In all reported cases, the different *TBCK* mutations resulted in aberrant TBCK protein. The knowledge about the function of TBCK is still limited. The protein contains a Tre-2/Bub2/Cdc16 (TBC) domain, a rhodanase-like domain and a kinase domain, which has been proposed to be inactive due to a lack of essential

* Correspondence: keber@med.uni-marburg.de
†Stefanie Beck-Wödl and Klaus Harzer contributed equally to this work.
^Deceased
[4]Department of Neuropathology, Philipps University and University Hospital of Marburg, Baldingerstrasse, 35043 Marburg, Germany
Full list of author information is available at the end of the article

catalytic subdomains [7, 29, 42]. The TBCK protein is expressed in most organs (https://www.proteinatlas.org/). It has been shown to suppress cell proliferation [29, 50] and to play a role in cell growth and actin organization by enhancing the signalling pathways of mammalian target of rapamycin (mTOR), presumably at a transcriptional or post-transcriptional level [29]. Interestingly, an autophagosomal-lysosomal dysfunction has been described recently in patients with TBCK deficiency [35] that is attributed to the disturbed activation of the mTOR complex 1 (mTORC1), which regulates autophagy [6]. In addition, it has been suggested that *TBCK* encodes a Rab GTPase-activating protein [9].

Despite these data, the actual mechanisms linking *TBCK* gene mutation to the clinical phenotype remain elusive, thus impeding the establishment of potential therapeutic strategies. This study provides the first autopsy reports of two siblings, who suffered from homozygous *TBCK* mutation. Macroscopic, histological and ultrastructural investigations give insights into the cellular changes in the disorder and provide compelling evidence for classification of TBCK deficiency disorder (TBCK-DD) as a novel type of lysosomal storage disease (LSD).

## Materials and methods

### General study design

Two siblings born in 1972 and 1974 suffered from the same severe and at that time unknown disease. Clinical examinations of both patients rendered no definite diagnosis. Autopsies were done immediately after death of patient 1 in 1978 and of patient 2 in 1985. Investigations included macroscopic, histological and biochemical analysis, but no definite diagnosis could be made. With the recent advent of modern genetic techniques it became possible to pinpoint the cause of the disorder. Subsequently, intense re-evaluation of tissue samples including completive immunohistochemical and ultrastructural studies was performed. Written informed consent to participate in the study and for publication of the clinical photographs (Fig. 2) was obtained from the parents of the siblings.

### Molecular gene analysis

Genomic DNA was isolated from spleen tissue of patient 2 using the QIAamp Mini Kit (Qiagen NV, Hilden, Germany) following the manufacturer's instructions. Mutations in the *TBCK* gene were uncovered by whole exome sequencing. Target regions were enriched using the SureSelectXT Human All Exon Kit V5 (Agilent, Böblingen, Germany) according to the manufacturer's protocol. Sequencing was performed on a HiSeq2500 instrument (Illumina, San Diego, CA; USA). On average 100 million paired-end reads with a length of 125 bp were produced per exome. The conversion of the sequence data in the FASTA format was done by Illumina bcl2fastq. Adapter sequences were removed with SeqPurge (https://github.com/imgag/ngs-bits) and the trimmed reads were mapped to the human reference genome hg19 (GRCh37) using Burrows Wheeler Aligner (http://bio-bwa.sourceforge.net). PCR-duplicates were removed with samblaster (https://github.com/GregoryFaust/samblaster). Deletions and insertions were realigned with ABRA (https://github.com/mozack/abra). Variants were detected using freebayes (https://github.com/ekg/freebayes) and transcript/protein information was annotated with SnpEff / SnpSift (http://snpeff.sourceforge.net).

Filtering of variants for pathogenicity was performed with an in-house tool (MS, unpublished). Calls with an allele frequency ≥ 1% in the 1000 Genomes, ExAC or Kaviar databases were excluded. In addition, frequently observed variants in our in-house database (≥ 20x) were removed. All exonic non-synonymous variants including splice sites which potentially change the protein were taken into account (other intronic and UTR mutations were eliminated). Finally the remaining SNVs and INDELs of the index patient were checked for the three modes of inheritance: Autosomal dominant (de novo?), autosomal recessive, X-linked recessive or dominant and the coverage (minimum 20x).

Sanger sequencing of the *TBCK* gene was performed on genomic DNA from spleen and paraffin-embedded brain tissue of patient 2. Genomic DNA was also isolated from peripheral blood leukocytes of both parents by standard methods in order to confirm the pathogenic variants and exclude de novo mutations. The following primer sequences were used: *TBCK*-Ex3F: AGCCCTTTCGTGGAAGAACC, *TBCK*-Ex3R: GCCC TGATCCCAGTTGCT, chr4: 107183639–107183188. *TBCK* reference sequence was NM_001163435.2, ENST00000394708.6 and all genomic positions are denoted according to GRCh37/hg19.

### Biochemical analysis

Enzymatic, cytochemical and thin-layer chromatographic lipid analyses screening more than 20 LSDs were performed on white blood cells, cultured fibroblasts and frozen tissue samples of brain, spinal cord and liver obtained from autopsy of both patients. Additionally, urine of patient 2 was tested for oligosaccharide concentration and spleen tissue of patient 2 was examined regarding its content of carbohydrate positive (CHp) material. For this, buffer extract from 200 mg spleen tissue was delipidated by phase partitioning with chloroform/ methanol 2:1 by volumes. The aqueous upper phase was dialyzed against water, concentrated and applied to a BioGel P-4 column [25]. The buffer-eluted fractions were monitored for CHp material by spotting aliquots to a thin-layer plate and reacting the spots with anisaldehyde/sulfuric acid reagent (characteristic colour for carbohydrates, glucose as a reference). CHp material was detected only in some fractions eluted with the void volume. These fractions were also positive with a mucopolysaccharide reagent [13]. Positive fractions were pooled and centrifuged. The resulting sediment and supernatant were again tested for CHp material as follows: The test spots were applied to a start line 1 cm above the lower edge of a thin-layer plate. Water-soluble, low-molecular-weight contaminations were removed from the start line by running the plate upwards with a polar solvent system for 2 h. Finally, the run plate was sprayed with anisaldehyde reagent to visualize CHp material. The entire procedure was also applied to spleen tissue from two control individuals.

### Histological and immunohistochemical analysis

Autopsies were done immediately after death of patient 1 in 1978 and of patient 2 in 1985. Visceral and central nervous tissue was formalin fixed and paraffin embedded according to standard protocols. Multiple stained sections of all relevant brain regions and of the spinal cord were available from patient 1 and re-evaluated for this study. From patient 2, both the stained sections and archived paraffin blocks of the central nervous system and peripheral organs were re-evaluated and used for new histological and immunohistochemical stains, respectively. Hematoxylin and eosin, Klüver Barrera (luxol fast blue and cresyl violet), Sudan black and red, periodic acid-Schiff (PAS), Alcian blue, Shimizu and Heidenhain-Woelcke stains as well as Gallyas silver impregnation were performed according to standard procedures. Investigation of sections was performed with normal or differential interference contrast microscopy and autofluorescence was evaluated with light excitation using ultraviolet (excitation wavelength 340–380 nm), blue (460–500 nm) and green (515–560 nm) light.

For immunohistochemistry, heat-induced epitope retrieval was performed either with citrate or EDTA according to the manufacturer's protocol of the respective primary antibody. Sections were incubated for one hour with the following primary antibodies: rabbit anti-GFAP (1:1000; Dako Z0334), mouse anti-ß-Amyloid (1:100; Dako M0872), rabbit anti-p62 (1:100; Enzo BML-PW9860), mouse anti-CD3 (1:50; Novocastra Laboratories NCL-CD3-PS1), mouse anti CD20 (1:400; Dako M0755), mouse anti-CD68 (1:100; Dako M0876) and mouse anti-CD138 (1:200; Dako M7228). Sections were washed and incubated with post-block solution and HRP-polymer reagent according to the manufacturer's protocol of ZytoChem-Plus HRP Polymer-Kit (Zytomed Systems).

### Ultrastructural analysis

For ultrastructural analysis, cylinders of 3 mm in diameter were punched out of paraffin embedded tissue of the neocortex, medulla oblongata and spinal cord anterior horn, respectively. We chose areas in which neuronal storage inclusions were histologically observed. The tissue was rehydrated and fixed in glutaraldehyde. Tissue preparation was performed as described previously [26]. In brief, the tissue cylinders were fixed in buffered glutaraldehyde, postfixed in osmiumtetroxide and embedded in Epon resin. Thin sections were contrasted with uranylacetate and lead citrate and analyzed using a Zeiss EM 902.

## Results

### Clinical report

The two sisters were born to healthy Caucasian German parents with distant consanguinity (Fig. 1). The third pregnancy was interrupted without a prenatal diagnosis. The clinical symptoms, age of onset and age of death of both patients are summarized in Table 1.

In detail, patient 1 started to suffer from hypotonia and loss of tendon reflexes at the age of about 4 months. The progressive hypotonia prevented any statomotor development except for lifting the head in prone position, an ability that was lost later on. At the age of 7, the body size was reduced (1.2 m, according to the 30. percentile of age-related WHO reference values), the body weight was regular (31.5 kg). X-ray examination revealed no signs of dysostosis. She had a short neck and mild facial dysmorphia with an open mouth, tented upper lip vermilion, macroglossia, furrowed tongue and right esotropia (Fig. 2). She was intellectually disabled, never able to speak and blind, but able to hear. At the age of 5 years, epilepsy with generalized onset motor seizures became manifest. Accordingly, electroencephalographic (EEG) waves of severely changed general activity and some hypersynchronous activity were observed. The patient died at the age of 7 years and 3 months from a bronchopneumonia with respiratory failure.

Patient 2, the younger sister, developed similar clinical features of a profound global developmental delay with a slightly later onset and longer survival. Her statomotor maximum was the all-fours position, when the symptoms with hypotonia started at the age of 10 months. The subsequent disease progress was faster compared to her sister and generalized onset motor seizures appeared soon. She was intellectually disabled, never able to speak and suffered from severely reduced visual acuity. Hearing was intact and she developed hyperacusis. The external appearance was comparable to her sister (Fig. 2, middle and right panel). Size and weight was normal at birth but severely reduced by the age of 11 years (size 1.24 m, according to < 1. percentile and weight 33 kg,

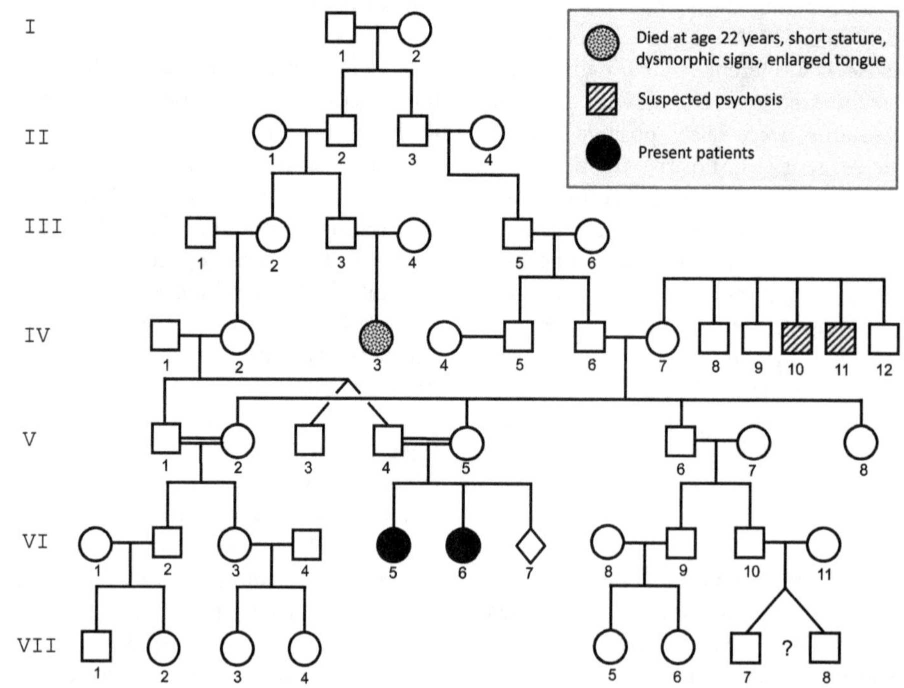


**Fig. 1** Family tree of the patients. The siblings (VI.5 and VI.6, black circles) were born to Caucasian, distantly consanguineous parents, who did not suffer from the disease. ◊, pregnancy with induced abortion. ?, twins with unknown zygosity

**Table 1** Clinic of siblings

| | Patient 1 | Patient 2 |
|---|---|---|
| Age of onset | 4 months | 10 months |
| Age of death | 7 years | 11 years |
| Cause of death | | |
| Respiratory failure | + | + |
| Main symptons | | |
| Severe Hypotonia | + | + |
| Global developmental delay | + | + |
| Intellectual disability | + | + |
| Generalized onset seizures | + | + |
| Reduced visual acuity | – | + |
| Blindness | + | – |
| Appearance | | |
| Undersize | + | + |
| Underweight | – | + |
| Short neck | + | + |
| Facial dysmorphia | + | + |
| Open mouth | + | + |
| Tented upper lip | + | + |
| Macroglossia | + | + |
| Furrowed tongue | + | + |
| Unilateral esotropia | + | + |

according to the 22. percentile of age-related WHO reference values, respectively). Electroneurographic and myographic measurements at the age of 9 years revealed reduced distal nerve conduction velocities and a complete absence of spontaneous and arbitrary muscular activity. Computer tomography showed a general cortical, frontally accentuated atrophy with slightly distended, deformed ventricles and a massive atrophy of the lower cerebellar vermis. The patient died at the age of 11 years from bronchopneumonia with respiratory failure.

### Genetic investigations

Whole exome sequencing of the DNA of patient 2 yielded 77 million mapped reads with a mean coverage of more than 94%. The analysis revealed a homozygous nonsense mutation in exon 3 of *TBCK*: NM_001163435.2:c.304C > T, p.Gln102* (Fig. 3a). This leads to a premature stop codon and affects the protein kinase domain. The mutation was confirmed by Sanger sequencing and accordingly heterogeneously present in both parents of the patients (Fig. 3b). Other gene mutations, especially of known metabolic diseases, were not detected.

### Biochemical investigations

Biochemical analyses were performed on white blood cells, cultured fibroblasts and frozen tissue samples of patient 2 and ruled out the following metabolic diseases: metachromatic leukodystrophy, multiple sulfatase deficiency,

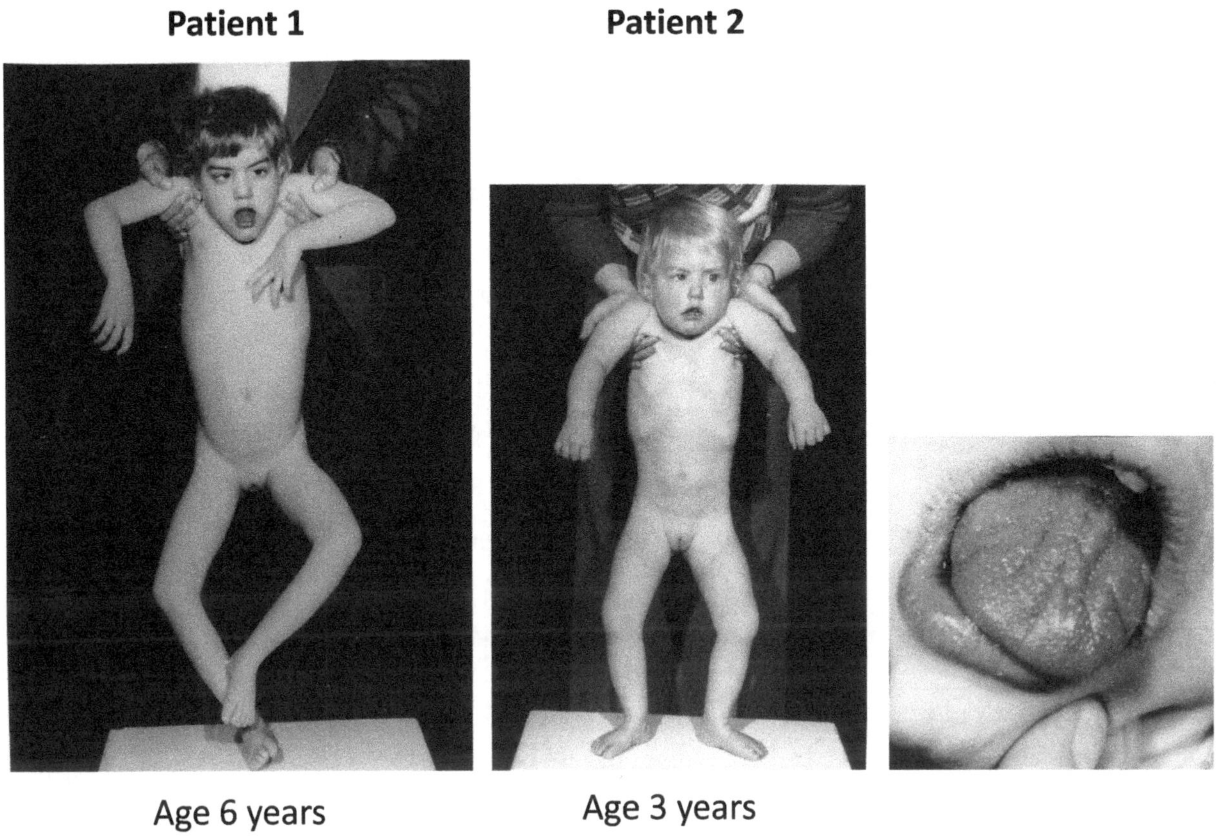


**Fig. 2** External appearance of the two patients. Severe hypotonia, a short neck and mild facial dysmorphia with open mouth, tented upper lip vermilion, macroglossia, furrowed tongues and right esotropia are seen

Krabbe disease, GM1 gangliosidosis I and II, GM2 gangliosidosis, galactosialidosis, sialidosis, Salla disease, Fabry disease, Schindler disease, Farber disease, Niemann-Pick disease, Gaucher disease, mucopolysaccharidoses (7 types), Wolman disease, cholesterylester storage disease and neuronal ceroid-lipofuscinosis (NCL). Thin-layer chromatographic lipid analyses of brain, spinal cord and liver tissues showed normal patterns of gangliosides including $GM_1$, $GM_2$ and $GM_3$, and of glucosylceramide, galactosylceramide, sulfatides, and sphingomyelins. Urinary oligo- and mucopolysaccharides were unremarkable.

Investigation of carbohydrate-positive material in spleen tissue of patient 2, on the thin-layer plate, detected carbohydrate-positive material at the start line suggestive of an accumulation of a carbohydrate-containing substance of high molecular weight. In contrast, the spleen tissue of two control individuals showed only small traces and thus distinctly less amounts of carbohydrate-positive material compared to the patient.

#### Visceropathological investigations

General autopsy of both patients revealed respiratory failure as cause of death, which was evident with multiple atelectases, recurrent small embolisms, pulmonary edema and single foci of pneumonia in patient 1 and with a fulminant bronchopneumonia in patient 2. Strikingly, in the obtained mesenterial lymph nodes few leucocytes contained large uniform bold vacuoles, which were pale in hematoxylin eosin staining, strongly PAS-positive and did not stain for chloracetate esterase (Fig. 4). They emitted a strong yellowish, green and red autofluorescence in light excitation with respective wave lengths. Immunohistochemical analysis characterized the vacuolated cells mainly as B-lymphocytes and as occasional plasma cells with an incomplete differentiation (Fig. 4e-f), whereas T-cells and macrophages were not affected. The vacuolated lymphocytes suggested an enhanced autophagosomal load, as indicated by p62 immunohistochemistry (Fig. 4d).

In both patients, the spleen showed subacute congestion. Here, single extracellular clusters of autofluorescent polymorphic structures suggestive of degraded material were seen (data not shown). The liver showed fatty degeneration, presenting as diffuse small lipid droplets in patient 1 and as centrolubular hypoxic fatty changes in patient 2. Neither in the spleen nor in the liver storage cells could be detected, but patient 2 exhibited

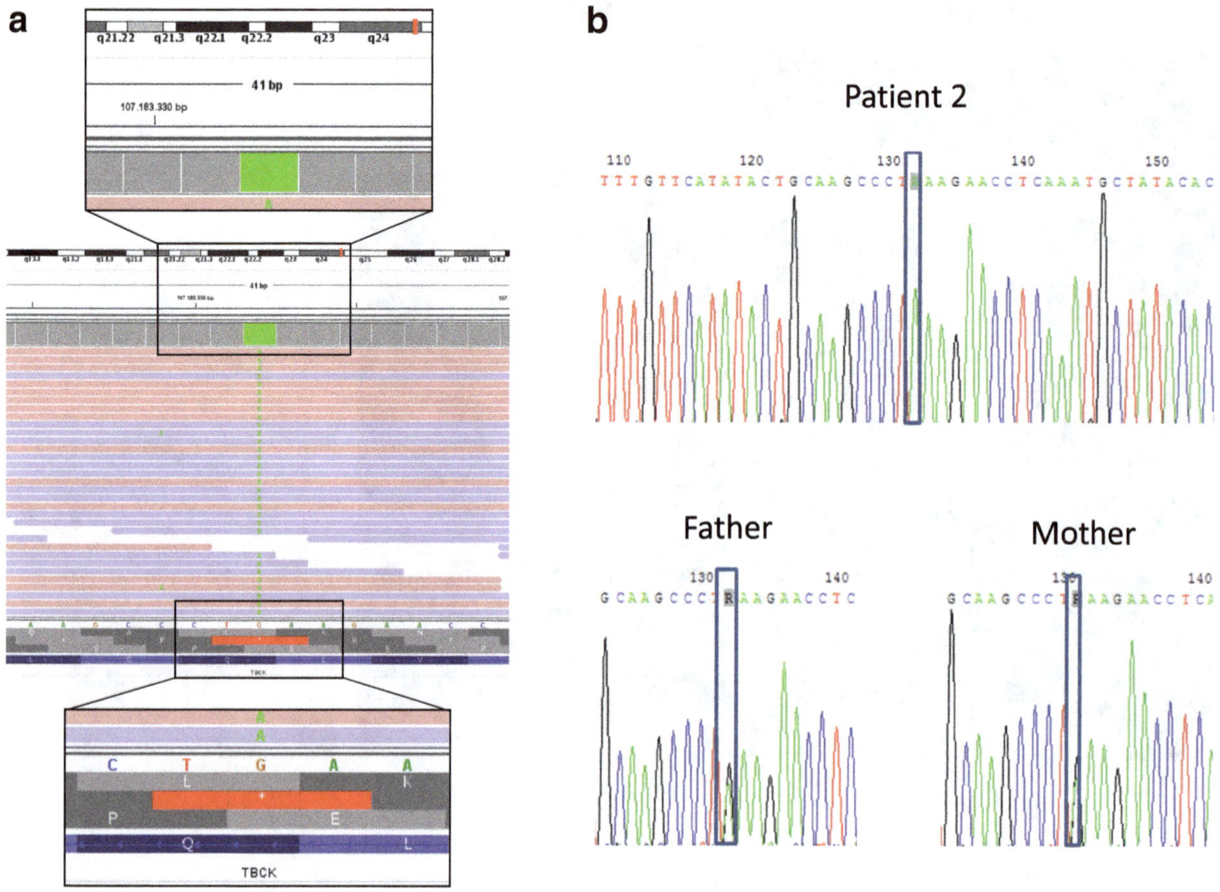


**Fig. 3** The TBCK defect in the genome of patient 2 and her parents. **a**, Integrative Genomics Viewer presentation of the homozygous stop mutation in the *TBCK* gene of patient 2. Below the green square, green dots show the base exchange (c.304C > T) in the multiple reads. **b**, Sanger sequencing of the *TBCK* gene of patient 2 and her parents. Sequencing was performed on the reverse strand, showing the base exchange G > A in our patient (grey boxes). Both parents carry the same mutation heterozygously, as seen in the R (grey boxes) that resembles an A and a G in each allele

PAS-positive material subendothelial to small arterioles in both organs. No lipopigments were seen in all investigated peripheral organs, including heart, lung, liver, spleen, kidneys, endocrine organs, gastrointestinal and urogenital tracts as well as skeletal musculature.

As individual pathologic changes, patient 1 showed a jejunal invagination with beginning impaired circulation and a reactive hyperplasia of single mediastinal, mesenterial and inguinal lymph nodes. Patient 2 had kidneys reduced in weight to 50% of the age related norm and a thoracolumbal scoliosis.

#### Neuropathological investigations

On autopsy, both brains showed a moderate global atrophy including a hydrocephalus internus and narrowed cortical gyri with dilated sulci in patient 1 and narrowing of white matter tracts in patient 2 (Fig. 5). Brain weights were appropriate to the age related norm (1490 g and 1350 g formalin fixed, respectively). The corpus callosum was thinned. Basal ganglia, thalami, hippocampi, brain stem and cerebellum appeared macroscopically unremarkable. The dorsal nerve roots of the spinal cord were partly thickened in patient 2. There was acute congestion with dilated capillaries. Singular microbleeds were found in the white matter of cerebrum, cerebellum and pons. In patient 1, individual hippocampal neurons of Sommer sector CA1 and of the nucleus dentatus were shrunken and hyperchromatic, indicating previous hypoxia. Patient 2 showed mild edematous changes in the cerebrum, a severe reduction of Purkinje cells with strong activation of Bergmann glia and a discrete fibrosis of leptomeninges. The white matter showed normal myelination.

Both patients showed a significant muscular atrophy, especially of the lower legs. Muscle specimens revealed a neurogenic atrophy with angular fibers and partial fiber groupings (data not shown).

Histological examination of the central nervous system (CNS) revealed one major pathological finding in both patients: cytoplasmic accumulation of granular storage

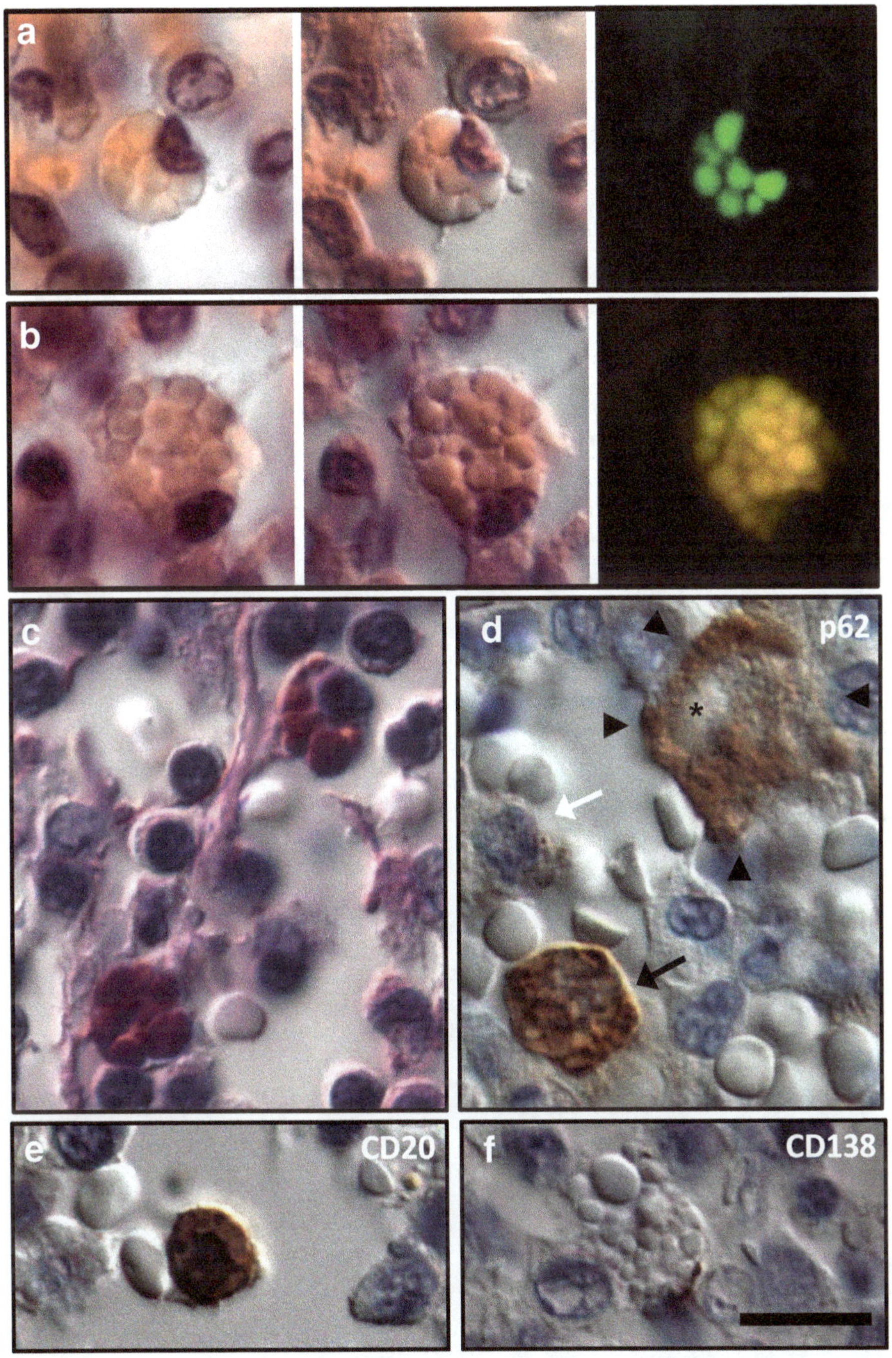


**Fig. 4** Vacuolated lymphocytes in lymph nodes of patient 1. A few lymphocytes with clear bold cytoplasmic vacuoles can be detected in the hematoxylin eosin staining in normal microscopy (**a** and **b**, first panel) and differential interference contrast (DIC) microscopy allowing for a three-dimensional illustration (**a** and **b**, second panel). The vacuoles exhibit a clear autofluorescence in different channels (**a** and **b**, right panel) and are strongly PAS-positive (**c**, DIC). An enhanced autophagosome formation is indicated by strong p62 immunoreactivity (**d**, black arrow), whereas normal lymphocytes are predominantly negative (white arrow). Note the positively stained larger macrophage (arrowheads) phagocytosing an erythrocyte (asterisk). Most of the vacuolated cells are $CD20^+$ B-lymphocytes (**e**, DIC), and single cells show a partial CD138 expression, likely pointing at immature plasma cells (**f**, DIC). Scale bar: 10 μm

material within neurons and to a lesser extent within glial cells. Interestingly, the number of neurons was normal to slightly reduced. The intracellular inclusions were distributed bihemispherically in many neurons of nearly all investigated brain regions. A detailed list is provided in Table 2. Most severely affected were the cerebral

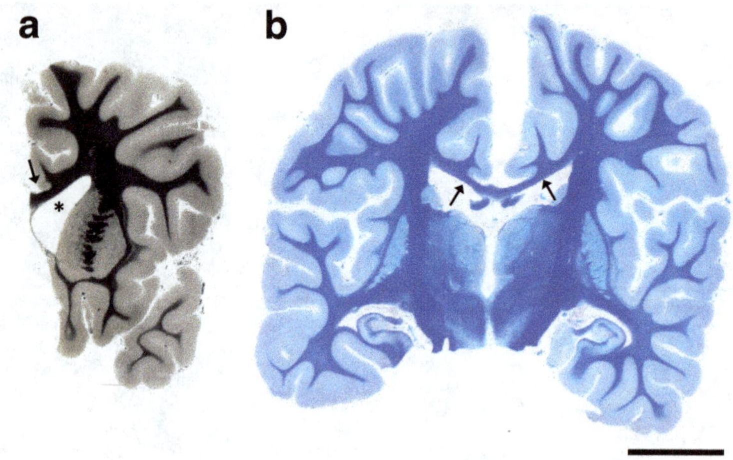


**Fig. 5** Whole mount coronar brain sections of patient 1 (**a**, Heidenhain-Woelcke stain) and patient 2 (**b**, luxol fast blue stain). The lateral ventricle is widened especially in patient 1 (**a**, asterisk). The brain of patient 2 shows narrowing of the white matter (**b**, blue staining of myelin). The corpus callosum is thinned in both patients (**a** and **b**, arrows). Scale bar: 2 cm

**Table 2** Distribution of neuronal storage material and PAS-positive granules in the central nervous system. Screening for neuronal inclusions was performed on sections stained with cresyl violet luxol fast blue (LFB) and sudan black (SB) or under ultraviolet light excitation for emission of autofluorescence (AF)

| Region | | | Neuronal storage material | | PAS + granules |
|---|---|---|---|---|---|
| | | | LFB/SB | AF | |
| Cerebrum | | | | | |
| | Basal ganglia | Neocortex I – IV | – | ++ | ++ |
| | | Neocortex V - VI | +++ | +++ | ++ |
| | | Nucleus caudatus | (+) | + | – |
| | | Putamen | – | ++ | (+) |
| | | Claustrum | +++ | +++ | – |
| | | Thalamus | ++ | +++ | – |
| | Hippocampus | CA 1 | ++ | +++ | + |
| | | CA 2–4 | + | ++ | + |
| | | Corpus geniculatum laterale | +++ | +++ | n. a. |
| | Cerebellum | Cortex | | | |
| | | Purkinje cells | – | – | – |
| | | Granule cells | – | – | – |
| | | Subcortical white matter | – | – | +++ |
| | | Nucleus dentatus | (+) | ++ | +++ |
| Brain stem | | | | | |
| | Mesencephalon | Substantia nigra | – | (+) | ++ |
| | | Nucleus oculomotorius | – | (+) | n. a. |
| | Pons | Pontine nuclei | (+) | + | +++ |
| | | Raphe nuclei | (+) | + | +++ |
| | Medulla oblongata | Olivary nuclei | +++ | +++ | (+) |
| | | Nucleus nervus vagus | +++ | +++ | – |
| | | Nucleus nervus hypoglossus | – | ++ | – |

Note the distinctly higher sensitivity of detection with autofluorescence. n. a., no available PAS-stained section or paraffin-embedded tissue cortex laminae V and VI, claustrum, corpus geniculatum laterale, olivary nuclei, nuclei nervi vagi and the anterior horn of the spinal cord. The mesencephalon and the lateral and posterior horns of spinal cord were mainly preserved, the Purkinje cells peculiarly spared. The occurrence of neurons with abnormal storage material was more pronounced in patient 1 as compared to patient 2, who showed significantly less affected neurons in the cortical laminae I-IV, striatum and hippocampus.

The neuronal inclusions were densely packed in the perikaryon and lay frequently adjacent to neuronal processes (Fig. 6). They had a round shape with an average diameter of 1 μm, varying from 0.3 to 2 μm. They stained strongly with luxol fast blue and sudan black and were argyrophilic. In unstained sections, they exhibited a bright silvery autofluorescence in ultraviolet light excitation and a weaker green and red autofluorescence in light excitation using respective lasers (Figs. 6 and 8 patient 1; Additional file 1: Supplement A patient 2). The detection of autofluorescent inclusions was most sensitive compared to other stains (Table 2). The PAS-reaction of the granules was heterogeneous and mainly weak (Fig. 6e), the alcian blue staining was entirely negative. A small proportion of the storage material was weakly immunoreactive for ß-amyloid, whereas a negative immunoreactivity was observed for ubiquitin, TDP-43 and the marker for autophagosomes p62 (Fig. 6h). In ultrastructural analysis, the inclusions presented as globular structures with a partially undulating border and a surrounding empty halo (Fig. 7). They consisted of amorphous osmiophilic, compact or granular material including high-density particles, lipid droplets (Fig. 7d-e) and sometimes membrane packages (Fig. 7d lower arrow), thus being highly suggestive of lipofuscin granules in lysosomal residual bodies. They furthermore showed a strong similarity to granular osmiophilic deposits (GRODs).

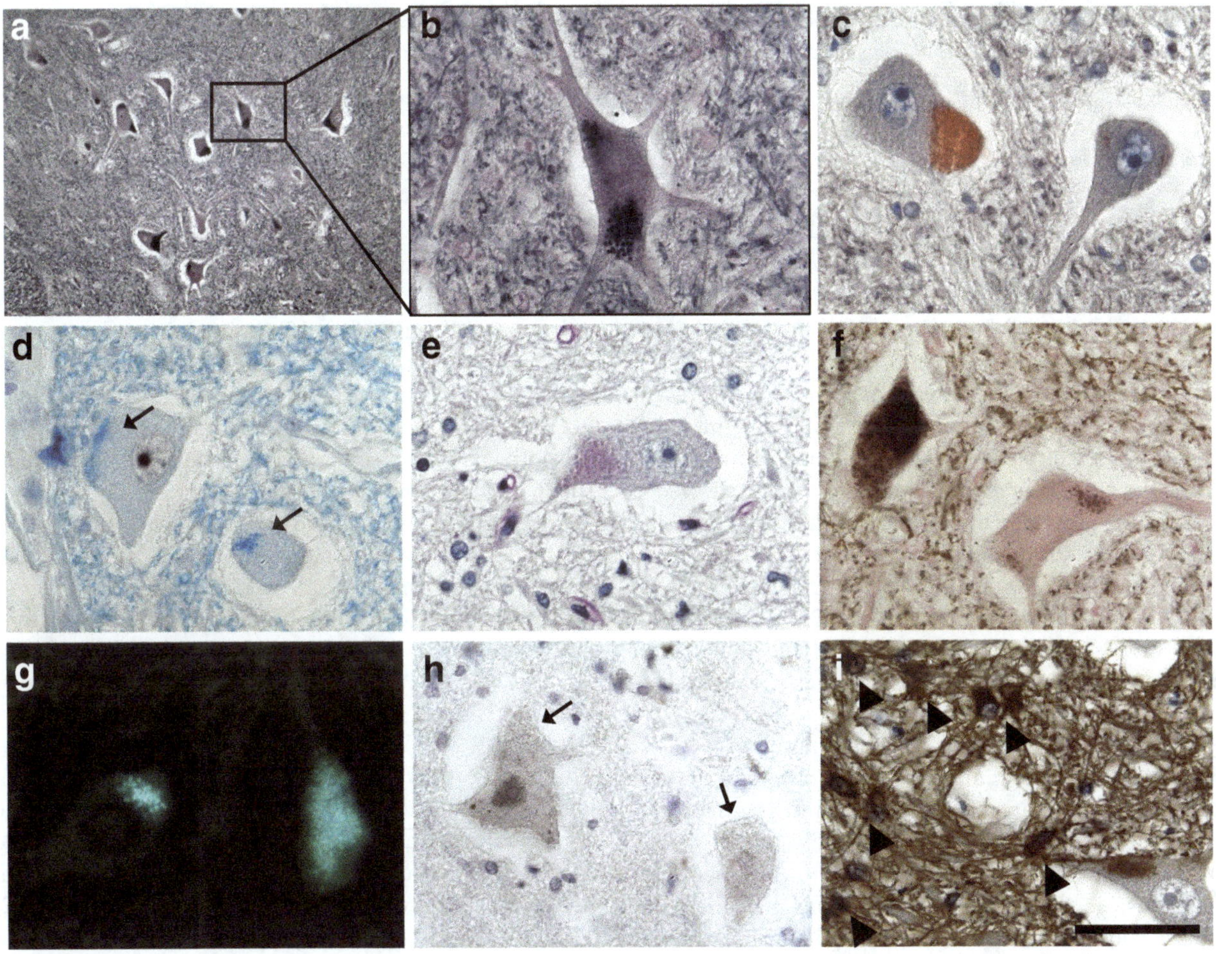


**Fig. 6** Neuronal inclusions in the spinal cord anterior horn of patient 2. Many neurons present with granular deposits in the perikaryon, which stain strongly with sudan black (**a** and **b**) and sudan red (**c**). Note the frequent localization adjacent to neuronal processes. The inclusions stain with luxol fast blue (**d**, arrows) and show a weak PAS-reaction (**e**). The storage material is moderately argyrophilic (**f**, Gallyas stain) and shows strong autofluorescence (**g**, unstained section). The storage material does not stain for p62 (**h**, arrows). Note the reactive GFAP$^{+}$ gliosis (**i**, arrowheads). GFAP, glial fibrillary acidic protein. Scale bar: 250 μm in **a**, 50 μm in **b**-**i**

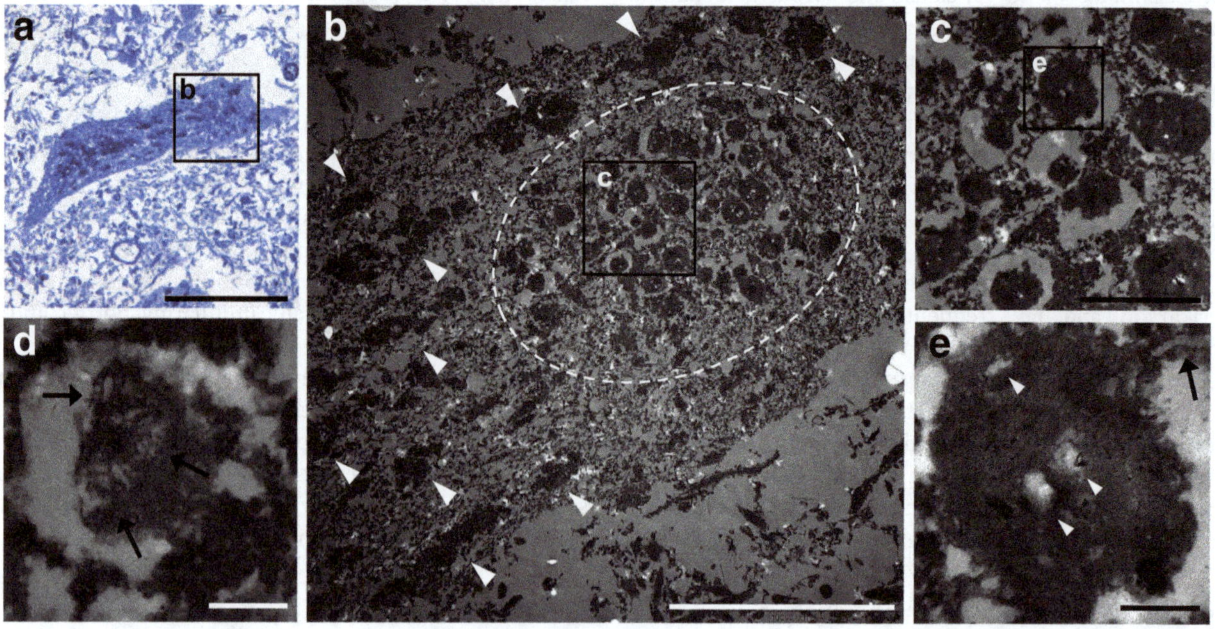


**Fig. 7** Ultrastructural morphology of neuronal storage material. Semi-thin section stained with toluidin blue of a neuron in the spinal cord anterior horn of patient 2 shows strongly stained storage material (**a**). Ultrastructural examination of the same neuron in a serial section (**b-e**) reveals a cluster of intracytoplasmic globular inclusions (delineated in **b**) consisting of amorphous osmiophilic material with high-density particles, lipid droplets (**e**; white arrowheads) and structures reminding of degraded membranous material (**d** and **e**; arrows). These inclusions correspond to lipofuscin granules in lysosomal residual bodies and remind of granular osmiophilic deposits (GRODs). Note the different polygonal shape of physiological Nissl substance (**b**; white arrowheads). Scale bar: 50 µm in **a**, 10 µm in **b**, 2 µm in **c**, 250 nm in **d** and **e**

Some neurons in addition contained vacuoles with membraneous structures resembling membranous cytoplasmic bodies (MCB) and zebra bodies (Additional file 1: Supplement B).

Intracellular storage material was not only present in neurons of both patients, but also in some glial cells. These inclusions varied in their features from those of neuronal storage material, as they showed a strong PAS reaction, no staining with luxol fast blue or sudan black/red and a silvery autofluorescence in ultraviolet light excitation of unstained sections (Fig. 8d-e). Double staining with PAS + GFAP and PAS + CD68 revealed a localization of the material in the cytoplasm mostly of astrocytes and to a lesser extent of microglia (Fig. 8f).

Finally, diffusely dispersed small granules of PAS- and Shimizu-positive material were observed in the neuropil of some areas in patient 1 and less frequent in patient 2. Affected regions were only partially concordant with the described areas showing neuronal inclusions, as the cerebellum and pons harbored the highest content of grains (Tab. 2, Fig. 9). The material lay diffusely in the grey and white matter of the mentioned regions with a notable dense perivascular accumulation (Fig. 9b). The remaining CNS showed isolated subendothelial aggregations. The deposits varied in size between 0.2 µm and 2 µm in diameter, the larger ones emitted autofluorescence. The granules were mainly globular, but large grains were often polygonal, allowing for discrimination against round corpora amylacea with a larger diameter. Considering the age of the patients, an excessive number of corpora amylacea was found in the brain and spinal cord of both patients, predominantly located in subpial, subependymal and perivascular areas.

An extensive reactive gliosis was present especially in the regions containing storage materials (Figs. 6i, 8c). Immunohistochemistry for CD68 revealed a moderate activation of microglia, other inflammatory changes were not seen.

## Discussion

This study provides a description of the morphological and biochemical pathology in the CNS and peripheral organs of patients with inherited TBCK-DD. The presence of 1) predominant lipofuscin-like storage material in CNS neurons, 2) storage deposits in astrocytes and to a lesser extent in microglia, 3) grainy PAS-positive deposits mostly in the pontine and cerebellar neuropil, spleen and liver, and 4) vacuolated lymphocytes support the classification of TBCK-DD as an LSD and give important evidence for the understanding of its pathogenesis.

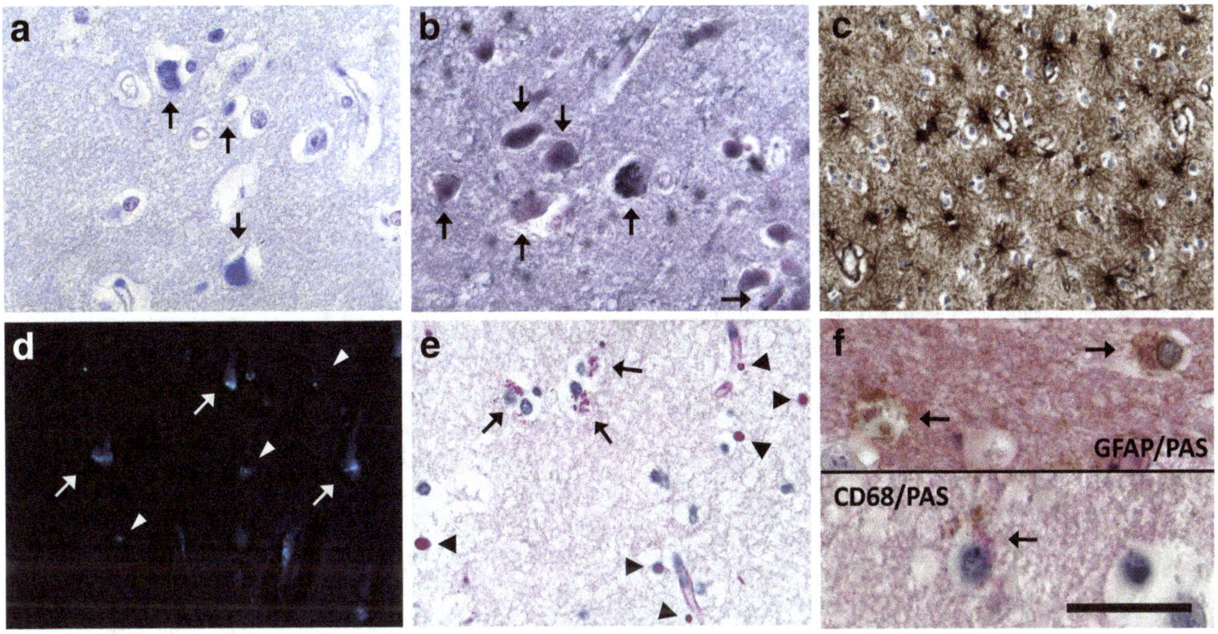


**Fig. 8** Morphological changes in the cortex of patient 2. Many cortical neurons in lamina V and VI incorporate storage material, which stains strongly with luxol fast blue in the Klüver Barrera staining (**a**, arrows) and with sudan black (**b**, arrows). A massive reactive astrocytosis is seen in GFAP immunohistochemistry (**c**). The intraneuronal inclusions (arrows) and glial inclusions (arrowheads) exert a strong autofluorescence (**d**, unstained section). Several cortical glia cells show cytoplasmatic PAS-positive granula (**e**, arrows). Note the numerous PAS-positive corpora amylacea (**e**, arrowheads). The laden glia cells are mainly astrocytes, as shown in double staining for PAS and GFAP (**f**, upper panel, arrows) and very few microglia cells, as shown in double staining for PAS and CD68 (**f**, lower panel, arrow). GFAP, glial fibrillary acidic protein. Scale bar: 50 μm in **a-e**, 20 μm in **f**

## Morphological classification of TCBK-DD

### *Neuronal inclusions correspond to lipofuscin granules*

The foremost observation were the frequent intraneuronal granular deposits spread throughout almost the whole central nervous system. Neuronal storage material is characteristic for LSDs, which comprise more than 50 diseases with a wide variation of storage products depending on defects in lysosomal enzymes, lysosomal membrane-associated proteins or non-lysosomal associated enzymes [33]. Here, positive staining for Sudan

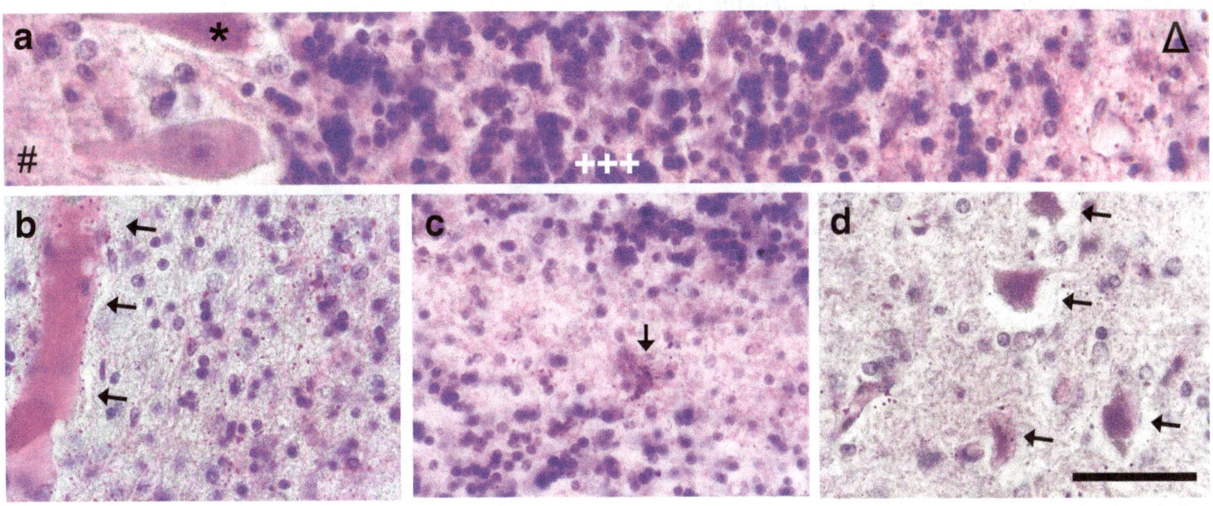


**Fig. 9** Diffuse PAS-positive material in the cerebellum of patient 1. The PAS-positive deposits are abundantly present in the subcortical cerebellar white matter (**a**, Δ; **b** and **c**) with sparing of molecular layer (#), Purkinje cell layer (*) and granular cell layer (+++). The deposits often accumulate perivascular (**b**, arrows) and are sometimes seen in glia cells (**c**, arrow). The nucleus dentatus is also affected (**d**). Note the shrunken and hyperchromatic neurons (arrows) as a sign of previous hypoxia. Scale bar: 65 μm in **a**, 50 μm in **b-d**

black and luxol fast blue, a moderate PAS reaction together with the absence of eosinophilia demonstrated that the inclusions consist predominantly of lipopigments with minor or no protein content [49]. In addition, the inclusion material showed strong autofluorescence, a characteristic feature of lipofuscin, the storage material in neuronal ceroid lipofuscinosis (NCL) and mucopolysaccharidosis type III (MPS III, Sanfilippo syndrome), respectively [12, 46, 52].

In concordance with the light microscopical characteristics, ultrastructurally the majority of storage material corresponded to lipofuscin granules in lysosomal residual bodies and in particular resembled granular osmiophilic deposits (GRODs) as seen in NCL types 1, 4, 5, 8–10, 12 and 14 [34]. Moreover, few zebra body- and MCB-like structures similar to inclusions in gangliosidoses and MPS were observed [16, 21]. In contrast to MPS, the neuronal deposits did not stain with Alcian blue and they showed strong autofluorescence distinguishing the disorder from gangliosidoses and all but one MPS (MPS III). Since the electron microscopical investigation was performed on material that was recovered from formalin fixed and paraffin embedded tissue, ultrastructural morphology was suboptimally preserved and therefore we cannot fully exclude the possibility that TBCK-DD pathology consists of further alterations.

The autofluorescent glial inclusions differed from the neuronal deposits in that they were PAS-positive and negative in luxol fast blue and Sudan black stains, suggesting that they contain a larger fraction of carbohydrates in addition to autofluorescent lipofuscin. The inclusions were mostly present in astrocytes, but also seen in few microglia.

#### *Diffuse accumulation of PAS-positive material in the CNS and in peripheral organs*

Moreover, PAS-positive granular deposits were observed diffusely in the neuropil. Interestingly, the spleen and liver contained PAS-positive granules in subendothelial areas, too. These deposits biochemically corresponded to increased concentration of carbohydrate-positive material in the spleen of patient 2 and indicate an insufficient degradation of saccharides or glycosylated substrates. Similarly, a recent study described enhanced oligosaccharide levels in fibroblasts and urine of patients with TBCK-DD [35]. The absence of urinary oligosaccharides in our patient 2 might be due to the lower sensitivity of the test used in 1987 as compared to the mass spectrometric analysis recently performed by Ortiz-Gonzalez et al. [35]. The distribution pattern of PAS-positive material was different in the two patients, indicating that these deposits might be a variable pathologic feature of TBCK-DD in different organs. The more severe brain affection of patient 1 correlated with the worse clinical course compared to that of her sister. All in all, storage of PAS-positive material was much less pronounced as in mucopoly-/oligosaccharidosis, gangliosidoses or polyglucosan body disease.

#### *Vacuolated lymphocytes*

Here, we discovered the presence of vacuolated B-cells and immature plasma cells in TBCK-DD. Vacuolated lymphocytes are a feature of several metabolic diseases including CLN3 [2, 3, 10, 27, 45] and CLN11 [8], Pompe's disease/adult acid maltase deficiency [2, 19, 36], GM1 gangliosidosis [2, 14, 15] and others as summarized by Anderson et al. [2].

The autofluorescence together with the strong PAS-reaction of the vacuoles in lymphocytes of our patients suggest an accumulation of both lipopigment and carbohydrates. PAS-positive vacuoles in lymphocytes have been reported in patients with Pompe's disease/adult acid maltase deficiency [2, 19] and Danon disease (LAMP2-deficient cardiomyopathy) [32]. At present it is unknown whether vacuolated lymphocytes are regularly present in the peripheral blood of patients with homozygous *TBCK* mutation. Should this be the case, peripheral blood film examination might represent a useful and simple diagnostic tool to support the diagnosis of TBCK-DD.

The vacuolated lymphocytes showed excessive p62-positive autophagosomes which have been previously described in TBCK-DD patients' fibroblasts [35]. This contrasted to neurons that showed no accumulation of p62 immunoreactive organelles. This variance may be explained either by cell type-specific effects of TBCK or by alternative pathways regulating autophagy in postmitotic neuronal cells as compared to dividing cells such as fibroblasts [11, 28].

#### *Synopsis of morphological changes*

In summary, our findings revealed characteristic morphological changes in both patients with TBCK-DD that are typical for an LSD. Subclassification into a specific group, however, is not straightforward since we observed aggregates with different morphological properties pointing at different storage materials. While the majority of neuronal inclusions in the CNS indicate an NCL, the PAS-positive vacuoles in lymphocytes are reminiscent of those seen in Pompe's disease and the PAS-positive aggregates in the CNS, spleen and liver as well as the occasional intraneuronal zebra bodies and MCB-like structures demonstrate carbohydrate-containing material as is stored in polyglycosan body diseases, mucopoly-/oligosaccharidosis or gangliosidosis. Together, TBCK-DD represents a new type of storage disorder, characterized by the occurrence of different storage products with predominance of lipofuscin.

Future studies will show whether a classification as a novel subtype of NCL (CLN15) is appropriate.

### Metabolic consequences of TBCK defects

A recent study demonstrated an autophagosomal-lysosomal dysfunction in TBCK-DD with accumulation of autophagosomes and impaired degradation of glycosylated proteins in cultured fibroblasts [35]. Mechanistically, TBCK can be linked to autophagy as a regulator of two distinct pathways including mTOR and small GTPases of the Rab-family. Knockdown of TBCK in vitro significantly downregulated the main inhibitor for autophagy initiation, mTORC1 [4, 6, 29], thus explaining an enhanced production of autophagosomes in case of defective TBCK. Importantly, disturbed mTORC1 signaling and lysosomal dysfunction have been observed in a mouse model of CLN11/progranulin deficiency, underpinning the concept of TBCK-DD being an NCL [40, 43, 48]. Furthermore, TBCK has been proposed a putative activator protein for small GTPases of the Rab-family [9], which regulate fusion of autophagosomes with lysosomes [18, 22, 24, 47]. In line with this interpretation, Rab-associated dysfunctional endocytic membrane trafficking was described in *CLN3* mammalian cells [30]. It is therefore likely that a TBCK defect leads to both, enhanced autophagosome formation and decreased fusion with lysosomes which in turn cause a disturbed clearance of cell components e.g. glycosylated substrates and an accumulation of non-degradable products such as lipofuscin.

In addition to the effects on autophagy, mTOR has been reported to mediate key endogenous neuroprotective mechanisms in motoneurons [41] and to contribute to peripheral axonal myelination and growth [44], thus possibly explaining the severe affection of the second motoneuron due to both CNS (storage inclusions) and peripheral (myelination and axonal growth) pathologies in TBCK-DD.

To date, few neurodevelopmental disorders have been linked to an aberrantly reduced mTOR signaling as seen in the herein described TBCK-DD, including Rett syndrome [38, 39], Phelan-McDermid syndrome with autism spectrum disorder [5] and Galloway-Mowat syndrome [23]. These diseases share the symptoms of cognitive deficits and epilepsy, but are not associated with an accumulation of storage products. Thus, the appearance of TBCK-DD as an LSD is likely to result from multifactorial TBCK-specific alterations, which need to be elucidated in further studies. So far, therapeutic mTORC1 activation may be a potential strategy to prevent disease progress in patients.

### Correlation of morphological changes to clinical symptoms

The presence of storage material in a large number of neurons in the absence of significant neuronal loss suggests neuronal dysfunction as the underlying cause of TBCK-DD. This is a clear difference to most other LSDs that are characterized by severe neuronal degeneration with marked brain atrophy in late stage disease. The distribution pattern of neuronal storage material fits well with the clinical phenotype: neurogenic atrophy of skeletal muscle is likely the consequence of secondary motoneurons in the spinal cord being severely affected and intellectual disability is consistent with the high amount of neuronal inclusions in the neocortex, archicortex and hippocampus. Those changes may not only explain neuronal deficits, but also account for uncontrolled neuronal excitations as a source of epileptic seizures. As the patients suffered from declining visual acuity or blindness, an involvement of the retina like in CLN1–3 and CLN5 [37] seems possible, although an electroretinogram in one patient with TBCK-DD was normal [9] and points to a cause by affected neurons in the central visual tract. Overall, the clinical symptoms with severe developmental delay and intellectual disability, hypotonia, severe visual deterioration and generalized seizures resemble those seen in infantile and late infantile CLN1 and CLN2, respectively.

## Conclusion

In conclusion, our investigations uncover TBCK-DD as a novel LSD. The predominant neuronal lipofuscin inclusions as well as the clinical symptoms are typical for an NCL and may indicate a novel subtype (CLN15). The accumulation of carbohydrate-related material and the PAS-positivity of lymphocytic vacuoles, however, exceed the pathological alterations seen in other NCL. Since our investigations are limited due to restrictedly archived tissue material, further studies, in particular ultrastructural analyses of the CNS and vacuolated lymphocytes are needed in order to come to a definite classification of this disorder. The underlying mechanism can be assigned to an autophagosomal-lysosomal dysfunction, including enhanced mTORC1-mediated autophagosome formation and reduced Rab-mediated autophagosome-lysosome fusion, thus implicating new targets for therapeutic approaches in TBCK-DD.

#### Abbreviations

CHp: Carbohydrate positive; CNS: Central nervous system; GROD: Granular osmiophilic deposit; IHPRF3: Infantile muscular hypotonia with psychomotor retardation and characteristic facies; LSD: Lysosomal storage disease; MCB: Membranous cytoplasmic body; MPS: Mucopolysaccharidosis; mTOR: mammalian target of rapamycin; mTORC1: mTOR complex 1; NCL: Neuronal ceroid lipofuscinosis; PAS: Periodic acid-Schiff; TBC: Tre-2/Bub2/Cdc16; TBCK: TBC1 domain-containing kinase; TBCK-DD: TBCK deficiency disorder; CLN1–15: type 1–15 of neuronal ceroid lipofuscinosis

**Acknowledgements**
We thank Dr. G. Spalke from the Department of Neurology, University of Marburg, Germany, and Dr. J. Rüschoff and the late Dr. C. Thomas from the Department of Pathology, University of Marburg, for essential neuropathological and pathologic reports. We thank Heike Geißel, Ruth Wassmuth, Heidi Jennemann, Petra Debelius-Rauch, Sylvia Stanek, Ginette Bortolussi and Petra Zschau for invaluable technical support.

**Funding**
This research received no specific grant from any funding agency.

**Author's contributions**
EL collected and provided all clinical data, autopsy and pathology protocols, she has long sustained the contact to the patient's parents. OR supervised the design of the genetic analyses. SB-W and RB did and supervised the whole exome analysis and complemented the manuscript. MS was responsible for the bioinformatic evaluations. KH provided the test materials, did the biochemical work, complemented and revised the manuscript. UK, AP and HDM did the neuropathological studies and AP revised the manuscript. UK wrote the manuscript. All authors read and approved the final manuscript.

**Competing interests**
The authors declare that they have no competing interest.

**Author details**
[1]Department of Medical Genetics and Applied Genomics, University of Tübingen, Tübingen, Germany. [2]Department of Neuropediatrics and Neurometabolic Laboratory, Children's Hospital of the University of Tübingen, Tübingen, Germany. [3]Department of Pediatrics, University Hospital of Marburg, Marburg, Germany. [4]Department of Neuropathology, Philipps University and University Hospital of Marburg, Baldingerstrasse, 35043 Marburg, Germany.

**References**

1. Alazami AM, Patel N, Shamseldin HE, Anazi S, Al-Dosari MS, Alzahrani F, Hijazi H, Alshammari M, Aldahmesh MA, Salih MA, Faqeih E, Alhashem A, Bashiri FA, Al-Owain M, Kentab AY, Sogaty S, Al Tala S, Temsah MH, Tulbah M, Aljelaify RF, Alshahwan SA, Seidahmed MZ, Alhadid AA, Aldhalaan H, AlQallaf F, Kurdi W, Alfadhel M, Babay Z, Alsogheer M, Kaya N, Al-Hassnan ZN, Abdel-Salam GM, Al-Sannaa N, Al Mutairi F, El Khashab HY, Bohlega S, Jia X, Nguyen HC, Hammami R, Adly N, Mohamed JY, Abdulwahab F, Ibrahim N, Naim EA, Al-Younes B, Meyer BF, Hashem M, Shaheen R, Xiong Y, Abouelhoda M, Aldeeri AA, Monies DM, Alkuraya FS (2015) Accelerating novel candidate gene discovery in neurogenetic disorders via whole-exome sequencing of prescreened multiplex consanguineous families. Cell Rep 10:148–161. https://doi.org/10.1016/j.celrep.2014.12.015
2. Anderson G, Smith VV, Malone M, Sebire NJ (2005) Blood film examination for vacuolated lymphocytes in the diagnosis of metabolic disorders; retrospective experience of more than 2,500 cases from a single Centre. J Clin Pathol 58:1305–1310. https://doi.org/10.1136/jcp.2005.027045
3. Baumann RJ, Markesbery WR (1978) Juvenile amaurotic idiocy (neuronal ceroid lipofuscinosis) and lymphocyte fingerprint profiles. Ann Neurol 4: 531–536. https://doi.org/10.1002/ana.410040609
4. Bhoj EJ, Li D, Harr M, Edvardson S, Elpeleg O, Chisholm E, Juusola J, Douglas G, Guillen Sacoto MJ, Siquier-Pernet K, Saadi A, Bole-Feysot C, Nitschke P, Narravula A, Walke M, Horner MB, Day-Salvatore DL, Jayakar P, Vergano SA, Tarnopolsky MA, Hegde M, Colleaux L, Crino P, Hakonarson H (2016) Mutations in TBCK, encoding TBC1-domain-containing kinase, lead to a recognizable syndrome of intellectual disability and hypotonia. Am J Hum Genet 98:782–788. https://doi.org/10.1016/j.ajhg.2016.03.016
5. Bidinosti M, Botta P, Kruttner S, Proenca CC, Stoehr N, Bernhard M, Fruh I, Mueller M, Bonenfant D, Voshol H, Carbone W, Neal SJ, McTighe SM, Roma G, Dolmetsch RE, Porter JA, Caroni P, Bouwmeester T, Luthi A, Galimberti I (2016) CLK2 inhibition ameliorates autistic features associated with SHANK3 deficiency. Science 351:1199–1203. https://doi.org/10.1126/science.aad5487
6. Bockaert J, Marin P (2015) mTOR in brain physiology and pathologies. Physiol Rev 95:1157–1187. https://doi.org/10.1152/physrev.00038.2014
7. Boudeau J, Miranda-Saavedra D, Barton GJ, Alessi DR (2006) Emerging roles of pseudokinases. Trends Cell Biol 16:443–452. https://doi.org/10.1016/j.tcb.2006.07.003
8. Canafoglia L, Morbin M, Scaioli V, Pareyson D, D'Incerti L, Fugnanesi V, Tagliavini F, Berkovic SF, Franceschetti S (2014) Recurrent generalized seizures, visual loss, and palinopsia as phenotypic features of neuronal ceroid lipofuscinosis due to progranulin gene mutation. Epilepsia 55:e56–e59. https://doi.org/10.1111/epi.12632
9. Chong JX, Caputo V, Phelps IG, Stella L, Worgan L, Dempsey JC, Nguyen A, Leuzzi V, Webster R, Pizzuti A, Marvin CT, Ishak GE, Ardern-Holmes S, Richmond Z, Bamshad MJ, Ortiz-Gonzalez XR, Tartaglia M, Chopra M, Doherty D (2016) Recessive inactivating mutations in TBCK, encoding a Rab GTPase-activating protein, cause severe infantile syndromic encephalopathy. Am J Hum Genet 98:772–781. https://doi.org/10.1016/j.ajhg.2016.01.016
10. Derwort A, Detering K (1959) Vacuolated lymphocytes in familial amaurotic idiocy and their diagnostic significance. Nervenarzt 30:442–448
11. Di Nardo A, Wertz MH, Kwiatkowski E, Tsai PT, Leech JD, Greene-Colozzi E, Goto J, Dilsiz P, Talos DM, Clish CB, Kwiatkowski DJ, Sahin M (2014) Neuronal Tsc1/2 complex controls autophagy through AMPK-dependent regulation of ULK1. Hum Mol Genet 23:3865–3874. https://doi.org/10.1093/hmg/ddu101
12. Dowson JH, Wilton-Cox H, Oldfors A, Sourander P (1989) Autofluorescence emission spectra of neuronal lipopigment in mucopolysaccharidosis (Sanfilippo's syndrome). Acta Neuropathol 77:426–429
13. Farndale RW, Buttle DJ, Barrett AJ (1986) Improved quantitation and discrimination of sulphated glycosaminoglycans by use of dimethylmethylene blue. Biochimica et Biophysica Acta (BBA)-General Subjects 883:173–177
14. Fricker H, O'Brien JS, Vassella F, Gugler E, Muhlethaler JP, Spycher M, Wiesmann UN, Herschkowitz N (1976) Generalized gangliosidosis: acid beta-galactosidase deficiency with early onset, rapid mental deterioration and minimal bone dysplasia. J Neurol 213:273–281
15. Giugliani R, Dutra JC, Pereira ML, Rotta N, Drachler Mde L, Ohlweiller L, Pina Neto JM, Pinheiro CE, Breda DJ (1985) GM1 gangliosidosis: clinical and laboratory findings in eight families. Hum Genet 70:347–354
16. Gonatas NK, Gonatas J (1965) Ultrastructural and biochemical observations on a case of systemic late infantile lipidosis and its relationship to Tay-Sachs disease and gargoylism. J Neuropathol Exp Neurol 24:318–340
17. Guerreiro RJ, Brown R, Dian D, de Goede C, Bras J, Mole SE (2016) Mutation of TBCK causes a rare recessive developmental disorder. Neurol Genet 2:e76. https://doi.org/10.1212/nxg.0000000000000076
18. Gutierrez MG, Munafo DB, Beron W, Colombo MI (2004) Rab7 is required for the normal progression of the autophagic pathway in mammalian cells. J Cell Sci 117:2687–2697. https://doi.org/10.1242/jcs.01114
19. Hagemans ML, Stigter RL, van Capelle CI, van der Beek NA, Winkel LP, van Vliet L, Hop WC, Reuser AJ, Beishuizen A, van der Ploeg AT (2010) PAS-positive lymphocyte vacuoles can be used as diagnostic screening test for Pompe disease. J Inherit Metab Dis 33:133–139. https://doi.org/10.1007/s10545-009-9027-4
20. Hartley T, Wagner JD, Warman-Chardon J, Tetreault M, Brady L, Baker S, Tarnopolsky M, Bourque PR, Parboosingh JS, Smith C, McInnes B, Innes AM, Bernier F, Curry CJ, Yoon G, Horvath GA, Bareke E, Gillespie M, Majewski J, Bulman DE, Dyment DA, Boycott KM (2018) Whole-exome sequencing is a valuable diagnostic tool for inherited peripheral neuropathies: outcomes from a cohort of 50 families. Clin Genet 93:301–309. https://doi.org/10.1111/cge.13101
21. Haust MD, Gordon BA (1986) Ultrastructural and biochemical aspects of the Sanfilippo syndrome,--type III genetic mucopolysaccharidosis. Connect Tissue Res 15:57–64
22. Jager S, Bucci C, Tanida I, Ueno T, Kominami E, Saftig P, Eskelinen EL (2004) Role for Rab7 in maturation of late autophagic vacuoles. J Cell Sci 117: 4837–4848. https://doi.org/10.1242/jcs.01370

23. Jinks RN, Puffenberger EG, Baple E, Harding B, Crino P, Fogo AB, Wenger O, Xin B, Koehler AE, McGlincy MH, Provencher MM, Smith JD, Tran L, Al Turki S, Chioza BA, Cross H, Harlalka GV, Hurles ME, Maroofian R, Heaps AD, Morton MC, Stempak L, Hildebrandt F, Sadowski CE, Zaritsky J, Campellone K, Morton DH, Wang H, Crosby A, Strauss KA (2015) Recessive nephrocerebellar syndrome on the Galloway-Mowat syndrome spectrum is caused by homozygous protein-truncating mutations of WDR73. Brain 138:2173–2190. https://doi.org/10.1093/brain/awv153
24. Kirisako T, Baba M, Ishihara N, Miyazawa K, Ohsumi M, Yoshimori T, Noda T, Ohsumi Y (1999) Formation process of autophagosome is traced with Apg8/Aut7p in yeast. J Cell Biol 147:435–446
25. Kobata A, Yamashita K, Takasaki S (1987) BioGel P-4 column chromatography of oligosaccharides: effective size of oligosaccharides expressed in glucose units. Methods Enzymol 138:84–94
26. Kraushaar T, Bruckner S, Veelders M, Rhinow D, Schreiner F, Birke R, Pagenstecher A, Mosch HU, Essen LO (2015) Interactions by the fungal Flo11 adhesin depend on a fibronectin type III-like adhesin domain girdled by aromatic bands. Structure 23:1005–1017. https://doi.org/10.1016/j.str.2015.03.021
27. Lake BD, Cavanagh NP (1978) Early-juvenile Batten's disease--a recognisable sub-group distinct from other forms of Batten's disease. Analysis of 5 patients. J Neurol Sci 36:265–271
28. Lipton JO, Sahin M (2014) The neurology of mTOR. Neuron 84:275–291. https://doi.org/10.1016/j.neuron.2014.09.034
29. Liu Y, Yan X, Zhou T (2013) TBCK influences cell proliferation, cell size and mTOR signaling pathway. PLoS One 8:e71349. https://doi.org/10.1371/journal.pone.0071349
30. Luiro K, Yliannala K, Ahtiainen L, Maunu H, Jarvela I, Kyttala A, Jalanko A (2004) Interconnections of CLN3, Hook1 and Rab proteins link batten disease to defects in the endocytic pathway. Hum Mol Genet 13:3017–3027. https://doi.org/10.1093/hmg/ddh321
31. Mandel H, Khayat M, Chervinsky E, Elpeleg O, Shalev S (2017) TBCK-related intellectual disability syndrome: case study of two patients. Am J Med Genet A 173:491–494. https://doi.org/10.1002/ajmg.a.38019
32. Maron BJ, Roberts WC, Arad M, Haas TS, Spirito P, Wright GB, Almquist AK, Baffa JM, Saul JP, Ho CY, Seidman J, Seidman CE (2009) Clinical outcome and phenotypic expression in LAMP2 cardiomyopathy. Jama 301:1253–1259. https://doi.org/10.1001/jama.2009.371
33. Menzies FM, Fleming A, Rubinsztein DC (2015) Compromised autophagy and neurodegenerative diseases. Nat Rev Neurosci 16:345–357. https://doi.org/10.1038/nrn3961
34. Nita DA, Mole SE, Minassian BA (2016) Neuronal ceroid lipofuscinoses. Epileptic Disord 18:73–88. https://doi.org/10.1684/epd.2016.0844
35. Ortiz-Gonzalez XR, Tintos-Hernandez JA, Keller K, Li X, Foley AR, Bharucha-Goebel DX, Kessler SK, Yum SW, Crino PB, He M, Wallace DC, Bonnemann CG (2018) Homozygous boricua TBCK mutation causes neurodegeneration and aberrant autophagy. Ann Neurol 83:153–165. https://doi.org/10.1002/ana.25130
36. Pralle H, Schroder R, Loffler H (1975) New kind of cytoplasmic inclusions of plasma cells in acid maltase deficiency. Acta Haematol 53:109–117. https://doi.org/10.1159/000208164
37. Radke J, Stenzel W, Goebel HH (2015) Human NCL neuropathology. Biochim Biophys Acta 1852:2262–2266. https://doi.org/10.1016/j.bbadis.2015.05.007
38. Rangasamy S, Olfers S, Gerald B, Hilbert A, Svejda S, Narayanan V (2016) Reduced neuronal size and mTOR pathway activity in the Mecp2 A140V Rett syndrome mouse model. F1000Res 5:2269. https://doi.org/10.12688/f1000research.8156.1
39. Ricciardi S, Boggio EM, Grosso S, Lonetti G, Forlani G, Stefanelli G, Calcagno E, Morello N, Landsberger N, Biffo S, Pizzorusso T, Giustetto M, Broccoli V (2011) Reduced AKT/mTOR signaling and protein synthesis dysregulation in a Rett syndrome animal model. Hum Mol Genet 20:1182–1196. https://doi.org/10.1093/hmg/ddq563
40. Roczniak-Ferguson A, Petit CS, Froehlich F, Qian S, Ky J, Angarola B, Walther TC, Ferguson SM (2012) The transcription factor TFEB links mTORC1 signaling to transcriptional control of lysosome homeostasis. Sci Signal 5: ra42. https://doi.org/10.1126/scisignal.2002790
41. Saxena S, Roselli F, Singh K, Leptien K, Julien JP, Gros-Louis F, Caroni P (2013) Neuroprotection through excitability and mTOR required in ALS motoneurons to delay disease and extend survival. Neuron 80:80–96. https://doi.org/10.1016/j.neuron.2013.07.027
42. Scheeff ED, Eswaran J, Bunkoczi G, Knapp S, Manning G (2009) Structure of the pseudokinase VRK3 reveals a degraded catalytic site, a highly conserved kinase fold, and a putative regulatory binding site. Structure 17:128–138. https://doi.org/10.1016/j.str.2008.10.018
43. Settembre C, Zoncu R, Medina DL, Vetrini F, Erdin S, Erdin S, Huynh T, Ferron M, Karsenty G, Vellard MC, Facchinetti V, Sabatini DM, Ballabio A (2012) A lysosome-to-nucleus signalling mechanism senses and regulates the lysosome via mTOR and TFEB. EMBO J 31:1095–1108. https://doi.org/10.1038/emboj.2012.32
44. Sherman DL, Krols M, Wu LM, Grove M, Nave KA, Gangloff YG, Brophy PJ (2012) Arrest of myelination and reduced axon growth when Schwann cells lack mTOR. J Neurosci 32:1817–1825. https://doi.org/10.1523/jneurosci.4814-11.2012
45. Stekhoven JH, van Haelst UJ, Joosten EM, Loonen MC (1977) Ultrastructural study of the vacuoles in the peripheral lymphocytes in juvenile amaurotic idiocy. Juvenile form of generalized ceroid lipofuscinosis Acta Neuropathol 38:137–142
46. Suzuki K (2008) Lysosomal storage diseases. In: Love S (ed) Greenfield's neuropathology. 8 edn. CRC press, p 562
47. Szatmari Z, Sass M (2014) The autophagic roles of Rab small GTPases and their upstream regulators: a review. Autophagy 10:1154–1166. https://doi.org/10.4161/auto.29395
48. Tanaka Y, Chambers JK, Matsuwaki T, Yamanouchi K, Nishihara M (2014) Possible involvement of lysosomal dysfunction in pathological changes of the brain in aged progranulin-deficient mice. Acta Neuropathol Commun 2: 78. https://doi.org/10.1186/s40478-014-0078-x
49. Terman A, Brunk UT (1998) Lipofuscin: mechanisms of formation and increase with age. Apmis 106:265–276
50. Wu J, Li Q, Li Y, Lin J, Yang D, Zhu G, Wang L, He D, Lu G, Zeng C (2014) A long type of TBCK is a novel cytoplasmic and mitotic apparatus-associated protein likely suppressing cell proliferation. J Genet Genomics 41:69–72. https://doi.org/10.1016/j.jgg.2013.12.006
51. Zapata-Aldana E, Kim DD, Remtulla S, Prasad C, Nguyen CT, Campbell C (2018) Further delineation of TBCK - infantile hypotonia with psychomotor retardation and characteristic facies type 3. Eur J Med Genet. https://doi.org/10.1016/j.ejmg.2018.08.004
52. Zeman W, Dyken P (1969) Neuronal ceroid-lipofuscinosis (Batten's disease): relationship to amaurotic family idiocy? Pediatrics 44:570–583

6

# Analysis of spinal and muscle pathology in transgenic mice overexpressing wild-type and ALS-linked mutant MATR3

Christina Moloney[1,2†], Sruti Rayaprolu[1,2†], John Howard[1,2], Susan Fromholt[1,2], Hilda Brown[1,2], Matt Collins[1,2], Mariela Cabrera[1,2], Colin Duffy[1,2], Zoe Siemienski[1,2], Dave Miller[1,2], David R. Borchelt[1,2,3*] and Jada Lewis[1,2,3*]

**Abstract**

Mutations in *MATR3* have been associated with amyotrophic lateral sclerosis (ALS) as well as a form of distal myopathy termed vocal cord pharyngeal distal myopathy (VCPDM). To begin to understand how mutations in *MATR3* may cause disease, here we provide initial characterization of transgenic (Tg) mice expressing human wild-type (WT) MATR3 ($MATR3^{WT}$) and ALS-mutant F115C MATR3 ($MATR3^{F115C}$) proteins under the control of the mouse prion promoter (MoPrP). For each construct, we established multiple independent lines of mice that stably transmitted the transgene. Unexpectedly, for all stably-transmitting lines examined, *MATR3* transgenic mRNA expression was more robust in muscle, with minimal expression in spinal cord. The levels of transgenic mRNA in muscle did not differ between mice from our lead $MATR3^{F115C}$ line and lead $MATR3^{WT}$ line, but mice from the lead $MATR3^{F115C}$ line had significantly higher levels of MATR3 protein in muscle over the lead $MATR3^{WT}$ line. Mice from the three independent, established lines of $MATR3^{F115C}$ mice developed weakness in both fore- and hind-limbs as early as < 1 months of age; whereas, $MATR3^{WT}$ mice aged to > 20 months were not overtly distinguishable from non-transgenic (NT) littermates based on basic motor phenotype. Muscle of both $MATR3^{WT}$ and $MATR3^{F115C}$ mice showed vacuoles by 2 months of age which worsened by ~ 10 months, but vacuolation was noticeably more severe in $MATR3^{F115C}$ mice. Overall, our results indicate that increasing the levels of MATR3 in muscle can cause pathologic changes associated with myopathy, with $MATR3^{F115C}$ expression causing overt muscle atrophy and a profound motor phenotype. The findings suggest that analysis of muscle pathology in individuals harboring ALS-linked MATR3 mutations should be routinely considered.

**Keywords:** MATR3, Transgenic mouse model, ALS, Distal myopathy

## Introduction

Amyotrophic lateral sclerosis (ALS) is a progressive neurodegenerative disease affecting both upper and lower motor neurons leading to progressive paresis and paralysis, with death occurring between three to five years from the diagnosis [18]. The majority of ALS cases appear sporadic (sALS), with around 10% of cases having a clear genetic link between family members (fALS) [18]. Superoxide dismutase 1 (*SOD1*) was the first gene to have mutations identified as causing ALS [17]. Since the late 2000s, there have been over a dozen genes in which mutations have been identified as causative for ALS, including Tar DNA binding protein (*TARDBP*) [21, 27], fused in sarcoma (*FUS*) [10, 22], and the GGGGCC hexanucleotide repeat expansion in chromosome 9 open reading frame 72 (*C9orf72*) [4, 16], with matrin 3 (*MATR3*) being one of the more recently discovered genes to have disease causing mutations [7].

Mutant MATR3 (S85C) had been previously associated with an autosomal dominant distal myopathy with vocal cord and pharyngeal weakness (VCPDM) [5, 19]; however, in 2014, three different mutations (F115C, P154S, or T622A) in *MATR3* were identified in cases of both fALS and sALS [7]. Patients harboring the S85C mutation in *MATR3* initially present with myopathy in the muscles of the hands and feet [5, 19] and have a slowly progressing disease that leads to respiratory

* Correspondence: drb1@ufl.edu; jada.lewis@ufl.edu
†Christina Moloney and Sruti Rayaprolu contributed equally to this work.
[1]Center for Translational Research in Neurodegenerative Disease, University of Florida, Gainesville, Florida, USA
Full list of author information is available at the end of the article

failure and death after 15 years of illness. The S85C *MATR3* mutation is associated with muscle pathology including rounded fibers, rimmed subsarcolemmal vacuoles and internalized nuclei [2, 5, 26]. In contrast, patients carrying the F115C mutation in *MATR3* develop dysarthria, dysphagia, weakness and variable degrees of dementia, with a typical course of 5 years before death [7]. Spinal cord tissue from F115C patients displayed intense staining of MATR3 within the motor neuron nuclei as well as occasional cytoplasmic immunostaining of MATR3 in neurons compared to spinal cords from control subjects [7]. Subsequent to the identification of ALS-linked *MATR3* mutations, Johnson and colleagues reclassified the original VCPDM S85C cases as ALS [7]; however, there have now been additional families with the S85C mutation that have been diagnosed with VCPDM, without indication of ALS [2, 12, 13, 19, 26], highlighting our lack of understanding of which disease(s) *MATR3* mutations cause.

In an effort to determine the natural regulation of MATR3 in the body, we previously found that murine MATR3 expression decreased with age from postnatal day 1 through 2 months of age in the central nervous system (CNS) [15]. Murine MATR3 was low in the spinal cord compared to several other regions of the CNS [15]. Additionally, MATR3 was difficult to detect in the skeletal muscle of adult mice [15]. It was interesting that both the spinal cord and muscle had such low levels of MATR3, given that they are pathologically affected in ALS or distal myopathy [15].

Given the low expression of MATR3 in the skeletal muscle and spinal cord of normal adult mice and that MATR3 gene trap mice were not reported to display a phenotype akin to ALS or distal myopathy [14], we sought to determine whether increasing expression of WT or mutant MATR3 through transgenesis would produce ALS or myopathic phenotypes. We drove expression of human MATR3 utilizing the mouse prion promoter (MoPrP), a promoter that is active in the spinal cord and muscle [3]. Our original intent was to determine if expression of ALS-linked F115C MATR3 or VCPDM- and ALS-linked S85C MATR3 in Tg mice would lead to distinct or overlapping phenotypes and pathologies. We attempted to control for the effects of Tg expression by also creating mice expressing WT human MATR3. Unexpectedly, transgene expression in these animals was highest in muscle with minimal expression in spinal cord, with the levels of MATR3$^{F115C}$ being significantly higher than that of mice expressing MATR3$^{WT}$ at the protein level in our lead lines. MATR3$^{S85C}$ mice did not robustly express MATR3 protein in either muscle or spinal cord compared to NT mice and were excluded from further study.

Both the MATR3$^{WT}$ and MATR3$^{F115C}$ mice developed myopathic changes that progressed with age from small vacuoles to large vacuolated fibers, rounded fibers, and fibers with internalized nuclei. The MATR3$^{F115C}$ mice developed obvious muscle weakness with a variable age of onset, between ~ 0.9 and 10 months of age, depending on the line. By contrast, MATR3$^{WT}$ mice typically did not show obvious weakness through 20 months of age. Data from lead MATR3$^{WT}$ and MATR3$^{F115C}$ lines indicate that increasing the levels of MATR3 protein in muscle produces myopathic changes. These mice provide new in vivo tools that can be used to dissect the role of MATR3 in muscle degeneration.

## Materials and methods

### Animal husbandry

Mice were kept on a 12-h light/12-h dark cycle with ad libitum access to food and water. All procedures were approved by the Institutional Animal Care and Use Committee of the University of Florida and complied with the National Institute of Health's "Guide for the Care and Use of Laboratory Animals."

### Generation of Tg animals

Tg mice expressing either WT or mutant human MATR3 were generated by cloning the human *MATR3* cDNA to drive expression of the full-length MATR3 protein, the predominant species in murine CNS [15]. pCMV-Sport6 (ThermoScientific, catalog #MHS6278–202757255) was used as the template to amplify human WT *MATR3* cDNA by PCR using primers 5′ attctctagggtcgaccaccATGtccaagtcattccagcag 3′ and 5′ tcactctagggtcgacTTAagtttccttc ttctgtctg 3′. This was cloned into the *Sal* I site of a modified pEF-BOS vector using the InFusion HD cloning kit, (Clontech, catalog #639649). No 5′ or 3′ untranslated region of the human MATR3 mRNA was included in the cDNA gene used to produce the mice; the untranslated sequences were derived from the MoPrP vector [3]. The upstream PCR primer includes an optimized Kozak sequence of CCACC immediately before the start codon. The pEF-BOS-MATR3 vector was digested with *Sal* I, the *MATR3* cDNA was gel purified, and ligated into the *Xho* I site of the MoPrP vector, which was then microinjected into fertilized FVB/NJ oocytes (Jackson Laboratory) and implanted into pseudopregnant females. The F115C and S85C mutations in the *MATR3* cDNA were created using the QuikChange II XL Site-directed Mutagenesis kit (Agilent, catalog #200522) and the mutant construct for each was prepared using the same procedure as the WT *MATR3* cDNA, as mentioned above. Seven MATR3$^{WT}$ founders were mated with FVB/NCr mice (Charles River), six of which transmitted the transgene (Lines 8, 9, 59, 60, 1554, 1563). Five MATR3$^{F115C}$ founders (70, 72, 1573, 1576, 1579) were mated with FVB/NCr mice (Charles River) to generate hemizygous F1 offspring, all of which transmitted the transgene. Five MATR3$^{S85C}$ founders (209,

212, 213, 257, 275) were mated with FVB/NCr mice (Charles River), all of which transmitted the transgene. Genotyping was performed on tail biopsy DNA from mice using the following primers: (PrP-sense) 5' GGGACTATG TGGACTGATGTCGG 3′, (PrP-antisense) 5' CCAA GCCTAGACCACGAGAATGC 3′, and (*MATR3*-sense) 5' AGCAAGAGCTTGGACGTGTG 3′. Mice were designated as Tg by the presence of a band approximately 1100 bp corresponding to the transgene and a 750 bp band produced by the endogenous *PrP* allele, while NT contained only the 750 bp endogenous *PrP* band.

#### Confirmation of *MATR3* allele in transgenic offspring

We verified the specific human *MATR3* allele by either sequencing or restriction digest of a human *MATR3* amplicon from tail biopsy DNA from the majority of the experimental mice (Additional file 1: Table S1, sequencing, asterisk; restriction digest, $). The MATR3$^{S85C}$ mice were discontinued before this verification process. In most cases, we confirmed the allele of *MATR3* present in the Tg mice using PCR to amplify *MATR3* transgene cDNA with the following primers: (sense) 5' ATTCTCTAGG*GTCGACC* ACC<u>ATG</u>TCCAAGTCTTCCAGCAG 3′ [complementary to 5′ elements of cDNA-*Xho*I cloning site italicized and start codon underlined] and (antisense) 5' CGTTGAAAATC CATGATGTCAACATCTCTGCTAGTTTCCACTCT 3′ [complementary to sequences spanning the junction of exons 4 and 5]; resulting in an 1200 bp PCR product. The PCR products were purified using a Monarch PCR & DNA cleanup kit (New England BioLabs catalog #T1030S) and then the purified PCR products were sent to GenScript for sequencing (Additional file 1: Table S1, asterisk) using the following primer which would allow for unambiguous identification of the sequences encoding both S85 and F115 positions: (antisense) 5' CCATAACTCAAGGTAGAGCCT TCTTCAGTTC 3′.

In some cases, restriction digestion of the PCR amplicon (generated as above) was used instead of sequencing (Additional file 1: Table S1, $) to confirm the presence or absence of the F115C mutation. 10 μL of the purified PCR product was then digested with *Pvu*II for 15 min at 37 °C and run on a 1% agarose gel. Since the F115C mutation creates a *Pvu*II site, MATR3$^{WT}$ mice have one band at 1.2 kb, and MATR3$^{F115C}$ mice have bands at 345 and 850 bp.

#### Phenotyping

Mice were phenotyped into two groups: mild-to-moderate (MM) or severe (S) phenotype based on cage behavior and escape extension. The MM phenotype displayed as moderate muscle weakness with no change to the escape extension, while the S phenotype appeared strikingly impaired when ambulating and an abnormal escape extension. In many cases, UF Animal Care Staff technicians initially identified animals that were developing a phenotype without knowledge of the genotype and informed the lab. In all cases, an observer unblinded to genotype assessed the levels of weakness, changes in body mass, and muscle size in phenotyping the affected mice. In some cases, an additional observer (J.L) validated phenotyping by blindly identifying mice with motor phenotypes.

#### Harvesting and tissue collection

Mice were euthanized by cervical dislocation or anesthetized with isoflurane, followed by exsanguination and perfusion with PBS. The right gastrocnemius, right quadriceps, and a small portion of the cervical spinal cord were snap frozen on dry ice and stored at − 80 °C until preparation of lysate or RNA. The remainder of the spinal cord and left hindlimb were dissected and immersion fixed in 10% formalin. After 24 h, fixed spinal cord and hindlimb muscles were transferred into PBS. All tissues were stored in PBS at 4 °C until processing.

#### Northern blotting

RNA was isolated from quadriceps and spinal cord using Trizol (Invitrogen, catalog #15596026) per manufacturer protocol. A DNA probe was made by digesting the PrP vector with *Eco*RI and *Xho*I, isolating a 450 bp fragment, which encompassed sequences in the 3′ untranslated segment of the transgene construct, and purifying it with Monarch Gel Extraction kit (New England BioLabs catalog #T1020S). This probe for the blots was labeled with α-$^{32}$P-dCTP using Rediprime II DNA Labeling System (GE Healthcare Amersham, catalog #RPN1633) and purified using ProbeQuant™ G-50 Micro Columns (GE Healthcare, catalog #28903408), both per manufacturer protocol. 5 μg of RNA was incubated with 3x volume of loading dye (360 μL formamide, 80 μL 10x MOPS buffer, 120 μL 37% formaldehyde, 50 μL glycerol, 10 μL 10% BPB) for 2–3 min at 100 °C, then cooled on ice. 1 μg of 0.5 mg/mL ethidium bromide was added to each sample, and then was resolved on the gel (1% agarose, 2% formaldehyde/MOPS buffer) at 120 V. The gel was soaked in de-ionized $H_2O$ for 40–60 min with three changes to remove formaldehyde and transferred to GreenScreen Plus nylon membrane (Perkin-Elmer, catalog #NEF976) by capillary action overnight using 10X SSC buffer. Next, cross-linking to membrane occurred using the autocrosslink function of the Stratalinker (UVP, model CL-1000). The following was completed at 65 °C. In the prehybridization step, the blot was incubated in hybridization buffer [1% BSA, (fraction V); 1 mM EDTA, pH 8; 0.5 M sodium phosphate, pH 7.2; 7% SDS; de-ionized $H_2O$] for two hours. The buffer was discarded, and the blot was hybridized in hybridization buffer with boiled probe ($0.5 \times 10^6$ cpm/mL) for ~ 18 h. The blot was rinsed and washed with wash buffer 1 (0.1% BSA, 1 mM EDTA, pH 8, 40 mM sodium phosphate, pH 7.2, 5% SDS) for 30 min twice in a hybridization bottle in the hybridization oven, then washed buffer 2 (1 mM EDTA, pH 8; 40 mM sodium phosphate, pH 7.2; 1% SDS) twice for 30 min, wrapped in saran wrap and exposed to film. Endogenous mouse prion was utilized as a control.

### Western blotting

To prepare lysate, frozen gastrocnemius and spinal cord were homogenized in six volumes of the weight in homogenization buffer [50 mM Tris pH 7.5, 300 mM NaCl, 5 mM EDTA, 1% Triton, 1x protease inhibitor (Sigma, catalog #8340), 1x phosphatase inhibitor #1 (Sigma, catalog #P0044), 1x phosphatase inhibitor #2 (Sigma, catalog #P5726)] and stored in aliquots at − 80 ° C to reduce freeze/thaw. An aliquot was further diluted to ten volumes of homogenization buffer. The samples were sonicated, and sodium dodecyl sulfate (SDS) was added to a final concentration of 2%. The samples were centrifuged for 20 min at 4 °C at 40,000 rpm. The supernatant was collected and protein concentration was determined using BCA protein assay (Pierce, Rockford, IL).

For MATR3 immunoblotting, 15 μg of protein from gastrocnemius or spinal cord were resolved on a 3–8% Tris-acetate gel and transferred onto a nitrocellulose membrane for 90 min at 200 mA. The blots were blocked in 5% milk in Tris-buffered saline (TBS) for an hour and were incubated overnight with rabbit α-MATR3 antibody (1:10,000, Novus Biologicals, catalog #NB100–1761) or mouse α-GAPDH antibody (1:5000, Meridian Life Sciences, catalog #H86504M) diluted in 5% milk/TBS. Following washes in TBS, blots were incubated with horseradish peroxidase-conjugated α-rabbit or α-mouse for one hour (1:5000, Jackson ImmunoResearch Laboratories Inc., α-rabbit catalog #711–036-125, α-mouse catalog #715–036-150). Membranes were then washed and incubated with ECL-Plus reagent (Fisher, catalog #509049326) and imaged on PXi using the GeneSys software (SynGene). When comparisons were performed across lines which had variable levels of degeneration, coomassie stain was used on 3–8% Tris-Acetate gels replicating the sample layout for gastrocnemius to confirm equivalent loading. When westerns were run within lines and age, immunoblotting for mouse α-GAPDH was utilized for a load control. Western analysis on spinal cord in the lead lines was run using GAPDH as the loading control.

### Immunohistochemistry

The formalin-fixed gastrocnemius and spinal cord were paraffin embedded and sectioned into 5 μm sections. Sections were deparaffinized and hydrated before antigen retrieval using either steaming in citrate buffer (10 mM citrate acid with 0.05% Tween-20, pH 6.0) for 30 min for MATR3 and GFAP or incubation in 10% formic acid for 10 min followed by a 20 min rinse under running water for Iba1. Following alternating washes in water and PBS, sections were blocked in 0.3% $H_2O_2$/PBS for 20 min. After thorough washes in Milli-Q $H_2O$, sections were blocked with 10% normal goat serum (Vector Labs, catalog #S1000) in PBS and 0.05% Tween-20 (PBS-T) for 30 min at room temperature. Sections were then incubated with primary antibody [rabbit α-MATR3 to detect both human and murine MATR3, 1:1000, Novus Biologicals, catalog #NB100–1761; rabbit α-GFAP, 1:1000, Dako, catalog #Z0334; rabbit α-Iba-1, 1:500, Wako, catalog #019–19,741] in 5% normal goat serum/PBS-T overnight at 4 °C. Subsequently, the sections were rinsed with PBS-T and incubated with biotinylated α-rabbit antibody (1:500, Vector Labs, catalog #BA-1000) in 5% normal goat serum/PBS-T for 30 min at room temperature. The signal was detected with a standard peroxidase ABC system (Vector Labs, catalog #PK6100) with DAB as the chromogen, counterstained with hematoxylin, dehydrated and cover-slipped using Cytoseal (Thermo Scientific, catalog #8310–4).

### Quantification

For Northern blot, boxes were drawn around each *MATR3* and *PrP* mRNA band three times using Alpha View SA software (Protein Simple). Tg samples were then normalized by dividing the *MATR3* signal by *PrP* signal, then averaged between the same sample. For muscle Western blots, boxes of equal size were drawn around MATR3 bands using GeneTools software (SynGene) and corrected for background. For spinal cord western blots, boxes of equal size were drawn around MATR3 and, when utilized, GAPDH bands using GeneTools software (SynGene), corrected for background, and densitometric values were normalized by dividing the MATR3 signal by GAPDH. Expression level values for ~ 120 doublet, 90, 75, and 55 kDa were summed to yield total MATR3 levels.

### Statistical analysis

GraphPad Prism 5 and GraphPad Prism 6 software were used for statistical analysis and graphing. One-way ANOVAs, two-way ANOVAs, or t-tests were used as indicated to compare NT, $MATR3^{WT}$, and $MATR3^{F115C}$ values. $p < 0.05$ was established as the threshold for statistically significance. Bonferroni's multiple comparison test was used. Error bars in figures show standard deviation.

## Results

We generated Tg mouse lines using a cDNA encoding either WT, F115C mutant, or S85C mutant MATR3 ($MATR3^{WT}$, $MATR3^{F115C}$, and $MATR3^{S85C}$ respectively) under the control of the MoPrP.Xho vector. Six Tg founders for $MATR3^{WT}$, five Tg founders for $MATR3^{F115C}$, and five Tg founders for $MATR3^{S85C}$ transmitted the transgene (Table 1); however, each line was mosaic with low

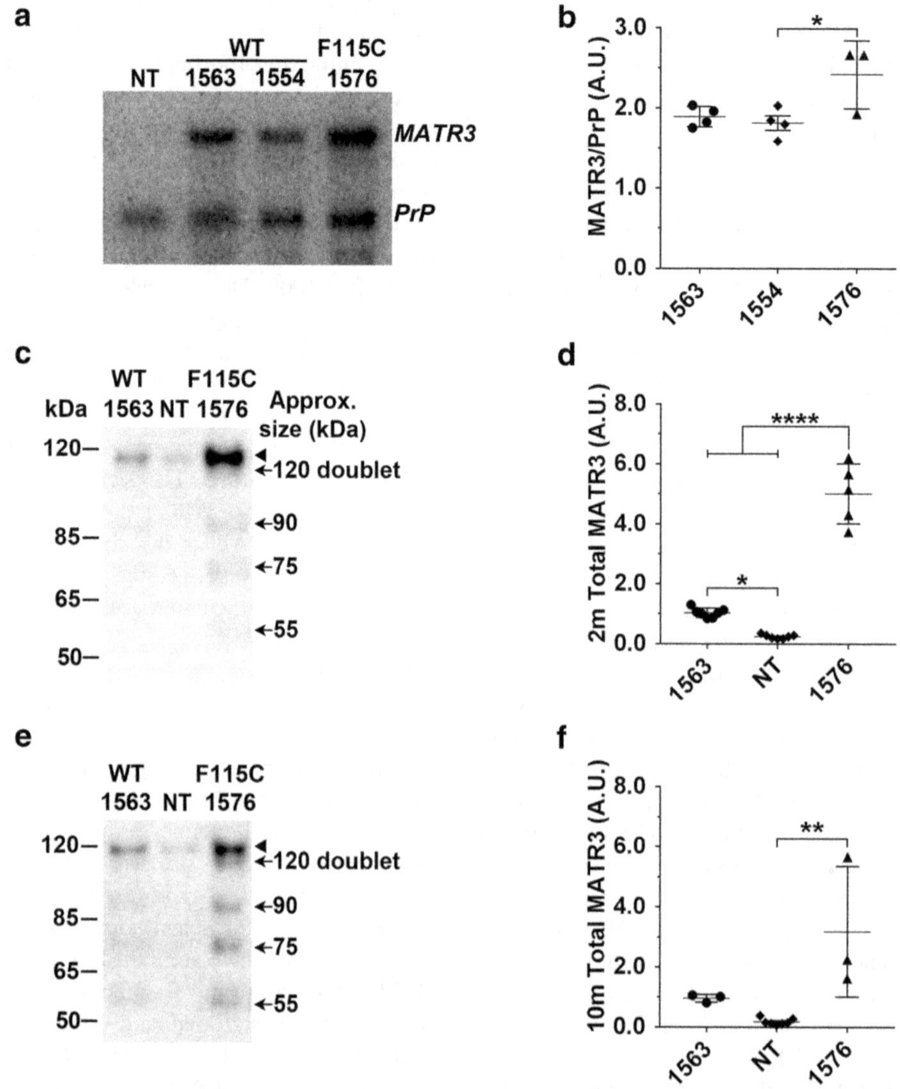


**Fig. 1** MATR3 is overexpressed in the muscle of $MATR3^{WT}$ and $MATR3^{F115C}$ transgenic mice. **a** Northern blot analysis of quadriceps showed transgenic *MATR3* RNA levels. Endogenous murine *PrP* mRNA, which is recognized by the same probe used to detect transgenic mRNA, was utilized as a loading control. **b** Quantification of Northern blots confirmed significant increases in MATR3 levels from lines 1563, 1554, and 1576. MATR3 values were normalized to PrP. One-way ANOVA, $p = 0.0308$. Bonferroni's multiple comparison test showed that lines 1576 and 1554 were significantly different ($p < 0.05$), while there was no difference between lines 1576 to 1563 and 1554 to 1563. **c** Representative western blot of gastrocnemius using an antibody that recognizes both human and murine MATR3 showed an increase in total MATR3 (120 doublet, 90, 75, and 55 kDa combined) in ~ 2 month old transgenic mice from $MATR3^{WT}$ lead line 1563 and $MATR3^{F115C}$ lead line 1576 compared to NT mice. **d** Quantification of western blot confirmed significant increase in total MATR3 levels (120 doublet, 90, 75, and 55 kDa combined) from $MATR3^{WT}$ and $MATR3^{F115C}$ lines compared to NT. One-way ANOVA, $p \leq 0.0001$. Bonferroni's multiple comparison test showed that total MATR3 levels from lines 1563 ($p \leq 0.05$) and 1576 ($p \leq 0.0001$) were statistically significant from NT. MATR3 levels from lead line 1576 were significantly elevated compared to 1563 ($p \leq 0.0001$). **e** Western blot analysis of gastrocnemius showed an increase in MATR3 levels in ~ 10 month old transgenic mice from $MATR3^{F115C}$ lead line 1576 compared to NT. **f** Quantification of western blot confirming significant increase in total MATR3 levels (120 doublet, 90, 75, and 55 kDa combined) from $MATR3^{F115C}$ mice compared to NT mice. One-way ANOVA, $p \leq 0.01$. Bonferroni's multiple comparison test showed that line 1576 ($p \leq 0.0001$) was statistically significant from NT. There is no significant difference between lead line 1576 compared to lead line 1563, as well as lead line 1563 compared to NT ($p > 0.05$). *, $p \leq 0.05$; **, $p \leq 0.01$, ****, $p \leq 0.0001$. Arrow head indicates expected MATR3 band at 120 kDa, arrows indicate lower molecular weight species as indicated

penetrance and required substantial breeding to establish consistent lines. To determine which lines of mice expressed the transgene, we initially relied on immunoblotting of spinal cord and muscle tissues. We quickly observed that a subset of mice transgenic for $MATR3^{WT}$ and $MATR3^{F115C}$ had elevated levels of MATR3 in muscle compared to NT mice and then used immunoblotting of muscle to screen mice towards establishing stable lines that

**Table 1** Founder lines of MATR3$^{WT}$ and MATR3$^{F115C}$ mice used in the study

| Transgene | Founder | Transmitting | Status | Use in paper | Reason for exclusion |
|---|---|---|---|---|---|
| MATR3$^{WT}$ | 8 | Yes | Extinct | None | No/low expression |
| | 9 | Yes | Extinct | None | No/low expression |
| | 59 | Yes | Back-up line | *Validation* | |
| | 60 | Yes | Extinct | None | No/low expression |
| | 66 | No | Extinct | None | Not transmitting |
| | 1554 | Yes | Extinct | *Validation* | |
| | **1563** | **Yes** | **Lead Line** | **Primary data** | |
| MATR3$^{F115C}$ | 70 | Yes | Extinct | None | No/low expression |
| | 72 | Yes | Extinct | None | X-Linked |
| | 1573 | Yes | Extinct | *Validation* | |
| | **1576** | **Yes** | **Lead Line** | **Primary data** | |
| | 1579 | Yes | Extinct | *Validation* | |
| MATR3$^{S85C}$ | 209 | Yes | Extinct | None | No/low expression |
| | 202 | Yes | Extinct | None | No/low expression |
| | 203 | Yes | Extinct | None | No/low expression |
| | 257 | Yes | Extinct | None | No/low expression |
| | 275 | Yes | Extinct | None | No/low expression |

Bold indicates lead lines

would be more thoroughly characterized (Table 1). In mice transgenic for MATR3$^{S85C}$, we could not identify mice with robust levels of MATR3 in muscle or spinal cord compared to NT mice and ultimately discontinued breeding all mice harboring the MATR3$^{S85C}$ transgene. Additionally, breeding patterns suggested that one of the MATR3$^{F115C}$ lines (line 72) was likely integrated on the X-chromosome; therefore, the line was excluded from the study.

In the MATR3$^{WT}$ and MATR3$^{F115C}$ lines we established, *MATR3* Tg mRNA was robustly expressed in the skeletal muscle (Fig. 1a). There was no statistically significant difference in human *MATR3* RNA levels between the lead MATR3$^{F115C}$ line (1576) compared to the lead MATR3$^{WT}$ line (1563) (Fig. 1a, b); however, *MATR3* Tg mRNA levels in the lead MATR3$^{F115C}$ line (1576) were modestly higher than the levels in one of the MATR3$^{WT}$ validation lines, 1554 (Fig. 1a, b; $p < 0.05$).

Total MATR3 protein levels in the skeletal muscle of ~ 2-month old mice from MATR3$^{WT}$ lead line 1563 ($p < 0.05$) and MATR3$^{F115C}$ (lead line 1576, $p < 0.0001$) were significantly elevated over that of NT mice (Fig. 1c-d). Compared to NT mice, MATR3 levels were increased ~ 4-fold ($p < 0.05$) in MATR3$^{WT}$ mice and ~ 20-fold ($p < 0.0001$) in MATR3$^{F115C}$ mice (Fig. 1c-d). At 10 months of age, total MATR3 protein levels were roughly 17-fold higher in MATR3$^{F115C}$ (lead line 1576) than NT mice (Fig. 1e, f; $p < 0.01$). Across all MATR3 Tg lines, MATR3$^{F115C}$ mice from line 1579 had the highest elevation of MATR3 protein levels at ~ 2 months of age compared to NT mice (Additional file 2: Figure S1a); however, line 1579 was only used for validation studies as they became moribund before breeding was possible.

During handling and while observing general cage behavior, Tg mice from MATR3$^{WT}$ and MATR3$^{F115C}$ lead lines initially were indistinguishable from NT littermates. At ~ 2 months of age, the escape extension in Tg mice from founder lines MATR3$^{WT}$ (1563) and MATR3$^{F115C}$ (1576) was generally comparable to NT mice (Fig. 2a-c). At ~ 10 months of age, the escape extension reflex in mice from MATR3$^{WT}$ lead line 1563 was visually equivalent to that of NT controls (Fig. 2d, e). By ~ 10 months of age, mice from MATR3$^{F115C}$ lead line 1576 typically presented with either no changes to escape extension (Fig. 2f) with observable mild-moderate impairment in walking behavior in home cage (not shown), or a severe change in escape extension (Fig. 2g) paired with striking difficulty while walking in the home cage (not shown). As early as ~ 4 months of age, a subset of MATR3$^{F115C}$ mice from lead line 1576 appeared smaller in body size, with muscles in the hind limbs appearing smaller. Furthermore, they presented with difficulty gripping the edge of the cage. Similar motor impairment was observed in a subset of transgenic MATR3$^{F115C}$ mice from validation lines 1573 (not shown) and 1579, which developed impairments as early as 0.9 months of age (Additional file 2: Figure S1c). In these young MATR3$^{F115C}$ mice from validation line 1579, motor impairment rapidly progressed to hindlimb paresis and paralysis.

The body weight of MATR3$^{WT}$ (lead line 1563) mice at ~ 2 and ~ 10 months of age was comparable to sex

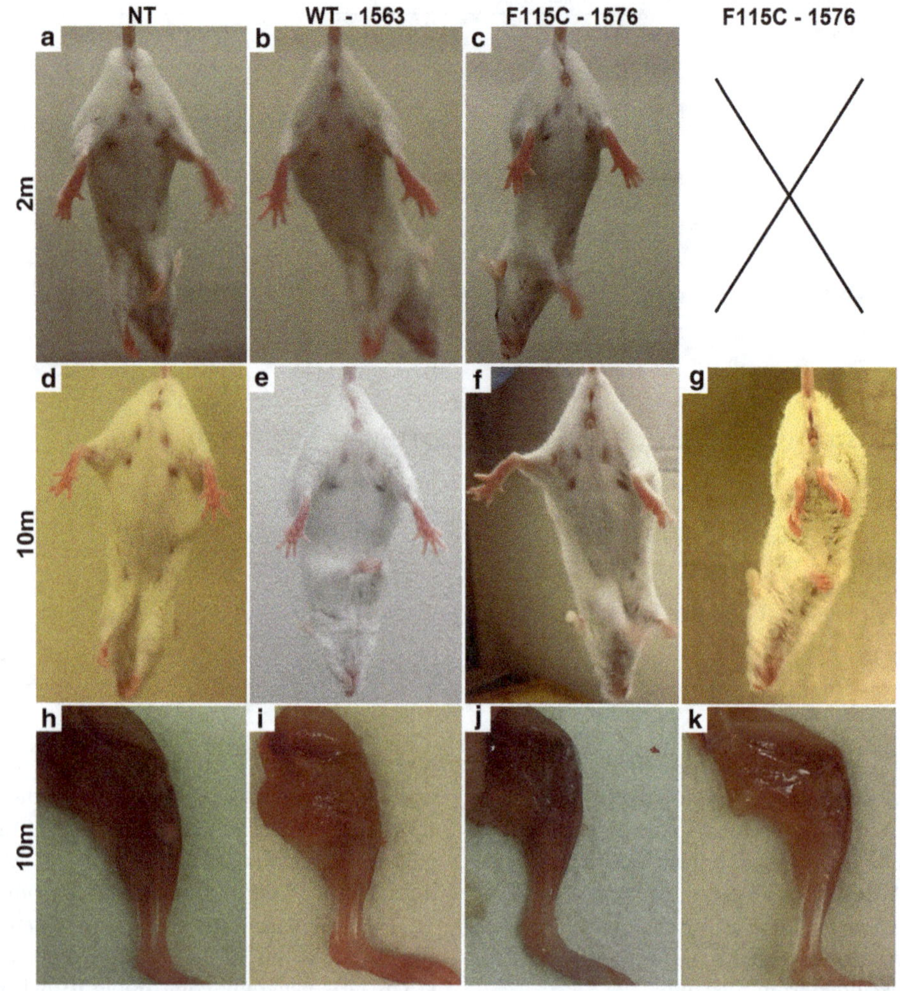


**Fig. 2** Severe phenotypic MATR3$^{F115C}$ transgenic mice develop profound motor phenotype and show gross muscle atrophy. Escape extension of mice at ~ 2 months showed no differences comparing **a** NT to **b** MATR3$^{WT}$ and **c** MATR3$^{F115C}$ (lines noted on figure). Escape extension of mice at ~ 10 months showed no difference comparing **d** NT to **e** MATR3$^{WT}$ displaying no obvious motor phenotype, and **f** MATR3$^{F115C}$ displaying a mild-to-moderate phenotype. A subset of ~ 10-month old **g** MATR3$^{F115C}$ mice lacked the normal escape reflex. Gross hindlimb muscle showed no difference between ~ 10 month old **h** NT and **i** MATR3$^{WT}$; however, muscles appeared grossly atrophied in **j** MATR3$^{F115C}$ displaying either a mild-to-moderate or **k** severe motor phenotype. Panels a-k are from female mice

and age-matched NT controls (Additional file 3: Table S2). In contrast, body weights were reduced in MATR3$^{F115C}$ mice from lead line 1576 compared to sex- and age-matched NT controls at both ~ 2 and ~ 10 months of age (Additional file 3: Table S2). Similarly, transgenic mice from MATR3$^{F115C}$ validation line 1579 had reduced body weights compared to age-matched NT mice, although measurements were only compared for phenotypic males, given the young age of disease-onset (Additional file 3: Table S2).

Although the gastrocnemii of 10-month-old NT and MATR3$^{WT}$ mice from lead line 1563 appeared grossly similar (Fig. 2h and i, respectively), gross muscle atrophy was apparent in ~ 10-month-old mice MATR3$^{F115C}$ from lead line 1576. MATR3$^{F115C}$ mice displaying the mild-to-moderate phenotype (Fig. 2j) showed moderate muscle atrophy, which was more pronounced in mice with the severe phenotype (Fig. 2k). MATR3$^{F115C}$ mice from validation line 1579 also developed pronounced muscle atrophy (Additional file 2: Figure S1e) compared to NT mice (Additional file 2: Figure S1d). Transgenic MATR3$^{F115C}$ mice (validation line 1579) which had severe motor abnormalities also showed severe myopathic changes (Additional file 2: Figure S1g) including rounded fibers, smaller fibers, centralized nuclei (white arrow head), and prominent vacuoles (white arrows) when compared to NT mice (Additional file 2: Figure S1f). To determine if myopathic changes were only present in mice with motor phenotypes, we examined muscle from MATR3$^{WT}$ lead line 1563 and MATR3$^{F115C}$ mice from lead line 1576 at ~ 2 and ~ 10 months of age (Fig. 3). The gastrocnemius of ~ 2-month-old MATR3$^{WT}$ (lead line 1563) and MATR3$^{F115C}$

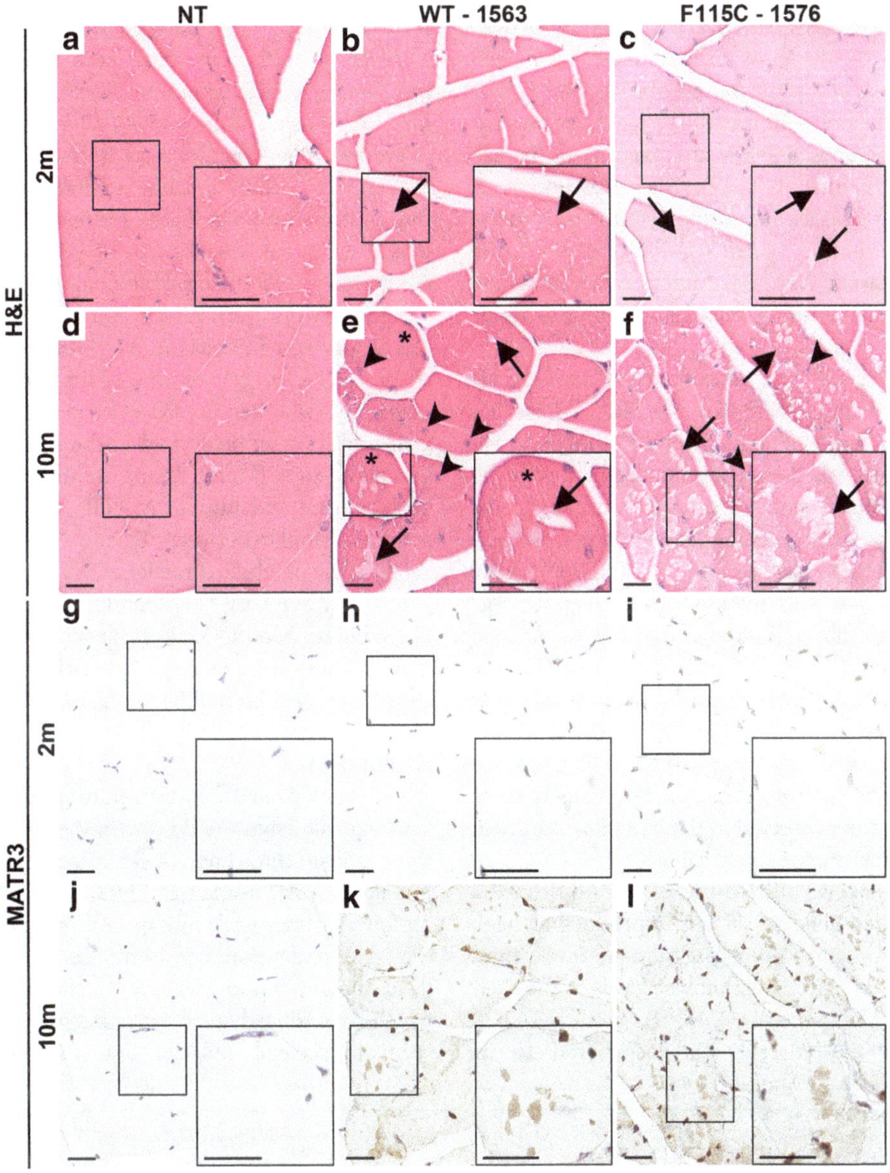


**Fig. 3** Muscle pathology is striking in ~ 10 month old MATR3$^{WT}$ (lead line 1563) and MATR3$^{F115C}$ (lead line 1576) transgenic mice. H&E of gastrocnemius at ~ 2 months of age from **a** NT, **b** MATR3$^{WT}$, and **c** MATR3$^{F115C}$ mice (lines noted on figure). Both the MATR3$^{WT}$ and MATR3$^{F115C}$ mice showed modest, early vacuolation in the fibers (arrow). H&E of the gastrocnemius at ~ 10 months of age from **d** NT, **e** MATR3$^{WT}$ and **f** MATR3$^{F115C}$ mice. Both MATR3$^{WT}$ and MATR3$^{F115C}$ mice showed striking pathology including vacuoles (arrow), internalized nuclei (arrow head), and rounded fibers (asterisks). MATR3 immunohistochemistry of the gastrocnemius at ~ 2 months of age from **g** NT, **h** MATR3$^{WT}$, and **i** MATR3$^{F115C}$. Both MATR3$^{WT}$ and MATR3$^{F115C}$ have increased immunostaining of MATR3 in the nucleus. MATR3 immunohistochemistry of the gastrocnemius ~ 10 months of age showed that compared to **j** NT mice, **k** MATR3$^{WT}$ and **l** MATR3$^{F115C}$ mice showed much more intense immunostaining of the nucleus, as well as robust cytoplasmic staining of MATR3. Scale bar measures 25 μm

(lead line 1576) showed vacuoles in the fibers compared to NT mice (Fig. 3a-c, black arrows) which appeared to worsen with age (Fig. 3d-f) based on the increased presence of rounded fibers (asterisks), internalized nuclei (black arrowheads), and larger and abundant vacuoles in the fibers when compared to NT gastrocnemii. The pathology was qualitatively more severe in MATR3$^{F115C}$ compared to MATR3$^{WT}$ mice, especially at ~ 10 months of age.

Next, we sought to determine whether immunohistochemical techniques would also show increased MATR3 levels within the gastrocnemii of Tg MATR3 mice compared to NT mice, as indicated in earlier immunoblotting data. NT mice could be easily distinguished from MATR3$^{WT}$ (lead line 1563) and MATR3$^{F115C}$ (lead line 1576 and validation line 1579) mice based on MATR3 immunostaining of the muscle (Fig. 3g-l, Additional file 2: Figure S1h, i). In the lead

$MATR3^{F115C}$ line (1576) and $MATR3^{WT}$ line (1563) at ~ 2 months of age, we observed MATR3 immunoreactivity heterogeneously in the nuclei of the gastrocnemius muscle fibers (Fig. 3h, i); however, in the muscle fibers of $MATR3^{WT}$ and $MATR3^{F115C}$ mice at ~ 10 months of age, there was extensive MATR3 immunostaining in the majority of the nuclei compared to NT mice (Fig. 3j-l). There was occasional MATR3 diffuse immunostaining to the cytoplasm in the ~ 2-month-old lead $MATR3^{WT}$ and $MATR3^{F115C}$ lines (not shown), but cytoplasmic MATR3 staining was robust and frequent in the ~ 10-month Tg muscles, seeming to reside within the vacuoles (Fig. 3k, l).

Although the $MATR3^{F115C}$ mice exhibited abbreviated life spans due to motor impairment, the $MATR3^{WT}$ mice live through 20 months of age without obvious motor abnormalities. To determine whether the muscle pathology in $MATR3^{WT}$ mice would eventually progress with age to the severity of that observed in the $MATR3^{F115C}$ mice, we performed H&E staining on gastrocnemii of $MATR3^{WT}$ mice from lead line 1563 at > 20 months of age (Fig. 4). Age matched NT muscle fibers showed occasional vacuolation consistent with aging (Fig. 4a, black arrows), but most of the 20-month-old $MATR3^{WT}$ mice examined showed extensive muscle pathology including internalized nuclei (black arrowheads) as well as rounded and vacuolated fibers that, in some cases, appeared almost destroyed (Fig. 4b). Surprisingly, these myopathic features were observed in the $MATR3^{WT}$ mice in the absence of obvious motor abnormalities.

In all MATR3 lines, we utilized the MoPrP to drive expression of the transgene as it has reproducibly been shown to drive transgene overexpression in the central nervous system [3, 11, 24, 25] with lower levels in the skeletal muscle [3]. Unexpectedly, MoPrP-driven MATR3 overexpression in the current study appeared to be minimal in the spinal cord of Tg mice from all lines examined. Northern blots showed minimal expression of the *MATR3* Tg mRNA in spinal cord from $MATR3^{WT}$ (lead line 1563 and validation line 1554) and $MATR3^{F115C}$ (lead line 1576), using endogenous *PrP* mRNA as a comparison (Additional file 4: Figure S2a). RNA was not available from $MATR3^{F115C}$ validation line 1579; however, immunoblotting indicated no significant change in total MATR3 protein levels in the spinal cords of ~ 1.2-month-old Tg mice compared to NT mice (Additional file 4: Figure S2b, c).

Although northern and immuno- blot analyses did not reveal an overt increase in MATR3 levels in spinal cords of Tg MATR3 mice, we utilized immunohistochemistry to determine whether the MATR3 protein localization and glial profiles may be altered in the spinal cord of Tg mice compared to NT mice. Using an antibody that recognizes both murine and human MATR3, immunoreactivity was generally similar between Tg and NT mice, primarily localizing to spinal cord nuclei in NT, $MATR3^{WT}$ (lead line 1563), and $MATR3^{F115C}$ (lead line 1576) mice (Additional file 5: Figure S3a-c). Glial profiles in the spinal cords of Tg MATR3 lines were largely unremarkable compared to NT spinal cord (Additional file 5: Figure S3d-i).

## Discussion

We characterized three transmitting lines of Tg mice expressing full-length WT human MATR3 ($MATR3^{WT}$) and three transmitting lines of Tg mice expressing full-length mutant (F115C) human MATR3 ($MATR3^{F115C}$). All of our Tg founder lines were mosaic and required substantial outcrossing to develop consistent lead lines for $MATR3^{WT}$ (lead line 1563) and $MATR3^{F115C}$ (lead line 1576), both of which have robustly elevated levels of total MATR3 protein in their skeletal muscle, but not spinal cords. Both

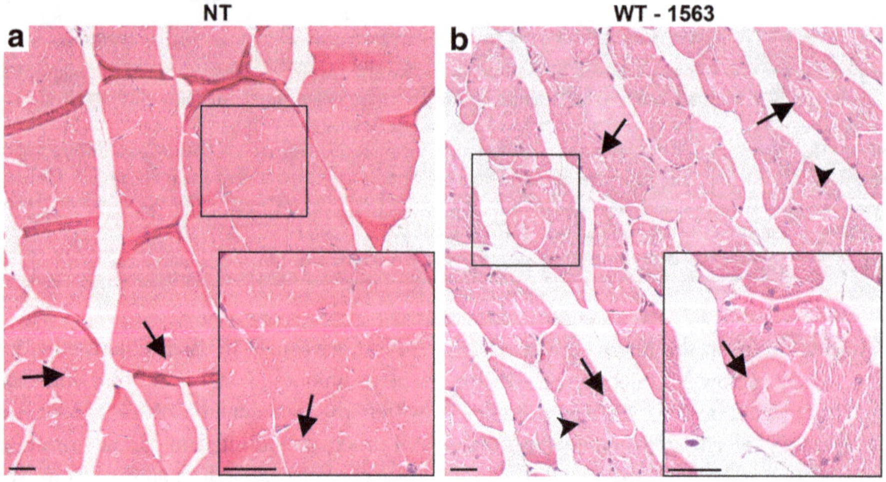


**Fig. 4** Striking muscle pathology in aged $MATR3^{WT}$ (lead line 1563) mice. H&E stain of gastrocnemii of **a** NT at 24.6 months and **b** $MATR3^{WT}$ from lead line 1563 at 22.7 months. While the NT muscle fibers showed some vacuoles (arrows), the $MATR3^{WT}$ muscle showed striking pathology with abundant subsarcolemmal vacuoles, internalized nuclei (arrow heads), and loss of fiber shape. Scale bar measures 25 μm

MATR3$^{WT}$ and MATR3$^{F115C}$ mice showed initial muscle pathology by 2 months of age that noticeably progressed by 10 months of age to include frequent, large vacuoles, rounded fibers, and internalized nuclei. Muscle pathology in the MATR3$^{WT}$ mice appeared to lag behind MATR3$^{F115C}$ mice, requiring additional aging to > 20 months of age before approximating the severity observed in the younger MATR3$^{F115C}$ counterparts. Only MATR3$^{F115C}$ mice develop a consistent, overt motor phenotype, which included paresis and paralysis. Motoric changes were accompanied by gross muscle atrophy, which could serve as one explanation for the body weight differences between NT mice and MATR3$^{F115C}$ mice and was not observed in the MATR3$^{WT}$ mice. Since MATR3$^{WT}$ and MATR3$^{F115C}$ lacked robust elevation or relocalization of MATR3 in the spinal cord and the overall glial profiles did not differ from NT mice, it appears that the transgenic MATR3 expression the in the muscle most likely led to myopathy rather than a primary motor neuron disease.

Although the human *MATR3* RNA expression levels in the skeletal muscle were not significantly different between the MATR3$^{F115C}$ lead line (1576) and MATR3$^{WT}$ lead line (1563), MATR3$^{F115C}$ mice (lead line 1576) have a ~ 4-fold elevation in total MATR3 protein levels over MATR3$^{WT}$ mice (lead line 1563) at ~ 2 months of age. Since the MATR3 antibodies that are commercially available detect both human and murine MATR3, it is impossible to know if the higher level of MATR3 protein in the mutant mice arise from induction of endogenous MATR3 expression or higher levels of human transgenic F115C MATR3 or an elevation of both murine and the transgenic MATR3. The elevation in the levels of MATR3 protein in the muscle MATR3$^{F115C}$ mice (lead line 1576) over MATR3$^{WT}$ mice (lead line 1563) was not proportional to the Tg mRNA levels between the two lead lines. This may suggest a disparity between translational regulation of WT versus F115C MATR3. Alternatively, it is possible that MATR3$^{F115C}$ may turnover more slowly than MATR3$^{WT}$, resulting in high steady-state levels of protein. Finally, it is possible that there is autoregulation of MATR3 expression, at some unknown level, in these lines and that WT and mutant MATR3 differ in their capacity to perform this function.

In immunoblots of skeletal muscle from younger NT and MATR3 Tg mice, we observed multiple MATR3-immunopositive bands (~ 120 doublet, 90, 75, 55 kDa). The origin of these bands is presently unclear. Since Tg MATR3 was expressed from a cDNA construct, the Tg *MATR3* RNA should not splice to produce alternative transcripts, and no such transcripts were observed on Northern blots. The ~ 120 kDa MATR3-immunopositive band is found in NT muscle as well as variety of other NT tissues [15]. Given these observations, the most likely origins of the lower MATR3-immunopositive species could be from either post-translational modification/proteolysis of the full-length protein or from alternative splicing of endogenous murine MATR3 that was induced by some means.

A surprising finding in these transgenic mice is that MATR3 was consistently elevated in the muscle, but not the spinal cord, despite the use of the MoPrP to drive transgene expression. The MoPrP-driven transgene overexpression is typically focused in the spinal cord and brain [3, 11, 24, 25] with lower levels in the skeletal muscle [3]. This is in direct opposition to our current results, which could indicate that muscle and spinal cord may have different abilities to regulate overexpression or different levels of tolerance for MATR3 expression. It is possible that we missed transgenic founders having high levels of MATR3 in the spinal cord because they did not survive until birth.

Given that the levels of MATR3 were consistently elevated only in muscle of both MATR3$^{WT}$ and MATR3$^{F115C}$ mice, it is not surprising that the pathology within mice is primarily confined to the muscle. We observed extensive structural changes within the muscle of multiple lines of MATR3$^{WT}$ and MATR3$^{F115C}$ mice including pronounced vacuolation of the muscle fibers, internalized nuclei, rounded and ring fibers, variation in muscle fiber size, and gross muscle atrophy. Each of these changes is generally associated with a form of muscular dystrophy rather than being neurogenic in origin [8]. The muscle pathology, gross muscle atrophy and motor phenotype that was present in our MATR3$^{F115C}$ Tg mice resembles that observed in the humans with VCPDM linked to mutant MATR3 [2, 5, 12, 13, 19, 26]. Interestingly, VCPDM has only been linked to the S85C mutation in MATR3 [2, 5, 12, 13, 19, 26]; whereas, the F115C mutation in MATR3 utilized in these transgenic mice has been linked to ALS. Muscle pathology in humans with S85C-linked VCPDM includes the presence of subsarcolemmal vacuoles, variable muscle fiber size, and an increase in internalize nuclei in the gastrocnemius or tibialis anterior [2, 5, 26]. We observed these features in muscle of MATR3$^{F115C}$ mice, and to a lesser degree in MATR3$^{WT}$ mice. The ability of ALS-linked F115C MATR3 to cause overlapping pathologies and phenotypes to human VCPDM indicates that humans bearing any *MATR3* mutation should be examined for myopathy.

One limitation of these Tg mice is that there are no reported cases of myopathy or ALS in humans caused by an overexpression of MATR3. Thus, phenotypes and pathology driven by the overexpression of MATR3 in mice may be caused by different mechanisms than diseases found in humans with MATR3 mutations. We note that heterozygous MATR3 gene-trap mice have not been reported to show ALS- or VCPDM-like phenotypes [14]. In these gene trap mice, the longer transcript of *Matr3* was disrupted; however, a shorter *Matr3* transcript, which is found in the developing heart, was produced [14]. Since the gene-trap mice may not accurately represent a complete MATR3 knockout model, additional attempts for knockout or knock-in models should be pursued in order to determine if the ALS or VCPDM mutations in *MATR3* could result from a loss of function of the protein. Regardless, we do see a similar pathology in muscles of MATR3$^{WT}$ and MATR3$^{F115C}$ mice compared to the muscle pathology in the VCPDM patients, indicating that MATR3 overexpression certainly affected muscle fiber biology. Another limitation to these Tg mice concerns muscle development by overexpressing human MATR3. RT-PCR of heart has shown that levels of *MATR3* during development decreases by embryonic day 16.5 through postnatal day 0, then remain consistent through adulthood [14]. It is possible that by overexpressing human MATR3 early in development, the normal developmental processing of MATR3 is disturbed, and the muscle pathology and phenotype we observe could be a case of inappropriate development.

It is not unusual for the first or even second-generation murine models to only partially mimic aspects of neurodegenerative diseases, even in the context of pathologies that may not initially seem disease-relevant. For example, many of the initial TDP-43 Tg models helped elucidate multiple biologically-relevant features of TDP-43 such as its role in mitochondrial biology [24], despite serving as incomplete models for the human condition. Similarly, homozygous progranulin knockout mice develop neuronal ceroid lipofuscinosis [1]; however, a link between progranulin deficiency and human neuronal ceroid lipofuscinosis was not discovered until two years after we reported the link in the mouse model [20]. We anticipate that the current MATR3 models could provide similar insights.

Our data suggest that MATR3-linked diseases may lie on a spectrum between ALS and distal myopathy, and this spectrum is not without precedent. Valosin-containing protein (*VCP*) is another gene that lies on this spectrum of ALS to myopathy. Mutations in *VCP* cause inclusion body myopathy associated with Paget disease of bone and frontotemporal dementia (IBMPFD) [9]. Individuals with *VCP* mutations present with proximal and distal muscle paresis, similar to limb girdle muscular dystrophy, and muscle biopsy showing myopathic features included a change in muscle fiber size and rimmed vacuoles [9]; however, mutations in *VCP* can also lead to ALS, including two of the same mutations that had been previously linked to IBMPFD [6, 23].

## Conclusions

In aggregate, our studies provide the first Tg mouse models expressing any form of human MATR3 and demonstrate that simple dysregulation of MATR3 can cause robust structural abnormalities of the muscle. Our data suggest that MATR3 may have regulatory mechanisms that are influenced by tissue type and/or mutation status. These novel MATR3 models will provide critical tools to explore MATR3 regulation and its role in normal and disease biology. Given that the F115C mutation in MATR3 has not been linked to myopathy in humans, our data support the possibility that *MATR3* mutations could cause diseases that lie in a spectrum between ALS and myopathy and that any individual containing a *MATR3* mutation should be assessed for myopathic changes, regardless of clinical diagnosis.

## Additional files

**Additional file 1: Table S1.** Animals used in the study. *Indicates genotype has been confirmed by sequencing. § indicates genotype has been confirmed by restriction digest. Bold indicates when data from animal is pictured within figure. Geno., genotype; Gen., generation; Pheno., phenotype; NP, no phenotype; MM, mild-to-moderate phenotype; S, severe phenotype; F, female; M, male; mo, month; Fig, Figure; SF, Supplementary Figure; T, Table; ST, Supplementary Table. (DOCX 37 kb)

**Additional file 2: Figure S1.** Muscle immunobloting and pathology show striking differences between MATR3$^{F115C}$ mice from validation line 1579 and NT mice. **a** Western blot analysis of gastrocnemius showed an increase in total MATR3 levels (~ 120 double, 90, 75, and 55 kDa combined) in mice ~ 1.5 months old transgenic mice from validation line 1579 compared to NT mice and mice from MATR3$^{F115C}$ lead line 1576 and 1573. Escape extension showed differences between **b** NT compared to **c** MATR3$^{F115C}$ transgenic mouse from validation line 1579 displaying a severe phenotype. Gross hindlimb muscle atrophy was apparent when comparing hindlimb of **d** NT to **e** MATR3$^{F115C}$ mice. H&E of **f** NT and **g** MATR3$^{F115C}$ where MATR3$^{F115C}$ gastrocnemius showed striking pathology including centralized nuclei (white arrow head), rounded fibers, smaller fibers, and subsarcolemmal vacuoles (white arrows). Immunohistochemistry of **h** NT gastrocnemius and **i** MATR3$^{F115C}$ showed that MATR3 immunoreactivity was elevated in the nucleus and cytoplasm of MATR3$^{F115C}$ mice. Panels b-e are from males. Scale bar measures 25 μm. (TIF 4722 kb)

**Additional file 3: Table S2.** Average body weights for lead MATR3$^{WT}$ and MATR3$^{F115C}$ lines. MATR3$^{WT}$ mice (lead line 1563) were not significantly different when compared to age-matched NT males (~ 2 mo.: two-way ANOVA, $p > 0.05$; ~ 10 mo.: t-test, $p > 0.05$) and females (~ 2 mo.: two-way ANOVA, $p > 0.05$). At ~ 2 months, MATR3$^{F115C}$ mice (lead line 1576) weighed significantly less compared to age-matched and sex-matched NT mice (two-way ANOVA, $p < 0.0001$) and at ~ 10 months, male (two-way ANOVA, $p < 0.0001$) and female (two-way ANOVA, $p < 0.05$) MATR3$^{F115C}$ mice (lead line 1576) weighed significantly less compared to age- and sex-matched NT mice. Not significant, n.s; *, $p \leq 0.05$; ****, $p \leq 0.0001$. (DOCX 16 kb)

**Additional file 4: Figure S2.** MATR3 is not robustly elevated in the spinal cords of MATR3$^{WT}$ and MATR3$^{F115C}$ mice. **a** Northern blot analysis of cervical spinal cord showed limited transgenic *MATR3* RNA expression in MATR3$^{WT}$ (lead line 1563 and validation line 1554) and MATR3$^{F115C}$ (lead line 1576) mice at ~ 4 months of age. Mouse prion (*PrP*) mRNA served as a loading control. **b** Western blot demonstrated that total MATR3 is not robustly elevated in spinal cord of MATR3$^{F115C}$ (validation line 1579) mice compared to NT mice at ~ 1.5 months of age. GAPDH was utilized as a loading control. **c** Quantification of Western blot showed no significant difference in total MATR3 levels in spinal cord of NT compared to MATR3$^{F115C}$ validation line 1579 mice (t-test, $p > 0.05$). (TIF 907 kb)

**Additional file 5: Figure S3.** Unremarkable spinal cord pathology in aged MATR3$^{WT}$ and MATR3$^{F115C}$ mice. MATR3 immunohistochemistry of spinal cord at ~ 10 months of age from **a** NT, **b** MATR3$^{WT}$ from lead line 1563, and **c** MATR3$^{F115C}$ from lead line 1576. Qualitatively, there appeared to be no difference in Iba-1 immunohistochemistry between **d** NT, **e** MATR3$^{WT}$, and **f** MATR3$^{F115C}$, or in GFAP immunohistochemistry of **g** NT, **h** MATR3$^{WT}$, and **i** MATR3$^{F115C}$ spinal cords. Scale bar measures 100 μm. (TIF 6303 kb)

**Abbreviations**

Mo: promoter; PrP: mouse prion; ALS: Amyotrophic lateral sclerosis; *C9orf72*: Chromosome 9 open reading frame gene; CNS: Central nervous system; F: Female; F115C: Phe115Cys. ALS causing mutation in MATR3; fALS: Familial ALS; Fig: Figure; *FUS*: fused in sarcoma gene; GAPDH: Glyceraldehyde 3-phosphatase dehydrogenase; Gen.: Generation; Geno.: Genotype; GFAP: Glial fibrillary acidic protein; H&E: Hematoxylin and eosin stain; Iba-1: allograft inflammatory factor 1, or ionized calcium-binding adapter molecule 1; IBMPFD: Inclusion body myopathy associated with Paget disease of bone and frontotemporal dementia; M: Male; *MATR3*: MATR3 gene; MATR3: Matrin 3, MATR3 protein; $MATR3^{F115C}$: Transgenic mice expressing F115C mutant human MATR3; $MATR3^{S85C}$: Transgenic mice expressing S85C mutant human MATR3; $MATR3^{WT}$: Transgenic mice expressing wild-type human MATR3; MM: Mild to moderate phenotype; mo.: Month; NLS: Nuclear localization sequence; NP: No phenotype; NT: Non-transgenic; PBS: Phosphate buffered saline; Pheno.: Phenotype; PrP: Mouse prion; S: Severe phenotype; S85C: Ser85Cys. ALS and VCPDM causing mutation in MATR3; sALS: Sporadic ALS; SDS: Sodium dodecyl sulfate; SF: Supplementary Figure; *SOD1*: Superoxide dismutase I gene; ST: Supplementary Table; T: Table; *TARDBP*: Tar-DNA binding protein gene; TBS: Tris-buffered saline; TDP-43: TAR DNA binding protein 43; Tg: Transgenic; UTR: Untranslated region; VCP: Valosin containing protein; *VCP*: Valosin containing protein gene; VCPDM: autosomal dominant distal myopathy with vocal cord and pharyngeal weakness; WT: Wild-type

**Acknowledgements**
We thank the UF Mouse Models Core for performing the microinjections, Marissa Ciesla for technical support and Dr. Maurice Swanson for thoughtful advice.

**Funding**
This study was funded by a grant from the McKnight Brain Institute to DRB, a grant from the ALS Association to JL and DRB, a grant from Barbara's Dream Fund for Frontotemporal Dementia research and education to JL and DRB, an NIH T32 NS082168 Predoctoral Interdisciplinary Training in Movement Disorders and Neurorestoration to SR and the University of Florida. The content is solely the responsibility of the authors and does not necessarily represent the official views of the National Institutes of Health.

**Authors' contributions**
All authors had full access to all the data in the study and take responsibility for the integrity of the data and the accuracy of the data analysis. Study concept and design: DRB, JL. Acquisition of data: CM, SR, JH, SF, HB, MC, MC, CD, ZS, DM. Analysis and interpretation of data: CM, SR, DRB, JL. Drafting of the manuscript: CM, SR, JL. Critical revision of the manuscript for important intellectual content: DRB, JL. Statistical analysis: CM, JH. Obtained funding: SR, DRB, JL. All authors read and approved the final manuscript.

**Competing interests**
The authors declare that they have no competing interests.

**Author details**
[1]Center for Translational Research in Neurodegenerative Disease, University of Florida, Gainesville, Florida, USA. [2]Department of Neuroscience, University of Florida, Gainesville, Florida, USA. [3]McKnight Brain Institute, Department of Neuroscience, University of Florida, Gainesville, Florida, USA.

**References**
1. Ahmed Z, Sheng H, Xu YF, Lin WL, Innes AE, Gass J, Yu X, Hou H, Chiba S, Yamanouchi K, Leissring M, Petrucelli L, Nishihara M, Hutton ML, McGowan E, Dickson DW, Lewis J (2010) Accelerated lipofuscinosis and ubiquitination in granulin knockout mice suggest a role for progranulin in successful aging. Am J Pathol 177:311–324. https://doi.org/10.2353/ajpath.2010.090915
2. Barp A, Malfatti E, Metay C, Jobic V, Carlier RY, Laforet P (2018) The first French case of MATR3 -related distal myopathy: clinical, radiological and histopathological characterization. Rev Neurol (Paris):8–11. https://doi.org/10.1016/j.neurol.2017.08.004
3. Borchelt DR, Davis J, Fischer M, Lee MK, Slunt HH, Ratovitsky T, Regard J, Copeland NG, Jenkins NA, Sisodia SS, Price DL (1996) A vector for expressing foreign genes in the brains and hearts of transgenic mice. Genet Anal Biomol Eng 13:159–163. https://doi.org/10.1016/S1050-3862(96)00167-2
4. DeJesus-Hernandez M, Mackenzie IR, Boeve BF, Boxer AL, Baker M, Rutherford NJ, Nicholson AM, Finch NA, Flynn H, Adamson J, Kouri N, Wojtas A, Sengdy P, Hsiung G-YR, Karydas A, Seeley WW, Josephs KA, Coppola G, Geschwind DH, Wszolek ZK, Feldman H, Knopman DS, Petersen RC, Miller BL, Dickson DW, Boylan KB, Graff-Radford NR, Rademakers R (2011) Expanded GGGGCC Hexanucleotide repeat in noncoding region of C9ORF72 causes chromosome 9p-linked FTD and ALS. Neuron 72:245–256. https://doi.org/10.1016/j.neuron.2011.09.011
5. Feit H, Silbergleit A, Schneider LB, Gutierrez JA, Fitoussi R-P, Réyès C, Rouleau GA, Brais B, Jackson CE, Beckmann JS, Seboun E (1998) Vocal cord and pharyngeal weakness with autosomal dominant distal myopathy: clinical description and gene localization to 5q31. Am J Hum Genet 63:1732–1742. https://doi.org/10.1086/302166
6. Johnson JO, Mandrioli J, Benatar M, Abramzon Y, Van Deerlin VM, Trojanowski JQ, Gibbs JR, Brunetti M, Gronka S, Wuu J, Ding J, McCluskey L, Martinez-Lage M, Falcone D, Hernandez DG, Arepalli S, Chong S, Schymick JC, Rothstein J, Landi F, Wang Y-D, Calvo A, Mora G, Sabatelli M, Monsurrò MR, Battistini S, Salvi F, Spataro R, Sola P, Borghero G, Galassi G, Scholz SW, Taylor JP, Restagno G, Chiò A, Traynor BJ (2010) Exome sequencing reveals VCP mutations as a cause of familial ALS. Neuron 68:857–864. https://doi.org/10.1016/j.neuron.2010.11.036
7. Johnson JO, Pioro EP, Boehringer A, Chia R, Feit H, Renton AE, Pliner HA, Abramzon Y, Marangi G, Winborn BJ, Gibbs JR, Nalls MA, Morgan S, Shoai M, Hardy J, Pittman A, Orrell RW, Malaspina A, Sidle KC, Fratta P, Harms MB, Baloh RH, Pestronk A, Weihl CC, Rogaeva E, Zinman L, Drory VE, Borghero G, Mora G, Calvo A, Rothstein JD, Drepper C, Sendtner M, Singleton AB, Taylor JP, Cookson MR, Restagno G, Sabatelli M, Bowser R, Chiò A, Traynor BJ (2014) Mutations in the Matrin 3 gene cause familial amyotrophic lateral sclerosis. Nat Neurosci 17:664–666. https://doi.org/10.1038/nn.3688
8. Joyce NC, Oskarsson B, Jin L (2012) Muscle biopsy evaluation in neuromuscular disorders. Phys Med Rehabil Clin N Am 23:609–631. https://doi.org/10.1016/j.pmr.2012.06.006
9. Kovach MJ, Waggoner B, Leal SM, Gelber D, Khardori R, Levenstien MA, Shanks CA, Gregg G, Al-Lozi MT, Miller T, Rakowicz W, Lopate G, Florence J, Glosser G, Simmons Z, Morris JC, Whyte MP, Pestronk A, Kimonis VE (2001) Clinical delineation and localization to chromosome 9p13.3–p12 of a unique dominant disorder in four families: hereditary inclusion body myopathy, Paget disease of bone, and Frontotemporal dementia. Mol Genet Metab 74:458–475. https://doi.org/10.1006/mgme.2001.3256
10. Kwiatkowski TJ, Bosco DA, LeClerc AL, Tamrazian E, Vanderburg CR, Russ C, Davis A, Gilchrist J, Kasarskis EJ, Munsat T, Valdmanis P, Rouleau GA, Hosler BA, Cortelli P, de Jong PJ, Yoshinaga Y, Haines JL, Pericak-Vance MA, Yan J, Ticozzi N, Siddique T, McKenna-Yasek D, Sapp PC, Horvitz HR, Landers JE, Brown RH (2009) Mutations in the FUS/TLS gene on chromosome 16 cause familial amyotrophic lateral sclerosis. Science (80-) 323:1205–1208. https://doi.org/10.1126/science.1166066
11. Lewis J, McGowan E, Rockwood J, Melrose H, Nacharaju P, Van Slegtenhorst M, Gwinn-Hardy K, Murphy MP, Baker M, Yu X, Duff K, Hardy J, Corral A, Lin W-L, Yen S-H, Dickson DW, Davies P, Hutton M (2000) Neurofibrillary tangles, amyotrophy and progressive motor disturbance in mice expressing mutant (P301L) tau protein. Nat Genet 25:402–405. https://doi.org/10.1038/78078
12. Müller TJ, Kraya T, Stoltenburg-Didinger G, Hanisch F, Kornhuber M, Stoevesandt D, Senderek J, Weis J, Baum P, Deschauer M, Zierz S (2014) Phenotype of matrin-3-related distal myopathy in 16 German patients. Ann Neurol 76:669–680. https://doi.org/10.1002/ana.24255
13. Palmio J, Evilä A, Bashir A, Norwood F, Viitaniemi K, Vihola A, Huovinen S, Straub V, Hackman P, Hirano M, Bushby K, Udd B (2016) Re-evaluation of the phenotype

caused by the common MATR3 p.Ser85Cys mutation in a new family. J Neurol Neurosurg Psychiatry 87:448–450. https://doi.org/10.1136/jnnp-2014-309349
14. Quintero-Rivera F, Xi QJ, Keppler-Noreuil KM, Lee JH, Higgins AW, Anchan RM, Roberts AE, Seong IS, Fan X, Lage K, Lu LY, Tao J, Hu X, Berezney R, Gelb BD, Kamp A, Moskowitz IP, Lacro RV, Lu W, Morton CC, Gusella JF, Maas RL (2015) MATR3 disruption in human and mouse associated with bicuspid aortic valve, aortic coarctation and patent ductus arteriosus. Hum Mol Genet 24:2375–2389. https://doi.org/10.1093/hmg/ddv004
15. Rayaprolu S, D'Alton S, Crosby K, Moloney C, Howard J, Duffy C, Cabrera M, Siemienski Z, Hernandez AR, Gallego-Iradi C, Borchelt DR, Lewis J (2016) Heterogeneity of Matrin 3 in the developing and aging murine central nervous system. J Comp Neurol 524:2740–2752. https://doi.org/10.1002/cne.23986
16. Renton AE, Majounie E, Waite A, Simón-Sánchez J, Rollinson S, Gibbs JR, Schymick JC, Laaksovirta H, van Swieten JC, Myllykangas L, Kalimo H, Paetau A, Abramzon Y, Remes AM, Kaganovich A, Scholz SW, Duckworth J, Ding J, Harmer DW, Hernandez DG, Johnson JO, Mok K, Ryten M, Trabzuni D, Guerreiro RJ, Orrell RW, Neal J, Murray A, Pearson J, Jansen IE, Sondervan D, Seelaar H, Blake D, Young K, Halliwell N, Callister JB, Toulson G, Richardson A, Gerhard A, Snowden J, Mann D, Neary D, Nalls MA, Peuralinna T, Jansson L, Isoviita V-M, Kaivorinne A-L, Hölttä-Vuori M, Ikonen E, Sulkava R, Benatar M, Wuu J, Chiò A, Restagno G, Borghero G, Sabatelli M, Heckerman D, Rogaeva E, Zinman L, Rothstein JD, Sendtner M, Drepper C, Eichler EE, Alkan C, Abdullaev Z, Pack SD, Dutra A, Pak E, Hardy J, Singleton A, Williams NM, Heutink P, Pickering-Brown S, Morris HR, Tienari PJ, Traynor BJ (2011) A Hexanucleotide repeat expansion in C9ORF72 is the cause of chromosome 9p21-linked ALS-FTD. Neuron 72:257–268. https://doi.org/10.1016/j.neuron.2011.09.010
17. Rosen DR, Siddique T, Patterson D, Figlewicz DA, Sapp P, Hentati A, Donaldson D, Goto J, O'Regan JP, Deng H-X, Rahmani Z, Krizus A, McKenna-Yasek D, Cayabyab A, Gaston SM, Berger R, Tanzi RE, Halperin JJ, Herzfeldt B, Van den Bergh R, Hung W-Y, Bird T, Deng G, Mulder DW, Smyth C, Laing NG, Soriano E, MA P–V, Haines J, Rouleau GA, Gusella JS, Horvitz HR, Brown RH (1993) Mutations in cu/Zn superoxide dismutase gene are associated with familial amyotrophic lateral sclerosis. Nature 362:59–62. https://doi.org/10.1038/362059a0
18. Rowland LP, Shneider NA (2001) Amyotrophic lateral sclerosis. N Engl J Med 344:1688–1700. https://doi.org/10.1056/NEJM200105313442207
19. Senderek J, Garvey SM, Krieger M, Guergueltcheva V, Urtizberea A, Roos A, Elbracht M, Stendel C, Tournev I, Mihailova V, Feit H, Tramonte J, Hedera P, Crooks K, Bergmann C, Rudnik-Schöneborn S, Zerres K, Lochmüller H, Seboun E, Weis J, Beckmann JS, Hauser MA, Jackson CE (2009) Autosomal-dominant distal myopathy associated with a recurrent missense mutation in the gene encoding the nuclear matrix protein, Matrin 3. Am J Hum Genet 84:511–518. https://doi.org/10.1016/j.ajhg.2009.03.006
20. Smith KR, Damiano J, Franceschetti S, Carpenter S, Canafoglia L, Morbin M, Rossi G, Pareyson D, Mole SE, Staropoli JF, Sims KB, Lewis J, Lin WL, Dickson DW, Dahl HH, Bahlo M, Berkovic SF (2012) Strikingly different clinicopathological phenotypes determined by progranulin-mutation dosage. Am J Hum Genet 90:1102–1107. https://doi.org/10.1016/j.ajhg.2012.04.021
21. Sreedharan J, Blair IP, Tripathi VB, Hu X, Vance C, Rogelj B, Ackerley S, Durnall JC, Williams KL, Buratti E, Baralle F, de Belleroche J, Mitchell JD, Leigh PN, Al-Chalabi A, Miller CC, Nicholson G, Shaw CE (2008) TDP-43 mutations in familial and sporadic amyotrophic lateral sclerosis. Science (80- ) 319:1668–1672. https://doi.org/10.1126/science.1154584
22. Vance C, Rogelj B, Hortobagyi T, De Vos KJ, Nishimura AL, Sreedharan J, Hu X, Smith B, Ruddy D, Wright P, Ganesalingam J, Williams KL, Tripathi V, Al-Saraj S, Al-Chalabi A, Leigh PN, Blair IP, Nicholson G, de Belleroche J, Gallo J-M, Miller CC, Shaw CE (2009) Mutations in FUS, an RNA processing protein, cause familial amyotrophic lateral sclerosis type 6. Science (80- ) 323:1208–1211. https://doi.org/10.1126/science.1165942
23. Watts GDJ, Wymer J, Kovach MJ, Mehta SG, Mumm S, Darvish D, Pestronk A, Whyte MP, Kimonis VE (2004) Inclusion body myopathy associated with Paget disease of bone and frontotemporal dementia is caused by mutant valosin-containing protein. Nat Genet 36:377–381. https://doi.org/10.1038/ng1332
24. Xu Y-F, Gendron TF, Zhang Y-J, Lin W-L, D'Alton S, Sheng H, Casey MC, Tong J, Knight J, Yu X, Rademakers R, Boylan K, Hutton M, McGowan E, Dickson DW, Lewis J, Petrucelli L (2010) Wild-type human TDP-43 expression causes TDP-43 phosphorylation, mitochondrial aggregation, motor deficits, and early mortality in transgenic mice. J Neurosci 30:10851–10859. https://doi.org/10.1523/JNEUROSCI.1630-10.2010
25. Xu Y-F, Zhang Y-J, Lin W-L, Cao X, Stetler C, Dickson DW, Lewis J, Petrucelli L (2011) Expression of mutant TDP-43 induces neuronal dysfunction in transgenic mice. Mol Neurodegener 6:73. https://doi.org/10.1186/1750-1326-6-73
26. Yamashita S, Mori A, Nishida Y, Kurisaki R, Tawara N, Nishikami T, Misumi Y, Ueyama H, Imamura S, Higuchi Y, Hashiguchi A, Higuchi I, Morishita S, Yoshimura J, Uchino M, Takashima H, Tsuji S, Ando Y (2015) Clinicopathological features of the first Asian family having vocal cord and pharyngeal weakness with distal myopathy due to a MATR3 mutation. Neuropathol Appl Neurobiol 41:391–398. https://doi.org/10.1111/nan.12179
27. Yokoseki A, Shiga A, Tan C-F, Tagawa A, Kaneko H, Koyama A, Eguchi H, Tsujino A, Ikeuchi T, Kakita A, Okamoto K, Nishizawa M, Takahashi H, Onodera O (2008) TDP - 43 mutation in familial amyotrophic lateral sclerosis. Ann Neurol 63:538–542. https://doi.org/10.1002/ana.21392

# 7

# Clinical significance of polyglutamylation in primary central nervous system lymphoma

Naoki Shinojima[1*†], Kenji Fujimoto[1†], Keishi Makino[1], Kohei Todaka[2], Kazumichi Yamada[1], Yoshiki Mikami[3], Kazutaka Oda[4], Kazumi Nakamura[4], Hirofumi Jono[4], Jun-ichi Kuratsu[1,5], Hideo Nakamura[1], Shigetoshi Yano[1] and Akitake Mukasa[1]

**Abstract**

The therapeutic response to high-dose methotrexate (HD-MTX) therapy for primary central nervous system lymphoma (PCNSL) varies. Polyglutamylation is a reversible protein modification with a high occurrence rate in tumor cells. MTX incorporated into cells is polyglutamylated and strongly binds to dihydrofolate reductase without competitive inhibition by leucovorin (LV). Tumor cells with high polyglutamylation levels are selectively killed, whereas normal cells with lower polyglutamylation are rescued by LV. We hypothesized that the extent of polyglutamylation in tumor cells determines treatment resistance. Here, we investigated the therapeutic response of PCNSL to HD-MTX therapy with LV rescue based on polyglutamylation status. Among 113 consecutive PCNSL patients who underwent HD-MTX therapy in our department between 2001 and 2014, polyglutamylation was evaluated by immunostaining in 82 cases, with relationships between polyglutamylation and therapeutic response retrospectively examined. Human malignant lymphoma lines were used for in vitro experiments, and folpolyglutamate synthetase (FPGS), which induces polyglutamylation, was knocked down with short-hairpin RNA, and a stable cell line with a low rate of polyglutamylation was established. Cell viability after MTX treatment with LV rescue was evaluated using sodium butyrate (NaBu), a histone-deacetylase inhibitor that induces polyglutamylation by elevating FPGS expression. The complete response rate was significantly higher in the group with polyglutamylation than in the non-polyglutamylation group [58.1% (25/43) and 33.3% (13/39), respectively] ($p < 0.05$), and progression-free survival was also significantly increased in the group with polyglutamylation ($p < 0.01$). In vitro, the relief effect of LV after MTX administration was significantly enhanced after FPGS knockdown in al cell lines, whereas enhancement of FPGS expression by NaBu treatment significantly reduced this relief effect. These findings suggested that polyglutamylation could be a predictor of therapeutic response to HD-MTX therapy with LV rescue in PCNSL. Combination therapy with HD-MTX and polyglutamylation-inducing agents might represent a promising strategy for PCNSL treatment.

**Keywords:** Polyglutamylation, Methotrexate, Primary central nervous system lymphoma, Leucovorin rescue

## Introduction

The standard treatment for primary central nervous system lymphoma (PCNSL) is high-dose methotrexate (HD-MTX)-based chemo-radiotherapies with leucovorin (LV) rescue [10, 16, 27]. The median overall survival of patients with PCNSL who undergo HD-MTX-based therapies is ~40 months [16, 27]; however, the therapeutic response to HD-MTX therapies varies in patients with PCNSL, with some cases showing poor therapeutic response or recurrence [21]. The established prognostic factors for therapeutic response to HD-MTX and for survival in PCNSL are age and performance status [2, 9], whereas no predictors have been identified for molecules supposedly targeted in this therapy. Polyglutamylation is a reversible post-translational modification of proteins that is thought to be involved in the stabilization of proteins, such as microtubules [7]. In contrast to normal cells, tumor cells show frequent occurrence of polyglutamylation [23]. Once the MTX

* Correspondence: nshinojima-kuh@umin.ac.jp
†Equal contributors
[1]Department of Neurosurgery, Kumamoto University Hospital, 1-1-1 Honjo Chuo-ku, Kumamoto 860-8556, Japan
Full list of author information is available at the end of the article

transported into the tumor cells is polyglutamylated, it is retained and strongly binds to dihydrofolate reductase (DHFR) in a process that is not subject to competitive inhibition by LV, resulting in long-lasting inhibition of thymidylate synthase [14, 22, 24]. Therefore, MTX treatment can selectively kill cancer cells in which polyglutamylation has occurred, whereas normal cells with lower levels of polyglutamylation are rescued with LV [8]. In this context, we hypothesized that the therapeutic response to HD-MTX therapy with LV rescue is dependent upon the extent of polyglutamylation in PCNSL. This study investigated whether the extent of polyglutamylation could predict the response to HD-MTX therapy in patients with PCNSL. To the best of our knowledge, this is the first study revealing that polyglutamylation could be a significant predictor of the therapeutic response to HD-MTX therapy with LV rescue in PCNSL.

## Materials and methods

### For clinical investigation

#### *Patients*

After screening to rule out systemic lymphoma by positron emission tomography (PET) or whole-body computed tomography (CT), the patients with preoperative diagnosis of PCNSL exclusively located within the CNS underwent biopsy at our department. After confirming the histological diagnosis of PCNSL based on criteria published by the World Health Organization [20], HD-MTX therapy was conducted between January 2001 and December 2014 at our institute and affiliated hospitals according to our PCNSL protocol (Fig. 1). Paraffin-embedded tissues were obtained from 82 of the 113 patients who were newly evaluated with consecutive immunocompetent PCNSL. Under the approval for genetic and molecular analysis using patient specimens by the Research Ethics Committee of the Institutional Review Board of Kumamoto University Hospital [30, 32], this study was conducted after obtaining written informed consent from all participating patients or their family members.

#### *PCNSL protocol*

HD-MTX-based chemotherapy with LV rescue was performed according to our previously reported protocol [21]. Induction therapy consisted of a cycle of high-dose MTX (3.5 g/m$^2$) delivered intravenously over 3 h on days 1, 22, and 43. LV rescue was initiated 24 h after the start of MTX infusion, and 15 mg of LV was intravenously administered nine times every 3 h, followed by five times every 6 h. The repeated intravenous administration of LV was continued until MTX clearance (< 0.1 μM). Procarbazine (60 mg/m$^2$) was administered orally on days 1 through 7, 22 through 28, and 43 through 49. The initial betamethasone treatment dose was

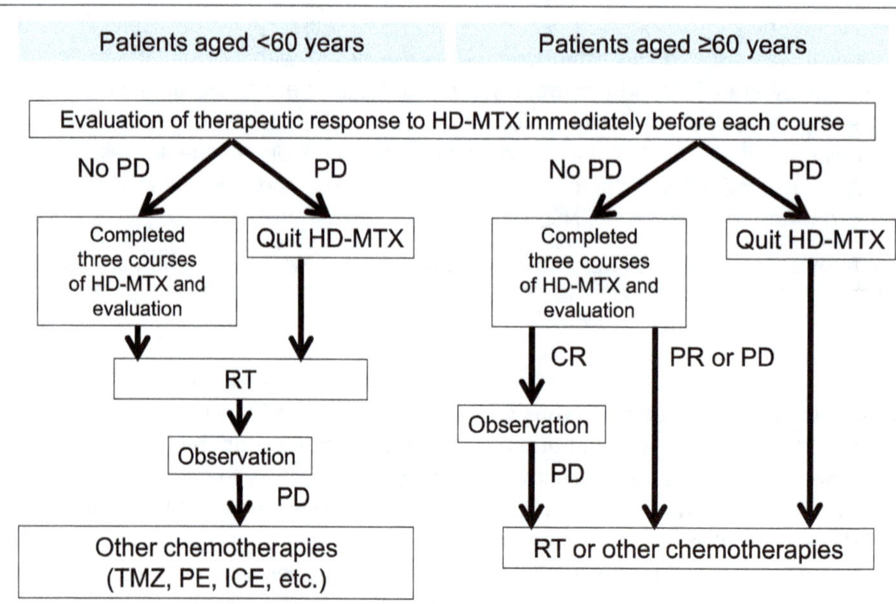


**Fig. 1** The PCNSL protocol used at our institute. A course of HD-MTX-based chemotherapy with LV rescue was administered every 3 weeks, with three such courses performed. Patients with PCNSL aged < 60 years were supposed to undergo RT from 4 weeks after the completion of three courses of HD-MTX treatment. Patients aged ≥60 years were monitored for CR to the therapy during follow-up evaluation after completion of the three courses. Alternatively, they underwent RT or other chemotherapies, such as temozolomide (TMZ), ICE (ifosphamide, cisplatin, and etoposide), or PE (carboplatin and etoposide). If PD occurred before the three courses of HD-MTX were completed, patients aged < 60 years underwent RT, whereas patients aged ≥60 years underwent RT or other chemotherapies. Second-line treatments were not uniform in cases of recurrence after HD-MTX therapies with or without RT. Patients who showed recurrence underwent TMZ, ICE, and PE treatment

tapered from 16 mg to 2 mg every 4 days. The first-line therapy did not include any rituximab therapy. One course was administered every 3 weeks, and three such courses were performed (Fig. 1). Patients with PCNSL and aged < 60 years were supposed to undergo radiotherapy (RT) from 4 weeks after the completion of three courses of HD-MTX therapy. By contrast, patients aged ≥60 years were monitored for complete response (CR) to the therapy during follow-up evaluation after completion of the three courses. Alternatively, they underwent RT or other chemotherapies. If the progressive disease (PD) occurred before the three courses of HD-MTX were completed, patients aged < 60 years underwent RT, whereas those aged ≥60 years underwent RT or other chemotherapies. The second-line therapy was not uniform in cases of recurrence after completing HD-MTX therapies with or without RT.

#### *Evaluation of therapeutic response to HD-MTX*

The therapeutic response to HD-MTX was evaluated using CT or magnetic resonance imaging (MRI), with contrast-enhancement according to the response criteria published by the International PCNSL Collaborative Group [1]. Evaluation of the therapeutic response to HD-MTX was performed just before the initiation of each course of HD-MTX, 3 weeks after the completion of the three courses, and during the follow-up period. We evaluated all patients every 3 months for the first 2 years and every 6 months thereafter. CR was assumed in cases of both CR and unconfirmed CR (CRu). For patients unable to complete the three courses of HD-MTX due to adverse events associated with MTX, MRI data obtained after the final HD-MTX treatment was used for the evaluation.

#### *Immunohistochemistry (IHC)*

IHC was performed on formalin-fixed paraffin-embedded (FFPE) tumor specimens with validation of positive and negative controls according to our previously reported protocol [29, 31]. The antibodies for polyglutamylation (mouse monoclonal; GT335; AdipoGen AG, Liestal, Switzerland) were used at 1:2000 dilution. A glioblastoma (GBM) specimen was used as a positive control for polyglutamylation, and specimens of meningioma and pituitary adenoma were used as negative controls, as was a GBM specimen without primary antibody treatment (Fig. 2a). Polyglutamylation positivity was quantified by manual counting. The antibodies for CD20 (rabbit monoclonal; SP32; Spring Bioscience, Pleasanton, CA, USA), a common B cell lymphoma marker, were used at 1:100 dilution. To classify the cell of origin of diffuse large B cell lymphoma into the germinal center B-cell-like (GCB) or non-GCB group using the algorithm established by Hans et al. [15], antibodies against the following proteins were used: CD10 (mouse monoclonal; 56C6; Leica Biosystems Newcastle Ltd., UK) at 1:25 dilution, Bcl-6 (mouse monoclonal; LN22; Leica Biosystems Newcastle Ltd., UK) at 1:100 dilution, and MUM1 (mouse monoclonal; MUM1p; Dako Cytomation, Glostrup Denmark) at 1:50 dilution.

#### *Immunofluorescence of tissue sections*

Multicolored immunofluorescence using different primary antibodies for polyglutamylation (AdipoGen) and CD20 (Spring Bioscience) was performed as reported previously [29]. To subtract the autofluorescence in FFPE tumor specimens, a Mantra system was used (PerkinElmer, Waltham, MA, USA) [25].

#### *Area under the concentration-time curve of MTX ($AUC_{MTX}$)*

According to population pharmacokinetic analysis using the nonlinear mixed-effects modeling program (NONMEM, version 7.3.0) [17], we examined $AUC_{MTX}$ in 67 patients with PCNSL whose plasma MTX concentrations were available. We also assessed the correlation between clinical response and $AUC_{MTX}$ according to polyglutamylation status.

### Survival analysis

As previously reported [21], overall survival (OS) was measured as the time from initial diagnosis to death from any cause, and progression-free survival (PFS) as the time from diagnosis to the first PD. Cases in which extracranial lesions were found by PET or contrast-enhanced CT after treatment were also considered PD. Patients whose day of death was uncertain and patients who were alive on the day of analysis were censored, with the time from the first diagnosis to the last physical interaction or clinic visit used as the censoring time. Patients whose day of PD was uncertain and patients without PD on the day of analysis were censored with the time from diagnosis to that of the last MRI/CT showing a response. We investigated whether polyglutamylation could be a predictor of OS and PFS using Kaplan-Meier survival curves and multivariate analysis. For survival analyses, we used the log-rank test to compare the Kaplan-Meier curves for OS or PFS in patients who did and did not manifest polyglutamylation. To estimate the treatment response to MTX, we applied the Cox proportional-hazards model. Univariate analysis was used to estimate the prognostic relevance of polyglutamylation status, a predictive marker for HD-MTX treatment, and of patient age, sex, preoperative Karnofsky performance status (KPS), MSKCC prognostic scoring [2], cell of origin (GCB vs non-GCB) [15], lactate dehydrogenase (LDH) levels, and tumor location, in which the tumors were divided into deep (corpus callosum, basal ganglia, brain stem, and cerebellum) or non-deep location included in the International Extranodal Lymphoma Study

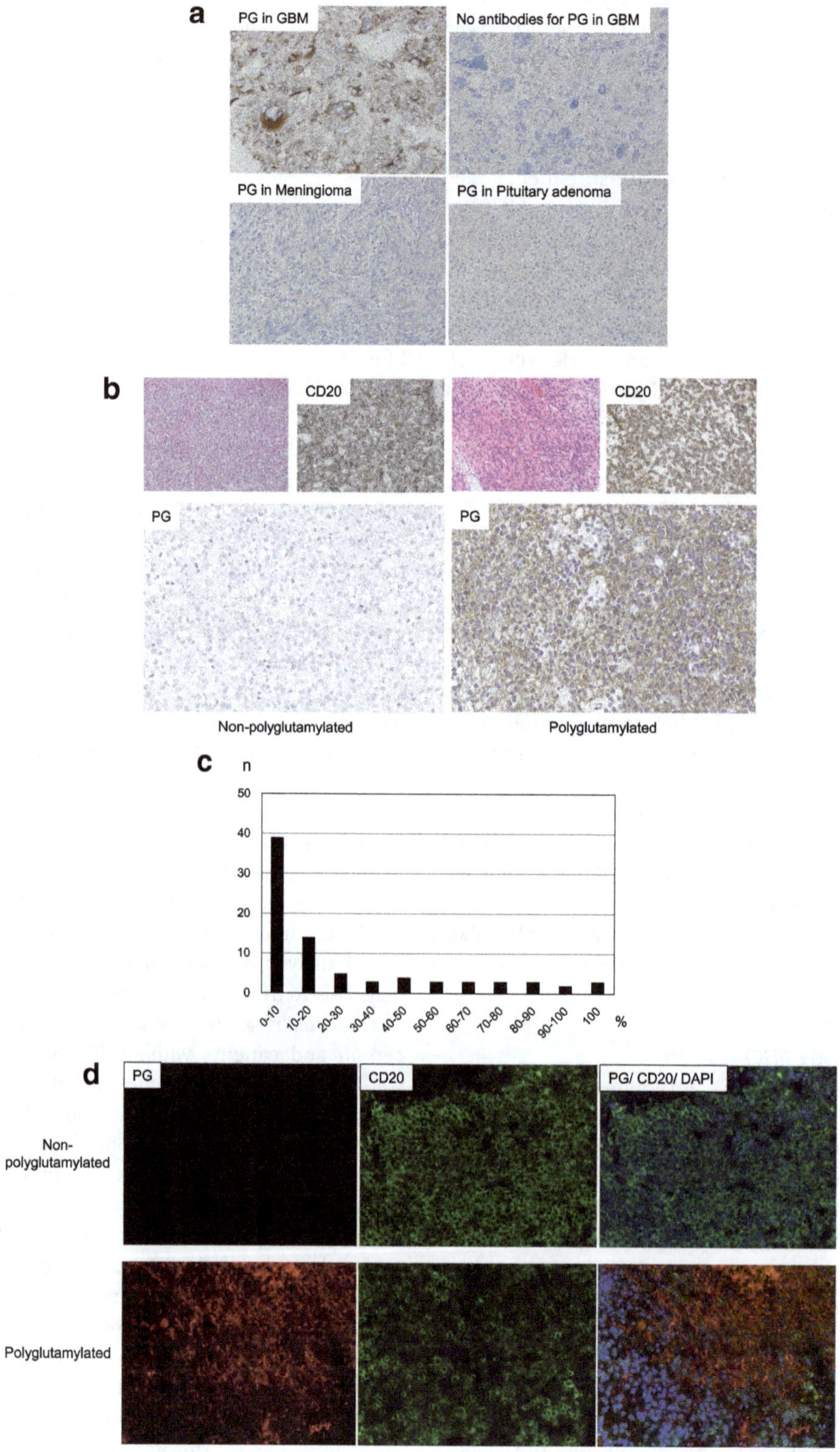


**Fig. 2** (See legend on next page.)

(See figure on previous page.)
**Fig. 2** Representative figures of IHC for polyglutamylation. **a** GBM specimen used as positive control and stained for polyglutamylation (PG). Specimens of meningioma and pituitary adenoma, and the GBM specimen without primary antibodies were used as negative controls, revealing no staining for PG. Magnification, 200×. **b** Each subset of panels (left and right) shows polyglutamylated and non- polyglutamylated tumor specimens, respectively. The left upper panels are stained with hematoxylin and eosin, and the right upper panels show IHC results for CD20. Magnification, 200×. The bottom panels show IHC results for PG. Magnification, 400×. **c** Histogram showing the percentage of stained cells (10% cut-off). **d** Each subset of panels (upper and lower) shows polyglutamylated and non-polyglutamylated tumor specimens, respectively. Multiple-fluorescence staining using two different antibodies was performed. PG (red; left), CD20 (green; middle), and the merged fluorescence image (right), including DAPI (blue). After subtraction of background of autofluorescence, double-positive staining for both PG and CD20 revealed cytoplasm with a yellow-to-orange color as a result of overlapping fluorescence in the merged image in the polyglutamylated group. The red-fluorescent region (lower right) in the merged image of the polyglutamylated tumor specimens was considered brain parenchyma

Group score [9]. The variables were included in the Cox model and subjected to multivariate analysis.

### For experimental investigation

#### *Cell lines*

Human lymphoma cell lines, namely, HKBML, a human PCNSL-derived cell line; RAJI, a Burkkit lymphoma cell line; and TL-1, a lymph node B-lymphoma cell line, were purchased from RIKEN BioResource Center (Tsukuba, Japan). These floating cells were maintained as previously reported [26].

#### Knockdown of folpolyglutamate synthetase (FPGS) in lymphoma cells

FPGS induces the accumulation of high levels of MTX polyglutamates in childhood leukemia [28]. To decrease this accumulation in lymphoma cell lines, we established stable, genetically modified cell lines in which FPGS was knocked down by a lentivirus system. Lentiviruses were prepared as reported previously [29]. PMD2.G (envelope vector) and psPAX2 (packaging vector) were purchased from Addgene (Cambridge, MA). FPGS-specific short-hairpin (sh)RNA constructs in pLKO.1 vectors were also obtained from Dharmacon (Lafayette, CO, USA), and an empty vector was used as a scrambled-sequence control. Cells were selected and maintained with puromycin (0.5–1 μg/mL).

#### Cell viability assay

We used the Cell Counting Kit-8 (Dojindo Molecular Technologies, Inc., Kumamoto, Japan) to evaluate cell viability after individual treatment, as previously reported [3, 4]. Cells were treated with 100 nM MTX (Wako Pure Chemical Industries, Ltd., Osaka, Japan) for 24 h, followed by the addition of LV (Pfizer Japan, Inc., Tokyo, Japan) at a final concentration of 3 μg/mL and culturing for an additional 24 h. Cell viability assay was performed 48 h later. Histone-deacetylase inhibitors (HDACIs) enhance the antitumor effect of MTX by up-regulating FPGS expression, thereby causing intracellular accumulation of long-chain MTX polyglutamates in childhood acute lymphoblastic leukemia (ALL) [19]. Sodium butyrate (NaBu; Sigma-Aldrich, St Louis, MO, USA), a pan-HDACI, was used in this study. Lymphoma cell lines were treated with 100 nM MTX with or without 1 mM NaBu for 24 h prior to the addition of LV. Cell viability was assessed 48 h later.

#### Western blot

Western blot was performed as previously described [29]. The primary antibodies used were anti-FPGS (1:1000; rabbit polyclonal; Spring Bioscience), anti-DHFR (1:10,000; rabbit monoclonal; EPR5285; Abcam, Cambridge, MA, USA), and anti-α-tubulin (1:5000; mouse monoclonal; Sigma-Aldrich).

#### Immunofluorescence of lymphoma cells

Lymphoma cells were collected, attached to glass slides using the cytospin method, and processed for immunofluorescence as previously reported [4, 29]. To evaluate polyglutamylation levels in cells, anti-polyglutamylation antibodies (AdipoGen) were used at 1:2000 dilution. 4′,6-Diamidino-2-phenylindole (DAPI; FluoroPure grade; Thermo Fisher Scientific, Waltham, MA, USA) was used for counterstaining.

#### Statistical analyses

Statistical differences were assessed by Mann-Whitney U test, chi-squared test, log-rank test, and Student's t test. Differences were determined to be statistically significant if $p < 0.05$. The data were represented as the mean ± standard deviation (SD) of at least three replicates for each experiment. The Statistical Package for the Social Sciences (SPSS version 19; IBM corp., Armonk, NY, USA) was used for all statistical analyses.

## Results

### Clinical investigation

Among 113 consecutive patients with PCNSL, sufficient tissue specimens were available from only 82 patients. There were no differences in the clinical characteristics of these 82 patients or the remaining 31 patients (data not shown). The 82 patients comprised 46 males and 36 females, with a median age of 67 years. The median KPS was 40 (range, 20–100). The rate of CR to HD-MTX was 46.4%, and median OS was 1275 days (~ 42.5 months).

Five patients who responded to HD-MTX therapy switched to RT before completing three courses of HD-MTX because HD-MTX caused adverse events. Six patients who showed new extracranial lesions after treatments were considered PD, although they showed no intracranial lesions. Two patients died due to adverse events associated with HD-MTX, such as hemophagocytic syndrome and interstitial pneumonia. One of them was a responder, as evidenced by MRI results, and was censored regarding PFS.

Representative figures of IHC for polyglutamylation are shown in Fig. 2b. The histogram categorizing the percentage of cells stained for polyglutamylation into every 10% is shown in Fig. 2c. In the specimens of 30 patients, 0% of the cells were stained, whereas 0.5 to 2.5% of the cells were stained in the specimens of 9 patients. In the specimens of the other 43 patients, ≥10% (the average was 45%, range was 10–100%) of the cells were stained. Next, we examined the distribution of patients with CR and non CR at different cut-off values for positivity of polyglutamylation (Table 1). There was a correlation between therapeutic response to HD-MTX and polyglutamylation positivity at 10% cut-off. We defined the polyglutamylation group as having ≥10% positivity and the non-polyglutamylation group as having < 10% positivity in this study. Because the brain parenchyma could contribute to the observed polyglutamylation staining, we utilized a multiple-fluorescence system using two different antibodies for polyglutamylation and CD20 in a subset of samples from 6 patients (one was non-polyglutamylation, 5 were polyglutamylation group). After subtraction of the autofluorescent background, double-positive stained cells for both polyglutamylation and CD20 (exhibiting cytoplasm with a yellow-to-orange color as a result of overlapping fluorescence in the merged fluorescent image) were observed in the polyglutamylated group (Fig. 2d). These results confirmed that the CD20-positive lymphoma cells had a high level of polyglutamylation in the samples from the polyglutamylation group (Fig. 2d).

**Table 1** Distribution of patients with CR and non CR at different cut-off values of polyglutamylation percentage

| | CR | No CR | *p* |
|---|---|---|---|
| 1% of cut-off value | | | |
| Polyglutamylation, ≧ 1% ($n = 48$) | 26 | 22 | |
| Non polyglutamylation, < 1% ($n = 34$) | 12 | 22 | 0.091[a] |
| 10% of cut-off value | | | |
| Polyglutamylation, ≧ 10% ($n = 43$) | 25 | 18 | |
| Non polyglutamylation, < 10% ($n = 39$) | 13 | 26 | 0.025[a] |
| 20% of cut-off value | | | |
| Polyglutamylation, ≧ 20% ($n = 28$) | 16 | 12 | |
| Non polyglutamylation, < 20% ($n = 54$) | 22 | 32 | 0.16[a] |
| 30% of cut-off value | | | |
| Polyglutamylation, ≧ 30% ($n = 24$) | 13 | 11 | |
| Non polyglutamylation, < 30% ($n = 58$) | 25 | 33 | 0.36[a] |

*CR* complete response
[a]Chi-squared test

The number of patients with CR, CRu, PR, and PD was seven, 18, five, and 13, respectively, in the polyglutamylation group and five, eight, seven, and 19, respectively, in the non-polyglutamylation group. The rate of GCB was 41.5% in the polyglutamylation group, which was significantly higher ($p < 0.05$) than that (17.9%) in the non-polyglutamylation group (Table 2).

The median PFS was 560 days in the polyglutamylation group and 95 days in the non-polyglutamylation group. Kaplan-Meier curves confirmed that PFS was significantly longer in the polyglutamylation group than in the non-polyglutamylation group ($p < 0.01$; Fig. 3a), whereas there was no difference in OS between the two groups (Fig. 3b). Multivariate analyses confirmed that polyglutamylation status was the only significant independent predictor for PFS ($p < 0.01$; Table 3), although it was not a prognostic factor for OS (Table 4). We then determined the prognostic value in patients with PCNSL aged < 60 years, because they had received similar treatments, i.e., RT following HD-MTX, as part of their first-line therapy with or without PD other than older patients. Similarly, PFS was significantly longer in the polyglutamylation group relative to the non-polyglutamylation group in patients aged < 60 years ($p < 0.01$; Fig. 3c). Moreover, we found a tendency toward a better median OS in the polyglutamylation group as compared with that in the non-polyglutamylation group for patients aged < 60 years ($p = 0.079$; Fig. 3d). These results suggest that the polyglutamylation status in PCNSL tissues could be a predictor of therapeutic response to HD-MTX.

#### Correlation of clinical response between polyglutamylation status and $AUC_{MTX}$

In the non-polyglutamylation group, 33.3% (13/39) of the patients had CR (Table 1). The MTX concentrations might be an underlying factor associated with the observed differences in clinical response, as $AUC_{MTX}$ is an important outcome predictor [18]. We examined the correlation between clinical response and the $AUC_{MTX}$ in 67 patients whose plasma MTX concentrations were available. The average $AUC_{MTX}$ was 1705.7 (range, 1074.2–5754.2) μmol/L/h in the 67 patients, and there was a tendency toward the average $AUC_{MTX}$ being higher in patients having CR as compared with those with no CR (1748.8 μmol/L/h vs.1568.3 μmol/L/h, respectively; $p = 0.091$; Fig. 3e) in the non-polyglutamylation group. However, in the polyglutamylation group, there was no correlation in

**Table 2** Clinical characteristics of patients based on polyglutamylation status

| | Polyglutamylation ($n = 43$) | Non polyglutamylation ($n = 39$) | $p$ |
|---|---|---|---|
| Age (y) | | | |
| Median (range) | 68 (37–84) | 67 (46–86) | 0.70* |
| Sex (# of pts) | | | |
| Male/ Female | 27/ 16 | 19/ 20 | 0.20** |
| KPS (%) | | | |
| Median (range) | 50 (20–100) | 40 (20–100) | 0.43* |
| (# of pts) High (≥70) / Low (≤60) | 12/ 31 | 10/ 29 | 0.82** |
| MSKCC prognostic score | | | |
| Median (range) | 3 (1–3) | 3 (1–3) | 0.76* |
| Cell of origin | | | |
| GCB/ non-GCB | 17/ 24[a] | 7/ 32 | 0.022** |
| LDH (# of pts) | | | |
| High/ Normal range | 16/ 27 | 15/ 24 | 0.91** |
| Location (# of pts) | | | |
| Deep/ No | 35/ 8 | 27/ 12 | 0.20** |

*KPS* Karnofsky performance status, *pts.* patients
* Mann-Whitney *U* test
** Chi-squared test
[a] data from two patients were not available

average $AUC_{MTX}$ between patients having CR and those having no CR (1863.4 μmol/L/h vs 1694.1 μmol/L/h, respectively; $p = 0.54$; Fig. 3e). This result might explain why one third of the patients showed CR in the non-polyglutamylation group.

**Experimental investigation**

To confirm the clinical results, we performed an in vitro study. To prevent the accumulation of polyglutamylation in lymphoma cells, we established a stable cell line in which FPGS was knocked down using shRNA constructs. Western blot results showed that FPGS expression was decreased in all cell lines treated with shRNA construct #3 (shFPGS#3), even after NaBu treatment, as compared with scrambled-sequence control cells (Fig. 4a). We used cell lines in which FPGS was knocked down by shFPGS#3 for all subsequent analyses and used immunofluorescence to confirm decreased polyglutamylation in FPGS-knockdown cells. The immunofluorescence level of polyglutamylation in the cytoplasm of FPGS-knockdown cells was lower than that in scrambled-sequence control cells (Fig. 4b). We then examined cell viability after MTX treatment and LV rescue. In HKBML and TL-1 cells, MTX-treated scrambled-sequence control cells were rescued by LV to the same level as control cells without treatment. However, the relief effect of LV after MTX treatment was significantly enhanced in cells exhibiting lower polyglutamylation levels by FPGS knockdown as compared with that in scrambled-sequence control cells (Fig. 4c). In RAJI cells after MTX and LV treatment, the viability of scramble control cells was significantly lower than that of controls without treatment. Additionally, the viability of cells in which FPGS was knocked down was restored to levels similar to that of controls without treatment. These results suggested that lymphoma cells with low levels of polyglutamylation were resistant to HD-MTX therapy with LV rescue. Although the tight binding of polyglutamylated MTX to DHFR is not subject to competitive inhibition by LV, resulting in long-lasting inhibition of DHFR [14, 22, 24], it is possible that DHFR expression is related to polyglutamylation levels in cells. We evaluated the expression of DHFR in control cells and in FPGS-knockdown cells, finding no difference in DHFR expression (Fig. 4d). Therefore, these findings suggest that DHFR activity might be regulated by polyglutamylated MTX.

HDACIs upregulate FPGS, causing intracellular accumulation of long-chain MTX polyglutamates and increasing the efficiency of MTX therapy with LV rescue in childhood ALL [19]. Here, we examined whether HDACIs could enhance the antitumor effect of MTX with LV rescue in lymphoma cells using NaBu. FPGS expression was upregulated by NaBu treatment in a concentration- and time-dependent manner (Fig. 5a), and the relief effect of LV after MTX treatment was significantly reduced after NaBu treatment, resulting in an increased antitumor effect (Fig. 5b). Therefore, combination therapy involving HDACIs and HD-MTX with LV rescue might be

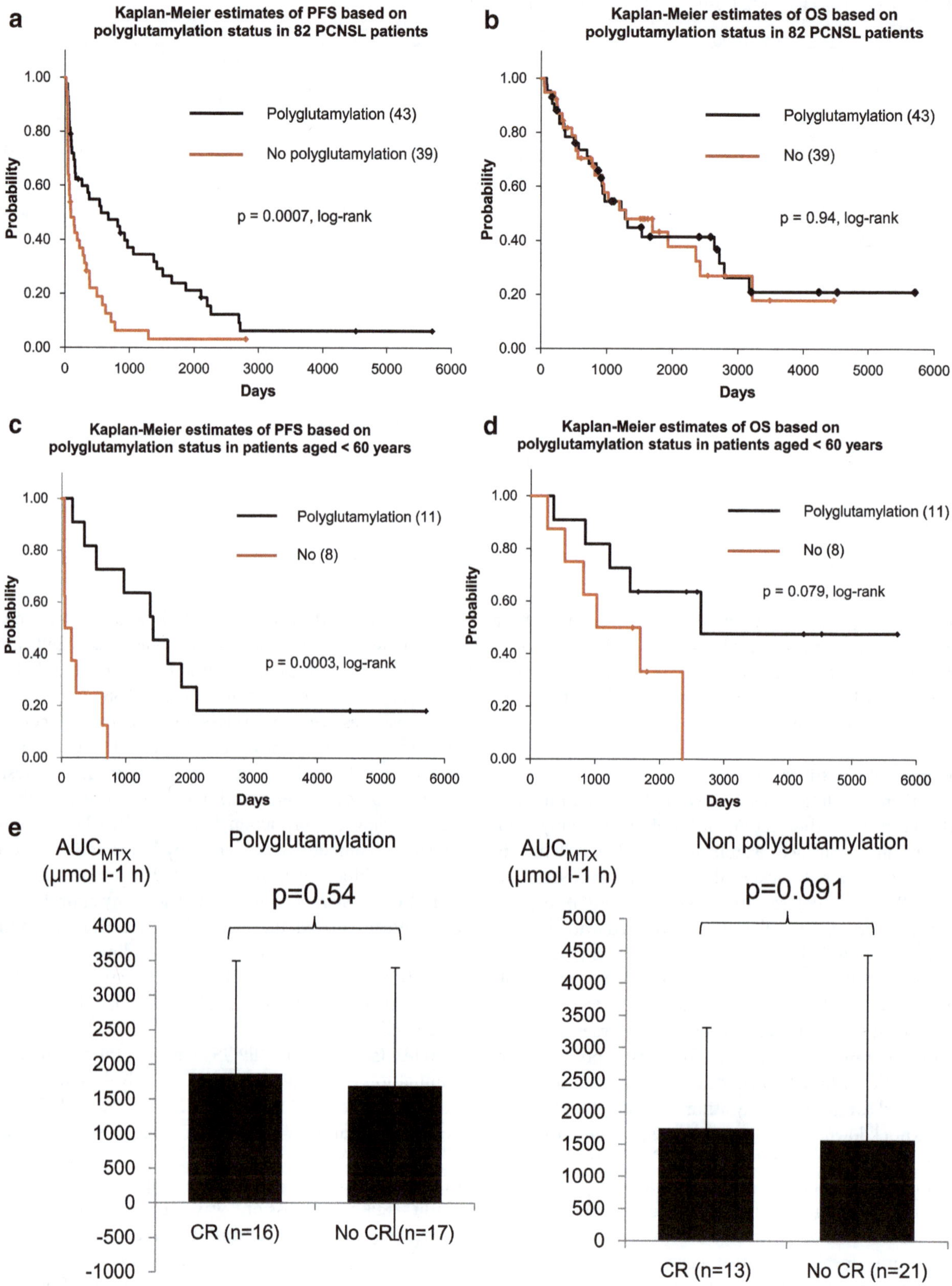


**Fig. 3** Kaplan-Meier curves of (**a**) PFS and (**b**) OS based on polyglutamylation status in 82 PCNSL patients. **c** PFS and (**d**) OS based on polyglutamylation status in 19 PCNSL patients aged < 60 years. **e** Correlation between clinical response and $AUC_{MTX}$ according to polyglutamylation status

**Table 3** Cox proportional hazard model for PFS

| | Univariate analysis | | Multivariate analysis | |
|---|---|---|---|---|
| Variable | HR (95% CI) | *p* | HR (95% CI) | *p* |
| Age | 1.015 (0.995–1.036) | 0.14 | 1.005 (0.972–1.038) | 0.79 |
| KPS (high vs. low) | 1.328 (0.784–2.250) | 0.29 | 0.717 (0.340–1.513) | 0.38 |
| Sex (M vs. F) | 1.531 (0.953–2.457) | 0.078 | 1.445 (0.820–2.545) | 0.20 |
| MSKCC score | 1.151 (0.819–1.619) | 0.42 | 0.782 (0.410–1.491) | 0.46 |
| Cell of origin (GCB vs. non-GCB) | 0.696 (0.407–1.191) | 0.19 | 1.086 (0.576–2.048) | 0.80 |
| LDH (high vs. normal range) | 1.306 (0.801–2.129) | 0.29 | 1.532 (0.860–2.731) | 0.15 |
| Location (deep vs. not deep) | 0.928 (0.531–1.622) | 0.79 | 1.377 (0.732–2.587) | 0.32 |
| Polyglutamylation vs. non-polyglutamylation | 0.439 (0.269–0.716) | 0.0010 | 0.461 (0.259–0.823) | 0.0087 |

*PFS* progression-free survival, *HR* hazard ratio, *CI* confidence interval, *KPS* Karnofsky performance status, *M* male, *F* female

more effective for patients with PCNSL via the FPGS/polyglutamate axis.

## Discussion

HD-MTX-based therapy with LV rescue is established as the standard treatment method for patients with PCNSL [10, 16, 27]. The therapeutic response to HD-MTX therapy varies, and no predictors for therapeutic response or survival have been identified in patients with PCNSL. MTX treatment with LV rescue can selectively kill tumor cells harboring high levels of polyglutamylation, whereas healthy cells with lower levels of polyglutamylation are rescued by LV [8]. We hypothesized that the therapeutic response to HD-MTX therapy with LV rescue depends upon the extent of polyglutamylation in PCNSL. We found that polyglutamylation is indeed a significant predictor of the response to HD-MTX therapy in patients with PCNSL. Additionally, our in vitro studies confirmed that the therapeutic response to HD-MTX treatment with LV rescue was dependent upon the extent of polyglutamylation in lymphoma cell lines, which was consistent with our clinical results. To the best of our knowledge, there have been no studies evaluating the correlation between therapeutic response and polyglutamylation in PCNSL. In other types of malignant neoplasms, high levels of MTX polyglutamylation (for example, in pediatric ALL, such as pediatric B cell lineage ALL) are correlated with therapeutic response, with pediatric B cell lineage ALL showing higher cure rates as compared with adult ALL and T cell lineage ALL [11]. The mechanism of resistance to MTX in leukemia possibly involves decreased uptake of the drug or lack of drug retention due mainly to low levels of polyglutamylation, increased polyglutamate breakdown, or increased DHFR activity [5, 6, 14]. Decreased expression of the reduced folate carrier, a transport protein, was associated with impaired MTX transport and was observed in relapsed acute lymphocytic leukemia after treatment with MTX therapy [13]. Low levels of DHFR gene amplification might also be an important cause of MTX resistance in ALL [12]. Such mechanisms of resistance to MTX aside from impaired polyglutamylation might explain why CR to MTX therapy was observed in only 60% of the patients with PCNSL who showed polyglutamylation in the present study. In contrast, one third of patients in the non-polyglutamylation group had CR. $AUC_{MTX}$ might be a predictor for therapeutic response [18], and here, we found higher $AUC_{MTX}$ values in

**Table 4** Cox proportional hazard model for OS

| | Univariate analysis | | Multivariate analysis | |
|---|---|---|---|---|
| Variable | HR (95% CI) | *p* | HR (95% CI) | *p* |
| Age | 1.027 (1.002–1.053) | 0.035 | 1.047 (1.005–1.092) | 0.028 |
| KPS (high vs. low) | 0.376 (0.182–0.779) | 0.0085 | 0.263 (0.096–0.724) | 0.0097 |
| Sex (M vs. F) | 1.096 (0.617–1.945) | 0.75 | 0.712 (0.369–1.374) | 0.31 |
| MSKCC score | 1.534 (0.982–2.394) | 0.060 | 0.607 (0.277–1.334) | 0.21 |
| Cell of origin (GCB vs. non-GCB) | 0.914 (0.483–1.730) | 0.78 | 1.129 (0.546–2.334) | 0.74 |
| LDH (high vs. normal range) | 1.029 (0.563–1.881) | 0.93 | 0.773 (0.391–1.528) | 0.46 |
| Location (deep vs. not deep) | 0.796 (0.419–1.514) | 0.49 | 0.603 (0.297–1.226) | 0.16 |
| Polyglutamylation vs. non-polyglutamylation | 0.978 (0.557–1.718) | 0.94 | 1.728 (0.716–4.171) | 0.22 |

*OS* overall survival, *HR* hazard ratio, *CI* confidence interval, *KPS* Karnofsky performance status, *M* male, *F* female

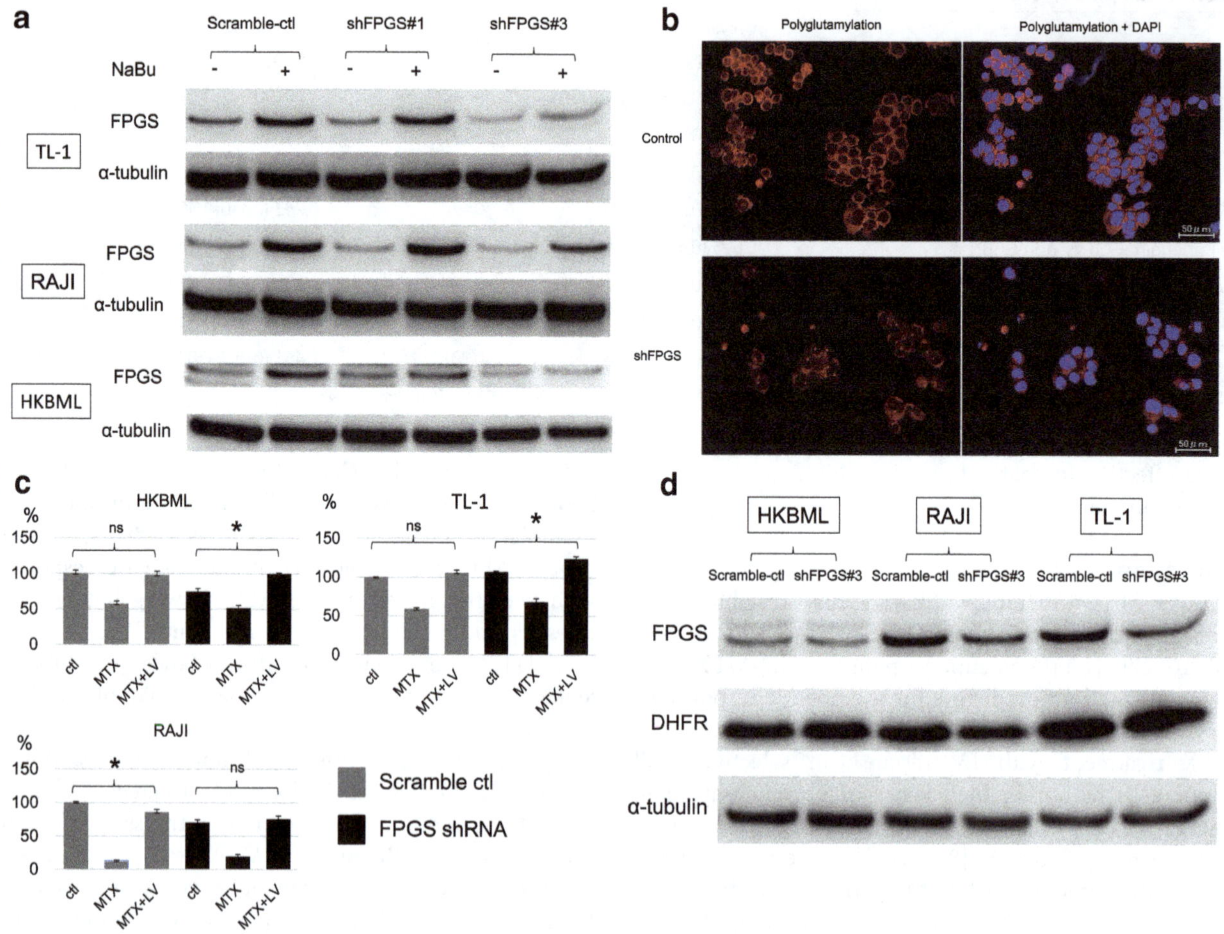


**Fig. 4 a** Immunoblotting for FPGS in different cell lines (scramble control and shFPGS#3) with or without exposure to 1 mM NaBu for 72 h. α-Tubulin was used as the internal control. **b** Immunofluorescence to identify polyglutamylation in TL-1 control and TL-1-shFPGS cells. Scale bar, 50 μm. **c** Cells were treated with MTX for 24 h, followed by the addition of LV and culturing for another 24 h. Cell viability assay was performed 48 h later. Error bars represent SDs. Viability of cells treated with MTX and MTX + LV as compared with that of control cells (no treatment). $^{*}p < 0.01$. ns, not statistically significant. **d** Immunoblotting for DHFR in different cell lines (scramble control and shFPGS#3). α-Tubulin was used as the internal control

patients with CR as compared with those with no CR. Therefore, the combination of polyglutamylation status and $AUC_{MTX}$ might be useful for prediction of MTX therapeutic response.

Regarding prognostic factors for survival in patients with PCNSL, polyglutamylation status was the only statistically significant prognostic factor for PFS, but did not qualify as a significant predictor of OS. Age and performance status, which have already been established as predictors of OS, were the only significant prognostic factors for OS in this study. These results might be explained by the fact that both the first- and second-line treatments were heterogeneous among differently aged groups in this study. Therefore, we examined the correlation between polyglutamylation status and clinical outcome in patients aged < 60 years, all of whom received radiation as part of their first-line therapy. We found a tendency toward better median OS in the polyglutamylation group than in the non-polyglutamylation group (Fig. 3c). To investigate whether polyglutamylation status predicts OS, further analysis of PCNSL patients who have previously undergone homogeneous therapies is needed.

The multiple-fluorescence system revealed that in addition to tumor cells expressing CD20 and exhibiting high levels of polyglutamylation, brain parenchyma also exhibited polyglutamylation, as revealed by red color resulting from non-overlapping fluorescence in the merged image (Fig. 2d). Although we used a 10% cut-off value based on IHC positivity, we might be able to identify a more accurate cut-off value for clinical use through the multiple-IHC-staining platform.

HDACIs improve the efficiency of MTX therapy with LV rescue in childhood ALL by upregulating FPGS

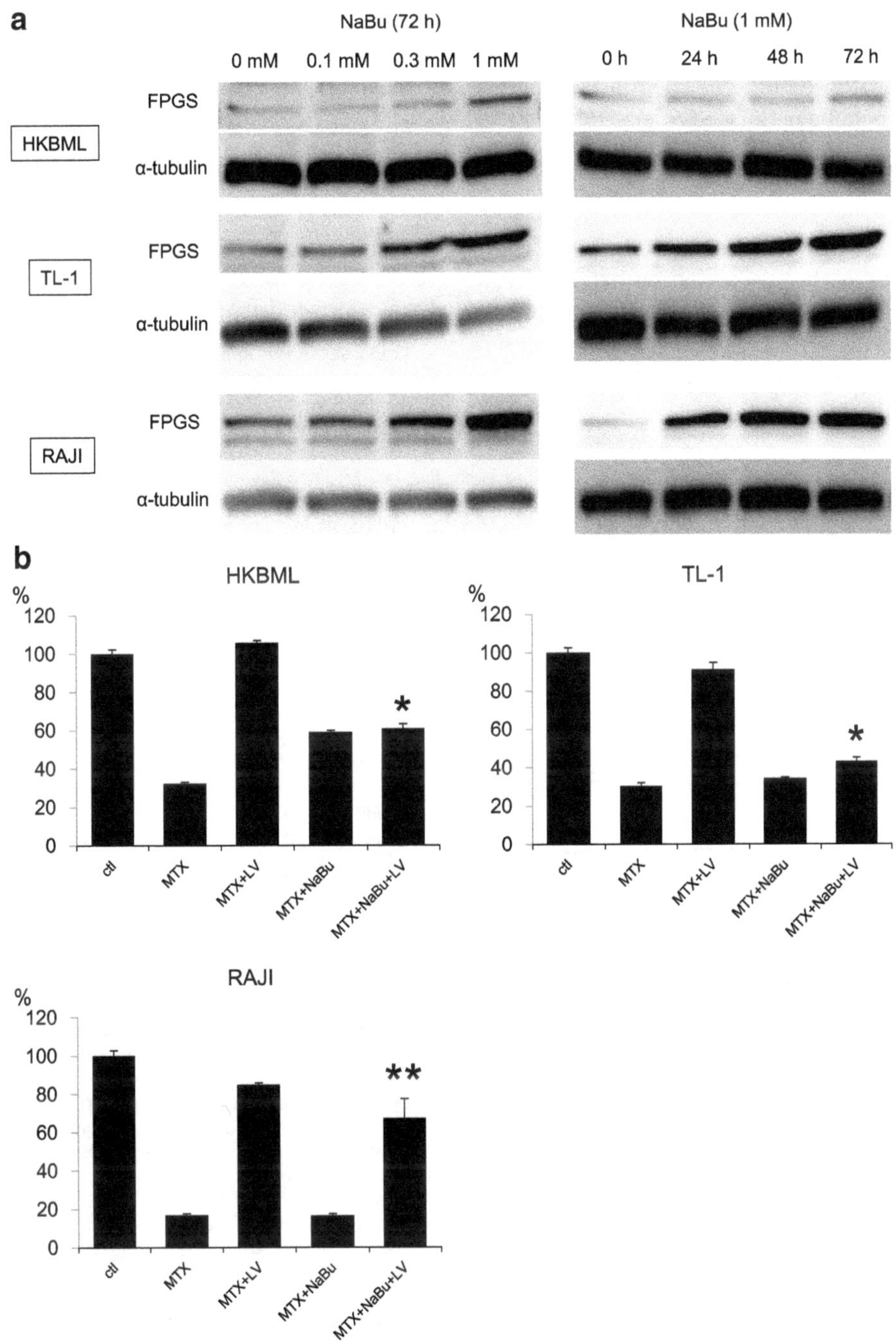


**Fig. 5** **a** Immunoblots showing upregulation of FPGS by NaBu treatment in a concentration- and time-dependent manner. α-Tubulin was used as the internal control. **b** Cells were treated with MTX with or without NaBu for 24 h, followed by addition of LV and culturing for another 24 h. Cell viability assay was performed 48 h later. Error bars represent the SD. Viability of cells treated with MTX + NaBu+LV as compared with that of control cells without NaBu treatment (MTX + LV). **p* < 0.001; ***p* < 0.05

expression and causing intracellular accumulation of long-chain MTX polyglutamates [19]. Our results revealed that HDACIs reduced the relief effect of LV after MTX therapy, thereby enhancing the antitumor effect. Therefore, modification of polyglutamylation levels could improve the antitumor effect of HD-MTX-based therapies for PCNSL. Identifying new drugs or subjecting known drugs to drug repositioning to specifically upregulate polyglutamylation in tumor cells could improve the efficacy of PCNSL treatment.

### Limitations

This was a retrospective study, therefore, prospective studies on the extent to which polyglutamylation levels predict the therapeutic response to HD-MTX treatment with LV rescue should be performed.

## Conclusions

Our findings suggest that polyglutamylation levels could represent a predictor of therapeutic response to HD-MTX therapy with LV rescue in PCNSL. Furthermore, combination therapy with HD-MTX and agents inducing polyglutamylation might be useful for treating PCNSL.

#### Funding

This work was supported by a Grant-in-Aid for Scientific Research (grant no. 25462272) from the Japan Society for the Promotion of Science.

#### Competing interests

The authors declare that they have no competing interests.

#### Author details

[1]Department of Neurosurgery, Kumamoto University Hospital, 1-1-1 Honjo Chuo-ku, Kumamoto 860-8556, Japan. [2]School of Medicine, Kumamoto University, Kumamoto, Japan. [3]Department of Diagnostic Pathology, Kumamoto University Hospital, Kumamoto, Japan. [4]Department of Pharmacy, Kumamoto University Hospital, Kumamoto, Japan. [5]Department of Neurosurgery, Sakurajuji Hospital, Kumamoto, Japan.

#### References

1. Abrey LE, Batchelor TT, Ferreri AJ, Gospodarowicz M, Pulczynski EJ, Zucca E et al (2005) Report of an international workshop to standardize baseline evaluation and response criteria for primary CNS lymphoma. J Clin Oncol 23:5034–5043
2. Abrey LE, Ben-Porat L, Panageas KS, Yahalom J, Berkey B, Curran W et al (2006) Primary central nervous system lymphoma: the Memorial Sloan-Kettering Cancer Center prognostic model. J Clin Oncol 24:5711–5715
3. Anai S, Hide T, Takezaki T, Kuroda J, Shinojima N, Makino K et al (2014) Antitumor effect of fibrin glue containing temozolomide against malignant glioma. Cancer Sci 105:583–591
4. Aoki H, Kondo Y, Aldape K, Yamamoto A, Iwado E, Yokoyama T et al (2008) Monitoring autophagy in glioblastoma with antibody against isoform B of human microtubule-associated protein 1 light chain 3. Autophagy 4:467–475
5. Banerjee D, Mayer-Kuckuk P, Capiaux G, Budak-Alpdogan T, Gorlick R et al (2002) Novel aspects of resistance to drugs targeted to dihydrofolate reductase and thymidylate synthase. Biochim Biophys Acta 1587:164–173
6. Bertino JR, Goker E, Gorlick R, Li WW, Banerjee D (1996) Resistance mechanisms to methotrexate in tumors. Stem Cells 14:5–9
7. Boucher D, Larcher JC, Gros F, Denoulet P (1994) Polyglutamylation of tubulin as a progressive regulator of in vitro interactions between the microtubule-associated protein tau and tubulin. Biochemistry 33:12471–12477
8. Fabre I, Fabre G, Goldman ID (1984) Polyglutamylation, an important element in methotrexate cytotoxicity and selectivity in tumor versus murine granulocytic progenitor cells in vitro. Cancer Res 44:3190–3195
9. Ferreri AJ, Blay JY, Reni M, Pasini F, Spina M, Ambrosetti A et al (2003) Prognostic scoring system for primary CNS lymphomas: the international Extranodal lymphoma study group experience. J Clin Oncol 21:266–272
10. Gabbai AA, Hochberg FH, Linggood RM, Bashir R, Hotleman K (1989) High-dose methotrexate for non-AIDS primary central nervous system lymphoma. Report of 13 cases. J Neurosurg 70:190–194
11. Goker E, Lin JT, Trippett T, Elisseyeff Y, Tong WP, Niedzwiecki D et al (1993) Decreased polyglutamylation of methotrexate in acute lymphoblastic leukemia blasts in adults compared to children with this disease. Leukemia 7:1000–1004
12. Goker E, Waltham M, Kheradpour A, Trippett T, Mazumdar M, Elisseyeff Y et al (1995) Amplification of the dihydrofolate reductase gene is a mechanism of acquired resistance to methotrexate in patients with acute lymphoblastic leukemia and is correlated with p53 gene mutations. Blood 86:677–684
13. Gorlick R, Goker E, Trippett T, Steinherz P, Elisseyeff Y, Mazumdar M et al (1997) Defective transport is a common mechanism of acquired methotrexate resistance in acute lymphocytic leukemia and is associated with decreased reduced folate carrier expression. Blood 89:1013–1018
14. Gorlick R, Goker E, Trippett T, Waltham M, Banerjee D, Bertino JR (1996) Intrinsic and acquired resistance to methotrexate in acute leukemia. N Engl J Med 335:1041–1048
15. Hans CP, Weisenburger DD, Greiner TC, Gascoyne RD, Delabie J, Ott G et al (2004) Confirmation of the molecular classification of diffuse large B-cell lymphoma by immunohistochemistry using a tissue microarray. Blood 103:275–282
16. Hiraga S, Arita N, Ohnishi T, Kohmura E, Yamamoto K, Oku Y et al (1999) Rapid infusion of high-dose methotrexate resulting in enhanced penetration into cerebrospinal fluid and intensified tumor response in primary central nervous system lymphomas. J Neurosurg 91:221–230
17. Joerger M, Ferreri AJ, Krahenbuhl S, Schellens JH, Cerny T, Zucca E et al (2012) Dosing algorithm to target a predefined AUC in patients with primary central nervous system lymphoma receiving high dose methotrexate. Br J Clin Pharmacol 73:240–247
18. Joerger M, Huitema AD, Krahenbuhl S, Schellens JH, Cerny T, Reni M et al (2010) Methotrexate area under the curve is an important outcome predictor in patients with primary CNS lymphoma: a pharmacokinetic-pharmacodynamic analysis from the IELSG no. 20 trial. Br J Cancer 102: 673–677
19. Leclerc GJ, Mou C, Leclerc GM, Mian AM, Barredo JC (2010) Histone deacetylase inhibitors induce FPGS mRNA expression and intracellular accumulation of long-chain methotrexate polyglutamates in childhood acute lymphoblastic leukemia: implications for combination therapy. Leukemia 24:552–562
20. Louis DN, Perry A, Reifenberger G, von Deimling A, Figarella-Branger D, Cavenee WK et al (2016) The 2016 World Health Organization classification of tumors of the central nervous system: a summary. Acta Neuropathol 131: 803–820
21. Makino K, Nakamura H, Hide T, Kuroda J, Yano S, Kuratsu J (2015) Prognostic impact of completion of initial high-dose methotrexate therapy on primary central nervous system lymphoma: a single institution experience. Int J Clin Oncol 20:29–34
22. Matherly LH, Barlowe CK, Goldman ID (1986) Antifolate polyglutamylation and competitive drug displacement at dihydrofolate reductase as important elements in leucovorin rescue in L1210 cells. Cancer Res 46:588–593
23. McGuire JJ (2003) Anticancer antifolates: current status and future directions. Curr Pharm Des 9:2593–2613
24. McGuire JJ, Mini E, Hsieh P, Bertino JR (1985) Role of methotrexate polyglutamates in methotrexate- and sequential methotrexate-5-fluorouracil-mediated cell kill. Cancer Res 45:6395–6400
25. Mlecnik B, Bindea G, Kirilovsky A, Angell HK, Obenauf AC, Tosolini M et al (2016) The tumor microenvironment and Immunoscore are critical determinants of dissemination to distant metastasis. Sci Transl Med 8:327ra326
26. Muta D, Makino K, Nakamura H, Yano S, Kudo M, Kuratsu J (2011) Inhibition of eIF4E phosphorylation reduces cell growth and proliferation in primary central nervous system lymphoma cells. J Neuro-Oncol 101:33–39
27. O'Brien PC, Roos DE, Pratt G, Liew KH, Barton MB, Poulsen MG et al (2006) Combined-modality therapy for primary central nervous system lymphoma: long-term data from a phase II multicenter study (trans-Tasman radiation oncology group). Int J Radiat Oncol Biol Phys 64:408–413
28. Rots MG, Pieters R, Peters GJ, Noordhuis P, van Zantwijk CH, Kaspers GJ et al (1999) Role of folylpolyglutamate synthetase and folylpolyglutamate hydrolase in methotrexate accumulation and polyglutamylation in childhood leukemia. Blood 93:1677–1683

29. Shinojima N, Hossain A, Takezaki T, Fueyo J, Gumin J, Gao F et al (2013) TGF-beta mediates homing of bone marrow-derived human mesenchymal stem cells to glioma stem cells. Cancer Res 73:2333–2344
30. Shinojima N, Nakamura H, Tasaki M, Kameno K, Anai S, Iyama K et al (2014) A patient with medulloblastoma in its early developmental stage. J Neurosurg Pediatr 14:615–620
31. Shinojima N, Tada K, Shiraishi S, Kamiryo T, Kochi M, Nakamura H et al (2003) Prognostic value of epidermal growth factor receptor in patients with glioblastoma multiforme. Cancer Res 63:6962–6970
32. Yamamoto T, Shinojima N, Todaka T, Nishikawa S, Yano S, Kuratsu J (2015) Meningioma in down syndrome. World Neurosurg 84:866 e861–866 e866

8

# Large inter- and intra-case variability of first generation tau PET ligand binding in neurodegenerative dementias

Melissa C. Wren[1,2], Tammaryn Lashley[2], Erik Årstad[1] and Kerstin Sander[1,3*]

**Abstract**

Imaging of pathological tau with positron emission tomography (PET) has the potential to allow early diagnosis of the dementias and monitoring of disease progression, including assessment of therapeutic interventions, in vivo. The first generation of tau PET tracers, including the carbazole flortaucipir and the 2-arylquinolines of the THK series, are now used in clinical research; however, concerns have been raised about off-target binding and low sensitivity.

With the aim to determine the nature of tau pathology depicted by structurally distinct tau ligands we carried out a microscopic neuropathological evaluation in *post-mortem* human brain tissue of cases with primary and secondary tauopathies. Carbazole and 2-arylquinoline binding was only observed in cases with Alzheimer's disease and one case with frontotemporal dementia and parkinsonism linked to chromosome 17 exhibiting a R406W *MAPT* mutation. In end stage Alzheimer's disease cases, fluorescent imaging with the carbazole T726 and the 2-arylquinoline THK-5117 revealed high inter- and intra-case variability of tracer binding, and this was corroborated by quantitative phosphorimaging with the PET tracer [$^{18}$F]THK-5117. Microscopic analysis of the pathological inclusions revealed that the fluorescent tracers preferentially bind to premature tau aggregates. Whilst T726 binding was limited to neuronal tau, THK-5117 additionally depicted neuritic tau. Neither tracer depicted tau in pre-symptomatic disease.

Our results highlight limitations of the first generation of tau PET tracers, in particular lack of correlation between pathological tau load and tracer binding, limited sensitivity to tau in early disease, and high variability in tracer binding between and within cases. Concerns remain that these limitations may also affect the next generation tracers as they target the same high affinity binding site. Therefore, it is crucial to assess inter- and intra-subject correlation of tracer binding with pathological tau load in *post-mortem* tissue studies, and to rigorously assess novel tau PET tracers before translation into clinical studies.

**Keywords:** Flortaucipir, THK, Positron emission tomography, Alzheimer's disease, Tauopathy

## Introduction

Dementia represents one of the most pressing public health challenges worldwide. A clinical diagnosis of the underlying disease causing the dementia remains challenging, particularly at the early stages, and a definite confirmation is usually only obtained *post-mortem* through histopathological examination of the brain.

Approximately 80% of dementia cases are associated with structural changes of the microtubule associated protein tau (*MAPT*), causing defective tau to aggregate in neurons and glial cells [48]. The shape and distribution of these inclusions are characteristic for the respective subtypes of tauopathy. In Alzheimer's disease, the most common dementia (50–70% of all clinical diagnoses), pathological tau load correlates closely with cognitive decline, suggesting that tau is a suitable biomarker for monitoring of disease progression [1, 14]. Quantitative assessment of tau pathology in vivo would have significant implications for medical research and for clinical practice, as it could potentially improve clinical diagnosis, predict disease progression, facilitate patient stratification and provide an outcome measure for putative disease-modifying interventions.

* Correspondence: k.sander@ucl.ac.uk
[1]Institute of Nuclear Medicine and Department of Chemistry, University College London, London, UK
[3]Radiochemistry, University College London, Kathleen Lonsdale Building, 5 Gower Place, London WC1E 6BS, UK
Full list of author information is available at the end of the article

The first generation of tau selective ligands for non-invasive imaging with positron emission tomography (PET) have recently entered clinical studies. The clinically most advanced compound [$^{18}$F]flortaucipir (formerly known as [$^{18}$F]AV-1451 or [$^{18}$F]T807), alongside the derivative [$^{18}$F]T808 and the fluorescent analogue T726, belong to the structural class of carbazoles, whereas the different compounds of the THK series ([$^{18}$F]THK-5105, [$^{18}$F]THK-5117 and [$^{18}$F]THK-5351) contain a 2-arylquinoline core. In patient studies, PET tracers from both compound classes have been reported to be suitable for staging of Alzheimer's disease [30, 39, 40], and for differential diagnosis of Alzheimer's disease and progressive supranuclear palsy [33, 47]. Some of these findings, in particular tracer binding to primary tauopathies, remain controversial, and are not supported by ex vivo studies on *post-mortem* brain tissue [13, 16, 22, 23, 29, 31, 37]. Furthermore, the first generation of tau PET tracers suffer from off-target binding, and in patient populations, where a signal is obtained, the sensitivity may be low [3, 36]. Efforts to develop and evaluate the next generation of tau selective tracers are ongoing [9, 15]. Pilot PET imaging studies with recently reported compounds, such as RO6958948, MK-6240 and PI-2620, suggest that these may have improved sensitivity and specificity for monitoring tau pathology in vivo. Yet, some, if not all, of the second generation tau ligands disclosed to-date display close structural similarities, and have an overlapping binding site with the first generation tau tracers. This highlights the importance of elucidating the interplay between the T808 binding site [50] and tau pathology.

We previously assessed binding of [$^{18}$F]flortaucipir, a structural analogue of T808, to human *post-mortem* brain tissue from cases with Alzheimer's disease and primary tauopathies, and observed a lack of correlation between PET tracer binding and total pathological tau load in the frontal and temporal cortices [37]. We also found evidence for tracer binding to a non-tau binding site. It has now been confirmed that flortaucipir exhibits strong off-target binding to monoamine oxidase isoforms and pigment containing cells, predominantly expressed in the striatum and the substantia nigra, respectively [15, 23, 46]. A similar off-target binding profile has been demonstrated for the compounds of the THK series [28, 31]. However, this does not fully explain the discrepancy between tracer binding and total tau load in the cortical brain areas.

The macroscopically observed lack of correlation between [$^{18}$F]flortaucipir binding and total tau load [37] prompted us to investigate what tau tracers depict on a cellular level. With the aim of determining whether this discrepancy can be attributed to the binding properties of specific compounds, different compound classes, or to the tau binding site(s), we carried out a microscopic neuropathological evaluation in *post-mortem* human brain tissue of cases with Alzheimer's disease, a range of primary tauopathies and non-demented controls with and without tau pathology. We used a combination of histology and nuclear imaging techniques to reveal ligand–tau interaction in a qualitative as well as in a quantitative manner. In particular, we aimed to answer the following questions: 1) what is the nature of tau pathology that the first generation tau ligands depict in vivo; 2) do carbazoles and 2-arylquinolines differ in their binding profiles; 3) is the T808 binding site an appropriate target for the development of tau PET tracers?

## Materials and methods

### Experimental design

Tau selective ligands were chosen to cover the most prominent compound classes of the first generation of tau PET tracers. We included the carbazoles flortaucipir and T726 as well as the 2-arylquinoline THK-5117, which is inherently fluorescent. As flortaucipir is not inherently fluorescent, we used the fluorescent structural analogue T726. T726 was used for screening purposes in the development process of flortaucipir and was shown to target the same tau binding site as flortaucipir [49]. We carried out a histopathological evaluation in human *post-mortem* brain tissue from neuropathologically well-characterised cases, selected to cover a range of tauopathies as well as controls (cf. 'Case selection' below). In order to assess the nature of tau pathology that the different compound classes depict, we used fluorescence microscopy with T726 and THK-5117 in conjunction with immunofluorescence. Where further clarification of tau ligand binding was required (THK-5117 binding to plaque like structures; *vide infra*), high resolution autoradiography in conjunction with immunohistochemistry was carried out. Due to the high concentration of fluorescent tau ligands needed for imaging experiments, we corroborated our results using quantitative phosphorimaging. PET tracer [$^{18}$F]THK-5117 binding was carried out at nanomolar concentrations that would be relevant for in vivo imaging.

### Case selection

We evaluated tissue from brains donated for research to the Queen Square Brain Bank for Neurological Disorders, Institute of Neurology, University College London. All cases had undergone standard neuropathological assessment and were diagnosed according to standard criteria. Demographic data are summarised in Table 1, and additional information on tissue processing can be found in the Additional file 1: Table S1.

Controls were cases without a clinical history of dementia, psychiatric or neurological diseases at the time of brain donation to the Queen Square Brain Bank. Although not showing any signs of cognitive impairment at the time of death, control cases can have a

**Table 1** Demographic Data of Cases Included in the Study

| Case | Sex | AAO | AAD | Brain Weight (g) | Braak Stage | Thal Phase | ABC Score |
|---|---|---|---|---|---|---|---|
| CTRL1 | F | – | 68 | 1330 | 0 | 0 | A0B0C0 |
| CTRL2 | M | – | 71 | 1480 | I | 0 | A0B1C0 |
| CTRL3 | F | – | 80 | 1242 | II | 0 | A0B1C0 |
| CTRL4 | M | – | 89 | 1448 | III | 3 | A2B2C1 |
| AD1 | F | 50 | 66 | 906 | VI | 5 | A3B3C3 |
| AD2 | M | 63 | 73 | 1269 | VI | 5 | A3B3C3 |
| AD3 | M | 52 | 68 | 1234 | VI | 5 | A3B3C3 |
| AD4 | M | 63 | 74 | 1022 | VI | 5 | A3B3C3 |
| FTDP1[a)] | M | 55 | 66 | 1208 | 0 | 0 | A0B0C0 |
| FTDP2[b)] | M | 68 | 74 | 1048 | II | 2 | A1B1C1 |
| FTDP3[c)] | M | 59 | 66 | 1399 | 0 | 0 | A0B0C0 |
| PICK1 | M | 57 | 62 | 1166 | III | 1 | A1B2C1 |
| PICK2 | M | 54 | 64 | 1040 | 0 | 3 | A2B0C1 |
| PSP1 | M | 62 | 74 | 1580 | 0 | 2 | A1B0C1 |
| PSP2 | F | 60 | 68 | 1177 | 0 | 1 | A1B0C1 |
| CBD | F | 62 | 69 | 1100 | 0 | 0 | A0B0C0 |

Abbreviations: CTRL, control; AD, Alzheimer's disease; FTDP, frontotemporal dementia with parkinsonism linked to chromosome 17; PICK, Pick's disease; PSP, progressive supranuclear palsy; CBD, corticobasal degeneration; MAPT, microtubule associated protein tau gene locus; M/F, male/female; AAO, age at onset; AAD, age at death

Genetic variants: a) MAPT R406W; b) MAPT Δ280K; c) MAPT 10 + 16

considerable burden of amyloid and tau pathology (up to Thal phase 4 and Braak & Braak stage IV, respectively). The control cases included in our study had absent pathology (CTRL1), or low levels of tau and/or amyloid pathology (Braak & Braak tau stage I–III and Thal phase 1–3; CTRL 2–4). All cases with neurodegenerative diseases had dementia in life. The selected Alzheimer's disease cases showed a high neuropathological change (CERAD frequent neuritic plaques, Braak & Braak tau stage VI and Thal phase 5 amyloid plaque pathology) using the National Institute on Aging-Alzheimer's Association guidelines [4, 25, 26, 44]. Differential diagnosis of the FTLD-tau cases was carried out following the criteria described by the consortium for Frontotemporal Lobar Degeneration [8]. The chosen FTDP-17 cases included exonic *MAPT* mutation variants (R406W and Δ280K), and one case with an intronic 10 + 16 *MAPT* mutation. Brain areas in the disease cases were selected due to the presence of abundant tau deposits. Frontal and temporal cortices as well as the hippocampus were examined in Alzheimer's disease, FTDP-17 and control cases. Frontal and temporal cortices were examined in Pick's disease, frontal cortex and cerebellum in progressive supranuclear palsy, and frontal and parietal cortex in corticobasal degeneration. The frontal area used corresponded to Brodman area 9, the temporal cortex and hippocampus were taken from the level of the lateral geniculate body. The choroid plexus was not attached to the hippocampus. Cerebellum sections contained cerebellar folia as well as white matter exhibiting the dentate nuclei. Parietal cortex samples were taken from the superior parietal lobule.

**Immunohistochemistry on flash frozen tissue sections**

Immunohistochemistry staining was carried out in flash frozen tissue on sequential sections to those used for autoradiography and fluorescence imaging. Tissue sections were cryosectioned at 10 μm, mounted on superfrost microscope slides and post-fixed in 4% paraformaldehyde for 30 min. Endogenous peroxidase activity was blocked using 0.3% hydrogen peroxide in methanol (10 min, room temperature). Non-specific binding was blocked and tissue permeabilised, using 10% dried non-fat milk under addition of 0.3% Triton X-100 (30 min, room temperature). Tissue sections were incubated with either AT8 (Thermoscientific, 1:600) or Aβ-XP (Cell Signaling, 1:200) for one hour at room temperature, followed by biotinylated anti-mouse or anti-rabbit IgG (DAKO, 1:200; 30 min), respectively, and avidin-biotin complex (Vector Laboratories; 30 min). Colour was developed with 3,3′-diaminobenzidine and hydrogen peroxide. Counterstaining was carried out using Mayer's haematoxylin.

Pathological phosphorylated tau burden was detected using AT8 immunostaining. AT8 recognises the two earliest phosphorylation sites on tau and highlights all levels of neurofibrillary pathology, including intra- and extracellular tangles, pre-tangles and neuropil threads [10]. Similarly, the amyloid antibody Aβ-XP detects several isoforms of amyloid beta, including the pathogenic species Aβ-42. Moreover, the combination of AT8 (raised in mouse) and Aβ-XP (raised in rabbit) allowed double immunofluorescence staining to be carried out [51]. Immunostained slides were scanned on an Aperio ScanScope slide scanner, producing high resolution digital histology images. Regions of interest were extracted using Aperio ImageScope software. Image quantification was performed using the analysis software packages ImageJ (version 1.48) [38] and Python (version 3.6.1). Macroinstructions processing of immunohistochemistry images was conducted firstly by random box generation of 10 squares within a dedicated region of interest, and secondly by setting thresholds for the 3,3′-diaminobenzidine chromogen. Tau load was quantified in adjacent sections to those exposed to [$^{18}$F]THK-5117, as percentage of positively stained tissue detected in regions of interest.

## Fluorescence microscopy

Tissue cryosections (10 μm) on superfrost microscope slides were post-fixed in 4% paraformaldehyde for 30 min. Autofluorescence was largely quenched by treating the sections with sudan black (0.1% in 70% ethanol) for ten minutes, followed by washing with 30% ethanol and tris buffered saline containing 0.05% Tween 20.

### *Fluorescent tau ligand binding studies*

Non-specific binding was blocked and tissue permeabilised, using 10% dried non-fat milk under addition of 0. 3% Triton X-100 (30 min, room temperature) [19]. Sections were incubated with either T726 (100 μM) [49] or THK-5117 (100 μM) [29] for one hour at room temperature, in a humidified chamber and under exclusion of light. Sections incubated with T726 were mounted with DAPI-containing fluorescent mounting medium (Vector Laboratories), and sections with THK-5117 were incubated with Nissl Neurotrace 640 (Molecular Probes; 1:100 for 20 min) to highlight neuronal nuclei within tissue samples.

The use of blocking buffer (composed of milk and Triton X-100) did not affect the binding of the fluorescent small molecule tau ligands (control experiments not shown), yet it helped to reduce auto fluorescence of the basal tissue extracellular matrix. In addition, comparability of results obtained from experiments in directly adjacent tissue sections (AT8 immunohistochemistry, AT8 immunofluorescence and co-staining with a tau ligand, staining with a tau ligand alone) was ensured. Nuclei markers were selected according to their compatibility with imaging of the respective tau ligand. Whilst T726 ($\lambda_{ex}$ 414 nm; $\lambda_{em}$ 500 nm) was imaged in conjunction with DAPI ($\lambda_{ex}$ 358 nm; $\lambda_{em}$ 461 nm), the excitation maxima of DAPI and THK-5117 ($\lambda_{ex}$ 362 nm; $\lambda_{em}$ 510 nm) were too close to allow for separate micrographs to be taken, and therefore, the neuronal nuclei marker Nissl Neurotrace 640 ($\lambda_{ex}$ 640 nm; $\lambda_{em}$ 660 nm) was used.

### *Fluorescent immunohistochemical co-staining with tau tracers*

Tissue sections were treated as described above. An additional blocking step before the addition of milk was used to reduce endogenous peroxidase activity, using methanol containing 0.3% hydrogen peroxide. Sections were incubated with the respective primary antibody, AT8 (Thermoscientific, 1:600), AT100 (Thermoscientific, 1:500), AT180 (Thermoscientific, 1:500), PHF1 (source: Peter Davies; 1:500) or Aβ-XP (Cell Signaling, 1:200), prior to tracer labelling. Incubation with a secondary biotinylated antibody (either rabbit anti-mouse IgG or swine anti-rabbit IgG; Dako, 1:200, 30 min) was followed by treatment with avidin-biotin complex (Vector Laboratories; 30 min). Tyramine signal amplification (red or green; 1:200) was used as a substrate for horseradish peroxidase. Sections were mounted with either DAPI-containing fluorescent mounting medium or Nissl Neurotrace 640, as described above.

### *Fluorescence imaging*

Fluorescence imaging was performed on a Leica epifluorescent microscope. Z-stacks of images were taken with a 63× oil objective. Fluorescent images were observed within specific wavelengths for maximal excitation and emission of each fluorophore. Images were subjected to three-dimensional (3D) deconvolution with the Leica LASAF image processing software. Deconvolution parameters used the Blind Method, detecting X, Y and Z volumes, with 5 iterations of each z-stack in each fluorescent channel. Using the same software, deconvoluted images were subjected to 3D projection processing, producing the final image of tau tracer and antibody binding fluorescence, as average 2D projected images of the original z-stack. Frequencies of fluorescent tau ligands binding to protein aggregates were semi-quantitatively recorded as 'very high', 'high', 'moderate', 'low', and 'absent', relating to pathological tau load determined by AT8 immunohistochemistry in directly adjacent tissue sections. Morphological characteristics of tau inclusions were used to differentiate pre-tangles, neurofibrillary tangles and ghost tangles. Pre-tangles were defined by their immature, small, amorphous and loosely compacted perinuclear structure [45]. Neurofibrillary tangles were classified by their larger and more densely packed mature fibrillar structure that clearly delineated the cytosolic neuronal compartments. Ghost tangles cannot reliably be detected by fluorescence microscopy; they are distinguished from neurofibrillary tangles by their lack of a nucleus and stainable cytoplasm as depicted by haemotoxylin and eosin, or by reactivity to silver. Both of these staining methods rely on detection by light microscopy [5]. Given their specific morphological characteristics, tau aggregates could clearly be differentiated from lipofuscin pigment granules, which were observed during fluorescent tracer imaging (this is pertaining to the comparably long exposure times required for imaging of T726 and THK-5117). The lipofuscin triggered fluorescence was not taken into account during the semi-quantitative assessment of tracer binding to tau pathology.

#### Synthesis of compounds and radiolabelling

Flortaucipir was synthesised in house following previously published synthetic routes [43], whilst the fluorescent analogue T726 was obtained through custom synthesis (AFChemPharm). THK-5117, and the labelling precursor THK-5119 were kindly provided by Prof N. Okamura, Department of Pharmacology, Tohoku University School of Medicine, Japan.

[$^{18}$F]THK-5117 was prepared as described previously [29]. Briefly, fluoride-18 was dissolved in 0.5 ml of a solution of potassium carbonate (15 mM) and Kryptofix (30 mM) in acetonitrile containing 15% water. The mixture was dried under a stream of nitrogen at 90 °C, followed by azeotropic drying with two subsequent additions of acetonitrile (0.5 ml). The labelling precursor THK-5119, dissolved in dimethyl sulfoxide (2 mg in 0.5 ml), was added, and the resulting mixture stirred at 110 °C for ten minutes. Hydrochloric acid (3 M, 0.5 ml) was added, and stirring was continued for five minutes. The reaction was quenched using sodium hydroxide (1 M, 1 ml) under cooling (ice bath). The radioactive product was purified on a semi-preparative Chromolith® Performance RP-18e column (Merck Millipore; 100 × 4.6 mm) at a flow rate of 5 ml/min, using a mixture of water and methanol containing 0.5% trifluoroacetic acid as mobile phase. Stepwise isocratic elution with 10% methanol in water for five minutes, followed by 38% methanol in water for ten minutes allowed isolation of the radioactive product (retention time 13 min). Reformulation in tris buffered saline (pH 7.4, containing < 10% ethanol) was carried out on a Sep-Pak C18 Plus Light cartridge (Waters). When starting with approximately 2 GBq of fluoride-18, [$^{18}$F]THK-5117 was obtained with a decay-corrected radiochemical yield (end of synthesis) of 48% ± 8, with a radiochemical purity of > 99%, and with a specific activity of 6.3 ± 1.2 GBq/μmol.

#### Quantitative phosphorimaging

Thawed and air-dried sections (10 μm) from flash frozen tissue were post-fixed in methanol (20 min), rehydrated in tris buffered saline (30 min) and incubated with a solution of [$^{18}$F]THK-5117 in tris buffered saline (2 MBq/ml) for 15 min (1 ml per slide). After incubation, unbound [$^{18}$F]THK-5117 was removed by washing the sections in water (five minutes) and 50% ethanol (five minutes). Internal standards were prepared by serial dilution of the [$^{18}$F]THK-5117 solution that was used for the incubation of the brain sections. Brain sections, and internal standards absorbed on filter paper, were left to air-dry and subsequently exposed to a phosphor screen (BAS-IP MS, GE Healthcare) overnight. Phosphorimaging was performed on a Typhoon Trio scanner (GE Healthcare), at a resolution of 50 μm.

For blocking studies, sections were rehydrated in tris buffered saline containing chlorgiline and L-deprenyl (1 μM each). Incubation with [$^{18}$F]THK-5117 was carried out under concomitant addition of different concentrations of either non-labelled THK-5117 or flortaucipir.

Phosphor images were analysed using the software ImageJ (version 1.48) [38]. Quantification of [$^{18}$F]THK-5117 binding in manually drawn regions of interest (mean ± standard deviation in kBq/cm$^2$) was based on correlation curves generated from the internal standards.

#### Nuclear emulsion autoradiography

Sections were treated with [$^{18}$F]THK-5117 as described above (Phosphorimaging). After tracer incubation, the air-dried sections were dipped in nuclear photographic emulsion K.5 (Ilford; 1:4 dilution in water) and exposed overnight under exclusion of light. Slides were washed in phenisol developer (Ilford; 20%, four minutes), acetic acid (1%, two minutes), hypam fixative solution (Ilford; 20%, four minutes) and water. Immunohistochemistry was subsequently performed as described above. The concentration of the primary antibodies was as follows: AT8 (Thermoscientific; 1:100), Aβ-XP (Cell Signalling; 1:100) and PHF-1 (source: Peter Davies; 1:100). Immunostaining controls not subject to silver dipping were carried out on adjacent tissue sections.

Nuclear emulsion autoradiography photomicrographs were assessed for accumulation of silver clusters over entire areas of brain tissue for each case assessed, including grey and white matter.

## Results

#### Case characterisation

The human *post-mortem* brain tissue used for this study was characterised using immunohistochemistry with the phospho-tau selective antibody AT8. Control cases had absent (Braak & Braak stage 0), or mild tau pathology (Braak & Braak stage I–III) in the medial temporal lobe.

Alzheimer's disease cases were classified as Braak & Braak stage VI and had pronounced tau pathology in the grey matter accounting for 25–35% of the surface of the respective flash frozen tissue sections (Fig. 1). In all Alzheimer's disease cases, dense neurofibrillary tangles, pre-tangles, as well as a meshwork of neuropil threads were observed in all brain areas investigated (Fig. 1a–d). In the FTDP-17 cases, small neurofibrillary tangles and abundant threads were identified (Fig. 1e and Additional file 1: Figure S1). Pick's disease cases displayed Pick's bodies in the cortical areas. Cases with progressive supranuclear palsy had pre-tangles, globose tangles, tufted astrocytes and neuropil threads in the frontal cortex and frequent coiled bodies in the cerebellum. Frequent astrocytic plaques, globose tangles and coiled bodies were identified in the case with corticobasal degeneration (Additional file 1: Figure S1).

#### Microscopic assessment of the nature of pathology depicted by tau ligands

In order to assess the binding profiles of tau PET tracers from distinct compound classes, we carried out fluorescence microscopy with the carbazole T726 and the 2-arylquinoline THK-5117. This revealed tracer binding to tissue from cases with Alzheimer's disease (Fig. 2–5) and the FTDP-17 case with the R406W *MAPT* mutation (Fig. 6), but not to cases with Pick's disease, progressive supranuclear palsy, corticobasal degeneration, and FTDP-17 with Δ280K or 10 + 16 *MAPT* mutation (Additional file 1: Figure S2). No fluorescent tracer binding was observed in the control cases; although tau inclusions were confirmed in the medial temporal lobe of control cases CTRL3 and CTRL4 that had clear signs of pathological aging (A0B1C0 and A2B2C1, respectively), these were not depicted by T726 and THK-5117 (Additional file 1: Figure S3).

In the Alzheimer's disease cases AD1–AD4, both fluorescent tau ligands depicted neurofibrillary tangles, pre-tangles and neuropil threads (Fig. 2a–o and Fig. 3a–t). On selected neurofibrillary tangles, we observed fluorescent ligand binding alongside immunoreactivity with the phospho-tau specific antibody AT8 (Fig. 2p–s, Fig. 3u–x and Additional file 1: Figure S4). Overall, the fluorescent tracers bound to fewer pathological inclusions than were depicted by antibodies: following semiquantitative assessment of the fluorescence microscopy images, T726 depicted approximately 20–30% of total pathological tau burden, as determined by AT8 immunohistochemistry, whereas THK-5117 labelled 50–80% of tau inclusions. However, both T726 and THK-5117 depicted neurons that were negative not only for the phospho-tau specific antibody AT8 (Fig. 2t and Fig. 3y), but also for antibodies detecting epitopes that are typically phosphorylated at later disease stages (AT100, AT180, PHF1) and that are therefore considered to be markers for mature neurofibrillary tangles (Additional file 1: Figure S5).

The fluorescent ligands showed high variability in depicting tau pathology across Alzheimer's disease cases, despite all cases having reached Braak & Braak stage VI and Thal phase 5. Regional differences in tracer binding were observed, yet there was no consistency in the binding pattern of the different compound classes (Fig. 4). T726 depicted low amounts of neurofibrillary tangles, pre-tangles and neuropil threads in the hippocampus, frontal and temporal cortices of case AD1. Similarly, in the case AD2, only a low percentage of neurofibrillary tangles was detected, but moderate to high degree of tracer binding to pre-tangles and threads was observed. Surprisingly, T726 binding to mature neurofibrillary tangles was absent in the cases AD3 and AD4. Pre-tangles and neuropil threads were identified by T726 in these cases, albeit in low amounts. Using THK-5117 in the case AD1, very high amounts of neurofibrillary tangles, pre-tangles and neuropil threads were identified in the three brain areas investigated. In this case, the tau load depicted by the fluorescent tracer was comparable to that found by immunohistochemistry with AT8 in the directly adjacent brain sections. In the case AD2, THK-5117 only depicted low amounts of tau pathology, compared to those found with AT8. High, and very high, percentage of neurofibrillary tangles, pre-tangles and threads was observed throughout brain areas in the cases AD3 and AD4, respectively.

Only THK-5117 (Fig. 3z), but not T726 (Fig. 2u), visualised plaque-like structures in the Alzheimer's disease cases. Using nuclear emulsion autoradiography with [$^{18}$F]THK-5117, in conjunction with immunohistochemistry, the nature of these plaque-like structures was further characterised (Fig. 5). [$^{18}$F]THK-5117 binding to neurofibrillary tangles that were immunoreactive for the phospho-tau specific antibodies AT8 and PHF1 was observed in all four Alzheimer's disease cases (Fig. 5a/b). Additionally, silver clusters co-localised with dystrophic neurites surrounding the core of neuritic plaques, following the same distribution pattern that was detected with the fluorescent tracer (Fig. 5c–f). The dense silver deposits surrounded by amyloid, as indicated by Aβ-XP staining (Fig. 5g/h), are likely to be ghost tangles or the cores of plaques.

Both T726 and THK-5117 bound to tissue from the FTDP-17 case with the R406W *MAPT* mutation (FTDP1), but not to cases with the Δ280K or the 10 + 16 variant (FTDP2/3). In FTDP1 we observed fluorescent T726 and THK-5117 labelling of a high amount of neurofibrillary tangles, pre-tangles and neuropil threads in the hippocampus (Fig. 6a). In the cortical areas, both

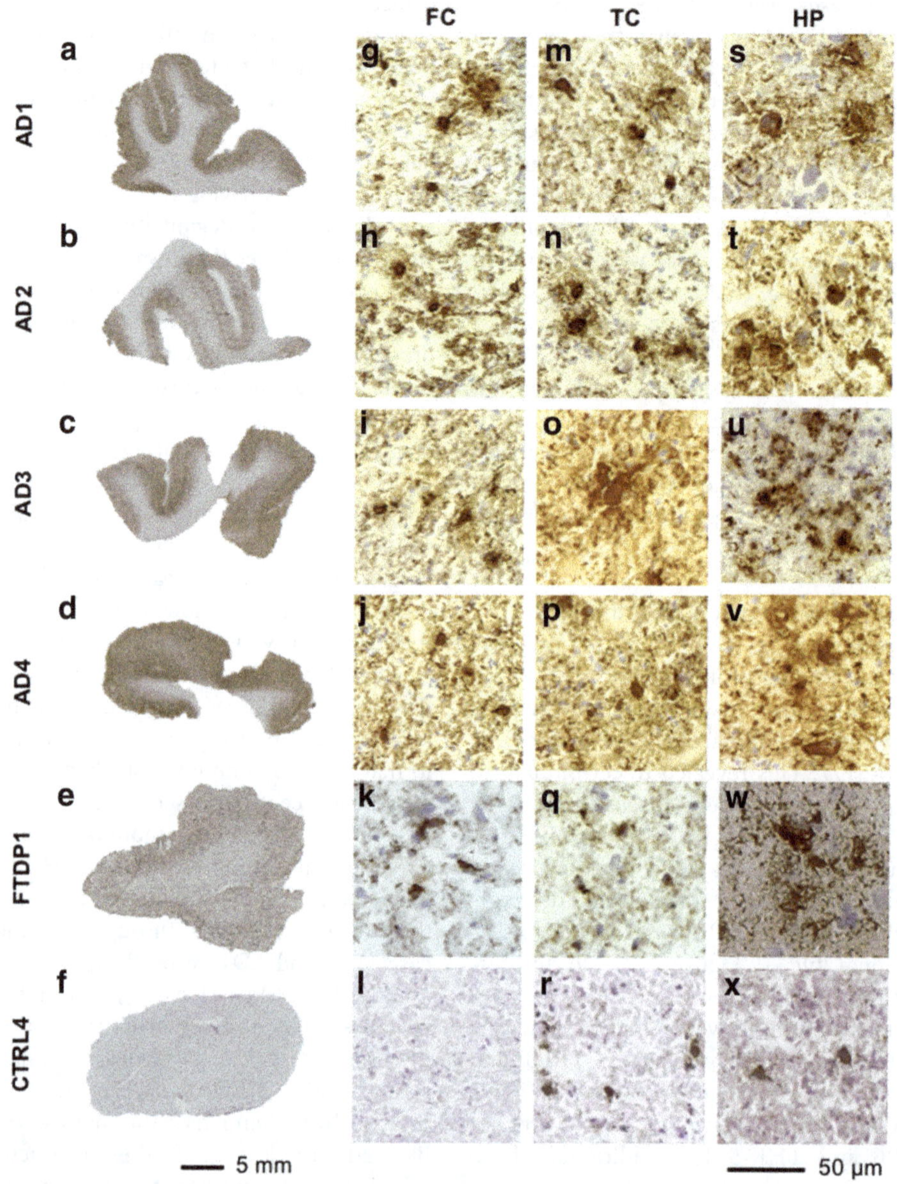


**Fig. 1** Tau immunohistochemistry in Alzheimer's disease cases. **a**–**f**) Representative images from frontal cortex, showing macroscopic AT8 distribution in the Alzheimer's disease cases AD1–AD4, the FTDP-17 case with a R406W *MAPT* mutation (FTDP1) and the control case CTRL4. **g**–**x**) Typical microscopic AT8 positive neurofibrillary tau aggregates in frontal cortex, temporal cortex and hippocampus. Abbreviations: AD, Alzheimer's disease; FTDP, frontotemporal dementia with parkinsonism linked to chromosome 17; CTRL, control; FC, frontal cortex; TC, temporal cortex; HP, hippocampus

tracers depicted tau inclusions with a lower frequency. Whereas THK-5117 binding reflected pathological tau load as determined by AT8, T726 lacked binding to neurofibrillary tangles in the temporal and frontal cortices of this case (Fig. 6b).

### Quantitative phosphorimaging with [$^{18}$F]THK-5117

In order to corroborate the high inter- and intra-case variability of tau tracer binding, as observed with fluorescent imaging, we carried out quantitative phosphorimaging with [$^{18}$F]THK-5117 in disease groups that had shown fluorescent tracer binding, i.e. Alzheimer's disease and FTDP-17, as well as control cases (Fig. 7 and Additional file 1: Figure S6).

Total [$^{18}$F]THK-5117 binding (Fig. 7a) in control cases with and without brain pathology was low, ranging between 0.6 and 0.9 kBq/cm$^2$ in the three brain areas investigated. In particular, there was no difference in tracer binding to the medial temporal lobe of cases with and without signs of pathological aging, despite existing pathology in the hippocampus and entorhinal cortex of the control case CTRL4 (Supporting Fig. 3). The

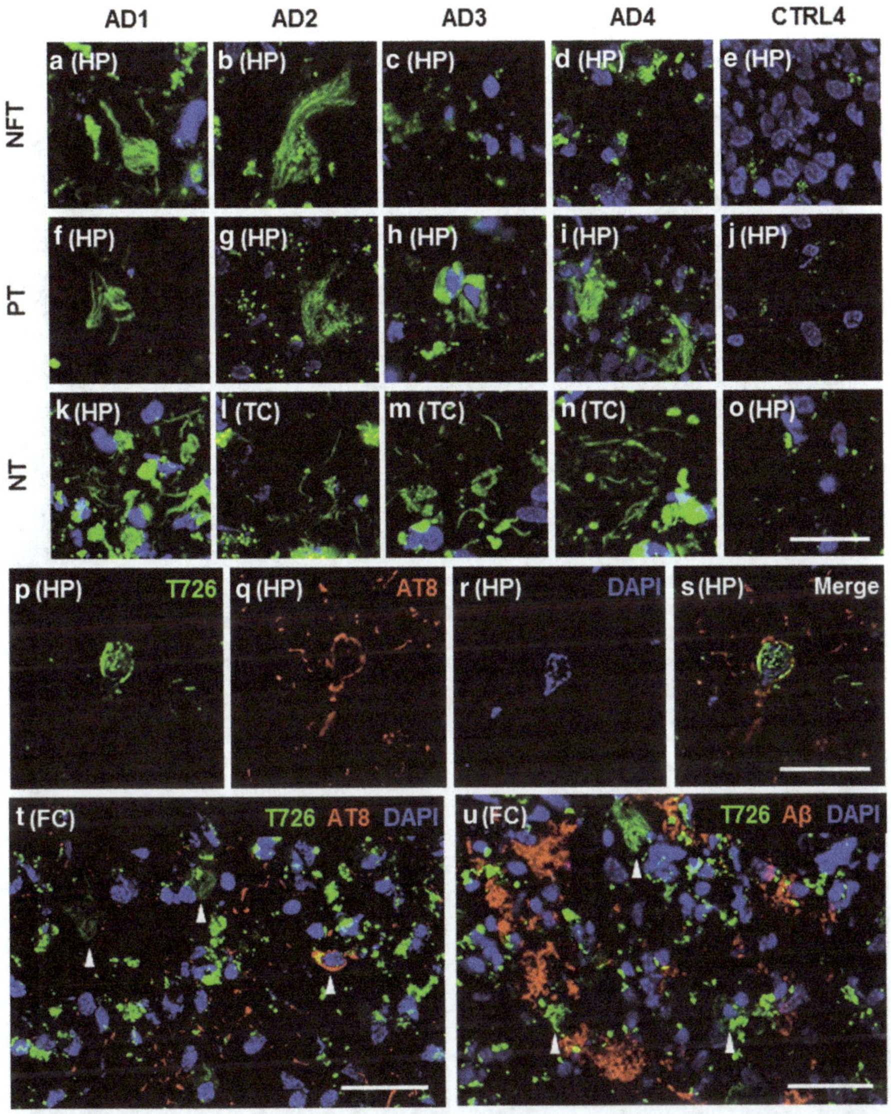


**Fig. 2** Fluorescence imaging with T726 in Alzheimer's disease cases and controls. **a–o**) T726 bound pathology in green, nuclear marker DAPI in blue; scale bar inset 50 μm. **a–d**) T726 bound mature tangle structures in individual Alzheimer's disease cases. **f–i**) Pre-tangle inclusions bound by T726. **k–n**) Neuropil threads bound by T726. **e/j/o**) Representative images from the control case CTRL4 depict the absence of T726 binding in control cases. **p–s**) T726 labelling of an AT8 immunoreactive hippocampal neurofibrillary tangle (Alzheimer's disease case AD1); T726 in green, AT8 in red, DAPI in blue; scale bar inset 25 μm. **t**) Representative image of T726 labelled structures negative for AT8, and AT8 immunodecorated tangles not labelled with T726 (Alzheimer's disease case AD1); T726 in green, AT8 in red, DAPI in blue; scale bar inset; 50 μm. **u**) Representative immunofluorescence image showing distinct binding patterns of T726 and Aβ-XP to cortical pathology (Alzheimer's disease case AD1); T726 in green, Aβ-XP in red, DAPI in blue; scale bar inset 50 μm. Abbreviations: AD, Alzheimer's disease; CTRL, control; NFT, neurofibrillary tangles; PT, pre-tangles; NT, neuropil threads; FC, frontal cortex; TC, temporal cortex; HP, hippocampus; Aβ, amyloid-beta

Alzheimer's disease case 1 (AD1) showed strong [$^{18}$F]THK-5117 binding in the grey matter of frontal and temporal cortices as well as in the hippocampus (9.9, 7.8 and 5.0 kBq/cm$^2$, respectively). AD2 showed a comparably high total binding in the frontal cortex (10.3 kBq/cm$^2$), but lower uptake in temporal cortex and hippocampus (3.8 and 1.5 kBq/cm$^2$, respectively). Total binding in tissue sections of the case AD3 was approximately half of that observed in AD1, but still delineated well from control cases (4.1, 5.3 and 2.5 kBq/cm$^2$ in frontal, temporal cortex and hippocampus, respectively). Interestingly, the case AD4 showed low [$^{18}$F]THK-5117 binding in the frontal cortex (3.2 kBq/cm$^2$), and particularly low uptake in temporal cortex and hippocampus (1.3 and 1.4 kBq/cm$^2$, respectively). The correlation of total tau load, as determined by immunohistochemistry with the phospho-tau specific antibody AT8, and total [$^{18}$F]THK-5117 binding to

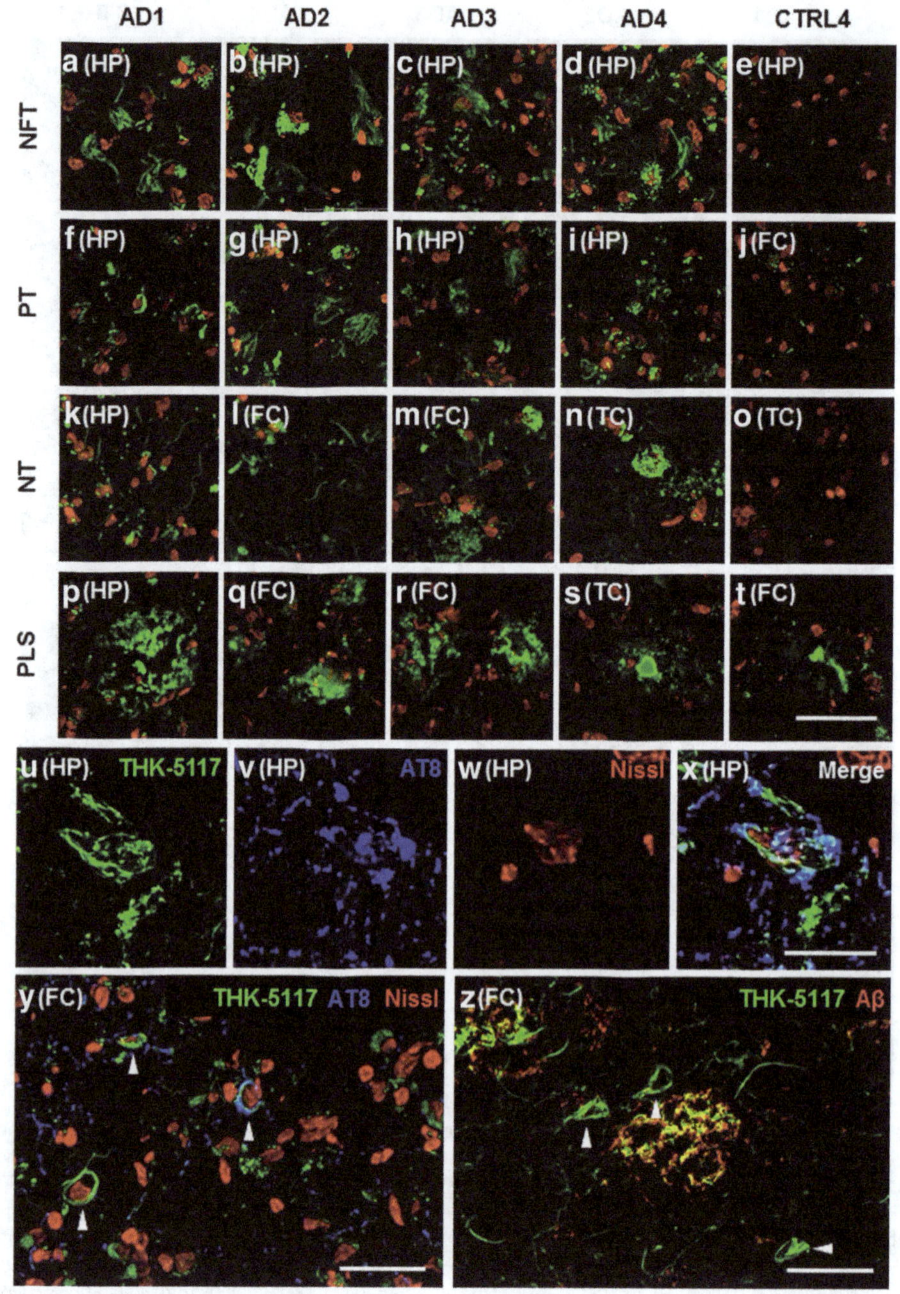


**Fig. 3** Fluorescence imaging with THK-5117 in Alzheimer's disease cases and controls. **a–t**) THK-5117 bound pathology in green, neuronal nuclear marker, Nissl Neurotrace 640, in red; scale bar inset 50 μm. **a–d**) Images showing neurofibrillary tangle structures detected by THK-5117 in individual AD cases. **f–i**) Images that present pre-tangles bound by THK-5117. **k–n**) THK-5117 bound neuropil threads were observed only in distinct regions of each AD case. **p–s**) THK-5117 labelling of plaque-like structures in all AD cases in distinct brain regions. **e/j/o**) Representative images of THK-5117 labelling in the control case CTRL4 depict the absence of THK-5117 binding to any pathological tau structures. **t**) THK-5117 binding to plaque-like structures in control tissue. **u–x**) THK-5117 fluorescent labelling of a hippocampal neurofibrillary tangle (Alzheimer's disease case AD1); THK-5117 in green, AT8 in blue, Nissl Neurotrace 640 in red; scale bar inset 25 μm. **y**) Representative immunofluorescence image showing THK-5117 labelled structures in absence of AT8 co-staining (Alzheimer's disease case AD1); THK-5117 in green, AT8 in blue, Nissl Neurotrace 640 in red; scale bar inset 50 μm. **z**) Representative image of THK-5117 and Aβ-XP immunofluorescence showing distinct and co-incidental binding of THK-5117 and amyloid beta to cortical pathology; THK-5117 in green, Aβ-XP in red; scale bar inset 50 μm. Abbreviations: AD, Alzheimer's disease; CTRL, control; NFT, neurofibrillary tangles; PT, pre-tangles; NT, neuropil threads; PLS, plaque-like structures; FC, frontal cortex; TC, temporal cortex; HP, hippocampus; Aβ, amyloid-beta

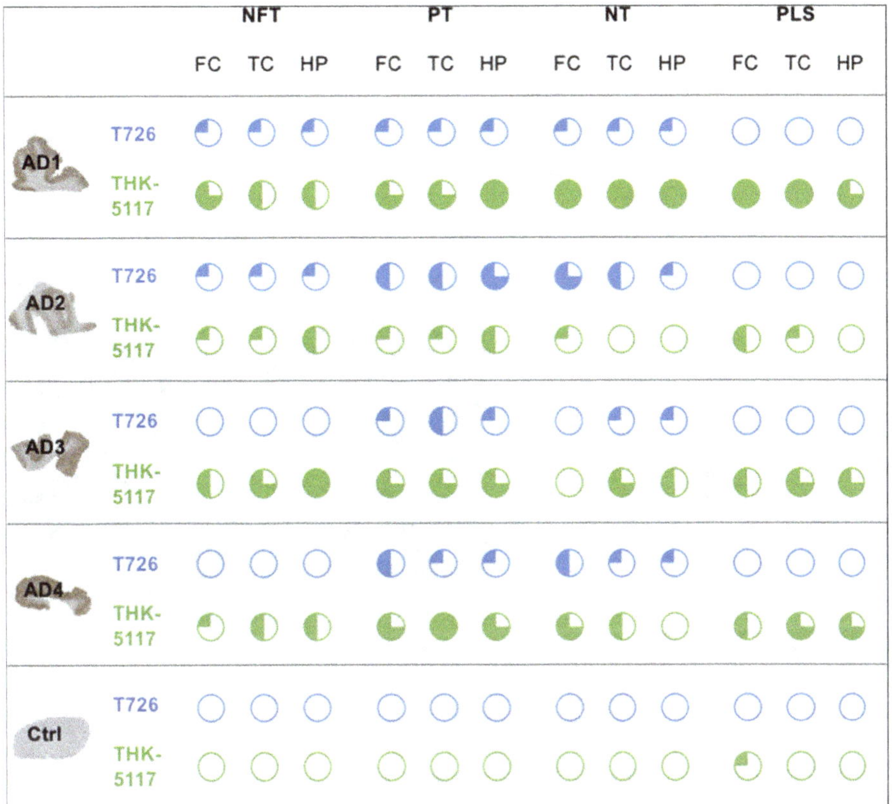


**Fig. 4** Frequency of pathology depicted by T726 (blue charts) and THK-5117 (green charts) in Alzheimer's disease and control cases. Frequencies: ●, extremely frequent; ◕, very frequent; ◑, frequent; ◔, infrequent; ○, absent; as compared to the amount of pathology depicted by the phospho-tau specific antibody AT8. Abbreviations: AD, Alzheimer's disease; Ctrl, control cases (averaged tracer uptake in normal and pathologically aged controls); NFT, neurofibrillary tangles; PT, pre-tangles; NT, neuropil threads; PLS, plaque like structures; FC, frontal cortex; TC, temporal cortex; HP, hippocampus

the grey matter of all Alzheimer's disease and control cases was low ($R^2$ of 0.27; Fig. 7b).

The FTDP-17 case harbouring the R406W mutation (FTDP1) showed slightly increased [$^{18}$F]THK-5117 binding in both frontal cortex and hippocampus (1.9 kBq/cm$^2$) when compared to control cases. FTDP2 with a 10 + 16 mutation showed similar uptake in the frontal cortex (1.9 kBq/cm$^2$), whereas in the temporal cortex and the hippocampus of this case as well as in all brain areas of case FTDP3 (Δ280K mutation) total binding was comparable to that in controls (< 1.1 kBq/cm$^2$).

In order to probe the specificity of the [$^{18}$F]THK-5117 binding we carried out blocking studies to determine the degree of non-specific, as well as off-target binding, using the frontal cortex of Alzheimer's disease case AD1 (Fig. 7c). In these experiments, both isoforms of monoamine oxidases, A and B, were blocked using chlorgiline and L-deprenyl, respectively, leading to an overall reduction of [$^{18}$F]THK-5117 binding from 9.9 to 6.9 kBq/cm$^2$ (30%). Non-specific [$^{18}$F]THK-5117 binding was high, and could only be reduced to < 20% of total binding when the concentration of the blocking agent exceeded 1000 times the value of the dissociation constant ($K_d$ of THK-5117 = 5.2 nM). Displacement of [$^{18}$F]THK-5117 with flortaucipir was observed in the micromolar concentration range (40% of total [$^{18}$F]THK-5117 binding at a blocking concentration of 1000 x $K_d$ (AV-1451) = 14.6 nM).

## Discussion

Tau ligand binding in the Alzheimer's disease cases used in this study did not reflect the high, and coherent, pathological tau load as determined by immunohistochemistry. Using fluorescent as well as radiolabelled tau ligands, we observed a large inter- and intra-case variability in tracer binding, and there was no dominant or consistent uptake pattern shared by the structurally different compounds. In contrast, staining with the phospho-tau specific antibody AT8 confirmed all Alzheimer's disease cases to be affected by severe tau pathology (Braak & Braak stage VI) throughout the brain areas investigated. In life, all cases had been diagnosed with the sporadic variant, and magnetic resonance imaging had shown generalised cortical atrophy typical for late stage disease.

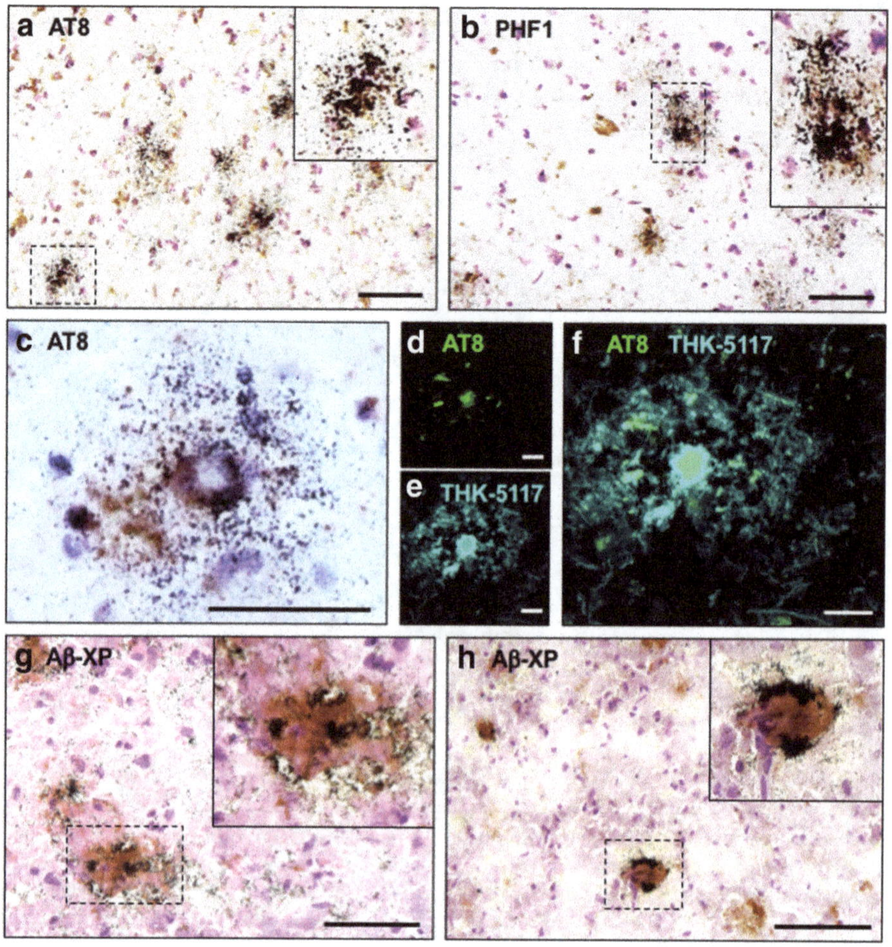


**Fig. 5** Nuclear emulsion autoradiography with [$^{18}$F]THK-5117 in the Alzheimer's disease case AD1. **a/b**) Silver deposition induced by [$^{18}$F]THK-5117 binding to tau inclusions co-stained with AT8 and PHF1, respectively. **c–f**) Neuritic plaques labelled with [$^{18/19}$F]THK-5117 and co-stained with AT8. **g/h**) Neuritic tau labelled with [$^{18}$F]THK-5117 surrounding plaques visualised with the amyloid beta antibody Aβ-XP. Scale bar insets 100 μm

Total [$^{18}$F]THK-5117 binding to the grey matter of the Alzheimer's disease cases ranged from 1.3 to 10.3 kBq/cm$^2$, and the lower uptake value barely delineated from that found in control tissue. In particular, one case (AD2) showed low frequency of tau pathology depicted by THK-5117 compared to that found in the other Alzheimer's disease cases, whereas the cases AD3 and AD4 appeared to be low-affinity binders for T726. Using fluorescence microscopy with THK-5117 and T726, we noted that not only the frequency, but also the type of the pathological inclusions depicted by the different compounds varied. Surprisingly, T726 binding to mature neurofibrillary tangles was only observed in the cases AD1 and AD2, but not in the cases AD3 and AD4; THK-5117 depicted neurofibrillary tangles with moderate to high frequency in all cases and brain areas investigated. Both tracers seemed to preferentially depict premature tau inclusions, such as pre-tangles and neuropil threads. Apart from the case AD2, i.e. the low-affinity binder for THK-5117, pre-tangles were found consistently throughout cases and brain areas using both tracers, whilst there were particular brain areas that exhibited a low frequency of threads, such as the frontal cortex of AD3 and the hippocampus of AD4. Interestingly, the 2-arylquinoline THK-5117 showed preferential binding to neuritic tau, whereas carbazole T726 binding was limited to neuronal tau. [$^{18}$F]THK-5117 binding was partially displaced by flortaucipir, confirming that the binding sites for the 2-arylquinoline and the carbazole overlap. Differences in the binding profile of the two compound classes may pertain to an additional binding site found for the 2-arylquinolines [6, 20].

The large variability in T726 and [$^{18/19}$F]THK-5117 binding to tissue from Alzheimer's disease cases is consistent with results from our previous study with [$^{18}$F]flortaucipir, which demonstrate a lack of correlation between tau ligand binding to *post-mortem* brain tissue and pathological tau load [37]. PET imaging in patients

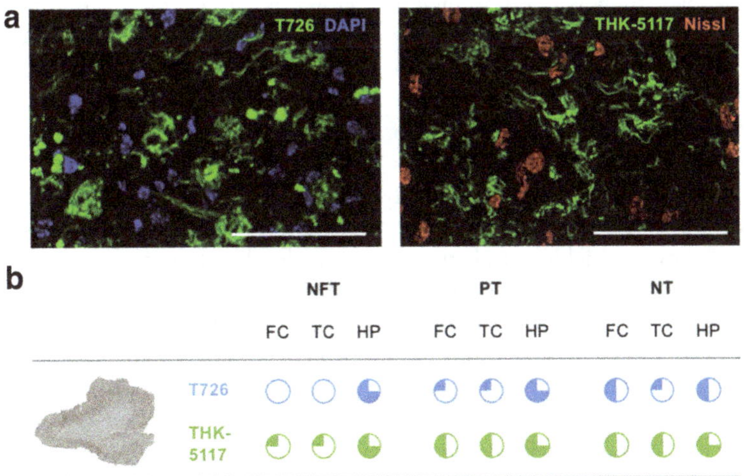


**Fig. 6** T726 and THK-5117 fluorescent labelling of the FTDP-17 case with a R406W MAPT mutation. **a)** T726 and THK-75117 binding to the CA1 section of the hippocampus; fluorescent tracers in green, DAPI in blue, Nissl Neurotrace 640 in red; scale bar inset 100 µm. **b)** Frequencies of tau pathology depicted by the fluorescent tau ligands as compared to the amount of pathology immunodecorated by the phospho-tau specific antibody AT8. Frequencies: ●, extremely frequent; ◕, very frequent, ◑, frequent; ◔, infrequent; ○, absent. Abbreviations: NFT, neurofibrillary tangles; PT, pre-tangles; NT, neuropil threads; FC, frontal cortex; TC, temporal cortex; HP, hippocampus; IHC, immunohistochemistry

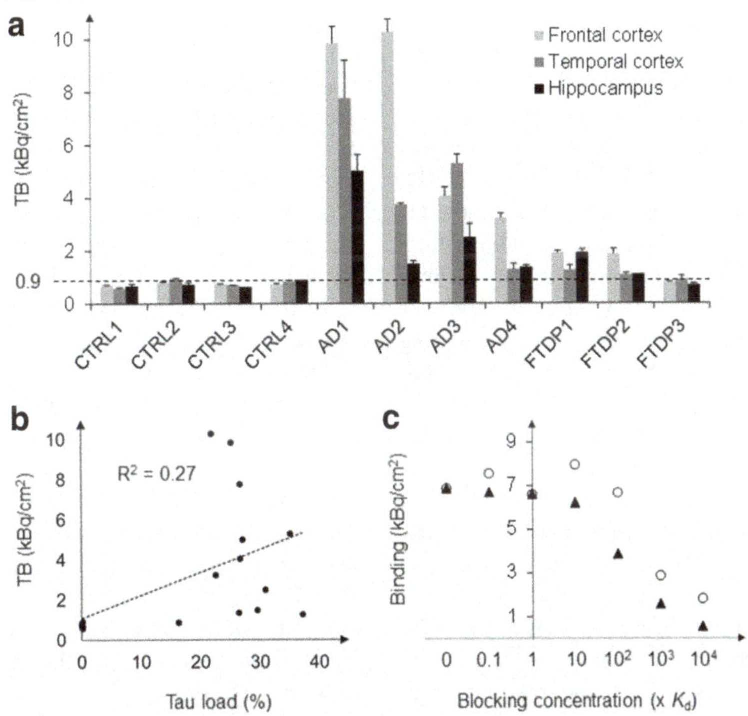


**Fig. 7** Quantitative phosphorimaging with [$^{18}$F]THK-5117 **a)** Total binding of [$^{18}$F]THK-5117 to the grey matter of control and tauopathy cases. Experiments were carried out in triplicates. **b)** Correlation of total [$^{18}$F]THK-5117 binding in the grey matter, as determined by quantitative phosphorimaging, and tau total load, as determined by AT8 immunohistochemistry in adjacent brain sections. **c)** [$^{18}$F]THK-5117 binding to the frontal cortex of case AD1 under constant inhibition of the monoamine oxidases A and B (using 1 µM chlorgylin and L-deprenyl, respectively) and with block of tracer binding using increasing concentrations of flortaucipir (circles) or THK-5117 (triangles) ranging from 0.1–10,000 times $K_d$. Abbreviations: CTRL, control; AD, Alzheimer's disease; FTDP, frontotemporal dementia with parkinsonism linked to chromosome 17 (microtubule-associated protein tau mutation); TB, total binding; FC, frontal cortex; TC, temporal cortex; HP, hippocampus

with Alzheimer's disease has shown [$^{18}$F]flortaucipir binding to be closely linked to brain areas affected by neurodegeneration, and tracer uptake to correlate with the degree of cognitive impairment [17, 32, 34]. However, in some Alzheimer's disease patients, who were positively tested for amyloid, [$^{18}$F]flortaucipir retention in the cortical areas was found to be low, and comparable to that observed in age-matched controls. Other study participants showed highly focal tracer binding in limited cortical areas [35]. A similar variability – despite smaller patient cohorts – was observed when using PET tracers from the THK series [13, 21]. These studies support the notion that PET tracer binding is dependent on the strain of tau pathology in the respective patient [7, 18, 27] and that there may be populations expressing tau inclusions with a particularly high, or low, affinity to the first generation tau PET tracers.

[$^{18}$F]Flortaucipir binding was recently reported to correlate with neurofibrillary tangle load, as determined by PHF1 antibody staining in *post-mortem* brain tissue from cases representing the different Braak & Braak stages (I–VI) [24]. In our hands, neither the structural analogue T726, nor the 2-arylquinoline THK-5117, depicted tau inclusions observed in the control cases with pathology (Braak & Braak stages II and III). Furthermore, the tau tracers did not exclusively bind to neurofibrillary tangles, but predominantly to premature tau inclusions such as pre-tangles and neuropil threads (*vide supra*). This is in contrast to observations made by others, which support the notion that flortaucipir [22, 31] and THK-5117 [11, 12] primarily depict mature tau inclusions. Methodological differences, in particular the use of paraffin embedded tissue that requires dewaxing and antigen retrieval methods before staining, as well as inter-case variability may explain different interpretations. Given the strong evidence of our fluorescence microscopy study for tau tracer binding to both premature and mature inclusions, we used the phospho-tau specific antibody AT8 to determine total pathological tau load in the tissue used for this study, as it detects the earliest phosphorylation sites on tau, resulting in the development of neurofibrillary structures. The low sensitivity for tau inclusions in prodromal disease cases, as reflected by the ratio of pathological tau depicted by the small molecule ligands to that depicted by AT8, may preclude detection of disease in vivo at the earliest stages. Over the course of disease, maturation of the tau inclusions may affect the accessibility of the binding site(s) for tau tracers, or the avidity of binding, for instance through gradual changes to the three-dimensional structure and density of the aggregates.

In this study, we did not observe any fluorescent tau tracer binding to inclusions predominantly composed of either three- or four-repeat tau isoforms. However, tau tracer binding was detected in the FTDP-17 case with a R406W *MAPT* mutation (case FTDP1), which produces pathological inclusions that closely resemble those found in Alzheimer's disease. Tau load in the hippocampus of the case FTDP1, as determined by immunohistochemistry with AT8, was comparable to that found in the Alzheimer's disease cases (ca. 30%), whereas in the cortical areas it was considerably lower (ca. 15%). This was corroborated using fluorescence microscopy and nuclear emulsion autoradiography. The results also reflect findings from [$^{18}$F]flortaucipir PET scans in patients with *MAPT* mutations that cause tau inclusions with mixed three- and four-repeat pathology (R406W and V337 M) [41, 42]. Although overall tau ligand binding in patients with the R406W and V337 M variants, as well as in the case included in our study, was lower than observed in subjects and cases with Alzheimer's disease, the distribution pattern differed in that tracer uptake is highly focal (hippocampus and surrounding temporal cortex) in the mutation carriers. Therefore, the first generation tau PET tracers may be suitable for monitoring disease progression in patients who carry the mentioned MAPT mutations; however, further studies are needed to clarify the specificity of this technique. In particular, contradictory findings of flortaucipir binding to patients and cases with *MAPT* mutations resulting in predominantly four-repeat pathology have been reported [2, 22, 24, 37].

In summary, our results highlight the limitations of first generation tau ligands, bearing carbazole and 2-arylquinoline core structures, for some clinical applications. In particular, the high variability of tau PET tracer binding within and between late-stage sporadic Alzheimer's disease, and the relatively low sensitivity to tau in earliest Braak stages may limit these tracers' use for early diagnosis, monitoring of disease progression or assessment of therapeutic interventions. These limitations may be overcome by the next generation of tau PET tracers. However, it remains a concern that several of the newer tracers also target the T808 binding site, and therefore may be affected by some of the drawbacks associated with the first generation tracers. Future studies in human *post-mortem* brain tissue are crucial to address this concern.

Our study highlights the importance of applying a range of research techniques to the non-clinical assessment of tau PET tracers. Despite the different tracer concentrations used for fluorescence and nuclear tissue imaging, the results obtained with the different techniques demonstrated the same tracer binding patterns and could therefore be used to obtain complementary information about the nature of tau pathology depicted by the structurally distinct tau ligands at the cellular level. Using this unique combination of nuclear imaging and histological methods allowed us to qualitatively and quantitatively assess tracer binding at different levels of resolution. Importantly, we were able to detect tracer binding patterns resembling those observed in clinical PET studies, in particular the high variability in tracer binding between and within cases and patients, respectively. In the future, novel PET tracers should be subject to rigorous non-clinical assessment before being translated into clinical studies.

## Additional files

**Additional file 1: Table S1.** Extended demographic data of cases included in the study. **Figure S1.** Tau immunohistochemistry in cases with primary tauopathies. **Figure S2.** Lack of fluorescent tau tracer binding in cases with primary tauopathies. **Figure S3.** Lack of tau tracer binding to the medial temporal lobe of control cases CTRL1–CTRL4 with and without tau pathology. **Figure S4.** Representative immunofluorescence images showing AT8 immunoreactive tau inclusions depicted by fluorescent tau tracers. **Figure S5.** Concomitant labelling of tissue from Alzheimer's disease cases with fluorescent tau tracers and phospho-tau specific antibodies. **Figure S6.** Quantitative phosphorimaging with [$^{18}$F]THK-5117. (PDF 2092 kb)

**Acknowledgements**
We thank Prof Nobuyuki Okamura (Department of Pharmacology, Tohoku University School of Medicine, Japan) for kindly providing THK-5117 and the respective labelling precursor, and Prof Peter Davies for gifting the antibody PHF1. We are grateful to Prof Nick C Fox (Dementia Research Centre, Institute of Neurology, University College London, UK) for his support of the study, and his advice on the manuscript.

**Funding**
We acknowledge funding by the Leonard Wolfson Experimental Neurology Centre (MCW, KS), Alzheimer's Research UK Senior Fellowship (TL) and the NIHR Queen Square Dementia Biomedical Research Unit. This work was undertaken at UCLH/UCL, which is funded in part by the Department of Health's NIHR Biomedical Research Centres funding scheme. The Queen Square Brain Bank is supported by the Reta Lila Weston Institute for Neurological Studies and the Progressive Supranuclear Palsy (Europe) Association.

**Authors' contributions**
TL, EÅ and KS conceptualised the study. TL selected the cases included in the study. MCW conducted immunohistochemistry and fluorescence imaging experiments. MCW and KS carried out phosphorimaging and nuclear emulsion autoradiography. MCW, TL and KS analysed the data. MCW and KS wrote the manuscript. All authors read and approved the final manuscript.

**Competing interests**
The authors declare that they have no competing interests.

**Author details**
[1]Institute of Nuclear Medicine and Department of Chemistry, University College London, London, UK. [2]Institute of Neurology, Department of Molecular Neuroscience, Queen Square Brain Bank for Neurological Disorders, University College London, London, UK. [3]Radiochemistry, University College London, Kathleen Lonsdale Building, 5 Gower Place, London WC1E 6BS, UK.

**References**

1. Arriagada PV, Growdon JH, Hedley-Whyte ET, Hyman BT (1992) Neurofibrillary tangles but not senile plaques parallel duration and severity of Alzheimer's disease. Neurology 42(3):631–639. https://doi.org/10.1212/WNL.42.3.631
2. Bevan Jones WRB, Cope TE, Passamonti L, Fryer TD, Hong YT, Aigbirhio F, Kril JJ, Forrest SL, Allinson K, Coles JP, Jones PS, Spillantini MG, Hodges JR, O'Brien JT, Rowe JB (2016) [$^{18}$F]AV-1451 PET in behavioural variant frontotemporal dementia due to MAPT mutation. Ann Clin Transl Neurol 3(12):940–947 https://doi.org/10.1002/acn3.366
3. Bischof GN, Endepols H, van Eimeren T, Drzezga A (2017) Tau-imaging in neurodegeneration. Methods 130:114–123 https://doi.org/10.1016/j.ymeth.2017.08.003
4. Braak H, Braak E (1991) Neuropathological stageing of Alzheimer-related changes. Acta Neuropathol 82(4):239–259 https://doi.org/10.1007/BF00308809
5. Braak H, Braak E (1994) Morphological criteria for the recognition of Alzheimer's disease and the distribution pattern of cortical changes related to this disorder. Neurobiol Aging 15(3):355–356 https://doi.org/10.1016/0197-4580(94)90032-9
6. Cai L, Qu B, Hurtle BT, Dadiboyena S, Diaz-Arrastia R, Pike VW (2016) Candidate PET radioligand development for neurofibrillary tangles: two distinct radioligand binding sites identified in postmortem Alzheimer's disease brain. ACS Chem Neurosci 7(7):897–911 https://doi.org/10.1021/acschemneuro.6b00051
7. Castillo-Carranza DL, Guerrero-Muñoz MJ, Sengupta U, Gerson JE (in press) Kayed R (2018) α-Synuclein oligomers induce a unique toxic tau strain. Biol Psychiatry https://doi.org/10.1016/j.biopsych.2017.12.018
8. Dickson DW, Hauw JJ, Agid Y, Litvan I (2011) Progressive supranuclear palsy and corticobasal degeneration. In: Dickson DW, Weller RO (eds) Neurodegeneration: the molecular pathology of dementia and movement disorders. Wiley-Blackwell, City, pp 135–155 https://doi.org/10.1002/9781444341256
9. Gobbi LC, Knust H, Körner M, Honer M, Czech C, Belli S, Muri D, Edelmann MR, Hartung T, Erbsmehl I, Grall-Ulsemer S, Koblet A, Rueher M, Steiner S, Ravert HT, Mathews WB, Holt DP, Kuwabara H, Valentine H, Dannals RF, Wong DF, Borroni E (2017) Identification of three novel radiotracers for imaging aggregated tau in Alzheimer's disease with positron emission tomography. J Med Chem 60(17):7350–7370 https://doi.org/10.1021/acs.jmedchem.7b00632
10. Goedert M, Jakes R, Vanmechelen E (1995) Monoclonal antibody AT8 recognises tau protein phosphorylated AT both serine 202 and threonine 205. Neurosci Lett 189(3):167–169 https://doi.org/10.1016/0304-3940(95)11484-E
11. Harada R, Okamura N, Furumoto S, Furukawa K, Ishiki A, Tomita N, Hiraoka K, Watanuki S, Shidahara M, Miyake M, Ishikawa Y, Matsuda R, Inami A, Yoshikawa T, Tago T, Funaki Y, Iwata R, Tashiro M, Yanai K, Arai H, Kudo Y (2015) [(18)F]THK-5117 PET for assessing neurofibrillary pathology in Alzheimer's disease. Eur J Nucl Med Mol Imaging 42(7):1052–1061 https://doi.org/10.1007/s00259-015-3035-4
12. Harada R, Okamura N, Furumoto S, Furukawa K, Ishiki A, Tomita N, Tago T, Hiraoka K, Watanuki S, Shidahara M, Miyake M, Ishikawa Y, Matsuda R, Inami A, Yoshikawa T, Funaki Y, Iwata R, Tashiro M, Yanai K, Arai H, Kudo Y (2016) $^{18}$F-THK5351: a novel PET radiotracer for imaging neurofibrillary pathology in Alzheimer disease. J Nucl Med 57(2):208–214 https://doi.org/10.2967/jnumed.115.164848

13. Harada R, Okamura N, Furumoto S, Tago T, Yanai K, Arai H, Kudo Y (2016) Characteristics of tau and its ligands in PET imaging. Biomol Ther 6(1):7 https://doi.org/10.3390/biom6010007
14. Haroutunian V, Davies P, Vianna C, Buxbaum JD, Purohit DP (2007) Tau protein abnormalities associated with the progression of Alzheimer disease type dementia. Neurobiol Aging 28(1):1–7 https://doi.org/10.1016/j.neurobiolaging.2005.11.001
15. Hostetler ED, Walji AM, Zeng Z, Miller P, Bennacef I, Salinas C, Connolly B, Gantert L, Haley H, Holahan M, Purcell M, Riffel K, Lohith TG, Coleman P, Soriano A, Ogawa A, Xu S, Zhang X, Joshi E, Della Rocca J, Hesk D, Schenk DJ, Evelhoch JL (2016) Preclinical characterization of $^{18}$F-MK-6240, a promising PET tracer for *in vivo* quantification of human neurofibrillary tangles. J Nucl Med 57(10):1599–1606 https://doi.org/10.2967/jnumed.115.171678
16. Ishiki A, Harada R, Okamura N, Tomita N, Rowe CC, Villemagne VL, Yanai K, Kudo Y, Arai H, Furumoto S, Tashiro M, Furukawa K (2017) Tau imaging with [$^{18}$F]THK-5351 in progressive supranuclear palsy. Eur J Neurol 24(1):130–136 https://doi.org/10.1111/ene.13164
17. Johnson KA, Schultz A, Betensky RA, Becker JA, Sepulcre J, Rentz D, Mormino E, Chhatwal J, Amariglio R, Papp K, Marshall G, Albers M, Mauro S, Pepin L, Alverio J, Judge K, Philiossaint M, Shoup T, Yokell D, Dickerson B, Gomez-Isla T, Hyman B, Vasdev N, Sperling R (2016) Tau positron emission tomographic imaging in aging and early Alzheimer disease. Ann Neurol 79(1):110–119 https://doi.org/10.1002/ana.24546
18. Kaufman SK, Sanders DW, Thomas TL, Ruchinskas AJ, Vaquer-Alicea J, Sharma AM, Miller TM, Diamond MI (2016) Tau prion strains dictate patterns of cell pathology, progression rate, and regional vulnerability in vivo. Neuron 92(4):796–812 https://doi.org/10.1016/j.neuron.2016.09.055
19. Lashley T, Rohrer JD, Bandopadhyay R, Fry C, Ahmed Z, Isaacs AM, Brelstaff JH, Borroni B, Warren JD, Troakes C, King A, Al-Saraj S, Newcombe J, Quinn N, Ostergaard K, Schrøder HD, Bojsen-Møller M, Braendgaard H, Fox NC, Rossor MN, Lees AJ, Holton JL, Revesz T (2011) A comparative clinical, pathological, biochemical and genetic study of fused in sarcoma proteinopathies. Brain 134(Pt 9):2548–2564 https://doi.org/10.1093/brain/awr160
20. Lemoine L, Saint-Aubert L, Marutle A, Antoni G, Eriksson JP, Ghetti B, Okamura N, Nennesmo I, Gillberg PG, Nordberg A (2015) Visualization of regional tau deposits using $^{3}$H-THK5117 in Alzheimer brain tissue. Acta Neuropathol Commun 3(40) https://doi.org/10.1186/s40478-015-0220-4
21. Lockhart SN, Baker SL, Okamura N, Furukawa K, Ishiki A, Furumoto S, Tashiro M, Yanai K, Arai H, Kudo Y, Harada R, Tomita N, Hiraoka K, Watanuki S, Jagust WJ (2016) Dynamic PET measures of tau accumulation in cognitively normal older adults and Alzheimer's disease patients measured using [$^{18}$F]THK-5351. PLoS One 11(6):e0158460 https://doi.org/10.1371/journal.pone.0158460
22. Lowe VJ, Curran G, Fang P, Liesinger AM, Josephs KA, Parisi JE, Kantarci K, Boeve BF, Pandey MK, Bruinsma T, Knopman DS, Jones DT, Petrucelli L, Cook CN, Graff-Radford NR, Dickson DW, Petersen RC, Jack CR Jr, Murray ME (2016) An autoradiographic evaluation of AV-1451 tau PET in dementia. Acta Neuropathol Commun 4(1):58 https://doi.org/10.1186/s40478-016-0315-6
23. Marquié M, Normandin MD, Vanderburg CR, Costantino IM, Bien EA, Rycyna LG, Klunk WE, Mathis CA, Ikonomovic MD, Debnath ML, Vasdev N, Dickerson BC, Gomperts SN, Growdon JH, Johnson KA, Frosch MP, Hyman BT, Gómez-Isla T (2015) Validating novel tau positron emission tomography tracer [F-18]-AV-1451 (T807) on postmortem brain tissue. Ann Neurol 78(5):787–800 https://doi.org/10.1002/ana.24517
24. Marquié M, Normandin MD, Meltzer AC, Siao Tick Chong M, Andrea NV, Antón-Fernández A, Klunk WE, Mathis CA, Ikonomovic MD, Debnath M, Bien EA, Vanderburg CR, Costantino I, Makaretz S, DeVos SL, Oakley DH, Gomperts SN, Growdon JH, Domoto-Reilly K, Lucente D, Dickerson BC, Frosch MP, Hyman BT, Johnson KA, Gómez-Isla T (2017) Pathological correlations of [F-18]-AV-1451 imaging in non-alzheimer tauopathies. Ann Neurol 81(1):117–128 https://doi.org/10.1002/ana.24844
25. Mirra SS, Heyman A, McKeel D, Sumi SM, Crain BJ, Brownlee LM, Vogel FS, Hughes JP, van Belle G, Berg L, neurologists p CERAD (1991) The consortium to establish a registry for Alzheimer's disease (CERAD). Part II. Standardization of the neuropathologic assessment of Alzheimer's disease. Neurology 41(4):479–486 https://doi.org/10.1212/WNL.41.4.479
26. Montine TJ, Phelps CH, Beach TG, Bigio EH, Cairns NJ, Dickson DW, Duyckaerts C, Frosch MP, Masliah E, Mirra SS, Nelson PT, Schneider JA, Thal DR, Trojanowski JQ, Vinters HV, Hyman BT, National Institute on Aging; Alzheimer's Association (2012) National Institute on Aging-Alzheimer's Association guidelines for the neuropathologic assessment of Alzheimer's disease: a practical approach. Acta Neuropathol 123(1):1–11 https://doi.org/10.1007/s00401-011-0910-3
27. Narasimhan S, Guo JL, Changolkar L, Stieber A, McBride JD, Silva LV, He Z, Zhang B, Gathagan RJ, Trojanowski JQ, Lee VMY (2017) Pathological tau strains from human brains recapitulate the diversity of tauopathies in nontransgenic mouse brain. J Neurosci 37(47):11406–11423 https://doi.org/10.1523/JNEUROSCI.1230-17.2017
28. Ng KP, Pascoal TA, Mathotaarachchi S, Therriault J, Kang MS, Shin M, Guiot MC, Guo Q, Harada R, Comley RA, Massarweh G, Soucy JP, Okamura N, Gauthier S, Rosa-Neto P (2017) Monoamine oxidase B inhibitor, selegiline, reduces $^{18}$F-THK5351 uptake in the human brain. Alzheimers Res Ther 9(1): 25 https://doi.org/10.1186/s13195-017-0253-y
29. Okamura N, Furumoto S, Harada R, Tago T, Yoshikawa T, Fodero-Tavoletti M, Mulligan RS, Villemagne VL, Akatsu H, Yamamoto T, Arai H, Iwata R, Yanai K, Kudo Y (2013) Novel $^{18}$F-labeled arylquinoline derivatives for noninvasive imaging of tau pathology in Alzheimer disease. J Nucl Med 54(8):1420–1427 https://doi.org/10.2967/jnumed.112.117341
30. Okamura N, Harada R, Furumoto S, Arai H, Yanai K, Kudo Y (2014) Tau PET imaging in Alzheimer's disease. Curr Neurol Neurosci Rep 14(11):500 https://doi.org/10.1007/s11910-014-0500-6
31. Ono M, Sahara N, Kumata K, Ji B, Ni R, Koga S, Dickson DW, Trojanowski JQ, Lee VM, Yoshida M, Hozumi I, Yoshiyama Y, van Swieten JC, Nordberg A, Suhara T, Zhang MR, Higuchi M (2017) Distinct binding of PET ligands PBB3 and AV-1451 to tau fibril strains in neurodegenerative tauopathies. Brain 140(3):764–780 https://doi.org/10.1093/brain/aww339
32. Ossenkoppele R, Schonhaut DR, Schöll M, Lockhart SN, Ayakta N, Baker SL, O'Neil JP, Janabi M, Lazaris A, Cantwell A, Vogel J, Santos M, Miller ZA, Bettcher BM, Vossel KA, Kramer JH, Gorno-Tempini ML, Miller BL, Jagust WJ, Rabinovici GD (2016) Tau PET patterns mirror clinical and neuroanatomical variability in Alzheimer's disease. Brain 139(Pt 5):1551–1567 https://doi.org/10.1093/brain/aww027
33. Passamonti L, Vázquez Rodríguez P, Hong YT, Allinson KS, Williamson D, Borchert RJ, Sami S, Cope TE, Bevan-Jones WR, Jones PS, Arnold R, Surendranathan A, Mak E, Su L, Fryer TD, Aigbirhio FI, O'Brien JT, Rowe JB (2017) $^{18}$F-AV-1451 positron emission tomography in Alzheimer's disease and progressive supranuclear palsy. Brain 140(3):781–791 https://doi.org/10.1093/brain/aww340
34. Phillips JS, Das SR, McMillan CT, Irwin DJ, Roll EE, Da Re F, Nasrallah IM, Wolk DA, Grossman M (2017) Tau PET imaging predicts cognition in atypical variants of Alzheimer's disease. Hum Brain Mapp:1–18 https://doi.org/10.1002/hbm.23874
35. Pontecorvo MJ, Devous MD Sr, Navitsky M, Lu M, Salloway S, Schaerf FW, Jennings D, Arora AK, McGeehan A, Lim NC, Xiong H, Joshi AD, Siderowf A, Mintun MA; $^{18}$F-AV-1451-A05 investigators (2017) Relationships between flortaucipir PET tau binding and amyloid burden, clinical diagnosis, age and cognition. Brain 140 (3): 748–763. https://doi.org/10.1093/brain/aww334
36. Saint-Aubert L, Lemoine L, Chiotis K, Leuzy A, Rodriguez-Vieitez E, Nordberg A (2017) Tau PET imaging: present and future directions. Mol Neurodegener 12(1):19 https://doi.org/10.1186/s13024-017-0162-3
37. Sander K, Lashley T, Gami P, Gendron T, Lythgoe MF, Rohrer JD, Schott JM, Revesz T, Fox NC, Årstad E (2016) Characterization of tau positron emission tomography tracer [$^{18}$F]AV-1451 binding to postmortem tissue in Alzheimer's disease, primary tauopathies, and other dementias. Alzheimers Dement 12(11):1116–1124 https://doi.org/10.1016/j.jalz.2016.01.003
38. Schneider CA, Rasband WS, Eliceiri KW (2012) NIH image to ImageJ: 25 years of image analysis. Nat Meth 9(7):671–675 https://doi.org/10.1038/nmeth.2089
39. Schöll M, Lockhart SN, Schonhaut DR, O'Neil JP, Janabi M, Ossenkoppele R, Baker SL, Vogel JW, Faria J, Schwimmer HD, Rabinovici GD, Jagust WJ (2016) PET imaging of tau deposition in the aging human brain. Neuron 89(5):971–982 https://doi.org/10.1016/j.neuron.2016.01.028
40. Schwarz AJ, Yu P, Miller BB, Shcherbinin S, Dickson J, Navitsky M, Joshi AD, Devous MD Sr, Mintun MS (2016) Regional profiles of the candidate tau PET ligand $^{18}$F-AV-1451 recapitulate key features of Braak histopathological stages. Brain 139: 1539–1550. https://doi.org/10.1093/brain/aww023
41. Smith R, Puschmann A, Schöll M, Ohlsson T, van Swieten J, Honer M, Englund E, Hansson O (2016) $^{18}$F-AV-1451 tau PET imaging correlates strongly with tau neuropathology in MAPT mutation carriers. Brain 139: 2372–2379 https://doi.org/10.1093/brain/aww163
42. Spina S, Schonhaut DR, Boeve BF, Seeley WW, Ossenkoppele R, O'Neil JP, Lazaris A, Rosen HJ, Boxer AL, Perry DC, Miller BL, Dickson DW, Parisi JE,

Jagust WJ, Murray ME, Rabinovici GD (2017) Frontotemporal dementia with the V337M MAPT mutation: tau-PET and pathology correlations. Neurology 88(8):758–766 https://doi.org/10.1212/WNL.0000000000003636

43. Szardenings AK, Kolb HC, Walsh JC, Chen G, Gangadharmath UB, Kasi D, Liu C, Sinha A, Wang E, Yu C, Zhang W, Chen K, Mocharla VP, Scott PJH (2012) Imaging agents for detecting neurological dysfunction. Patent Application US20120302755 A1 (Siemens Medical Solutions USA, Inc.)
44. Thal DR, Rueb U, Orantes M, Braak H (2000) Phases of a beta-deposition in the human brain and its relevance for the development of AD. Neurology 58(12):1791–1800 https://doi.org/10.1212/WNL.58.12.1791
45. Uchihara T, Nakamura A, Yamazaki M (2001) Mori O (2001) evolution from pretangle neurons to neurofibrillary tangles monitored by thiazin red combined with Gallyas method and double immunofluorescence. Acta Neuropathol 101(6):535–539 https://doi.org/10.1007/s004010000306
46. Vermeiren C, Motte P, Viot D, Mairet-Coello G, Courade JP, Citron M, Mercier J, Hannestad J, Gillard M (2018) The tau positron-emission tomography tracer AV-1451 binds with similar affinities to tau fibrils and monoamine oxidases. Mov Disord 33(2):273–281 https://doi.org/10.1002/mds.27271
47. Vettermann F, Brendel M, Schaenecker S, Haeglinger G, Danek A, Levin J, Bartenstein P, Okamura N, Rominger A (2016) [$^{18}$F]THK-5351 PET in patients with clinically diagnosed progressive supranuclear palsy. J Nucl Med 57 (supplement 2): 457
48. Wang Y, Mandelkow E (2016) Tau in physiology and pathology. Nat Rev Neurosci 17:5–21 https://doi.org/10.1038/nrn.2015.1
49. Xia CF, Arteaga J, Chen G, Gangadharmath U, Gomez LF, Kasi D, Lam C, Liang Q, Liu C, Mocharla VP, Mu F, Sinha A, Su H, Szardenings AK, Walsh JC, Wang E, Yu C, Zhang W, Zhao T, Kolb HC (2013) [(18)F]T807, a novel tau positron emission tomography imaging agent for Alzheimer's disease. Alzheimers Dement 9(6):666–676 https://doi.org/10.1016/j.jalz.2012.11.008
50. Zhang W, Arteaga J, Cashion DK, Chen G, Gangadharmath U, Gomez LF, Kasi D, Lam C, Liang Q, Liu C, Mocharla VP, Mu F, Sinha A, Szardenings AK, Wang E, Walsh JC, Xia C, Yu C, Zhao T, Kolb HC (2012) A highly selective and specific PET tracer for imaging of tau pathologies. J Alzheimers Dis 31(3):601–612 https://doi.org/10.3233/JAD-2012-120712
51. Zhao Z, Sagare AP, Ma Q, Halliday MR, Kong P, Kisler K, Winkler EA, Ramanathan A, Kanekiyo T, Bu G, Owens NC, Rege SV, Si G, Ahuja A, Zhu D, Miller CA, Schneider JA, Maeda M, Maeda T, Sugawara T, Ichida JK, Zlokovic BV (2015) Central role for PICALM in amyloid-β blood-brain barrier transcytosis and clearance. Nat Neurosci 18(7):978–987 https://doi.org/10.1038/nn.4025

# 9

# A new TAO kinase inhibitor reduces tau phosphorylation at sites associated with neurodegeneration in human tauopathies

Caterina Giacomini[1], Chuay-Yeng Koo[1], Natalia Yankova[2], Ignatius A. Tavares[1], Selina Wray[3], Wendy Noble[2], Diane P. Hanger[2] and Jonathan D. H. Morris[1*]

**Abstract**

In Alzheimer's disease (AD) and related tauopathies, the microtubule-associated protein tau is highly phosphorylated and aggregates to form neurofibrillary tangles that are characteristic of these neurodegenerative diseases. Our previous work has demonstrated that the thousand-and-one amino acid kinases (TAOKs) 1 and 2 phosphorylate tau on more than 40 residues in vitro. Here we show that TAOKs are phosphorylated and active in AD brain sections displaying mild (Braak stage II), intermediate (Braak stage IV) and advanced (Braak stage VI) tau pathology and that active TAOKs co-localise with both pre-tangle and tangle structures. TAOK activity is also enriched in pathological tau containing sarkosyl-insoluble extracts prepared from AD brain. Two new phosphorylated tau residues (T123 and T427) were identified in AD brain, which appear to be targeted specifically by TAOKs. A new small molecule TAOK inhibitor (Compound 43) reduced tau phosphorylation on T123 and T427 and also on additional pathological sites (S262/S356 and S202/T205/S208) in vitro and in cell models. The TAOK inhibitor also decreased tau phosphorylation in differentiated primary cortical neurons without affecting markers of synapse and neuron health. Notably, TAOK activity also co-localised with tangles in post-mortem frontotemporal lobar degeneration (FTLD) brain tissue. Furthermore, the TAOK inhibitor decreased tau phosphorylation in induced pluripotent stem cell derived neurons from FTLD patients, as well as cortical neurons from a transgenic mouse model of tauopathy (Tau35 mice). Our results demonstrate that abnormal TAOK activity is present at pre-tangles and tangles in tauopathies and that TAOK inhibition effectively decreases tau phosphorylation on pathological sites. Thus, TAOKs may represent a novel target to reduce or prevent tau-associated neurodegeneration in tauopathies.

**Keywords:** Alzheimer, Tauopathy, Dementia, TAOK, Tau, Phosphorylation, Kinase

## Introduction

Pathological aggregation of highly phosphorylated tau and the formation of neurofibrillary tangles (NFTs) in the brain provide one of the main characteristic pathological features of a subgroup of neurodegenerative disorders termed tauopathies. Alzheimer's disease (AD) is the most prevalent tauopathy but similar tangle-like features are also displayed in frontotemporal lobar degeneration (FTLD), Pick's disease, progressive supranuclear palsy and corticobasal degeneration [17, 19]. The presence of extracellular plaques of beta-amyloid (Aβ) provides an additional hallmark for AD. However, the emergence of tau pathology appears to correlate more closely than plaques with the progression of cognitive impairment in AD [26].

Human tau is encoded by the *MAPT* gene located on chromosome 17 and alternative splicing of exons 2, 3 and 10 produces six tau isoforms containing up to two inserts at the N terminus (0 N, 1 N or 2 N) and three or four repeated sequences (3R or 4R) at the C terminus of the protein [8, 36]. Tau is expressed predominantly in neurons and is a major microtubule-associated protein (MAP) involved in the regulation of microtubule dynamics and organisation [13, 58]. Tau splicing is developmentally regulated and only the shortest 0N3R tau isoform is expressed in the foetal brain, whereas all six tau isoforms are present in the adult central nervous

* Correspondence: jonathan.morris@kcl.ac.uk
[1]King's College London, School of Cancer and Pharmaceutical Sciences, New Hunt's House, Guy's Campus, London SE11UL, UK
Full list of author information is available at the end of the article

system (CNS) [8, 36]. In AD and related tauopathies, aberrant tau phosphorylation results in its dissociation from microtubules and the aggregation of tau in the cytosol to form NFTs [23, 34]. The relative importance of individual or combinations of phosphorylated tau residues remains to be determined. Phosphorylation of the KXGS repeated motifs (notably S262 and S356) located in the C-terminal microtubule binding domain are involved in regulating tau microtubule-binding, as are additional phosphorylation sites flanking this region [1–3, 22].

A number of protein kinases have been shown to target tau, at least in vitro, including microtubule-affinity regulating kinase (MARK), glycogen synthase kinase 3 (GSK-3), cyclin-dependent kinase 5 (CDK5), Fyn and also extracellular signal regulated kinase 2 (ERK2), c-Jun N-terminal kinase (JNK) and p38 mitogen-activated protein kinases (MAPKs) [3, 24, 33, 40, 48, 61]. An important challenge for dementia is to identify kinases that are catalytically active, associated with tangles, and are therefore likely to contribute directly to the development of tau pathology [20]. Previously, we have reported that the thousand-and-one amino acid kinases (TAOKs, also referred to as prostate-derived sterile 20-like kinases (PSKs)) phosphorylate tau on multiple disease-associated sites and that these kinases are activated in AD brain [55]. TAOKs belong to the sterile 20 group of mammalian protein kinases, with family members including TAOKs 1–3 [9, 25, 44, 69]. TAOK1 and TAOK2 can regulate MAPKs and stimulate JNK and p38 MAPK signalling pathways [9, 25, 44, 68, 69]. TAOK1 and TAOK2 also induce apoptotic changes via activation of JNK, MAPK and caspases; however, a key feature of TAOKs is their ability to regulate microtubule dynamics and organisation [38, 43, 56, 68]. TAOK1 induces microtubule instability through its direct activation of MARK and phosphorylation of MAPs, including tau, which dissociate from microtubules, resulting in their disassembly [55–57]. TAOK2 binds to microtubules directly through its C terminus (amino acids 745–1235), leading to stabilisation of perinuclear microtubules, which contain increased acetylated α–tubulin and are resistant to nocodazole-induced depolymerisation [43].

Although very little is known about the relationship of TAOKs to neurodegenerative diseases, the TAOK2 gene is located on chromosome 16p11.2, a region that carries significant susceptibility for autism spectrum disorders and schizophrenia [41, 62]. In the developing mouse brain, TAOK2 is required for basal dendritic development and callosal axon projection in cortical neurons, where it acts downstream of the neuropilin-1 receptor for semaphorin 3A, to regulate dendrite arborisation and axon elongation through JNK [10]. Phosphorylation of TAOK1 (pT440) and TAOK2 (pT475) by mammalian sterile 20-like kinase 3 (MST3) results in myosin Va binding and subsequent localisation of these kinases to dendrites, where they regulate spine and synapse development [59]. TAOK2 also mediates post-synaptic density protein 95 (PSD95) stability and dendritic spine maturation via phosphorylation and relocation of the cytoskeletal GTPase septin 7 [65]. A recent study has also identified three missense mutations in *TAOK2* in autism spectrum disorder subjects and shown that the expression of mutated forms of TAOK2 or increased expression of wild type TAOK2 impairs dendritic spine development in primary neurons [49]. These studies demonstrate important functions for TAOK2 during early brain development; however, the potential roles for TAOKs in the adult brain and in the aberrant phosphorylation of tau in tauopathies have not yet been explored.

In this study, we have investigated the effects of tau phosphorylation resulting from TAOK activity and inhibition using a new small molecule inhibitor. We found that TAOK activity was present in pre-tangles and tangles in AD and FTLD brain, whereas it was only weakly detectable in control human brain. TAOKs phosphorylated tau on pathological sites in human cell lines in addition to murine and human neurons, and this was reduced by the TAOK inhibitor. Our findings implicate the TAOKs as important contributors to the development of tau pathology in AD and FTLD.

## Materials and methods

### Plasmids, antibodies and reagents

Plasmids pRK5-TAOK1, pRK5-TAOK2, pRK5-TAOK2 (K57A) and pRK5-TAOK2 (amino acids 1–349) were generated as described previously [44, 69] and subcloned into pCAGGS-IRES-EGFP or pCAGGS-IRES-Tomato vectors (gift from Dr. L. Gasparini, Italian Institute of Technology, Genoa, Italy). PLenti-lox3.7 vectors expressing TAOK2-shRNA or non-targeting-shRNA and enhanced green fluorescent protein (EGFP) using an alternative promoter were a gift from Dr. S. Ultanir (Crick Institute, London, UK). Tau-pT123, tau-pT427 and TAOK-pS181 affinity-purified rabbit antibodies and peptides were produced by Eurogentec. Mouse tau-pS262/S356 antibody (12E8) was a gift from Dr. P. Seubert (Prothena, USA). Commercially available mouse monoclonal antibodies were obtained to detect TAOK1 (BD), tau-pS202/T205/S208 (AT8, Thermo Fisher Scientific), total tau (Tau5, Thermo Fisher Scientific), synaptophysin (SP15, Enzo), Myc (9E10, Sigma-Aldrich) and glyceraldehyde 3-phosphate dehydrogenase (GAPDH) (Merck Millipore). Rabbit antibodies were obtained to recognise TAOK1 and TAOK2 (Proteintech), BIII Tubulin (Sigma-Aldrich), total tau (Dako), synapsin 1 (Merck Millipore) and active cleaved caspase III (R&D Systems). GST-TAOK1 (amino acids 1–314) and GST-TAOK2 (amino acids1–314) were obtained from

SignalChem. Reagents and chemicals were purchased from Sigma-Aldrich and cell culture reagents were obtained from Thermo Fisher Scientific, unless otherwise stated. Compound 43 was made by Evotec as described previously [29].

#### Immunostaining of human brain tissue

Clinically and pathologically confirmed post-mortem human AD, FTLD and control brains (Additional file 1: Table S1) were obtained from the MRC London Neurodegenerative Disease Brain Bank (King's College London). Tissue sections (7 μm) were cut from formalin-fixed paraffin-embedded blocks of human brain. Sections were deparaffinised and endogenous peroxidase activity inhibited by incubating samples in 3% (*v*/v) hydrogen peroxide (30 min) followed by antigen retrieval using enhanced microwaving in 10 mM sodium citrate buffer (20 min) (pH 6.0). Sections were blocked for 1 h in 10% (v/v) goat serum before incubation overnight with TAOK-pS181, tau-pT123 or tau-pT427 antibodies (4 °C). Sections were incubated with goat anti-rabbit-biotinylated secondary antibodies (45 min, Dako) and developed using the VECTASTAIN Elite ABC kit (Vector Laboratories) and 0.5 mg/ml 3, 3′-diaminobenzidine chromogen (Vector Laboratories). All sections were counterstained with hematoxylin. For double immunofluorescence labelling, sections were pre-treated as described above, and incubated overnight with phospho-tau antibodies (4 °C) followed by secondary goat anti-rabbit 568 or goat anti-mouse 488 Alexa Fluor antibodies (Thermo Fisher Scientific). Autofluorescence was quenched by Sudan black (0.1% Sudan black in 70% ethanol) and images were acquired using a CSU-X1 inverted spinning-disk confocal microscope (Nikon) equipped with EM-CCD camera (Andor iXon3) and a 60×/1.40 NA oil objective (Nikon).

#### Extraction of sarkosyl-insoluble tau

Sarkosyl extraction of tau from brain tissue was performed as described previously [30]. Briefly, brain tissues were homogenised in 50 mM Tris buffered saline (TBS, pH 7.4) containing 2 mM EGTA, 1 mM $Na_3VO_4$, 10 mM NaF and 1 mM phenylmethylsulfonyl fluoride. Samples were centrifuged at 20,000 *g* for 20 min (4 °C) and sarkosyl (10% *v*/v) was added to the resultant supernatant to give a final concentration of 1% (*v*/v). Samples were mixed for 30 min at ambient temperature, then centrifuged at 100,000 *g* for 1 h at ambient temperature. The supernatant was collected and the pellet washed twice with 1% (v/v) sarkosyl before solubilisation in 2× sodium dodecyl sulphate (SDS) sample buffer (National Diagnostics). The three fractions produced comprised (i) low speed supernatant, (ii) sarkosyl-soluble tau, and (iii) sarkosyl-insoluble tau. Proteins in the samples were resolved by SDS gel electrophoresis (SDS-PAGE) and processed for immunoblotting.

#### In vitro kinase assays

3 μg human recombinant tau (2N4R isoform, Sigma-Aldrich) and 30 ng purified glutathione S-transferase (GST)-TAOK1 (1–314) or GST-TAOK2 (1–314) were incubated in kinase buffer (20 mM $MgCl_2$, 2 mM $MnCl_2$, 3 mM ATP and 30 mM Tris, pH 7.4) for 6 h at 30 °C. Reactions were terminated in 5× Laemmli gel sample buffer (10% SDS, 50% glycerol, 0.05% bromophenol blue, 350 mM dithiothreitol and 1 M Tris, pH 6.8). Samples were resolved by SDS-PAGE and protein phosphorylation was analysed on immunoblots probed with appropriate antibodies.

#### Culture of HEK293T cells and primary cortical neurons

Human embryonic kidney (HEK) 293 T cells were cultured in Dulbecco's Modified Eagle's Medium (DMEM, Sigma-Aldrich), supplemented with 10% (*v*/v) foetal calf serum (FCS, Thermo Fisher Scientific) and antibiotics, at 37 °C in an atmosphere of 5% $CO_2$. Cells were transfected using Lipofectamine 2000 (Thermo Fisher Scientific) according to the manufacturer's instructions. Cultured HEK293T cells were incubated with TAOK inhibitor compound 43 (Cp 43), or equivalent concentrations of vehicle dimethyl sulfoxide (DMSO and to a maximum of 0.3%), for 24 h. Treated cells were collected, lysed and analysed on western blots. Rat primary cortical neurons were prepared from embryonic (E) day 18.5 brains as described previously [16] and neurons were seeded onto poly-L-lysine–coated coverslips or 6 well plates at $3–8 \times 10^4$ cells per coverslip (18 mm) or at $5 \times 10^5$ cells per well. Neurons in neurobasal medium containing B-27, GlutaMAX and antibiotics (Thermo Fisher Scientific) were cultured at 37 °C, in an atmosphere of 5% $CO_2$. Primary cortical neurons were prepared from Tau35 transgenic mice [4] and cultured as described above. Neurons were treated with Cp 43 or vehicle for the indicated times and concentrations, adding fresh inhibitor daily for longer time points. Cells were either lysed for analysis on western blots or stained for immunofluorescence analysis. Neurons transfected with Lipofectamine 2000 were fixed and stained for immunofluorescence analysis. All methods were carried out in accordance with the UK Animals (Scientific Procedures) Act 1986.

#### Culture of induced pluripotent stem cell-derived neurons

Induced pluripotent stem cells (iPSCs) from control and FTLD patients carrying the MAPT 10 + 16 mutation were prepared as described previously [53]. IPSCs were differentiated into cortical neurons using dual SMAD inhibition followed by in vitro neurogenesis, as described previously [52, 53]. After culture for 28–30 days in vitro (DIV), when a substantial amount of neurogenesis had occurred, cells were plated onto poly-ornithine and laminin coated plates (Sigma-Aldrich) or on eight-well chamber slides for immunofluorescence (Ibidi) and fed every two days with neuronal maintenance media (N-2 medium and B-27 medium, ratio 1:1). N-2 medium consists of DMEM/F-12 GlutaMAX containing 1 x N-2, 5 μg/ml insulin, 1 mM L-glutamine, 100 μM non-essential amino acids, 100 units M2-mercaptoethanol, 50 U/ml penicillin and 50 mg/ml streptomycin. B-27 medium consists of Neurobasal medium containing 1 x B-27, 20 mM L-glutamine, 50 U/ml penicillin and 50 mg/ml streptomycin (Thermo Fisher Scientific). Neurons were treated with Cp 43 or vehicle, and cultures were either lysed for immunoblotting or stained for immunofluorescence analysis at 60 DIV.

### Immunofluorescence

Primary cortical neurons were fixed with 4% (*w/v*) paraformaldehyde (PFA) in phosphate-buffered saline (PBS, pH 7.4) for 15 min, permeabilised with 0.2% (w/v) Triton X-100 in PBS for 5 min, and blocked with 10% (*v/v*) goat serum and 0.25% (w/v) Triton X-100 in PBS for 30 min. Neurons were incubated sequentially overnight at 4 °C with appropriate primary antibodies followed by Alexa Fluor 488-, 568- or 647-conjugated secondary antibodies (2 h). Coverslips were mounted using Prolong Gold (Thermo Fisher Scientific) containing 4′, 6′-diamidino-2-phenylindole (DAPI) to label nuclei. To quantify tau phosphorylation on threonine 427 (T427) in neurons transfected with TAOK2 and treated with Cp 43 or vehicle, z-stack confocal images were acquired using fixed laser and scanning settings. Mean immunofluorescence intensity was measured using ImageJ software [50]. Results are expressed as the amount of tau-pT427/tau5 (total tau) immunofluorescence intensity.

### Cytotoxicity assays

Rat primary neurons were treated with Cp 43 (6 h) and cytotoxicity assessed by measuring LDH release into the culture medium using a Cytotox 96 assay kit (Promega, Madison, WI, USA), according to the manufacturer's instructions. Optical density was measured at 492 nm and LDH release from neuronal cultures was expressed as a percentage of total LDH in each sample. Cytotoxicity was also assessed by quantifying through immunofluorescence staining the number of active caspase 3-positive cells following treatment with Cp 43 (72 h). Quantification was carried out on blind-coded sample images using ImageJ software.

### Western blotting

HEK293T cells, primary and iPSC derived neurons were lysed in RIPA buffer (1% NP-40, 0.1% SDS, 150 mM NaCl and 50 mM Tris pH 7.5) supplemented with protease and phosphatase inhibitors (Sigma-Aldrich). Lysed cells were sonicated for 5 min and clarified by centrifugation at 10,000 g for 10 min at ambient temperature. Protein concentrations were determined using a bicinchoninic acid assay (Thermo Fisher Scientific). Equal amounts of protein (15–30 μg) in 5× Laemmli sample buffer were resolved by SDS-PAGE and transferred to 0. 2 μm nitrocellulose membranes (GE Healthcare). Membranes were blocked in 5% (*w/v*) skimmed milk in buffer (150 mM NaCl, 0.1% Tween 20 and 10 mM Tris, pH 7.5), incubated with appropriate primary antibodies overnight at 4 °C, followed by horse radish peroxidase (HRP)-conjugated secondary antibodies (Dako) for 1 h at ambient temperature. Protein bands were visualised using SuperSignal West Pico Chemiluminescent Substrate (Thermo Fisher Scientific) and Hyperfilm ECL (GE Healthcare) and densitometric analysis was carried out using ImageJ software.

### Statistical analysis

Statistical analysis of data was performed using Student's *t*-test for two groups or ANOVA followed by the Holm-Sidak post hoc test in case of multiple comparisons (Sigma Plot 13.0 Software). Differences between groups were considered statistically significant when $p < 0.05$. Results are reported as mean values ± SEM, except when specified otherwise.

## Results

### Active TAOK-pS181 associates with tau pathology in AD and FTLD brain

Previously, we have used a phospho-antibody (TAOK-pS181) to detect forms of TAOK1 and TAOK2 that are catalytically active and phosphorylated on serine residue 181 (S181) as part of their conformational activation [63, 66, 68]. To investigate the contribution of TAOKs to the development of tau pathology and disease progression in AD, serial sections were prepared from the entorhinal cortex of AD brain displaying mild (Braak stage II, $n = 3$), moderate (Braak stage IV, $n = 3$) or severe (Braak stage VI, $n = 4$) pathology alongside control brain ($n = 4$) (Additional file 1: Table S1) [5]. Sections (× 12 per brain sample) were immunostained with the TAOK-pS181 antibody, and strong positive immunoreactivity was observed in tangles and pre-tangle structures in all sections from AD brains with mild, moderate or severe Braak stages (Fig. 1a, Braak stages II, IV, VI). In contrast, no tangle-like structures were apparent with TAOK-pS181 staining in control brain (Fig. 1a). The accumulation of highly phosphorylated tau aggregates at tangles not only provides a key feature for AD but is also characteristic for a number of related tauopathies, including frontotemporal lobar degeneration with tau-immunoreactive inclusions (FTLD-tau)

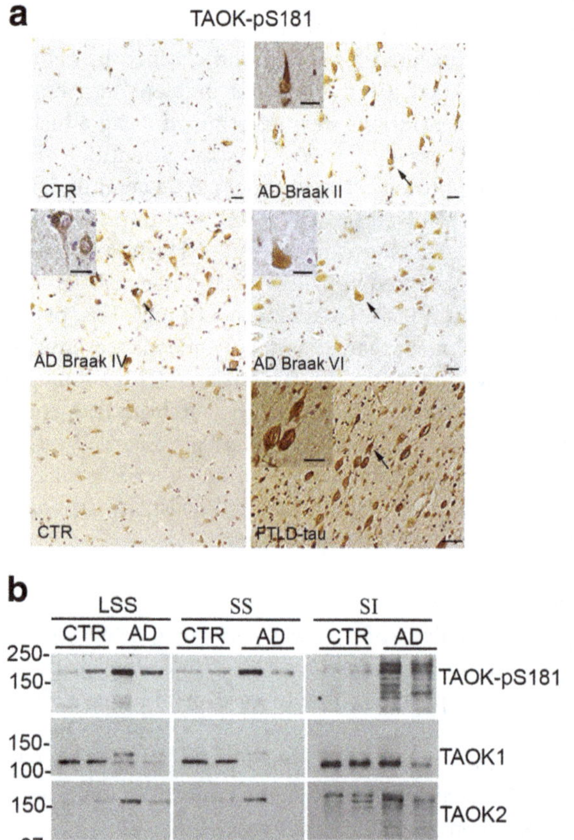


**Fig. 1** TAOK-pS181 associated with tau pathology in AD and FTLD-tau brain. **a** Formalin-fixed sections from the entorhinal cortex of AD (Braak stages II, IV and VI), FTLD-tau or control brains were immunostained with antibody to detect phosphorylated and active TAOKs (TAOK-pS181). Strong positive antibody immunoreactivity was observed on NFTs in AD brain sections from early and late disease stages and in FTLD brain sections (arrows indicate magnified NFTs). **b** AD (Braak VI) or control (CTR) entorhinal cortex brain samples were extracted with sarkosyl and low speed supernatants (LSS) or sarkosyl-soluble (SS) or sarkosyl-insoluble (SI, insoluble tau) fractions immunoblotted with antibodies to detect TAOK1, TAOK2, TAOK-pS181 and GAPDH or tau-pS262/S356 (12E8), tau-pS202/T205/S208 (AT8), total tau and GAPDH. Representative images and immunoblots are shown. Scale bar = 20 μm

[17]. Consequently, entorhinal cortex sections (× 12 per brain sample) from two individuals with FTLD-tau were immunostained with the TAOK-pS181 antibody and positive immunoreactivity was detected in tangle-like structures in all sections (Fig. 1a, Additional file 1: Table S1). These results imply that TAOK activity may also contribute to tau pathology and tangle formation in additional tauopathies such as FTLD-tau.

The association between TAOK expression and activity and tau pathology was investigated further by preparing extracts from the entorhinal cortex of two Braak stage VI AD and two control brains. Low speed supernatants (LSS), sarkosyl-soluble (SS) and sarkosyl-insoluble (SI, insoluble tau) brain fractions were analysed on western blots probed with antibodies recognising active TAOKs, TAOK1, TAOK2 or GAPDH (Fig. 1b). TAOK1 (~ 110 kDa) and TAOK2 (~ 175 kDa) displayed apparent molecular weights that were similar to those reported previously for TAOK1 and TAOK2 [25, 44] and their expression levels in AD and control samples were comparable in the SI fraction (Fig. 1b). Phosphorylated and active TAOK1 and TAOK2 are recognised by the TAOK-pS181 antibody [63] and these phosphorylated proteins are increased in SI fractions prepared from AD brain compared to control brain (Fig. 1b). Additional immunoblotting with phospho-tau and total tau antibodies showed that tau-pS202/S205/S208 (AT8) and tau-pS262/S356 (12E8) were enriched in the sarkosyl-insoluble fraction of AD brain, in which active TAOK-pS181 was also increased (Fig. 1b). Taken together, these results demonstrate that TAOK activity is increased in AD brain compared to controls and this kinase activity co-localises with mild, moderate and severe tau pathology during disease progression. Furthermore, while both TAOK1 and TAOK2 were apparent in the SI fraction of both control and AD brain, active TAOKs appeared to be enriched in SI fraction containing pathological aggregated tau species in AD brain.

### Compound 43 inhibits tau phosphorylation by TAOK2 in vitro and in cells

We have identified a small molecule inhibitor of TAOKs, termed compound 43 (Cp 43) [29]. Cp 43 has an $IC_{50}$ of 11–15 nM, is ATP-competitive and targets TAOKs selectively [29]. In vitro kinase assays were used to determine whether Cp 43 could inhibit the phosphorylation of tau by TAOK2. Purified recombinant TAOK2 (amino acids 1–314) containing the catalytic domain, was incubated with recombinant human tau (htau, 2N4R isoform) in vitro in the presence of increasing concentrations of Cp 43 (5–60 μM) and samples were analysed by immunoblotting with 12E8 and AT8 phospho-tau antibodies. Cp 43 inhibited phosphorylation of tau by TAOK2 in a dose-dependent manner (Fig. 2a).

To investigate the effects of TAOK2 on tau phosphorylation in cells, HEK293T cells were transfected with constructs to express Myc-TAOK2 (1–349) or kinase-defective Myc-TAOK2 (1–349, K57A) and htau (2N4R), and cell lysates were probed with AT8 antibody. Figure 2b shows that exogenous TAOK2, but not kinase-defective TAOK2

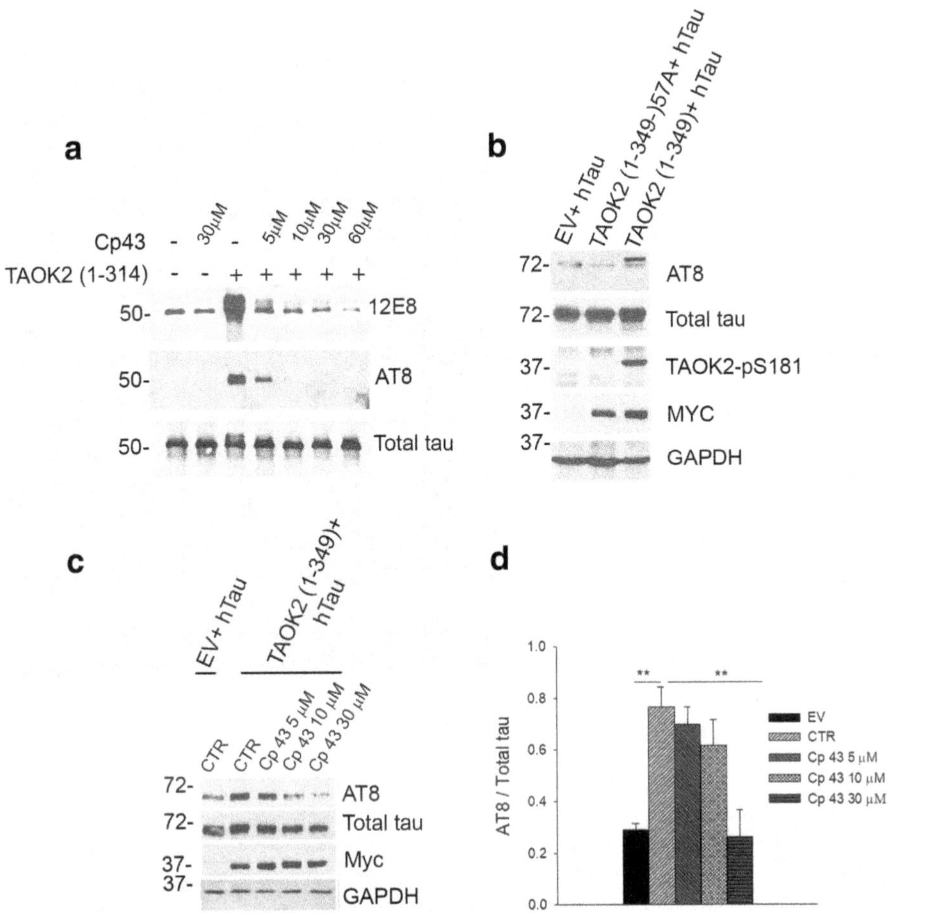


**Fig. 2** Cp 43 reduced tau phosphorylation by TAOK2. **a** In vitro kinase assays were carried out using GST-TAOK2 (1–314) and/or recombinant htau (2N4R) in the presence or absence of Cp 43 as indicated. Samples were immunoblotted with antibodies to detect tau-pS262/S356 (12E8), tau-pS202/T205/S208 (AT8) or total tau. **b** HEK293T cells were co-transfected with empty vector (EV), kinase-deficient TAOK2 (1–349, K57A) or TAOK2 (1–349) and htau (2N4R) as indicated, and cell lysates immunoblotted with antibodies to detect, TAOK-pS181, tau-pS202/T205/S208 (AT8), total tau, Myc or GAPDH. **c** HEK293T cells were co-transfected with empty vector (EV) or TAOK2 (1–349) and htau (2N4R), and treated with or without Cp 43 as indicated. After 24 h, cell lysates were immunoblotted with antibodies to detect tau-pS202/T205/S208 (AT8), total tau, Myc or GAPDH. **d** Quantitative analysis of the relative levels of tau-pS202/T205/S208 versus total tau in transfected HEK293T cells is shown. The data are normalised to total tau and the bars represent the average ratio ± SEM ($n = 4$); $^{**}p < 0.01$, one-way ANOVA followed by multiple comparison with the Holm-Sidak method

(K57A), enhanced tau phosphorylation on the AT8 epitope. HEK293T cells expressing TAOK2 and htau were also incubated with increasing concentrations of Cp 43 (5–30 μM) to determine whether this small molecule was able to inhibit tau phosphorylation by TAOK2 in cells. Figure 2c-d shows that Cp 43 (30 μM) significantly reduced TAOK2-mediated tau phosphorylation on the AT8 epitope. Taken together, these results demonstrate that Cp 43 can inhibit tau phosphorylation by TAOK2 in vitro and in cells.

### TAOKs are expressed and active in differentiating cortical neurons

Previous studies have demonstrated that TAOK2 is expressed in the brains of developing mouse embryos [10, 59]. Therefore, we investigated TAOK expression and activity during differentiation of rat primary cortical neurons. Lysates prepared from cortical neurons at 3, 7, 10, and 14 days in vitro (DIV) were immunoblotted with antibodies to detect TAOK-pS181, TAOK2, or TAOK1. The activity and expression of TAOKs increased between 3 and 14 DIV relative to βIII-tubulin, in parallel with increases in total and phosphorylated tau recognised by AT8 and 12E8 (Fig. 3a).

To further investigate the activity of TAOKs during differentiation, cortical neurons at 5 DIV were transfected with a bicistronic vector expressing EGFP as a reporter, together with Myc-TAOK1, Myc-TAOK2, the catalytic domain of TAOK2 (amino acids 1–349) or full-length kinase-defective TAOK2 (K57A). Neurons were

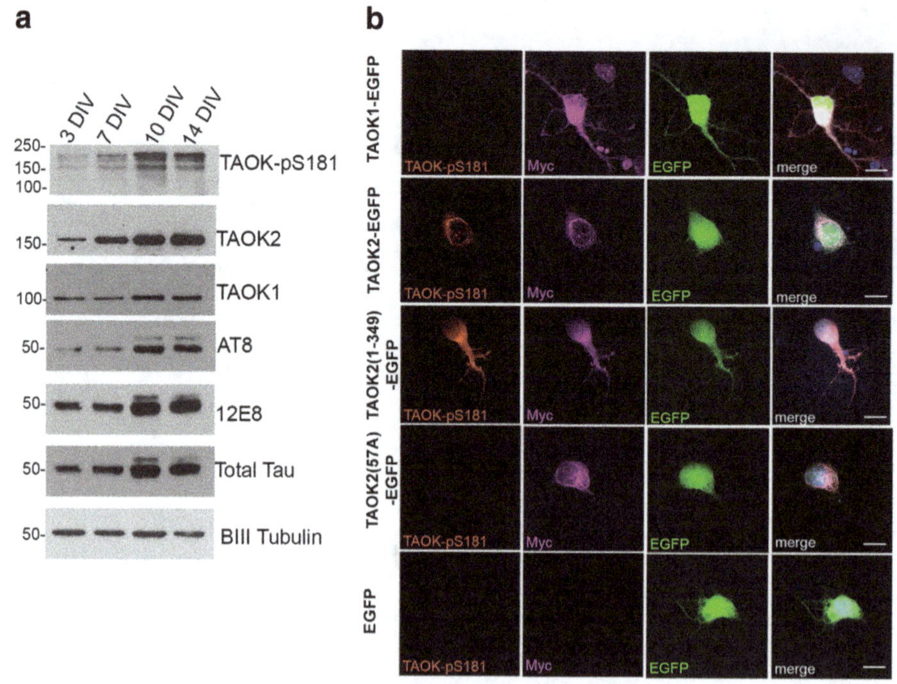


**Fig. 3** Primary cortical neurons expressed active TAOK-pS181. **a** Neurons were cultured for 3, 7, 10 or 14 DIV and lysates immunoblotted with antibodies to detect TAOK-pS181, TAOK1, TAOK2, tau-pS202/T205/S208 (AT8), tau-pS262/S356 (12E8), total tau or BIII tubulin as indicated. **b** Neurons were transfected with pCAGS-Myc-TAOK1-IRES-EGFP (TAOK1-GFP), pCAGS-Myc-TAOK2-IRES-EGFP (TAOK2-EGFP), pCAGS-Myc-TAOK2–1-349-IRES-EGFP (TAOK2–1-349-EGFP), pCAGS-Myc-TAOK2-K57A-IRES-EGFP (TAOK2 K57A-EGFP) or pCAGS-IRES-EGFP (EGFP) plasmids, as indicated. 7 DIV transfected neurons were fixed and immunostained with antibodies to detect active TAOK-pS181 (red) and Myc (magenta). Nuclei were counterstained with DAPI (blue) and representative maximal projection of confocal z-stack images is shown. Scale bar = 10 μm

fixed 48 h after transfection and immunostained with antibodies to detect either Myc (TAOKs) or active TAOK-pS181. Exogenous expression of both TAOK1 and TAOK2 was confirmed by detection of the Myc tag in transfected neurons, however, only TAOK2 was active, as detected by the TAOK-pS181 antibody (Fig. 3b). Full-length TAOK2 (both wild-type and K57A) localised to the perinuclear microtubule cage in differentiating neurons (Fig. 3b), as described previously [43]. In contrast, the catalytic domain of TAOK2 (1–349), which lacks the microtubule binding region (amino acids 745–1235) [43], was distributed throughout the cytoplasm and neurites (Fig. 3b). Expression of full-length and kinase-defective TAOK2 (K57A) in cortical neurons provided a negative control, which was detected by the Myc antibody but not the TAOK-pS181 antibody (Fig. 3b). Exogenous TAOK2 was therefore expressed and catalytically active in transfected cortical neurons.

#### TAOK inhibition reduces tau phosphorylation in rat primary cortical neurons

To evaluate the effects of TAOK inhibition on tau phosphorylation in primary rat cortical neurons, cultures at 7 and 17 DIV were treated with Cp 43 (5, 10, 30 μM) for 72 h prior to analysis on western blots. Cp 43 (30 μM) caused significant reductions in tau phosphorylation at the 12E8 and AT8 epitopes, relative to total tau, in neurons cultured for both 7 and 17 DIV (Fig. 4a-d). TAOK inhibition did not increase the number of active caspase-3 positive 7 or 17 DIV neurons treated with Cp 43 (30 μM) for 72 h or affect the expression of the pre-synaptic proteins synapsin 1 and synaptophysin in 17 DIV neurons (Additional file 2: Figure S1 A-C). Cp 43 was able to reduce tau phosphorylation significantly after 6 h of incubation even at a lower concentration of 10 μM (Additional file 2: Figure S1 D-E). The release of lactate dehydrogenase (LDH) into the culture medium was also used to assess cytotoxicity. 7 and 17 DIV neurons were incubated with increasing concentrations of Cp 43 (6 h) and the release of LDH into the culture medium determined. Cp 43 did not affect LDH levels in the media or appear to be cytotoxic under these conditions (Additional file 2: Figure S1F). Taken together, these results show that TAOK inhibition can reduce tau phosphorylation in differentiating neurons without inducing significant cytotoxicity.

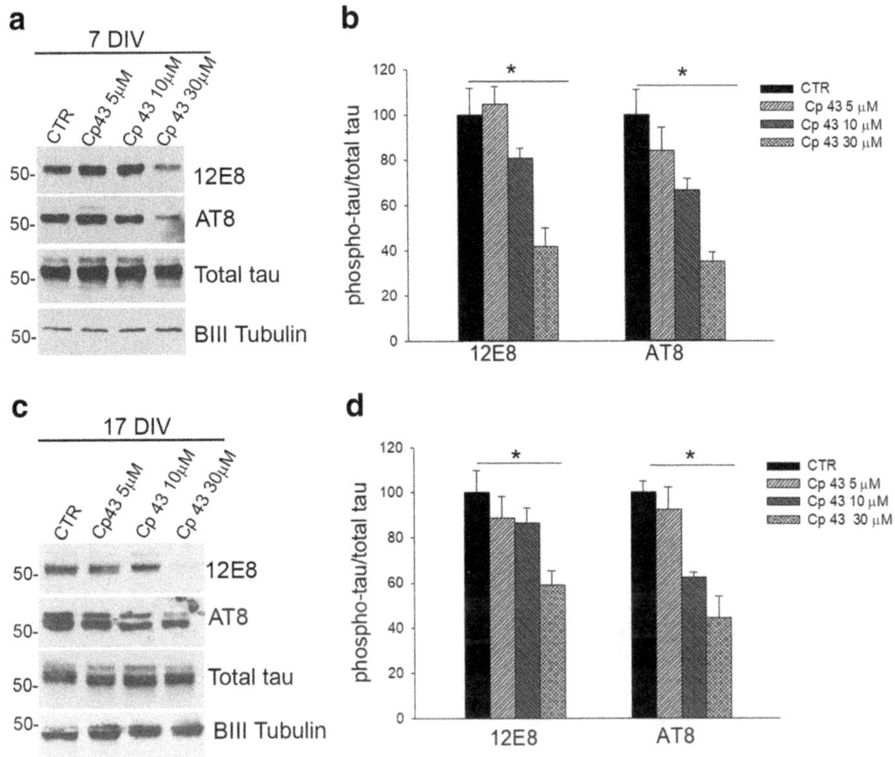


**Fig. 4** Cp 43 reduced tau phosphorylation in primary cortical neurons. **a**, **c** Lysates were prepared from 7 DIV (**a**) or 17 DIV(**c**) neurons treated with or without Cp 43 for 72 h as indicated and immunoblotted with antibodies to detect tau-pS262/S356 (12E8), tau-pS202/T205/S208 (AT8), total tau or BIII Tubulin. **b**, **d** Quantitative analysis of the effects of increasing Cp 43 concentration on the levels of phosphorylated tau, 12E8 and AT8 epitopes, in 7 DIV (**b**) and 17 DIV neurons (**d**). The data are normalised to total tau and the bars represent the average ratio ± SEM ($n = 7$). *$p < 0.05$, one-way ANOVA followed by multiple comparison with the Holm-Sidak method

### Two new tau residues (T123 and T427) are phosphorylated by TAOK2 and associate with tangles in AD and FTLD-tau brain

Mass spectrometric analysis has identified 49 tau residues that are phosphorylated by TAOK1 and TAOK2 in vitro, including several sites that are phosphorylated aberrantly in AD brain [55]. The phosphorylation of two of these AD-tau residues, T123 and T427, has not yet been attributed to the activity of any alternative kinases and may therefore be specific to TAOKs (https://bit.ly/1SpzgoL). Therefore, we generated two new phospho-tau antibodies to detect tau-pT123 and tau-pT427, and these were used to monitor TAOK activity in human brain and cell experimental models.

In vitro kinase assays were carried out using recombinant htau (2N4R) and purified TAOK1 (1–314) or TAOK2 (1–314), and phosphorylation of tau on both sites was detected on western blots using antibodies tau-pT123, tau-pT427 and 12E8 (Fig. 5a). Entorhinal cortex sections (× 12 per brain sample) from brains presenting mild (Braak stage II, $n = 3$), moderate (Braak stage IV, $n = 3$) or severe (Braak stage VI, $n = 4$) AD pathology, or from FTLD-tau brains ($n = 2$) or control brains ($n = 4$), were immunostained with the tau-pT123 and tau-pT427 antibodies. Tangle-like structures were labelled with both the tau-pT123 and tau-pT427 antibodies in all AD (Braak stages II, IV and VI) and FTLD-tau sections (Fig. 5b-c). Immunoreactivity was also detected in some nuclei in AD and FTLD-tau brain and to a lesser extent in controls (Fig. 5b-c).

Epitope specificity for the tau-pT123, tau-pT427 and TAOK-pS181 antibodies was confirmed by pre-treating these reagents with their appropriate phospho-peptides, which blocked antibody recognition of their target epitopes in immunostained AD sections and in immunoblotted in vitro kinase assays (Additional file 3: Figure S2A-B). Tau-pT123 and tau-pT427 antibody labelling co-localised with 12E8 and AT8 in AD sections, confirming labelling of tangles by both of the new phospho-dependent tau antibodies (Fig. 5d). Extracts from the entorhinal cortex of AD (Braak VI; $n = 2$) and control brains ($n = 2$) showed that tau-pT123 and tau-pT427 were enriched in the sarkosyl insoluble (SI) fractions extracted from AD but not control brains (Fig. 5e). The results presented here confirm that both of these tau residues are targeted by TAOKs and show that tau is phosphorylated

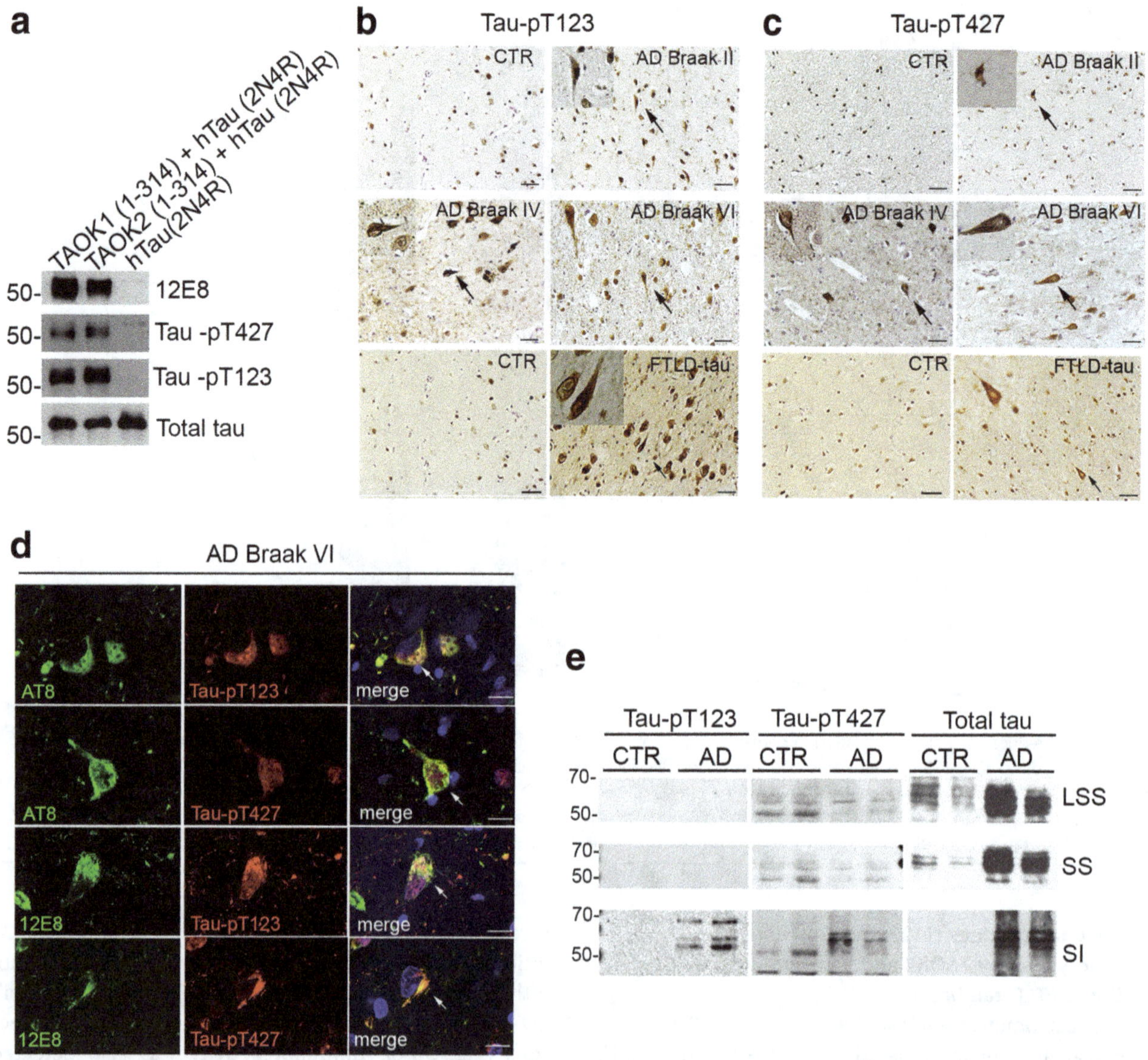


**Fig. 5** Tau-pT123 and tau-pT427 are targeted by TAOKs and are associated with tangles in AD and FTLD-tau brain. **a** In vitro kinase assays were carried out using GST-TAOK1 (1–314), GST-TAOK2 (1–314) and/or htau (2N4R) as indicated and samples immunoblotted with antibodies to detect tau-pS262/S356 (12E8), tau-pT427, tau-pT123 or total tau. **b-c** Entorhinal cortices from control (CTR), AD (Braak stage II-VI) or FTLD-tau brains were immunostained with antibodies to detect tau-pT123 (**b**) or tau-pT427 (**c**). Strong positive antibody immunoreactivity was observed for tau-pT123 and tau-pT427 at NFTs in each stage of AD and in FTLD-tau (arrows indicate magnified NFTs). **d** Sections from the entorhinal cortex of advanced AD (Braak stage VI) brains were immunostained with antibodies to detect tau-pS202/T205/S208 (AT8, green) or tau-pS262/S356 (12E8, green) and tau-pT123 or tau-pT427 (red) as indicated. Nuclei were counterstained with DAPI (blue). **e** AD (Braak VI) or control (CTR) hippocampal and entorhinal cortex brain samples were extracted with sarkosyl and low speed supernatants (LSS) or sarkosyl-soluble (SS) or sarkosyl-insoluble fractions (SI, insoluble tau) immunoblotted with antibodies to detect tau-pT123, tau-pT427 or total tau as indicated. Representative images and immunoblots are shown. Scale bar = 20 μm

on T123 and T427 in early and late-stage AD and also in FTLD-tau brain.

### TAOK2 activity is required to phosphorylate tau on T427 in cortical neurons

Tau phosphorylation on T123 and T427 was investigated next in rat primary cortical neurons using a bi-cistronic IRES vector to express Myc-TAOK2 together with EGFP to provide a reporter protein. 7 DIV transfected neurons expressing exogenous active TAOK2 were strongly immunoreactive with the tau-pT427 antibody (Fig. 6a). In contrast, untransfected neurons or transfected neurons expressing kinase-defective TAOK2 (K57A) or EGFP alone were not recognised by the tau-pT427 antibody (Fig. 6a).

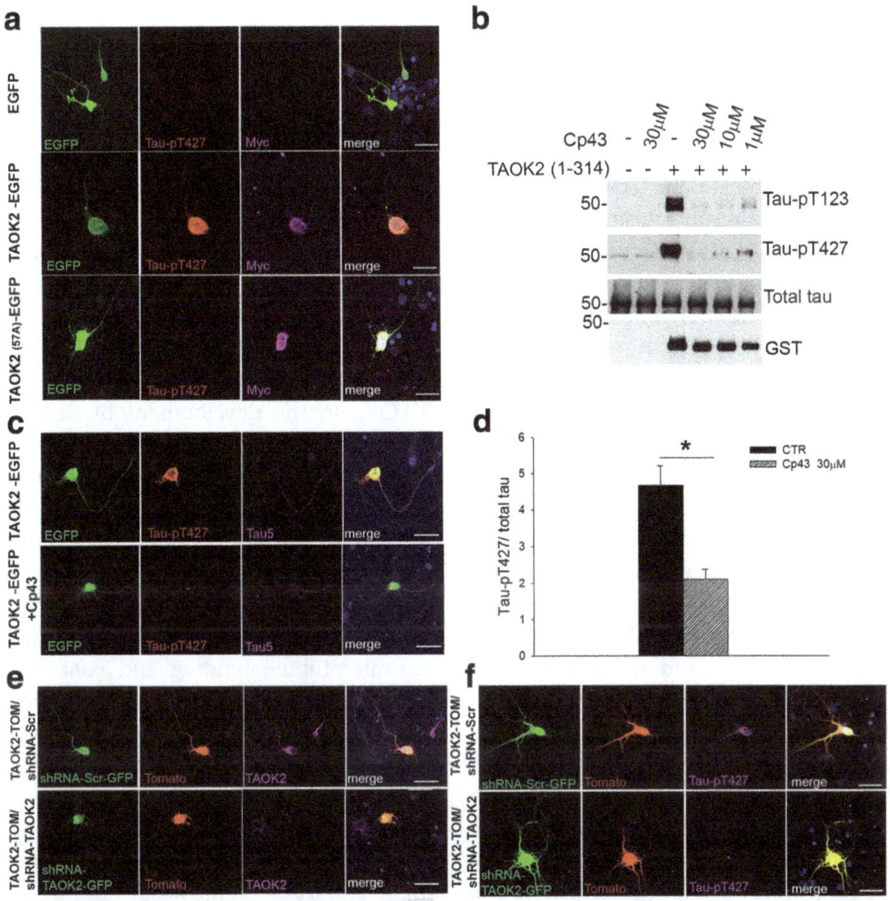

**Fig. 6** Cp 43 reduced tau phosphorylation on T427 by TAOK2 in primary neurons. **a** IRES-EGFP and TAOK2-EGFP transfected neurons (7 DIV) were fixed and immunostained with antibodies to detect tau-pT427 (red) and Myc (magenta). **b** In vitro kinase assays were carried out using GST-TAOK2 (1–314) and/or recombinant htau (2N4R) in the presence or absence of Cp 43 as indicated. Samples were immunoblotted with antibodies to detect tau-pT123, tau-pT427, total tau or GST. **c** TAOK2-EGFP transfected neurons (7 DIV) were incubated with or without Cp 43 (30 μM) for 24 h as indicated and immunostained with antibodies to detect tau-pT427 (red) or total tau (tau-5, magenta). **d** Quantitative analysis of tau-pT427 immunoreactivity in TAOK2-EGFP transfected neurons incubated with or without Cp 43. Bars represent the average immunofluorescence intensity ± SEM of tau-pT427 normalised to total tau. > 65 neurons were analysed for each group ($n = 4$). *$p < 0.05$, student t-test. **e-f** TAOK2-IRES-Tomato and TAOK2-shRNA-EGFP or scrambled-shRNA-EGFP were co-transfected into neurons as indicated and after 72 h cells were fixed and immunostained for TAOK2 (magenta, **e**) or tau-pT427 (magenta, **f**). Nuclei were counterstained with DAPI (blue). Representative maximal projection of z-stack images and immunoblots are shown. Scale bar = 10 μm

These results demonstrate that tau is not phosphorylated physiologically on T427 in differentiating cortical neurons. The ability of Cp 43 to inhibit tau phosphorylation on T123 and T427 by TAOK2 was initially tested using in vitro kinase assays, which showed that tau phosphorylation on these epitopes was decreased by the inhibitor compound (Fig. 6b). Treatment of TAOK2 transfected cortical neurons with Cp 43 (30 μM, 24 h) also reduced tau phosphorylation on T427, and tau-pT427 immunoreactivity was decreased by 55% in neurons incubated with the inhibitor compared to controls (Fig. 6c-d, Cp 43 $n = 70$, controls $n = 65$). In addition, co-transfection of Myc-TAOK2-IRES-Tomato together with TAOK2-shRNAs to knockdown expression of exogenous TAOK2 in cortical neurons (Fig. 6e) also decreased tau-pT427 immunoreactivity (Fig. 6f). These results show that tau phosphorylation on T427 was stimulated by expression of exogenous TAOK2 in transfected neurons and that this effect can be inhibited by treating cells with Cp 43 or by silencing TAOK2 expression using shRNAs.

Although we did not observe any positive immunoreactivity in lysates from rat primary cortical neurons immunoblotted with tau-pT123 and tau-pT427 antibodies, tau-pT123 immunostaining showed a positive signal in untransfected neurons that was restricted to the nuclear compartment. However, this signal was not increased following transfection and over-expression of TAOK2 (Additional file 4: Figure S3A).

### Cp 43 decreased tau phosphorylation in murine and human neuronal cell models of tauopathy

The positive immunoreactivity for TAOK-pS181, tau-pT123 and tau-pT427 antibodies observed in the tangle structures in FTLD-tau-brain suggests that TAOK activity may contribute to tau pathology in this disease. Therefore, we decided to evaluate the effect of TAOK inhibition on tau phosphorylation in murine and human neuronal cell models of FTLD-tau. Previous studies have demonstrated the presence of an N-terminally truncated form of tau in tauopathy brains [64]. This human brain derived tau fragment, tagged with HA to provide an epitope tag, has recently been used to generate the Tau-35 mouse model, which displays key disease associated features including enhanced tau phosphorylation and the presence of tangle like structures in the brain [4, 54]. The activity of TAOKs and their potential contribution to tau phosphorylation was investigated here by preparing primary cortical neurons from Tau35 transgenic mouse embryos and incubating these cultures in the presence or absence of Cp 43 (10 or 30 μM for 6 h). Cell lysates were prepared at 14 DIV and western blotting analysis detected active TAOK-pS181 and demonstrated that treatment with Cp 43 caused significant reductions in tau phosphorylation on the 12E8 and AT8 epitopes (Fig. 7a-b). Tau did not appear to be phosphorylated on T123 or T427 in these lysates prepared from Tau35 mouse neurons and this result was similar to our observations in wild-type rat primary cortical neurons.

To investigate the effects of TAOKs on tau phosphorylation in human neurons, induced pluripotent stem cells (iPSCs) from two control iPSC lines and one iPSC line generated from an individual with the FTLD-associated 10 + 16 *MAPT* mutation, were differentiated into cortical neurons [53]. Cells were cultured for 60 DIV and neuronal morphology was analysed by expression of MAP2, total tau, unphosphorylated tau (Tau1) and phosphorylated tau (12E8) (Additional file 5: Figure S4). Lysates prepared from these cells showed similar levels of expression of TAOK1, TAOK2 and active TAOK-pS181 were detected in control and FTLD-tau samples (Fig. 7c). Tau phosphorylation on the 12E8 epitope was comparable in control and FTLD-tau neurons at 60 DIV (Fig. 7c). Treatment with Cp 43 (30 μM, 6 h) caused a significant reduction in 12E8 immunoreactivity in both control and FTLD-tau human neurons (Fig. 7c-d). These results show that endogenous TAOKs are active in these murine and human neuronal models for tauopathy and that tau phosphorylation was decreased by Cp 43.

## Discussion

An important objective for dementia research is the identification of tau kinases that are catalytically active at tangle structures in tauopathies and therefore likely to contribute directly to the aberrant phosphorylation and aggregation of tau. In this study, active TAOK-pS181 was present and detected at pre-tangles and tangles in AD brain sections displaying mild, intermediate and advanced tau pathology (Braak stages II-VI). In contrast, we were unable to detect significant TAOK activity in control brain sections. Sarkosyl-insoluble extracts of AD brain tissues (Braak stage VI) also demonstrated the presence of active TAOK-pS181 in those fractions which contained aggregated and pathologically phosphorylated tau, whereas TAOK activity and phosphorylated tau were largely absent in extracts prepared from control brain.

These results are consistent with potential roles for TAOKs in the development of early and late-stage tau pathology in AD brain. The association between aberrant phosphorylation and self-aggregation of tau in pathological conditions has been well documented, however, the precise phosphorylation events resulting in tau toxicity are not well defined [14, 37]. KXGS motifs located within the tau repeat domain are of special interest because tau phosphorylation on the 12E8 epitope (S262/S356) reduces tau-microtubule binding and contributes to the pathogenic cascade, where tau is phosphorylated on additional residues associated with tangle formation [22, 45]. A recent study has also shown that tau phosphorylation on the AT8 epitope (S202/T205/S208), located within the proline rich domain, is sufficient to promote tau aggregation and relocalisation of pathogenic tau in the dendrite compartment, and these events occur during early neurodegeneration in AD [11, 27]. Attenuation of tau phosphorylation on these sites, through inhibition of appropriate tau kinases, could provide a suitable strategy for the treatment of early stage AD and related tauopathies.

Abnormal tau phosphorylation can result in aberrant pathology via several different mechanisms, and these appear to include changes in tau degradation pathways and cleavage. For example, tau phosphorylated on S262/S356 is not recognised by the C terminus of HSP70-interacting protein-heat shock protein 90 (CHIP–HSP90) complex and is therefore protected from proteasomal degradation [12]. In addition, tau phosphorylation on S422 can prevent tau cleavage by Caspase 3 at T421 [18]. We have demonstrated previously that TAOKs can phosphorylate tau on more than 40 residues in vitro, and 29 of these sites are modified in PHF-tau extracted from AD brain [55]. Two of these PHF-tau residues, T123 and T427, were investigated here because they are uncharacterised and could be targeted by TAOKs specifically. Immunohistochemical analysis of early and late stage AD brain sections (Braak II-VI) detected tau-pT123 and tau-pT427 at pre-tangles and tangles, where TAOK activity also occurred. Furthermore, sarkosyl-insoluble tau from AD brain was also phosphorylated on T123 and T427 and this fraction also contained active TAOK-pS181.

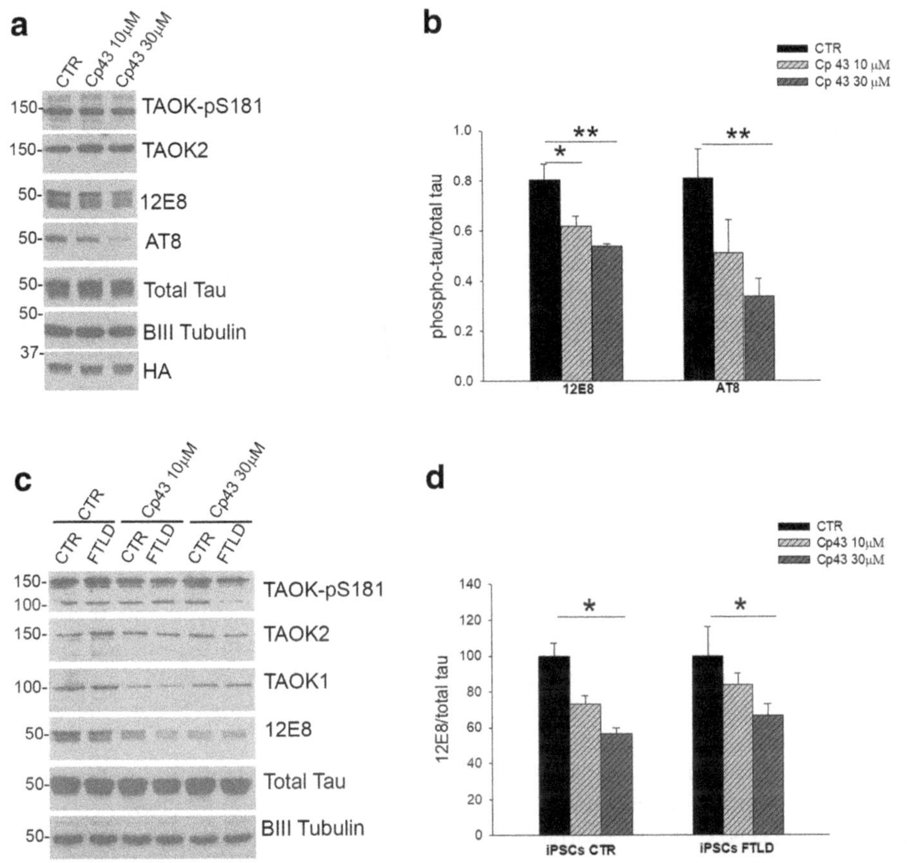


**Fig. 7** Cp 43 decreased tau phosphorylation in murine and human neuronal models of tauopathy. **a** Neurons were prepared from Tau35 transgenic mouse embryos and incubated at 14 DIV with or without Cp 43 (10, 30 μM, 6 h) and lysates immunoblotted with antibodies to detect TAOK-pS181, TAOK2, tau-pS262/S356 (12E8), tau-pS202/T205/S208 (AT8), total tau, BIII Tubulin or HA. **b** Quantitative analysis of the relative levels of phosphorylated tau (12E8 and AT8) in Tau-35 primary neurons. The data are normalised to total tau and the bars represent the average ratio ± SEM ($n = 6$). **c** CTR or FTLD (10 + 16 *MAPT* mutation) iPSC derived neurons (60 DIV) were incubated with or without Cp 43 (10, 30 μM, 6 h) and lysates immunoblotted with antibodies to detect TAOK-pS181, TAOK1, TAOK2, tau-pS262/S356 (12E8), total tau or BIII Tubulin. **d** Quantitative analysis of the relative levels of phosphorylated tau (12E8) present in Cp 43 treated iPSC derived neurons. Data are normalised to total tau and are expressed as mean percentages ± SEM of the controls ($n = 6$). *$p < 0.05$; **$p < 0.01$, one-way ANOVA followed by multiple comparison using the Holm-Sidak method

The presence of TAOK activity at pre-tangles and tangles in early stage AD brain correlates with the appearance of tau phosphorylated on multiple epitopes recognised by the 12E8, AT8, tau-pT123 and tau-pT427 antibodies. The ability of TAOKs to phosphorylate tau on pathogenic epitopes was investigated here using a recently characterised TAOK inhibitor compound, which inhibited tau phosphorylation in vitro and in HEK293 cells expressing exogenous TAOK2 and human tau. Cp 43 also decreased basal levels of tau-12E8 and tau-AT8 in differentiating rat neurons without inducing cytotoxicity or causing significant changes in pre-synaptic protein expression levels in primary neurons.

The normal physiological functions of TAOKs in adult brain remain to be determined but TAOK2 can regulate dendrite arborisation, spine maturation and axonal outgrowth in the developing mouse brain [10, 49, 59, 65]. Here we have shown that endogenous TAOK activity and tau-12E8 and tau-AT8 are increased as primary cortical neurons undergo differentiation and that TAOK2, but not TAOK1, is active catalytically when over-expressed in transfected neurons. Furthermore, TAOK-pS181 immunoreactivity in lysates prepared from rat cortical neurons was observed and this antibody recognised a protein band that appeared to migrate with the same mobility as TAOK2. These observations are consistent with a role for TAOK2 in regulating neuronal maturation during early murine brain development as reported previously [10, 49, 59, 65]. TAOK expression and activity were also detected in differentiating Tau35 primary neurons and in FTLD-tau and control human iPSC-derived neurons. However, only limited immunoreactivity with the TAOK-pS181 antibody was observed in adult human asymptomatic brain sections when compared to AD and FTLD brains, where strong TAOK-pS181 immunoreactivity occurred at tangle structures. These results suggest that appropriate levels of TAOK activity are required for neuronal maturation in the developing brain whereas increased TAOK activity in the adult brain may result in pathogenic effects.

In differentiating primary cortical neurons tau was not phosphorylated on T427 unless these cells were transfected with TAOK2. Tau was however phosphorylated on T123 where immunoreactivity was located in the nucleus of differentiating neurons and phosphorylation levels on this epitope were not increased by over-expression of TAOK2. Previous studies have demonstrated enriched expression of the 1N4R tau isoform in the neuronal nucleus but not in the cytoplasm or neurites, where the 0N3R fetal tau isoform is predominantly expressed at this stage of differentiation [6, 35, 42]. The absence of mature tau isoform expression in the cytoplasm and neurites in differentiating neurons and the lack of TAOK2 expression in the nucleus, may account for the inefficient phosphorylation of tau on T123 by TAOK2 observed here.

Tau phosphorylation and TAOK activity were also examined in an additional tauopathy. Immunohistochemical analysis of FTLD-tau brain sections showed that active TAOK-pS181, tau-pT123 and tau-pT427 each localised to pre-NFTs and NFT structures. Primary cortical neurons were also prepared from brains from Tau35 transgenic mice, which overexpress a C-terminally truncated 35 kDa htau fragment that is associated with tauopathies [4]. Treatment of these Tau35 mouse neurons with Cp 43 reduced tau phosphorylation on the 12E8 and AT8 epitopes. Human neurons were also produced using iPSCs derived from control and individual with the 10 + 16 *MAPT* mutation which is associated with FTLD and these differentiated cells expressed active TAOKs and tau phosphorylated on S262/S356. Addition of Cp 43 decreased tau phosphorylation on the 12E8 epitope in these FTLD iPSC derived neurons but we were unable to detect tau-pT123 or tau-pT427. A previous study has shown that these FTLD neurons express the foetal 0N3R tau isoform at this time point (60 DIV) and it is possible that adult tau isoform expression and enhanced TAOK activity are required for tau phosphorylation on T123 and T427 [53]. In contrast, T123 and T427 were phosphorylated under pathogenic conditions in FTLD-tau brain sections, where all six tau isoforms are expressed, and tau-pT123 and tau-pT427 localised to pre-tangles and tangles, where TAOK activity occurred.

A number of kinases can phosphorylate tau in vitro and to date GSK-3, MARK, JNK, p38, AMPK, Nuak1 and TAOKs have been shown to be active catalytically at tangles in AD brain tissues [15, 21, 31, 57, 60, 67]. TAOKs can stimulate the catalytic activity of several of these tangle-associated kinases, including MARK, JNK and p38, and TAOKs could potentially phosphorylate tau on additional pathological sites via such pathways [25, 44, 56]. Indeed, TAOKs can phosphorylate and activate MARK directly and both of these kinases can phosphorylate tau on the 12E8 epitope [3, 56]. The appearance of TAOK activity at pre-tangle and tangle structures during early AD (Braak stage II) and their phosphorylation of tau on multiple residues, including pathogenic sites such as T123 and T427, are consistent with potential roles for TAOKs during early disease development. Therefore, inhibitors of TAOK activity may reduce aberrant tau phosphorylation and tau pathology. In a previous study using breast cancer cell models, we have shown that abnormal TAOK activity can contribute to clustering of supernumerary-amplified centrosomes in malignant cells and prevents multipolar mitoses and associated cell death [29]. Cp 43 can stimulate centrosome declustering, multipolarity and mitotic catastrophe in these centrosome amplified cancer cells selectively, whereas normal bipolar cells continue to divide and proliferate in the presence of this compound [29]. Aberrant TAOK activity can therefore induce clustering of supernumerary-amplified centrosomes in malignant breast cells as well as stimulating pathological tau phosphorylation in neurons and tauopathies and TAOKs may therefore offer suitable therapeutic targets for both diseases. To date, TAOKs are not reported to be involved in any other diseases.

Tau kinase inhibitors have been used already to treat tau transgenic mice, in order to slow or prevent the development of tau pathology in these animals [28, 32, 46]. Previous studies have shown that inhibiting GSK3 reduces tau phosphorylation and ameliorates memory deficits in transgenic mouse models of AD [7, 46, 47, 51]. Initial studies targeting GSK-3 produced encouraging results in pre-clinical studies but failed during clinical trials due to off-target toxicity and the requirement for GSK-3 activity to sustain normal cell function [39]. The appearance of TAOK activity at NFTs in AD and FTLD, and their phosphorylation of tau on multiple pathological sites, suggests that these proteins could offer novel and suitable alternative drug targets for the treatment of neurodegenerative disorders.

## Conclusions

In summary, we have shown that TAOKs are active and co-localise with tangle structures in AD and FTLD brain. We have used a new TAOK inhibitor to reduce tau phosphorylation on sites associated with neurodegeneration in human tauopathies and examined two new phosphorylation sites on tau (T123 and T427) that are targeted by TAOKs and detected in AD and FTLD brain. TAOK activity and tau phosphorylation on pathological sites are also shown to be decreased by Cp 43 in vitro and in neuronal and disease cell models. Our results suggest compounds that inhibit the activity of these kinases could reduce tau pathology and potentially delay associated cognitive decline with such effects providing significant benefits for individuals with early symptoms of dementia.

## Additional files

**Additional file 1: Table S1.** Characteristics of the subjects whose brain tissues were used in this study. PMD refers to post-mortem delay in hours before samples were processed. (DOCX 16 kb)

**Additional file 2: Figure S1.** Cp 43 decreased tau phosphorylation in rat primary cortical neurons. **A.** Quantitative analysis of cleaved active Caspase 3 positive neurons (7 DIV or 17 DIV) treated with or without 30 μM Cp 43 (72 h). > 800 neurons were counted for each experimental condition and bars represent mean percentages ± SEM ($n = 4$). **B.** Neurons (14 DIV) were incubated without or with Cp 43 (5, 10 or 30 μM, 72 h) and lysates immunoblotted with antibodies to detect Synapsin 1, Synaptophysin or BIII tubulin. **C.** Quantitative analysis of the effects of Cp 43 on synaptic protein expression levels normalised to BIII tubulin. Bars represent the average ratio ± SEM ($n = 7$). **D.** Neurons (7 DIV) were treated with or without Cp 43 for 6 h as indicated and lysates immunoblotted with antibodies to detect tau-pS262/S356 (12E8), tau-pS202/T205/S208 (AT8), total tau or BIII Tubulin. **E.** Quantitative analysis of the effects of increasing Cp 43 concentration on the levels of phosphorylated tau (12E8 and AT8 epitopes). Data are normalised to total tau and are expressed as mean percentages ± SEM of the controls ($n = 5$). ** $p < 0.01$ *$p < 0.05$, one-way ANOVA followed by multiple comparison with the Holm-Sidak method. **F.** 7 and 17 DIV neurons were incubated with or without Cp 43 (1–30 μM) for 6 h. Bars represent the average ratio of the percentages of LDH released versus total LDH ± SEM ($n = 24$; collected in 3 independent experiments). Representative immunoblots and images are shown. Scale bar = 10 μm. (TIF 815 kb)

**Additional file 3: Figure S2.** Blocking phospho-peptides abolished epitope recognition by TAOK-pS181, tau-pT123 and tau-p427 antibodies. **A.** Entorhinal cortex sections from AD (Braak VI) brains were immunostained with antibodies to detect TAOK-pS181, tau-pT123 or tau-pT427 in the presence (left side) or absence (right side) of their appropriate blocking phospho-peptide epitopes (1 μM). **B.** In vitro kinase assays were carried out using GST-TAOK1 (1–314) or GST-TAOK2 (1–314) and recombinant htau (2N4R), and samples immunoblotted with tau-pT123 or tau-pT427 antibodies in the presence (right side) or absence (left side) of their appropriate blocking phospho-peptide. Representative images and immunoblots are shown. Scale bar = 20 μm. (TIF 7890 kb)

**Additional file 4: Figure S3.** Tau phosphorylated on T123 was present in the nuclei of rat primary neurons. **A** Neurons (7 DIV) were transfected with IRES-GFP, TAOK2-IRES-GFP or TAOK2 K57A-IRES-GFP, fixed and immunostained with antibodies to detect tau-pT123 (red) and Myc (magenta). Nuclei were counterstained with DAPI (blue). Representative images are shown. Scale bar = 10 μm. (TIF 409 kb)

**Additional file 5 Figure S4** FTLD and control iPSC-derived neurons expressed phosphorylated tau. **A-D.** FTLD (10 + 16 *MAPT* mutation) and control iPSC-derived neurons (60 DIV) were fixed and immmunostained with antibodies to detect total tau (red, A-B), tau-12E8 (green, A-B), tau-1 (green, C-D) and Map2 (red, C-D). Nuclei were counterstained with DAPI (blue). Representative images are shown. Scale bar = 10 μm. (TIF 4365 kb)

### Abbreviations

AD: Alzheimer's disease; CDK5: cyclin-dependent kinase 5; Cp 43: Compound 43; DAPI: 4′, 6′-diamidino-2-phenylindole; DMEM: Dulbecco's modified Eagles medium; DMSO: dimethyl sulfoxide; ERK: extracellular-signal regulated kinase; FTLD: Frontotemporal lobar degeneration; GAPDH: glyceraldehyde-3-phosphate dehydrogenase; GFP: green fluorescent protein; GSK-3: Glycogen synthase kinase-3; GST: glutathione-S-transferase; HRP: horse radish peroxidase; iPSC: induced pluripotent stem cell; JNK: c-Jun N-terminal kinase; LDH: lactate dehydrogenase; LSS: low speed supernatant; MAP: microtubule-associated protein; MAPK: mitogen-activated protein kinase; MARK: microtubule-regulated protein kinase; NFT: neurofibrillary tangles; PBS: phosphate buffered saline; PSD95: post synaptic density protein 95; SI: sarkosyl insoluble; SS: sarkosyl soluble; TAOK: thousand-and-one amino acid kinase

### Acknowledgements

We thank the MRC London Neurodegenerative Diseases Brain Bank (King's College London) and Brains for Dementia Research for providing tissues. We also thank Elizabeth Chan, Mideia Kotsogianni, Juan Burrone, Istvan Bodi, Claire Troakes and members of the Hanger and Noble laboratories for many helpful discussions and technical assistance during this project. We thank Laura Price for a donation to support this work.

### Funding

The study was supported by Alzheimer's Research UK Project Grant (IRG2014–06) awarded to J.D.H. Morris and D.P. Hanger. Additional funding was obtained from a King's College London Alzheimer's Research UK Network pump priming grant awarded to CG. SW is supported through an Alzheimer's Research UK Senior Research Fellowship (SFR2016B-2).

### Authors' contributions

CG, IT, WN, DH and JM oversaw and designed the study. CG, CK and NY designed and performed the experiments. CG, CK, SW, WN, DH and JM analysed and interpreted the data. CG, SW, WN, DH and JM drafted and wrote the manuscript. All authors read, reviewed, helped to edit, and approved the final manuscript.

### Competing interests

The authors declare that they have no competing interests.

### Author details

[1]King's College London, School of Cancer and Pharmaceutical Sciences, New Hunt's House, Guy's Campus, London SE11UL, UK. [2]King's College London, Department of Basic and Clinical Neuroscience, Maurice Wohl Clinical Neuroscience Institute, Institute of Psychiatry, Psychology & Neuroscience, 5 Cutcombe Road, London SE59RX, UK. [3]UCL Institute of Neurology, Department of Molecular Neuroscience, University College London, 1 Wakefield Street, London WC1N1PJ, UK.

### References

1. Biernat J, Gustke N, Drewes G, Mandelkow EM, Mandelkow E (1993) Phosphorylation of Ser262 strongly reduces binding of tau to microtubules: distinction between PHF-like immunoreactivity and microtubule binding. Neuron 11:153–163
2. Biernat J, Mandelkow EM (1999) The development of cell processes induced by tau protein requires phosphorylation of serine 262 and 356 in the repeat domain and is inhibited by phosphorylation in the proline-rich domains. Mol Biol Cell 10:727–740
3. Biernat J, Wu YZ, Timm T, Zheng-Fischhofer Q, Mandelkow E, Meijer L, Mandelkow EM (2002) Protein kinase MARK/PAR-1 is required for neurite outgrowth and establishment of neuronal polarity. Mol Biol Cell 13:4013–4028. https://doi.org/10.1091/mbc.02-03-0046

4. Bondulich MK, Guo T, Meehan C, Manion J, Rodriguez Martin T, Mitchell JC, Hortobagyi T, Yankova N, Stygelbout V, al BJP (2016) Tauopathy induced by low level expression of a human brain-derived tau fragment in mice is rescued by phenylbutyrate. Brain 139:2290–2306. https://doi.org/10.1093/brain/aww137
5. Braak H, Braak E (1991) Neuropathological stageing of Alzheimer-related changes. Acta Neuropathol 82:239–259
6. Brion JP, Octave JN, Couck AM (1994) Distribution of the phosphorylated microtubule-associated protein tau in developing cortical neurons. Neuroscience 63:895–909
7. Caccamo A, Oddo S, Tran LX, LaFerla FM (2007) Lithium reduces tau phosphorylation but not a beta or working memory deficits in a transgenic model with both plaques and tangles. Am J Pathol 170:1669–1675. https://doi.org/10.2353/ajpath.2007.061178
8. Caillet-Boudin ML, Buee L, Sergeant N, Lefebvre B (2015) Regulation of human MAPT gene expression. Mol Neurodegener 10:28. https://doi.org/10.1186/s13024-015-0025-8
9. Chen Z, Hutchison M, Cobb MH (1999) Isolation of the protein kinase TAO2 and identification of its mitogen-activated protein kinase/extracellular signal-regulated kinase kinase binding domain. J Biol Chem 274:28803–28807
10. de Anda FC, Rosario AL, Durak O, Tran T, Graff J, Meletis K, Rei D, Soda T, Madabhushi R, Ginty DD et al (2012) Autism spectrum disorder susceptibility gene TAOK2 affects basal dendrite formation in the neocortex. Nat Neurosci 15:1022–1031. https://doi.org/10.1038/nn.3141
11. Despres C, Byrne C, Qi H, Cantrelle FX, Huvent I, Chambraud B, Baulieu EE, Jacquot Y, Landrieu I, Lippens G et al (2017) Identification of the tau phosphorylation pattern that drives its aggregation. Proc Natl Acad Sci U S A 114:9080–9085. https://doi.org/10.1073/pnas.1708448114
12. Dickey CA, Kamal A, Lundgren K, Klosak N, Bailey RM, Dunmore J, Ash P, Shoraka S, Zlatkovic J, Eckman CB et al (2007) The high-affinity HSP90-CHIP complex recognizes and selectively degrades phosphorylated tau client proteins. J Clin Invest 117:648–658. https://doi.org/10.1172/JCI29715
13. Drechsel DN, Hyman AA, Cobb MH, Kirschner MW (1992) Modulation of the dynamic instability of tubulin assembly by the microtubule-associated protein tau. Mol Biol Cell 3:1141–1154
14. Eidenmuller J, Fath T, Maas T, Pool M, Sontag E, Brandt R (2001) Phosphorylation-mimicking glutamate clusters in the proline-rich region are sufficient to simulate the functional deficiencies of hyperphosphorylated tau protein. Biochem J 357:759–767
15. Ferrer I, Blanco R, Carmona M, Puig B (2001) Phosphorylated mitogen-activated protein kinase (MAPK/ERK-P), protein kinase of 38 kDa (p38-P), stress-activated protein kinase (SAPK/JNK-P), and calcium/calmodulin-dependent kinase II (CaM kinase II) are differentially expressed in tau deposits in neurons and glial cells in tauopathies. J Neural Transm 108: 1397–1415. https://doi.org/10.1007/s007020100016
16. Giacomini C, Mahajani S, Ruffilli R, Marotta R, Gasparini L (2016) Lamin B1 protein is required for dendrite development in primary mouse cortical neurons. Mol Biol Cell 27:35–47. https://doi.org/10.1091/mbc.E15-05-0307
17. Goedert M, Spillantini MG (2011) Pathogenesis of the tauopathies. J Mol Neurosci 45:425–431. https://doi.org/10.1007/s12031-011-9593-4
18. Guillozet-Bongaarts AL, Cahill ME, Cryns VL, Reynolds MR, Berry RW, Binder LI (2006) Pseudophosphorylation of tau at serine 422 inhibits caspase cleavage: in vitro evidence and implications for tangle formation in vivo. J Neurochem 97:1005–1014. https://doi.org/10.1111/j.1471-4159.2006.03784.x
19. Guo T, Noble W, Hanger DP (2017) Roles of tau protein in health and disease. Acta Neuropathol 133:665–704. https://doi.org/10.1007/s00401-017-1707-9
20. Hanger DP, Anderton BH, Noble W (2009) Tau phosphorylation: the therapeutic challenge for neurodegenerative disease. Trends Mol Med 15: 112–119. https://doi.org/10.1016/j.molmed.2009.01.003
21. Hanger DP, Hughes K, Woodgett JR, Brion JP, Anderton BH (1992) Glycogen synthase kinase-3 induces Alzheimer's disease-like phosphorylation of tau: generation of paired helical filament epitopes and neuronal localisation of the kinase. Neurosci Lett 147: 58–62 doi 0304-3940(92)90774-2.
22. Hanger DP, Seereeram A, Noble W (2009) Mediators of tau phosphorylation in the pathogenesis of Alzheimer's disease. Expert Rev Neurother 9:1647–1666. https://doi.org/10.1586/ern.09.104
23. Hernandez F, Avila J (2007) Tauopathies. Cell Mol Life Sci 64:2219–2233. https://doi.org/10.1007/s00018-007-7220-x
24. Ho GJ, Hashimoto M, Adame A, Izu M, Alford MF, Thal LJ, Hansen LA, Masliah E (2005) Altered p59Fyn kinase expression accompanies disease progression in Alzheimer's disease: implications for its functional role. Neurobiol Aging 26:625–635. https://doi.org/10.1016/j.neurobiolaging.2004.06.016
25. Hutchison M, Berman KS, Cobb MH (1998) Isolation of TAO1, a protein kinase that activates MEKs in stress-activated protein kinase cascades. J Biol Chem 273:28625–28632
26. Ingelsson M, Fukumoto H, Newell KL, Growdon JH, Hedley-Whyte ET, Frosch MP, Albert MS, Hyman BT, Irizarry MC (2004) Early Abeta accumulation and progressive synaptic loss, gliosis, and tangle formation in AD brain. Neurology 62:925–931
27. Jin M, Shepardson N, Yang T, Chen G, Walsh D, Selkoe DJ (2011) Soluble amyloid beta-protein dimers isolated from Alzheimer cortex directly induce tau hyperphosphorylation and neuritic degeneration. Proc Natl Acad Sci U S A 108:5819–5824. https://doi.org/10.1073/pnas.1017033108
28. Kaufman AC, Salazar SV, Haas LT, Yang J, Kostylev MA, Jeng AT, Robinson SA, Gunther EC, van Dyck CH, Nygaard HB et al (2015) Fyn inhibition rescues established memory and synapse loss in Alzheimer mice. Ann Neurol 77:953–971. https://doi.org/10.1002/ana.24394
29. Koo CY, Giacomini C, Reyes-Corral M, Olmos Y, Tavares IA, Marson CM, Linardopoulos S, Tutt AN, Morris JDH (2017) Targeting TAO kinases using a new inhibitor compound delays mitosis and induces mitotic cell death in centrosome amplified breast Cancer cells. Mol Cancer Ther 16:2410–2421. https://doi.org/10.1158/1535-7163.MCT-17-0077
30. Kurbatskaya K, Phillips EC, Croft CL, Dentoni G, Hughes MM, Wade MA, Al-Sarraj S, Troakes C, O'Neill MJ, Perez-Nievas BG et al (2016) Upregulation of calpain activity precedes tau phosphorylation and loss of synaptic proteins in Alzheimer's disease brain. Acta Neuropathol Commun 4:34. https://doi.org/10.1186/s40478-016-0299-2
31. Lasagna-Reeves CA, de Haro M, Hao S, Park J, Rousseaux MW, Al-Ramahi I, Jafar-Nejad P, Vilanova-Velez L, See L, De Maio A et al (2016) Reduction of Nuak1 decreases tau and reverses phenotypes in a Tauopathy mouse model. Neuron 92:407–418. https://doi.org/10.1016/jneuron.2016.09.022
32. Le Corre S, Klafki HW, Plesnila N, Hubinger G, Obermeier A, Sahagun H, Monse B, Seneci P, Lewis J, Eriksen J et al (2006) An inhibitor of tau hyperphosphorylation prevents severe motor impairments in tau transgenic mice. Proc Natl Acad Sci U S A 103:9673–9678. https://doi.org/10.1073/pnas.0602913103
33. Lee C, Low CY, Francis PT, Attems J, Wong PT, Lai MK, Tan MG (2016) An isoform-specific role of FynT tyrosine kinase in Alzheimer's disease. J Neurochem 136:637–650. https://doi.org/10.1111/jnc.13429
34. Lee VM, Goedert M, Trojanowski JQ (2001) Neurodegenerative tauopathies. Annu Rev Neurosci 24:1121–1159. https://doi.org/10.1146/annurev.neuro.24.1.1121
35. Liu C, Gotz J (2013) Profiling murine tau with 0N, 1N and 2N isoform-specific antibodies in brain and peripheral organs reveals distinct subcellular localization, with the 1N isoform being enriched in the nucleus. PLoS One 8:e84849. https://doi.org/10.1371/journal.pone.0084849
36. Liu F, Gong CX (2008) Tau exon 10 alternative splicing and tauopathies. Mol Neurodegener 3:8. https://doi.org/10.1186/1750-1326-3-8
37. Liu F, Li B, Tung EJ, Grundke-Iqbal I, Iqbal K, Gong CX (2007) Site-specific effects of tau phosphorylation on its microtubule assembly activity and self-aggregation. Eur J Neurosci 26:3429–3436. https://doi.org/10.1111/j.1460-9568.2007.05955.x
38. Liu T, Rohn JL, Picone R, Kunda P, Baum B (2010) Tao-1 is a negative regulator of microtubule plus-end growth. J Cell Sci 123:2708–2716. https://doi.org/10.1242/jcs.068726
39. Lovestone S, Boada M, Dubois B, Hull M, Rinne JO, Huppertz HJ, Calero M, Andres MV, Gomez-Carrillo B, Leon T et al (2015) A phase II trial of tideglusib in Alzheimer's disease. J Alzheimers Dis 45:75–88. https://doi.org/10.3233/JAD-141959
40. Lund ET, McKenna R, Evans DB, Sharma SK, Mathews WR (2001) Characterization of the in vitro phosphorylation of human tau by tau protein kinase II (cdk5/p20) using mass spectrometry. J Neurochem 76:1221–1232
41. McCarthy SE, Makarov V, Kirov G, Addington AM, McClellan J, Yoon S, Perkins DO, Dickel DE, Kusenda M, Krastoshevsky O et al (2009) Microduplications of 16p11.2 are associated with schizophrenia. Nat Genet 41:1223–1227. https://doi.org/10.1038/ng.474
42. McMillan P, Korvatska E, Poorkaj P, Evstafjeva Z, Robinson L, Greenup L, Leverenz J, Schellenberg GD, D'Souza I (2008) Tau isoform regulation is region- and cell-specific in mouse brain. J Comp Neurol 511:788–803. https://doi.org/10.1002/cne.21867
43. Mitsopoulos C, Zihni C, Garg R, Ridley AJ, Morris JD (2003) The prostate-derived sterile 20-like kinase (PSK) regulates microtubule organization and stability. J Biol Chem 278:18085–18091. https://doi.org/10.1074/jbc.M213064200
44. Moore TM, Garg R, Johnson C, Coptcoat MJ, Ridley AJ, Morris JD (2000) PSK, a novel STE20-like kinase derived from prostatic carcinoma that activates

the c-Jun N-terminal kinase mitogen-activated protein kinase pathway and regulates actin cytoskeletal organization. J Biol Chem 275:4311–4322
45. Nishimura I, Yang Y, Lu B (2004) PAR-1 kinase plays an initiator role in a temporally ordered phosphorylation process that confers tau toxicity in drosophila. Cell 116:671–682
46. Noble W, Planel E, Zehr C, Olm V, Meyerson J, Suleman F, Gaynor K, Wang L, LaFrancois J, Feinstein B et al (2005) Inhibition of glycogen synthase kinase-3 by lithium correlates with reduced tauopathy and degeneration in vivo. Proc Natl Acad Sci U S A 102:6990–6995. https://doi.org/10.1073/pnas.0500466102
47. Onishi T, Iwashita H, Uno Y, Kunitomo J, Saitoh M, Kimura E, Fujita H, Uchiyama N, Kori M, Takizawa M (2011) A novel glycogen synthase kinase-3 inhibitor 2-methyl-5-(3-{4-[(S )-methylsulfinyl]phenyl}-1-benzofuran-5-yl)-1,3,4-oxadiazole decreases tau phosphorylation and ameliorates cognitive deficits in a transgenic model of Alzheimer's disease. J Neurochem 119: 1330–1340. https://doi.org/10.1111/j.1471-4159.2011.07532.x
48. Reynolds CH, Betts JC, Blackstock WP, Nebreda AR, Anderton BH (2000) Phosphorylation sites on tau identified by nanoelectrospray mass spectrometry: differences in vitro between the mitogen-activated protein kinases ERK2, c-Jun N-terminal kinase and P38, and glycogen synthase kinase-3beta. J Neurochem 74:1587–1595
49. Richter M, Murtaza N, Scharrenberg R, White SH, Johanns O, Walker S, Yuen RKC, Schwanke B, Bedurftig B, Henis M et al (2018) Altered TAOK2 activity causes autism-related neurodevelopmental and cognitive abnormalities through RhoA signaling. Mol Psychiatry. https://doi.org/10.1038/s41380-018-0025-5
50. Schneider CA, Rasband WS, Eliceiri KW (2012) NIH image to ImageJ: 25 years of image analysis. Nat Methods 9:671–675
51. Sereno L, Coma M, Rodriguez M, Sanchez-Ferrer P, Sanchez MB, Gich I, Agullo JM, Perez M, Avila J Guardia-Laguarta Cet al (2009) a novel GSK-3beta inhibitor reduces Alzheimer's pathology and rescues neuronal loss in vivo. Neurobiol Dis 35:359–367. https://doi.org/10.1016/jnbd2009.05.025
52. Shi Y, Kirwan P, Smith J, MacLean G, Orkin SH, Livesey FJ (2012) A human stem cell model of early Alzheimer's disease pathology in Down syndrome. Sci Transl Med 4:124ra129. https://doi.org/10.1126/scitranslmed.3003771
53. Sposito T, Preza E, Mahoney CJ, Seto-Salvia N, Ryan NS, Morris HR, Arber C, Devine MJ, Houlden H, Warner TT et al (2015) Developmental regulation of tau splicing is disrupted in stem cell-derived neurons from frontotemporal dementia patients with the 10 + 16 splice-site mutation in MAPT. Hum Mol Genet 24:5260–5269. https://doi.org/10.1093/hmg/ddv246
54. Tamagnini F, Walsh DA, Brown JT, Bondulich MK, Hanger DP, Randall AD (2017) Hippocampal neurophysiology is modified by a disease-associated C-terminal fragment of tau protein. Neurobiol Aging 60:44–56. https://doi.org/10.1016/j.neurobiolaging.2017.07.005
55. Tavares IA, Touma D, Lynham S, Troakes C, Schober M, Causevic M, Garg R, Noble W, Killick R, Bodi I et al (2013) Prostate-derived sterile 20-like kinases (PSKs/TAOKs) phosphorylate tau protein and are activated in tangle-bearing neurons in Alzheimer disease. J Biol Chem 288:15418–15429. https://doi.org/10.1074/jbc.M112.448183
56. Timm T, Li XY, Biernat J, Jiao J, Mandelkow E, Vandekerckhove J, Mandelkow EM (2003) MARKK, a Ste20-like kinase, activates the polarity-inducing kinase MARK/PAR-1. EMBO J 22:5090–5101. https://doi.org/10.1093/emboj/cdg447
57. Timm T, Matenia D, Li XY, Griesshaber B, Mandelkow EM (2006) Signaling from MARK to tau: regulation, cytoskeletal crosstalk, and pathological phosphorylation. Neurodegener Dis 3:207–217. https://doi.org/10.1159/000095258
58. Trinczek B, Biernat J, Baumann K, Mandelkow EM, Mandelkow E (1995) Domains of tau protein, differential phosphorylation, and dynamic instability of microtubules. Mol Biol Cell 6:1887–1902
59. Ultanir SK, Yadav S, Hertz NT, Oses-Prieto JA, Claxton S, Burlingame AL, Shokat KM, Jan LY, Jan YN (2014) MST3 kinase phosphorylates TAO1/2 to enable myosin Va function in promoting spine synapse development. Neuron 84:968–982. https://doi.org/10.1016/j.neuron.2014.10.025
60. Vingtdeux V, Davies P, Dickson DW, Marambaud P (2011) AMPK is abnormally activated in tangle- and pre-tangle-bearing neurons in Alzheimer's disease and other tauopathies. Acta Neuropathol 121:337–349. https://doi.org/10.1007/s00401-010-0759-x
61. Wang Y, Mandelkow E (2016) Tau in physiology and pathology. Nat Rev Neurosci 17:5–21. https://doi.org/10.1038/nrn.2015.1
62. Weiss LA, Shen Y, Korn JM, Arking DE, Miller DT, Fossdal R, Saemundsen E, Stefansson H, Ferreira MA, Green T et al (2008) Association between microdeletion and microduplication at 16p11.2 and autism. N Engl J Med 358:667–675. https://doi.org/10.1056/NEJMoa075974
63. Wojtala RL, Tavares IA, Morton PE, Valderrama F, Thomas NS, Morris JD (2011) Prostate-derived sterile 20-like kinases (PSKs/TAOKs) are activated in mitosis and contribute to mitotic cell rounding and spindle positioning. J Biol Chem 286:30161–30170. https://doi.org/10.1074/jbc.M111.228320
64. Wray S, Saxton M, Anderton BH, Hanger DP (2008) Direct analysis of tau from PSP brain identifies new phosphorylation sites and a major fragment of N-terminally cleaved tau containing four microtubule-binding repeats. J Neurochem 105:2343–2352. https://doi.org/10.1111/j.1471-4159.2008.05321.x
65. Yadav S, Oses-Prieto JA, Peters CJ, Zhou J, Pleasure SJ, Burlingame AL, Jan LY, Jan YN (2017) TAOK2 kinase mediates PSD95 stability and dendritic spine maturation through Septin7 phosphorylation. Neuron 93:379–393. https://doi.org/10.1016/j.neuron.2016.12.006
66. Zhou T, Raman M, Gao Y, Earnest S, Chen Z, Machius M, Cobb MH, Goldsmith EJ (2004) Crystal structure of the TAO2 kinase domain: activation and specificity of a Ste20p MAP3K. Structure 12:1891–1900. https://doi.org/10.1016/j.str.2004.07.021
67. Zhu X, Ogawa O, Wang Y, Perry G, Smith MA (2003) JKK1, an upstream activator of JNK/SAPK, is activated in Alzheimer's disease. J Neurochem 85:87–93
68. Zihni C, Mitsopoulos C, Tavares IA, Baum B, Ridley AJ, Morris JD (2007) Prostate-derived sterile 20-like kinase 1-alpha induces apoptosis. JNK- and caspase-dependent nuclear localization is a requirement for membrane blebbing. J Biol Chem 282:6484–6493. https://doi.org/10.1074/jbc.M608336200
69. Zihni C, Mitsopoulos C, Tavares IA, Ridley AJ, Morris JD (2006) Prostate-derived sterile 20-like kinase 2 (PSK2) regulates apoptotic morphology via C-Jun N-terminal kinase and Rho kinase-1. J Biol Chem 281:7317–7323. https://doi.org/10.1074/jbc.M513769200

10

# Testing of therapies in a novel nebulin nemaline myopathy model demonstrate a lack of efficacy

Tamar E. Sztal[1], Emily A. McKaige[1], Caitlin Williams[1], Viola Oorschot[2], Georg Ramm[2,3,4] and Robert J. Bryson-Richardson[1*]

**Abstract:** Nemaline myopathies are heterogeneous congenital muscle disorders causing skeletal muscle weakness and, in some cases, death soon after birth. Mutations in *nebulin*, encoding a large sarcomeric protein required for thin filament function, are responsible for approximately 50% of nemaline myopathy cases. Despite the severity of the disease there is no effective treatment for nemaline myopathy with limited research to develop potential therapies. Several supplements, including L-tyrosine, have been suggested to be beneficial and consequently self-administered by nemaline myopathy patients without any knowledge of their efficacy. We have characterized a zebrafish model for nemaline myopathy caused by a mutation in *nebulin*. These fish form electron-dense nemaline bodies and display reduced muscle function akin to the phenotypes observed in nemaline myopathy patients. We have utilized our zebrafish model to test and evaluate four treatments currently self-administered by nemaline myopathy patients to determine their ability to increase skeletal muscle function. Analysis of muscle pathology and locomotion following treatment with L-tyrosine, L-carnitine, taurine, or creatine revealed no significant improvement in skeletal muscle function emphasizing the urgency to develop effective therapies for nemaline myopathy.

**Keywords:** Nebulin, Nemaline myopathy, Zebrafish, Treatment

## Introduction

Nemaline myopathies are congenital muscle diseases characterized by the presence of nemaline (rod-like) bodies that form within the skeletal muscles. The disease presents with clinically heterogeneous phenotypes, ranging from adult onset mild muscle weakness to, in severe cases, death in utero or just after birth [43]. Causative mutations have now been identified in 11 different genes, encoding components that form or regulate the thin filament (*ACTA1* [27], *NEB* [31], α-tropomyosin [18], β-tropomyosin [8], troponin T1 [14], cofilin [1], *KBTBD13* [34], *KLHL40* [32], *KLHL41* [11], *leiomodin-3* [45], and *MYPN* [24]).

*Nebulin* (*NEB*) plays an important role in regulating thin filament length and is the most frequently affected gene in nemaline myopathy, accounting for approximately 50% of all cases [2]. Mutations in *NEB* result in nemaline bodies throughout the muscle combined with diminished contractile strength and force generation [21, 31]. Deletion of exon 55, causing a common form of autosomal recessive nemaline myopathy [19], results in shortened thin filaments, alterations in crossbridge cycling kinetics, and reduced calcium-sensitivity following loss of NEB [28, 30]. Similarly, a reduction in Nebulin in zebrafish recapitulates many of the clinical and pathological aspects of nemaline myopathy observed in patients [38, 39].

The lack of an effective treatment for nemaline myopathy has resulted in many patients and their families testing compounds on an ad-hoc basis, with a number of compounds listed on patient support websites (http://www.nemaline.org/resources/drugs.html). Perhaps the most promising of these is L-tyrosine, a non-essential amino acid, either derived from the diet or synthesised in the liver from phenylalanine, which functions as a precursor to several neurotransmitters and hormones including adrenaline and dopamine [5]. Kalita (1989) reported

* Correspondence: robert.bryson-richardson@monash.edu
[1]School of Biological Sciences, Monash University, Melbourne, Australia
Full list of author information is available at the end of the article

improvements in muscle strength and appetite and reductions in pharyngeal secretions after he and his son received daily supplementations of L-tyrosine. Within 10 days of L-tyrosine withdrawal there was a decrease in muscle strength suggesting that the improvement observed resulted from L-tyrosine treatment and was not sustained [15]. In a small-scale trial, five patients received L-tyrosine doses from 250 to 3000 mg/day for a period of 2 months to 5 years [33]. Following L-tyrosine treatment, all patients reported varying short-term improvements in muscle strength and 'energy' levels, however due to various limitations (no placebo group, large age variability, and variable disease mutations), no firm conclusions could be made as to efficacy [33]. L-tyrosine doses were also administered to a mouse model of nemaline myopathy (*ACTA1*$^{H40Y}$) for 4 weeks, and although treatment was reported to partially alleviate mobility deficits and decrease nemaline bodies [26], the long-term benefits of L-tyrosine supplementation were not determined.

We have established a zebrafish model of NEB nemaline myopathy to test the ability of existing supplements, currently self-administered by patients, to improve skeletal muscle function. We show that zebrafish *neb*$^{-/-}$ mutants exhibit a reduction in birefringence, resulting from disruption of muscle structure, the formation of electron dense nemaline bodies, as well as Actinin2 and F-actin positive aggregates throughout their muscle fibres, analogous to patient biopsies. The NEB nemaline myopathy model display decreased muscle function which cannot be improved by treatment by L-tyrosine, taurine, L-carnitine, or creatine. This suggests that existing treatments are ineffective in improving skeletal muscle performance in NEB nemaline myopathy, highlights the need for further research into novel therapies, and provides a model to assist in their identification.

## Methods

### Fish strains and maintenance

Zebrafish were maintained according to standard protocols [44]. Zebrafish strains used were Tg(*neb*$^{+/-}$; *Lifeact-eGFP*) [4] and an ENU-generated *neb* mutant line (sa906), obtained from the Zebrafish International Resource Centre. Allele specific PCR KASP technology (Geneworks) was used for *neb* genotyping.

### cDNA synthesis and RT-PCR

Total RNA was extracted using TRIzol reagent (Invitrogen Life Technologies). RNA samples were treated with RQ1 RNase-free DNase (Promega). cDNA was synthesized from 1 µg of each RNA sample in a 20 µl reaction using Protoscript first strand cDNA synthesis kit (New England Biosciences) and oligo(dT)20 primer following the supplier's instructions. Primers used for RT-PCR were (*neb*F: TGAGCACAACTACCGCACTC, *neb*R: GAACCTTTGAGGCCA TTTTG, *βAct*F: GCAT TGCTGACCGTATGCAG, *βAct*R: GA TCCACA TCTG CTGGAAGGTGG).

### Histology and antibody staining

For Gomori trichrome staining, 6 dpf zebrafish were anesthetized and heads were cut for genotyping. Tails were snap frozen and sections (10 µm) were cut using a Leica CM 1850 cryostat. Sections were then stained with modified Gomori trichrome and imaged using a 63× 1.4 numerical aperture oil immersion objective. Fiber area was measured using Fiji [35]. Antibody staining was performed as described in [38]. Antibodies used were anti-α-Actinin2 (Sigma clone A7811, 1:100), rhodamine tagged phalloidin (Molecular Probes, 1:200), and AlexaFlour-488-labelled secondary antibody (Molecular Probes, 1:200).

### Electron microscopy

Zebrafish were fixed according standard procedures in 2.5% glutaraldehyde, 2% paraformaldehyde in 0.1 M sodium cacodylate buffer. Post-fixed with 1% $OsO_4$, 1.5% $K_3Fe(III)(CN)_6$. Samples were dehydrated in ethanol and the zebrafish were flat embedded in Epon 812. Ultrathin sections of 70 nm were cut on a Leica Ultracut UCT7 and stained with uranyl acetate and lead citrate. Large area EM tile sets were taken on a FEI NovaNanoSEM 450 equipped with an ETD secondary electrons in-lens detector set at 10 kV and a STEM II (HAADF) detector set at 30 kV. MAPS 2.1 software was used to create the tile sets. High resolution EM imaging was done on a Hitachi 7500 TEM and a FEI Tecnai 12 TEM.

### Muscle function assays

Touch evoke and locomotion assays were performed on 2 and 6 dpf zebrafish respectively as per [37]. For dosage analyses on wildtype zebrafish, an inactivity threshold of 6 mm/s, detection threshold of 25 mm/s and maximum burst threshold of 30 mm/s were used. For the NEB nemaline myopathy zebrafish model, an inactivity threshold of 1 mm/s, detection threshold of 30 mm/s and maximum burst threshold of 30 mm/s were used. The total distance swum above the inactivity threshold and below maximum burst threshold in a 10-min period were extracted using the ZebraLab software (ViewPoint Life Sciences). Blinding of treatments groups was used in combination with randomization of both the position of the fish within the plates and screening order of plates to remove any bias. Once the testing and genotyping was completed the treatments groups were uncovered.

### Toxicology analyses

For dosage analyses, L-tyrosine disodium salt hydrate (T1145, Sigma), taurine (T0625, Sigma), L-carnitine inner salt (C0158, Sigma), and creatine monohydrate (C3630, Sigma) were all dissolved in water at a concentration of 250 mM and diluted appropriately to ensure that 1 ml of each chemical was added to 24 ml of embryo medium in a 90 cm petri dish. Thirty wildtype Tübingen embryos aged 28 h post fertilization (hpf) were dechorionated and placed in the petri dish. For control treatments, 1 ml of water alone was added to 24 ml of embryo medium. Zebrafish were treated from 28 hpf until 6 dpf. Treatments were changed daily and zebrafish were monitored for survival, heart rate, and swimming performance as indicators of toxicity. Four independent treatments were performed for tyrosine and three independent treatments were performed for taurine, L-carnitine, and creatine. The resting heart rates were measured at 2 dpf by counting the number of heart beats in 10 s. Heart rate measurements were performed in triplicate with 10 fish per experiment. For heart rate and swimming assays all treatments were blinded and randomized to avoid experimental bias. Once the testing and analyses were completed the treatments groups were revealed.

### Chemical treatments

For treatment of the NEB nemaline myopathy zebrafish model, Tg(*neb*$^{+/-}$; *Lifeact-eGFP*) or *neb*$^{+/-}$ adult fish were incrossed and the resultant progeny were dechorinated at 24 hpf and 30 embryos were placed in either chemically or water treated embryo at 28 hpf. Treatments were changed daily from 28 hpf water until 6 dpf at which time wildtype embryos were transferred to 24-well plates and NEB nemaline myopathy zebrafish were transferred into 48-well plates for locomotion assays. For distance assays, based on the SD (0.178±0.146) of the untreated *neb*$^{-/-}$ mutant and the smallest n for the drug treated mutant fish groups (206) fish this gave us 0.80 power at 0.05 significance to detect an improvement of 20%. For speed assays, based on the SD (0.496 ±0.176) of the untreated *neb*$^{-/-}$ mutant fish this gave us 0.80 power at 0.05 significance to detect an improvement of 9%.

### Statistics

For toxicology analyses on wildtype fish, all values were normalized to water supplemented wildtype fish in the same replicate. Normality of data was determined using a D'Agostino and Pearson test for normality. For toxicology analyses on wildtype fish, normal data (Additional file 1: Figures S2, S3, and S4a and b) was analysed by one-way ANOVA using Dunnett's correction for multiple comparisons. For data failing the normality test (Additional file 1: Figure S4C), the test was repeated after the data was logtransformed which did not result in a normal distribution of data. Therefore, data from the three replicates was pooled and a Kruskal-Wallis test was performed and correction for multiple comparisons conducted using Dunn's test. For swimming analyses and fiber area quantification on the NEB nemaline myopathy model, all values were normalized to the average water supplemented *neb*$^{+/+}$ siblings. Normality of data was determined using a D'Agostino and Pearson test for normality and normal data (Fig. 1e, g and 2b) was analysed using an unpaired t-test or one-way ANOVA using Dunnett's correction for multiple comparisons. For data failing the normality test (Fig. 1f, Fig. 4, Additional file 1: Figures S5 and S6), the test was repeated after the outliers were removed by the ROUT method (Q = 1%) or the data was logtransformed. In neither case did this result in a normal distribution of data. Therefore, in these cases the data from the three replicates was pooled and a Kruskal-Wallis test was performed and correction for multiple comparisons conducted using Dunn's test. For phenotypic analyses (Fig. 5b, c and Additional file 1: Figure S7), the results of the three replicates were used to determine the mean percentage of each phenotype and to plot the graphs. The proportion of the phenotypes was determined by pooling the data from all three replicates and conducting a Chi-square test for each treatment against its respective control. All statistical analyses were conducted using GraphPad Prism 7.

## Results

### *neb* mutants display a reduction in muscle function

We obtained a zebrafish mutant strain (sa906) which contains a point mutation in *neb* causing a nonsense mutation in exon 30 (of 134) of the transcript. We have verified the mutation in this strain and show, using RT-PCR, that this leads to a reduction in *neb* mRNA in *neb*$^{-/-}$*fish* compared to their wildtype siblings (Fig. 1c). Morphologically, *neb*$^{-/-}$ mutants are smaller than their wildtype siblings and display a thinner trunk region (Fig. 1a). *neb*$^{-/-}$ mutants also show a loss of birefringence at 4 days post fertilization (dpf) compared to wildtype siblings indicating that their sarcomeric muscle structure is disrupted (Fig. 1b). To determine whether loss of Neb results in impaired skeletal muscle function, we performed touch evoke and locomotion analyses to measure swimming performance. *neb*$^{-/-}$ mutants display a significant reduction in maximum acceleration (proportional to muscle force) at 2 dpf (*neb*$^{-/-}$ = 0.66±0.32 SEM, *neb*$^{+/-}$ = 0.92±0.49 SEM, *neb*$^{+/+}$ = 1.0±0.49 SEM; Fig. 1e), in distance travelled at 6 dpf (*neb*$^{-/-}$ = 0.16 ±0.08 SEM, *neb*$^{+/-}$ = 0.84±0.17 SEM, *neb*$^{+/+}$ = 1.0±0.17 SEM; Fig. 1f) and speed at 6 dpf (*neb*$^{-/-}$ = 0.49±0.10 SEM, *neb*$^{+/-}$ = 0.94±0.19 SEM, *neb*$^{+/+}$ = 1.0±0.14 SEM; Fig. 1g) compared to wildtype siblings. Interestingly, we observe that *neb*$^{-/-}$ mutants fail to inflate their swim bladder by 4 dpf (Fig. 1a&d), another indicator of impaired muscle function.

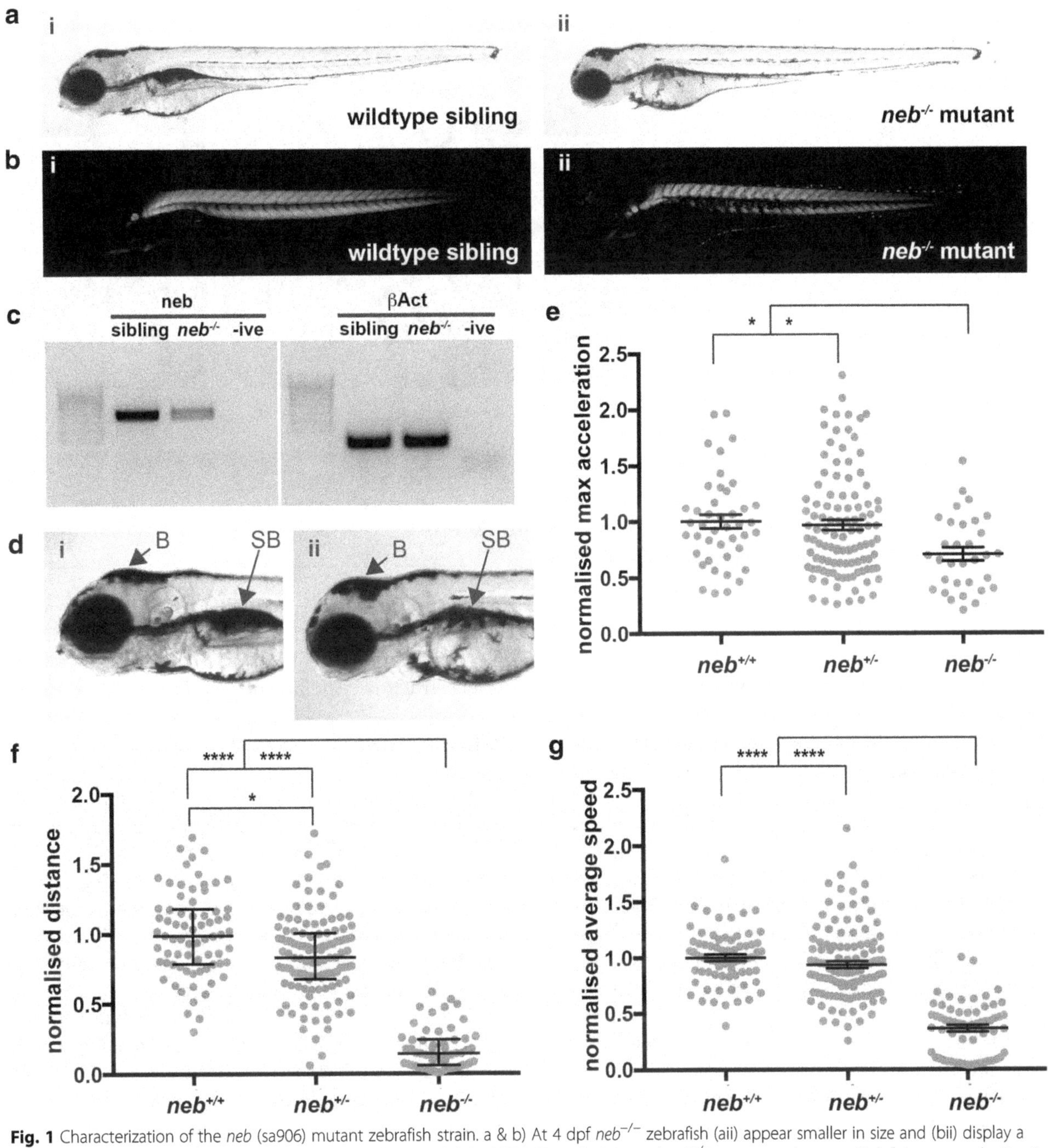


**Fig. 1** Characterization of the *neb* (sa906) mutant zebrafish strain. a & b) At 4 dpf $neb^{-/-}$ zebrafish (aii) appear smaller in size and (bii) display a loss of birefringence compared to their wildtype siblings (ai & bi). c) RT-PCR analysis in and $neb^{-/-}$ mutant embryos at 2 dpf shows a reduction in *neb* mRNA levels compared to wildtype siblings (sibling). *βAct* was used as a positive control. d) ii) $neb^{-/-}$ mutants display a smaller eye, brain region (B) and deflated swim bladder (SB) compared to their i) wildtype siblings. e) Quantification of the maximum acceleration recorded from touch-evoked response assays of $neb^{-/-}$ fish compared to wildtype siblings at 2 dpf. Error bars represent mean±SEM for three independent experiments ($n$ = 11,9,12 $neb^{-/-}$, 55,25,32 $neb^{+/-}$, 18,13,12 $neb^{+/+}$ zebrafish per experiment), $^{**}p < 0.01$. f & g) Quantification of the normalized (f) distance and (g) speed travelled by $neb^{-/-}$ mutants compared to wildtype siblings at 6 dpf. For f) error bars represent median±interquartile range for three independent experiments (for $n$ = 19,23,19 $neb^{-/-}$, 41,42,36 $neb^{+/-}$, 31,20,21 $neb^{+/+}$ zebrafish). For g) error bars represent mean±SEM range (for n = 19,23,14 $neb^{-/-}$, 41,42,36 $neb^{+/-}$, 30,20,21 $neb^{+/+}$ zebrafish per experiment). $^{*}p < 0.5$, **** $p < 0.001$

### $neb^{-/-}$ mutants display nemaline bodies and actin accumulation

NEB nemaline myopathy is characterized by the presence of electron-dense nemaline bodies and myofibrillar disorganization, which have been observed in both patient muscle biopsies [21, 30] and mice models carrying mutations in *Neb* [3, 29]. To test whether these are present in $neb^{-/-}$ zebrafish, we first stained sections of

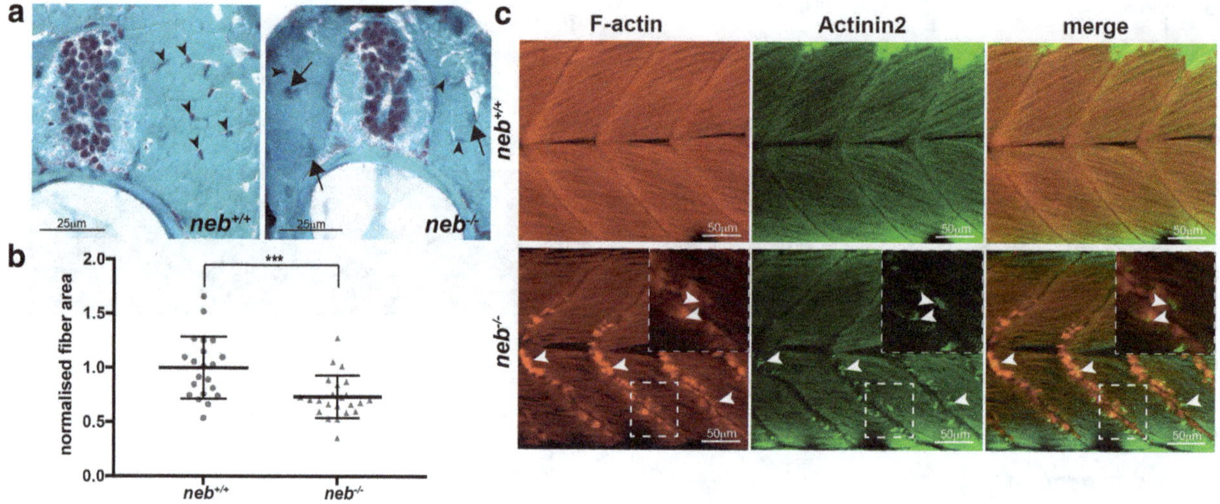


**Fig. 2** Characterisation of skeletal muscle pathology in $neb^{-/-}$ fish. **a** Gomori trichome staining of $neb^{-/-}$ skeletal muscle sections reveal the presence of dark regions (arrows) throughout the muscle indicative of nemaline bodies not observed in $neb^{+/+}$ fish. Nuclei (arrowhead) are evenly organized in $neb^{+/+}$, however, appear disorganized in $neb^{-/-}$ fish. **b** Quantification of normalized fiber area from Gomori trichome stained sections in $neb^{-/-}$ ($n = 23$ fibers) compared to $neb^{+/+}$ fish ($n = 21$ fibers). Error bars represent mean±SD, *** $p < 0.001$. **c** $neb^{-/-}$ mutants exhibit F-actin (red) and Actinin2 (green) positive aggregates at the myosepta (arrowheads) (and zoomed inset) compared to wildtype siblings at 2 dpf

skeletal muscle at 6 dpf with Gomori trichome. We observed large darkly stained patches throughout the muscle fibers, indicative of nemaline bodies which were not present in stained sections from $neb^{+/+}$ siblings (Fig. 2a). We also determined that $neb^{-/-}$ fish have a much smaller skeletal muscle fiber cross-sectional area than $neb^{+/+}$ siblings, reflecting a severe reduction in the diameter of muscle fibers ($neb^{-/-} = 0.73 \pm 0.20$ SD, $neb^{+/+} = 1.0 \pm 0.29$ SD) (Fig. 2b). We performed electron microscopy to analyze the muscle ultrastructure. As shown in Fig. 3a, we observed thickened Z-disks (Fig. 3ai) and an accumulation of electron dense nemaline bodies (Fig. 3aiii) in $neb^{-/-}$ zebrafish at 6 dpf which were not present in wildtype siblings (Fig. 3b). $neb^{-/-}$ mutant fibers also appeared disorganized and in many cases, there was a complete loss of structure with remnants of sarcomeric material (Fig. 3aii, aiv), suggesting a complete loss of muscle integrity.

We have previously shown that knockdown of Neb using two different antisense morpholinos produced Actinin2 and F-actin positive aggregates in the skeletal muscle [38]. We performed antibody staining for Actinin2 and F-actin and observed Actinin2 and F-actin positive aggregates along the vertical myosepta and scattered throughout $neb^{-/-}$ skeletal muscle fibers at 2 dpf, similar to those identified in Neb morphants [38], which are not present in $neb^{+/+}$ siblings (Fig. 2c). These actin accumulations do not result from broken fibers since the fibers in the same cell are intact (Fig. 2c inset). We also crossed our *neb* mutant strain to the Tg(*Lifeact-eGFP*) transgenic line, which labels actin in all of the thin filaments within the skeletal muscle. Unlike their wildtype siblings, Tg($neb^{-/-}$; *Lifeact-eGFP*) zebrafish show an accumulation of actin at the myosepta from 2 dpf and by 6 dpf, exhibit broken fibers greatly disrupting skeletal muscle structure (Additional file 1: Figure S1).

### Evaluation of nemaline myopathy treatments on *neb* mutants

We have established that the $neb^{-/-}$ mutant zebrafish closely mimics nemaline myopathy phenotypes observed in patients validating its use as a NEB nemaline myopathy model. We next wanted to use the model to determine the efficacy of a number of suggested treatments which are currently self-administered by patients to improve skeletal muscle function. We selected four treatments (L-tyrosine, L-carnitine, creatine, and taurine) based on anecdotal reports from the nemaline myopathy patient support website (http://www.nemaline.org/resources/drugs.html) and published studies on nemaline myopathy patients and mice models [15, 33].

Given that none of these compounds have been previously tested in zebrafish, we first determined a maximal dose to investigate therapeutic potential without affecting the health and viability of the fish. We chose six doses ranging from 0.1 μM to 10 mM, dissolved in water and added these to zebrafish embryo medium. For control treatments, we added the equivalent volume of water, which was used as the vehicle, to the zebrafish embryo medium instead of the compound. For each of the treatments, we recorded the survival from 24 hpf to 6 dpf as well as the resting heart rate of the embryos at 2 dpf. We also quantified the swimming performance at 6 dpf and, combined with the survival and heart rate

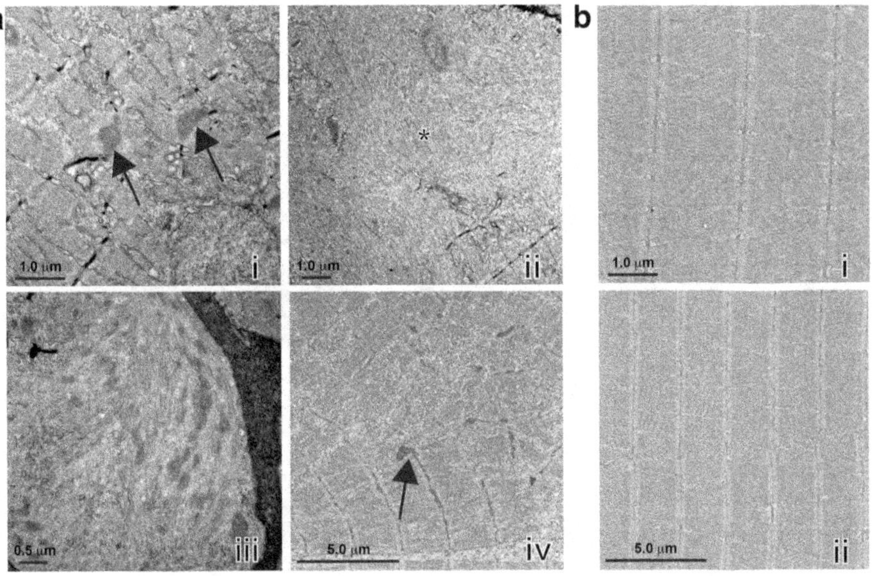


**Fig. 3** Examination of *neb*$^{-/-}$ skeletal muscle by electron microscopy. a) *neb*$^{-/-}$ mutant skeletal muscles display (i, iv) thickened Z-disks (arrows), (ii) fiber breakage (asterisks), (iii) accumulations of nemaline bodies and (iv) disruption of sarcomeric structures that are not observed in b) *neb*$^{+/+}$ wildtype siblings

results, determined that a L-tyrosine and L-carnitine concentration of 10 μM (for L-tyrosine: [23], for L-carnitine: Additional file 1: Figure S3), a taurine concentration of 1 mM (Additional file 1: Figure S2), and a creatine concentration of 100 μM (Additional file 1: Figure S4) are the maximal non-toxic doses for treatment.

To determine whether any of the treatments improved skeletal muscle function or pathology we quantified both the locomotion and phenotypic severity of the skeletal muscle in the treated NEB nemaline model fish at 6 dpf. We observed a significant decrease in swimming performance for *neb*$^{-/-}$ mutants compared to their wildtype siblings (*neb*$^{+/+}$ and *neb*$^{+/-}$) (Additional file 1: Figure S5 and S6). However, for all chemicals tested there was no significant difference in the distance or speed travelled by *neb*$^{-/-}$ mutants treated with the chemical supplements compared to water treated *neb*$^{-/-}$ fish (Fig. 4).

To assess pathology in treated *neb*$^{-/-}$ zebrafish as well as their wildtype siblings, we categorized the phenotypic severity of the skeletal muscle as wildtype, mild (less than five aggregates at the myosepta) and severe (fiber breakage and more than five aggregates at the myosepta and throughout the muscle fibers; Fig. 5a) and then genotyped the scored the embryos. We found no significant difference in the severity of the skeletal muscle phenotype of *neb*$^{-/-}$ mutants, nor for their wildtype siblings for all treatments tested (Fig. 5b+c), showing these therapies do not improve skeletal muscle function in our nemaline myopathy model. There was also no obvious difference in the appearance of facial muscles between

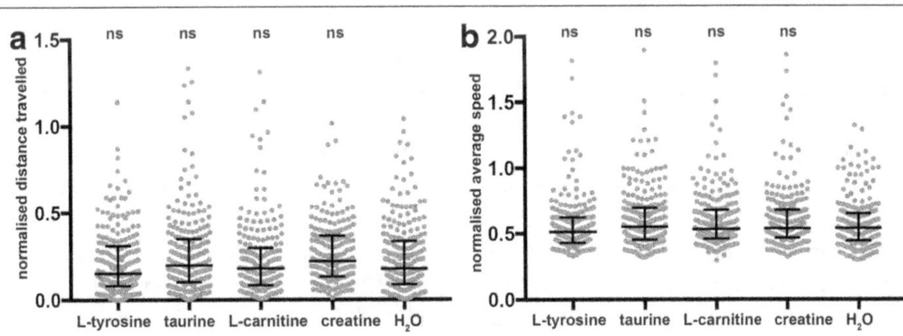


**Fig. 4** Quantification of muscle function in *neb*$^{-/-}$ mutants at 6 dpf. Quantification of the **a**) normalized distance and **b**) speed travelled by *neb*$^{-/-}$ mutants at 6 dpf supplemented with either L-tyrosine, taurine, L-carnitine, creatine, or water ($H_2O$). Error bars represent median±interquartile range for three independent experiments (for a; *n* = 81,79,51 *neb*$^{-/-}$ for L-tyrosine; *n* = 82,89,59 *neb*$^{-/-}$ for taurine; n = 82,82,42 *neb*$^{-/-}$ for L-carnitine; *n* = 87,79,46 *neb*$^{-/-}$ for creatine, and n = 87,96,42 *neb*$^{-/-}$ for water and for b; n = 81,79,51 *neb*$^{-/-}$ for L-tyrosine; n = 82,89,59 *neb*$^{-/-}$ for taurine; n = 82,82,42 *neb*$^{-/-}$ for L-carnitine; *n* = 92,79,46 *neb*$^{-/-}$ for creatine, and n = 87,96,42 *neb*$^{-/-}$ for water per experiment). ns = not significant

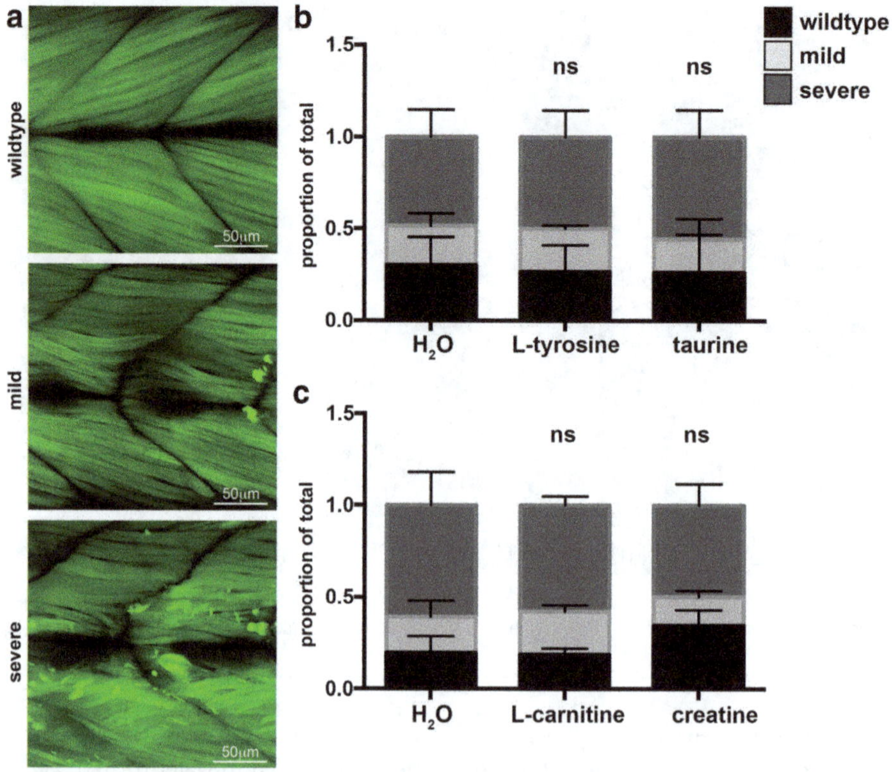


**Fig. 5** Quantification of the phenotypic severity of *neb*$^{-/-}$ mutants at 6 dpf. Quantification of the phenotypic severity of Tg(*neb*$^{-/-}$; *Lifeact-eGFP*) fish at 6 dpf supplemented with either L-tyrosine, taurine, L-carnitine, creatine, or water ($H_2O$). **a** Phenotypes were scored as either wildtype, mild (less than five Lifeact-eGFP positive aggregates at the myosepta or a mild disruption of muscle fibres), or severe (severely disorganised fibres or an accumulation of five or more Lifeact-eGFP positive aggregates within the muscle cell). **b** Quantification of the phenotypic severity of Tg(*neb*$^{-/-}$; *Lifeact-eGFP*) fish supplemented with either L-tyrosine, taurine, or water. **c** Quantification of the phenotypic severity of Tg(*neb*$^{-/-}$; *Lifeact-eGFP*) fish supplemented with either L-carnitine, creatine, or water ($H_2O$). **b** & **c** Error bars represent mean±SEM for three independent experiments. For **b**) *n* = 6,8,7 Tg(*neb*$^{-/-}$; *Lifeact-eGFP*) for L-tyrosine, n = 11,5,11 Tg(*neb*$^{-/-}$; *Lifeact-eGFP*) for taurine and n = 9,8,10 Tg(*neb*$^{-/-}$; *Lifeact-eGFP*) for water. For **c**) n = 8,10,4 Tg(*neb*$^{-/-}$; *Lifeact-eGFP*) for L-carnitine, n = 6,8,3 Tg(*neb*$^{-/-}$; *Lifeact-eGFP*) for creatine, and *n* = 10,9,5 Tg(*neb*$^{-/-}$; *Lifeact-eGFP*) for water per experiment). ns = not significant

*neb*$^{+/+}$ siblings and *neb*$^{-/-}$ mutants. (Additional file 1: Figure S8).

## Discussion

At present, there is no effective therapy for nemaline myopathies with limited research into treatments in vivo using animal systems. For individuals surviving through childhood, nemaline myopathy is a chronic condition requiring continued therapy throughout life to manage symptoms. Our main goal is to develop zebrafish nemaline myopathy models to find effective treatments that can improve skeletal muscle function.

Here, we have characterized and validated a new NEB nemaline myopathy model containing a mutation within the super repeat region of the nebulin protein [9], causing nonsense mediating decay of the resulting transcript. Unlike the previously published model containing a missense mutation in the super repeat region, also predicted to cause a loss of nebulin protein function, we show that *neb*$^{-/-}$ zebrafish mutants display darkly stained patches of muscle in Gomori trichome stained sections corresponding to nemaline bodies. Electron microscopy revealed the presence of electron dense nemaline bodies and thickened Z-disks consistent with those observed in patient biopsies [10, 21] which are not present in the previously published zebrafish *neb* mutant [39]. These pathological defects lead to a disruption in fiber integrity, indicated by the absence of sarcomeric structures by EM and loss of birefringence, resulting in reduced skeletal muscle function.

Akin to Neb KO mice models [3], *neb*$^{-/-}$ mutant zebrafish are indistinguishable from their wildtype siblings prior to 2 dpf, however, as development proceeds their growth is reduced. The reduced growth in Neb KO and Neb$^{\Delta Exon55}$ mice [20, 29] results from a significant reduction in thin filament length and fiber cross sectional area leading to a reduction in maximal force generating capacity [3, 20, 29] causing muscle weakness [30]. Similarly, sectioning of *neb*$^{-/-}$ zebrafish larvae at 6 dpf revealed significantly smaller fiber cross-sectional area compared to wildtype siblings, indicating a reduction in fiber size. Both our Neb morphant model [38] and *neb*$^{-/-}$ genetic mutants show an accumulation of actin at the myosepta suggesting that this may be an important pathological hallmark of nemaline myopathy. Thus, it is likely that the depletion of actin from the sarcomere, in addition to the loss of nebulin from the thin filament, may contribute to the reduction in myofiber size and the observed muscle weakness.

We evaluated a number of existing treatments for nemaline myopathy by quantifying their ability to reduce actin aggregation or improve skeletal muscle performance in our *neb*$^{-/-}$ zebrafish. Of the four treatments we examined, L-tyrosine has been tested in ACTA1$^{H40Y}$ mouse models [26] and in a limited patient study [15, 33] however no firm conclusions had been made as to its effectiveness to increase skeletal muscle function. Our results suggest that L-tyrosine treatment of *neb*$^{-/-}$ mutant zebrafish, as reported for ACTA1$^{D286G}$ zebrafish and mouse models [23], does not improve skeletal muscle performance. It is noted that L-tyrosine treatment may be beneficial to increase weight gain, appetite, and reduce pharyngeal secretions in nemaline myopathy patients [15, 33], however, this was not examined in the current study. We did however, examine the facial muscle structure in *neb*$^{-/-}$ zebrafish, and observed no difference in appearance compared to their wild type siblings preventing an assessment of the effect of treatments on facial musculature.

We also treated *neb*$^{-/-}$ mutants with either taurine, creatine, or L-carnitine, which are all naturally occurring compounds, present in many tissues including skeletal muscle, and are involved in modulating ion channel function, membrane stability, calcium homeostasis and energy metabolism [6, 7, 12, 13, 17, 22, 25, 42]. Taurine has been previously shown to improve muscle strength and reduce inflammation in mdx mice [40, 41] and in an analysis of six clinical trials for muscular dystrophy, 192 participants reported an increase in muscle strength when treated with creatine compared to the placebo group [16]. Unfortunately, chemical supplementation of *neb*$^{-/-}$ mutants with creatine, L-carnitine, or taurine also failed to restore skeletal muscle function or improve skeletal muscle pathology. Interestingly, of the four compounds tested, taurine showed the least toxicity at high concentrations, which is in line with previous reports from clinical trials [36]. However, toxic effects observed in wildtype zebrafish treated with high doses of creatine, and L-carnitine suggest caution when administering high doses to patients. Importantly, our study has highlighted the inadequacies of existing nemaline myopathy treatments. Nevertheless, the zebrafish NEB nemaline myopathy model we have characterized provides an excellent system in which to perform high-throughput chemical screens and find an effective treatment for nemaline myopathy.

#### Acknowledgements
We would like to thank Dr. Angela Finch (UNSW) for her advice.

#### Funding
The work was supported by an Australian National Health and Medical Research Council (NHMRC) Project Grant (APP1010110). TS is supported by an MDA Development Grant (APP381325) and an AFM Postdoctoral Fellowship (APP19853).

#### Authors' contributions
TES conceptualized, performed and analyzed the data as well as wrote, reviewed and edited the manuscript. EAM assisted with the *neb* Zebrabox screen and the Gomori trichome staining, as well as reviewed the manuscript. CW assisted with the *neb* Zebrabox screen and reviewed the manuscript. VO and GR performed the electron microscopy and edited the manuscript. RBR conceptualized the methodology, wrote, reviewed and edited the manuscript as well as supervised the project. TES and RBR obtained funding for the research. All authors read and approved the final manuscript.

#### Competing interests
The authors declare that they have no competing interests.

#### Author details
[1]School of Biological Sciences, Monash University, Melbourne, Australia. [2]Monash Ramaciotti Centre for Cryo Electron Microscopy, Monash University, Melbourne, VIC 3800, Australia. [3]Department of Biochemistry and Molecular Biology, Monash University, Melbourne, Australia. [4]Biomedicine Discovery Institute, Monash University, Melbourne, Australia.

#### References
1. Agrawal PB, Greenleaf RS, Tomczak KK, Lehtokari V-L, Wallgren-Pettersson C, Wallefeld W, Laing NG, Darras BT, Maciver SK, Dormitzer PR, Beggs AH (2006) Nemaline myopathy with minicores caused by mutation of the *CFL2* gene encoding the skeletal muscle actin-binding protein, cofilin-2. Am J Hum Genet 80:162–167. https://doi.org/10.1086/510402
2. Agrawal PB, Strickland CD, Midgett C, Morales A, Newburger DE, Poulos MA, Tomczak KK, Ryan MM, Iannaccone ST, Crawford TO, Laing NG, Beggs AH (2004) Heterogeneity of nemaline myopathy cases with skeletal muscle α-actin gene mutations. Ann Neurol 56:86–96. doi: https://doi.org/10.1002/ana.20157
3. Bang M-L, Li X, Littlefield R, Bremner S, Thor A, Knowlton KU, Lieber RL, Chen J (2006) Nebulin-deficient mice exhibit shorter thin filament lengths and reduced contractile function in skeletal muscle. J Muscle Res Cell Motil 173:905–916. https://doi.org/10.1083/jcb.200603119
4. Berger J, Hall TE, Currie PD (2015) Novel transgenic lines to label sarcolemma and myofibrils of the musculature. Zebrafish 12:124–125. https://doi.org/10.1089/zeb.2014.1065
5. Daubner SC, Le T, Wang S (2011) Tyrosine hydroxylase and regulation of dopamine synthesis. Arch Biochem Biophys 508:1–12. https://doi.org/10.1016/j.abb.2010.12.017

6. De Luca A, Pierno S, Camerino DC (2015) Taurine: the appeal of a safe amino acid for skeletal muscle disorders. J Transl Med:1–18. https://doi.org/10.1186/s12967-015-0610-1
7. De Luca A, Pierno S, Huxtable RJ, Falli P, Franconi F, Giotti A, Camerino DC (1992) Effects of taurine depletion on membrane electrical properties of rat skeletal muscle. Adv Exp Med Biol 315:199–205
8. Donner K, Ollikainen M, Ridanpää M, Christen H-J, Goebel HH, de Visser M, Pelin K, Wallgren-Pettersson C (2001) Mutations in the *β-tropomyosin* (*TPM2*) gene – a rare cause of nemaline myopathy. Neuromuscul Disord 12:151–158. doi: https://doi.org/10.1016/S0960-8966(01)00252-8
9. Donner K, Sandbacka M, Lehtokari V-L, Wallgren-Pettersson C, Pelin K (2004) Complete genomic structure of the human *nebulin* gene and identification of alternatively spliced transcripts. Eur J Hum Genet 12:744–751. https://doi.org/10.1038/sj.ejhg.5201242
10. Gajda A, Horvath E, Hortobagyi T, Gergev G, Szabo H, Farkas K, Nagy N, Szell M, Sztriha L (2013) Nemaline myopathy type 2 (NEM2): two novel mutations in the *Nebulin* (*NEB*) gene. J Child Neurol. https://doi.org/10.1177/0883073813494476
11. Gupta VA, Ravenscroft G, Shaheen R, Todd EJ, Swanson LC, Shiina M, Ogata K, Hsu C, Clarke NF, Darras BT, Farrar MA, Hashem A, Manton ND, Muntoni F, North KN, Sandaradura SA, Nishino I, Hayashi YK, Sewry CA, Thompson EM, Yau KS, Brownstein CA, Yu TW, Allcock RJN, Davis MR, Wallgren-Pettersson C, Matsumoto N, Alkuraya FS, Laing NG, Beggs AH (2013) Identification of *KLHL41* mutations implicates BTB-Kelch-mediated ubiquitination as an alternate pathway to Myofibrillar disruption in Nemaline myopathy. Am J Hum Genet 93:1108–1117. https://doi.org/10.1016/j.ajhg.2013.10.020
12. Huxtable RJ (1992) Physiological actions of taurine. Physiol Rev 72:101–163
13. J Jang J, Park J, Chang H, Lim K (2016) L-carnitine supplement reduces skeletal muscle atrophy induced by prolonged hindlimb suspension in rats. Appl Physiol Nutr Metab 41:1240–1247. doi: https://doi.org/10.1139/apnm-2016-0094
14. Johnston JJ, Kelley RI, Crawford TO, Morton DH, Agarwala R, Koch T, Schäffer AA, Francomano CA, Biesecker LG (2000) A novel nemaline myopathy in the Amish caused by a mutation in *troponin T1*. Am J Hum Genet 67:814–821. https://doi.org/10.1086/303089
15. Kalita D (1989) A new treatment for congenital nonprogressive nemaline myopathy. J Orthomol Med
16. Kley RA, Tarnopolsky MA, Vorgerd M (1996) Creatine for treating muscle disorders. https://doi.org/10.1002/14651858.CD004760.pub4
17. Koons S, Cooke R (1986) Function of creatine kinase localization in muscle contraction. Adv Exp Med Biol 194:129–137
18. Laing NG, Wilton SD, Akkari PA, Dorosz S, Boundy K, Kneebone C, Blumbergs P, White S, Watkins H, Love DR (1995) A mutation in the *alpha tropomyosin gene TPM3* associated with autosomal dominant nemaline myopathy NEM1. Nat Genet 10:249–249. https://doi.org/10.1038/ng0695-249
19. Lehtokari V-L, Greenleaf RS, DeChene ET, Kellinsalmi M, Pelin K, Laing NG, Beggs AH, Wallgren-Pettersson C (2009) The exon 55 deletion in the *nebulin* gene–one single founder mutation with world-wide occurrence. Neuromuscul Disord 19:179–181. https://doi.org/10.1016/j.nmd.2008.12.001
20. Li F, Buck D, De Winter J, Kolb J, Meng H, Birch C, Slater R, Escobar YN, Smith JE III, Yang L, Konhilas J, Lawlor MW, Ottenheijm C, Granzier HL (2015) Nebulin deficiency in adult muscle causes sarcomere defects and muscle-type-dependent changes in trophicity: novel insights in nemaline myopathy. Hum Mol Genet 24:5219–5233. https://doi.org/10.1093/hmg/ddv243
21. Malfatti E, Lehtokari V-L, Böhm J, De Winter JM, Schäffer U, Estournet B, Quijano-Roy S, Monges S, Lubieniecki F, Bellance R, Viou M, Madelaine A, Wu B, Taratuto A, Eymard B, Pelin K, Fardeau M, Ottenheijm CA, Wallgren-Pettersson C, Laporte J, Romero NB (2014) Muscle histopathology in nebulin-related nemaline myopathy: ultrastrastructural findings correlated to disease severity and genotype. Acta Neuropathol Commun 2:44. https://doi.org/10.1016/j.spen.2011.10.006
22. McGarry JD, Brown NF (1997) The mitochondrial carnitine palmitoyltransferase system. From concept to molecular analysis. Eur J Biochem 244:1–14
23. Messineo AM, Gineste C, Sztal TE, McNamara EL, Vilmen C, Ogier AC, Hahne D, Bendahan D, Laing NG, Bryson-Richardson RJ, Gondin J, Nowak KJ (2017) L-tyrosine supplementation is not therapeutic for skeletal muscle dysfunction in zebrafish and mouse models of dominant skeletal muscle α-actin nemaline myopathy. bioRxiv. https://doi.org/10.1101/218016
24. Miyatake S, Mitsuhashi S, Hayashi YK, Purevjav E, Nishikawa A, Koshimizu E, Suzuki M, Yatabe K, Tanaka Y, Ogata K, Kuru S, Shiina M, Tsurusaki Y, Nakashima M, Mizuguchi T, Miyake N, Saitsu H, Ogata K, Kawai M, Towbin J, Nonaka I, Nishino I, Matsumoto N (2017) Biallelic mutations in *MYPN*, encoding Myopalladin, are associated with childhood-Onset,Slowly progressive Nemaline myopathy. Am J Hum Genet 100:169–178. https://doi.org/10.1016/j.ajhg.2016.11.017
25. Montesano A, Senesi P, Luzi L, Benedini S, Terruzzi I (2015) Research ArticlePotential therapeutic role of L-carnitine in skeletal muscle oxidative stress and atrophy conditions. Oxidative Med Cell Longev:1–13. https://doi.org/10.1155/2015/646171
26. Nguyen MAT, Joya JE, Kee AJ, Domazetovska A, Yang N, Hook JW, Lemckert FA, Kettle E, Valova VA, Robinson PJ, North KN, Gunning PW, Mitchell CA, Hardeman EC (2011) Hypertrophy and dietary tyrosine ameliorate the phenotypes of a mouse model of severe nemaline myopathy. Brain 134: 3516–3529. https://doi.org/10.1093/brain/awr274
27. Nowak KJK, Wattanasirichaigoon DD, Goebel HHH, Wilce MM, Pelin KK, Donner KK, Jacob RLR, Hübner CC, Oexle KK, Anderson JRJ, Verity CMC, North KNK, Iannaccone STS, Müller CRC, Nürnberg PP, Muntoni FF, Sewry CC, Hughes II, Sutphen RR, Lacson AGA, Swoboda KJK, Vigneron JJ, Wallgren-Pettersson CC, Beggs AHA, Laing NGN (1999) Mutations in the skeletal muscle *alpha-actin* gene in patients with actin myopathy and nemaline myopathy. Nat Genet 23: 208–212. https://doi.org/10.1038/13837
28. Ottenheijm CAC, Granzier H (2010) New insights into the structural roles of Nebulin in skeletal muscle. J Biomed Biotechnol 2010:1–6. https://doi.org/10.1091/mbc.E07-07-0690
29. Ottenheijm CAC, Buck D, de Winter JM, Ferrara C, Piroddi N, Tesi C, Jasper JR, Malik FI, Meng H, Stienen GJM, Beggs AH, Labeit S, Poggesi C, Lawlor MW, Granzier H (2013) Deleting exon 55 from the *nebulin* gene induces severe muscle weakness in a mouse model for nemaline myopathy. Brain 136:1718–1731. https://doi.org/10.1093/brain/awt113
30. Ottenheijm CAC, Witt CC, Stienen GJ, Labeit S, Beggs AH, Granzier H (2009) Thin filament length dysregulation contributes to muscle weakness in nemaline myopathy patients with nebulin deficiency. Hum Mol Gen 18: 2359–2369. https://doi.org/10.1093/hmg/ddp168
31. Pelin KK, Hilpelä PP, Donner KK, Sewry CC, Akkari PAP, Wilton SDS, Wattanasirichaigoon DD, Bang MLM, Centner TT, Hanefeld FF, Odent SS, Fardeau MM, Urtizberea JAJ, Muntoni FF, Dubowitz VV, Beggs AHA, Laing NGN, Labeit SS, la Chapelle de AA, Wallgren-Pettersson CC (1999) Mutations in the *nebulin* gene associated with autosomal recessive nemaline myopathy. Proc Natl Acad Sci U S A 96:2305–2310. https://doi.org/10.2307/47056
32. Ravenscroft G, Miyatake S, Lehtokari V-L, Todd EJ, Vornanen P, Yau KS, Hayashi YK, Miyake N, Tsurusaki Y, Doi H, Saitsu H, Osaka H, Yamashita S, Ohya T, Sakamoto Y, Koshimizu E, Imamura S, Yamashita M, Ogata K, Shiina M, Bryson-Richardson RJ, Vaz R, Ceyhan O, Brownstein CA, Swanson LC, Monnot S, Romero NB, Amthor H, Kresoje N, Sivadorai P, Kiraly-Borri C, Haliloglu G, Talim B, Orhan D, Kale G, Charles AK, Fabian VA, Davis MR, Lammens M, Sewry CA, Manzur A, Muntoni F, Clarke NF, North KN, Bertini E, Nevo Y, Willichowski E, Silberg IE, Topaloglu H, Beggs AH, Allcock RJN, Nishino I, Wallgren-Pettersson C, Matsumoto N, Laing NG (2013) Mutations in *KLHL40* are a frequent cause of severe autosomal-recessive nemaline myopathy. Am J Hum Genet 93:6–18. https://doi.org/10.1016/j.ajhg.2013.05.004
33. Ryan MM, Sy C, Rudge S, Ellaway C, Ketteridge D, Roddick LG, Iannaccone ST, Kornberg AJ, North KN (2007) Dietary L-tyrosine supplementation in Nemaline myopathy. J Child Neurol 23:609–613. https://doi.org/10.1177/0883073807309794
34. Sambuughin N, Swietnicki W, Techtmann S, Matrosova V, Wallace T, Goldfarb L, Maynard E (2012) KBTBD13 interacts with Cullin 3 to form a functional ubiquitin ligase. Biochem Biophys Res Commun:1–7. https://doi.org/10.1016/j.bbrc.2012.04.074
35. Schindelin J, Arganda-Carreras I, Frise E, Kaynig V, Longair M, Pietzsch T, Preibisch S, Rueden C, Saalfeld S, Schmid B, Tinevez J-Y, White DJ, Hartenstein V, Eliceiri K, Tomancak P, Cardona A (2012) Fiji: an open-source platform for biological-image analysis. Nat Methods 9:676–682. https://doi.org/10.1038/nmeth.2019
36. Shao A, Hathcock JN (2008) Risk assessment for the amino acids taurine, L-glutamine and L-arginine. Regul Toxicol Pharmacol 50:376–399. https://doi.org/10.1016/j.yrtph.2008.01.004
37. Sztal TE, Ruparelia AA, Williams C, Bryson-Richardson RJ (2016) Using Touch-evoked Response and Locomotion Assays to Assess Muscle Performance and Function in Zebrafish. J Vis Exp 116:e54431.
38. Sztal TE, Zhao M, Williams C, Oorschot V, Parslow AC, Giousoh A, Yuen M, Hall TE, Costin A, Ramm G, Bird PI, Busch-Nentwich EM, Stemple DL, Currie PD, Cooper ST, Laing NG, Nowak KJ, Bryson-Richardson RJ (2015) Zebrafish models for nemaline myopathy reveal a spectrum of nemaline bodies

contributing to reduced muscle function. Acta Neuropathol 130:389–406. https://doi.org/10.1007/s00401-015-1430-3

39. Telfer WR, Nelson DD, Waugh T, Brooks SV, Dowling JJ (2012) Neb: a zebrafish model of nemaline myopathy due to *nebulin* mutation. Dev Biol 5: 389–396. https://doi.org/10.1242/dmm.008631
40. Terrill JR, Grounds MD, Arthur PG (2015) Taurine deficiency, synthesis and transport in the mdx mouse model for Duchenne muscular dystrophy. Int J Biochem Cell Biol 66:141–148. https://doi.org/10.1016/j.biocel.2015.07.016
41. Terrill JR, Pinniger GJ, Graves JA, Grounds MD, Arthur PG (2016) Increasing taurine intake and taurine synthesis improves skeletal muscle function in the mdx mouse model for Duchenne muscular dystrophy. J Physiol 594: 3095–3110. https://doi.org/10.1113/JP271418
42. Thompson CH, Kemp GJ, Sanderson AL, Dixon RM, Styles P, Taylor DJ, Radda GK (1996) Effect of creatine on aerobic and anaerobic metabolism in skeletal muscle in swimmers. Br J Sports Med 30:222–225
43. Wallgren-Pettersson C, Wallgren-Pettersson C, Sewry CA, Sewry CA, Nowak KJ, Nowak KJ, Laing NG, Laing NG (2011) Nemaline myopathies. YSPEN 18: 230–238. https://doi.org/10.1016/j.spen.2011.10.004
44. Westerfield M (2007) The Zebrafish Book.
45. Yuen M, Sandaradura SA, Dowling JJ, Kostyukova AS, Moroz N, Quinlan KG, Lehtokari V-L, Ravenscroft G, Todd EJ, Ceyhan-Birsoy O, Gokhin DS, Maluenda J, Lek M, Nolent F, Pappas CT, Novak SM, D'Amico A, Malfatti E, Thomas BP, Gabriel SB, Gupta N, Daly MJ, Ilkovski B, Houweling PJ, Davidson AE, Swanson LC, Brownstein CA, Gupta VA, Medne L, Shannon P, Martin N, Bick DP, Flisberg A, Holmberg E, Van den Bergh P, Lapunzina P, Waddell LB, Sloboda DD, Bertini E, Chitayat D, Telfer WR, Laquerrière A, Gregorio CC, Ottenheijm CAC, Bönnemann CG, Pelin K, Beggs AH, Hayashi YK, Romero NB, Laing NG, Nishino I, Wallgren-Pettersson C, Melki J, Fowler VM, MacArthur DG, North KN, Clarke NF (2014) Leiomodin-3 dysfunction results in thin filament disorganization and nemaline myopathy. J Clin Invest 124: 4693–4708. https://doi.org/10.1172/JCI75199

11

# Sequential stages and distribution patterns of aging-related tau astrogliopathy (ARTAG) in the human brain

Gabor G. Kovacs[1,2*], Sharon X. Xie[3], John L. Robinson[2], Edward B. Lee[2], Douglas H. Smith[4], Theresa Schuck[2], Virginia M.-Y. Lee[2] and John Q. Trojanowski[2*]

**Abstract**

Aging-related tau astrogliopathy (ARTAG) describes tau pathology in astrocytes in different locations and anatomical regions. In the present study we addressed the question of whether sequential distribution patterns can be recognized for ARTAG or astroglial tau pathologies in both primary FTLD-tauopathies and non-FTLD-tauopathy cases. By evaluating 687 postmortem brains with diverse disorders we identified ARTAG in 455. We evaluated frequencies and hierarchical clustering of anatomical involvement and used conditional probability and logistic regression to model the sequential distribution of ARTAG and astroglial tau pathologies across different brain regions. For subpial and white matter ARTAG we recognize three and two patterns, respectively, each with three stages initiated or ending in the amygdala. Subependymal ARTAG does not show a clear sequential pattern. For grey matter (GM) ARTAG we recognize four stages including a striatal pathway of spreading towards the cortex and/or amygdala, and the brainstem, and an amygdala pathway, which precedes the involvement of the striatum and/or cortex and proceeds towards the brainstem. GM ARTAG and astrocytic plaque pathology in corticobasal degeneration follows a predominantly frontal-parietal cortical to temporal-occipital cortical, to subcortical, to brainstem pathway (four stages). GM ARTAG and tufted astrocyte pathology in progressive supranuclear palsy shows a striatum to frontal-parietal cortical to temporal to occipital, to amygdala, and to brainstem sequence (four stages). In Pick's disease cases with astroglial tau pathology an overlapping pattern with PSP can be appreciated. We conclude that tau-astrogliopathy type-specific sequential patterns cannot be simplified as neuron-based staging systems. The proposed cytopathological and hierarchical stages provide a conceptual approach to identify the initial steps of the pathogenesis of tau pathologies in ARTAG and primary FTLD-tauopathies.

**Keywords:** Aging-related tau astrogliopathy, ARTAG, Astrocytic plaque, Brain barrier, Hierarchical involvement, Tufted astrocyte, Ramified astrocyte, Spreading, Tau, Tauopathy

## Introduction

Deposition of pathologically altered proteins in astrocytes has been increasingly detected in neurodegenerative diseases (NDD) leading to the concept of protein astrogliopathies [33]. One main group of NDDs is associated with abnormal accumulation of the microtubule-associated protein tau, hence called tauopathies [28]. Primary tauopathies are discussed in the context of frontotemporal lobar degeneration (FTLD) as well [22]. Primary FTLD-tauopathies show a wide range of astroglial tau immunoreactive morphologies, such as tufted astrocytes in progressive supranuclear palsy (PSP), astrocytic plaques in corticobasal degeneration (CBD), ramified astrocytes in Pick's disease (PiD) or globular astroglial inclusions in globular glial tauopathies (GGT) [22, 28]. Further tauopathies comprise argyrophilic grain disease (AGD) and neurofibrillary tangle (NFT) only dementia, which is included in the concept of primary age-related tauopathy (PART) [13, 28]. Recently, the importance of

* Correspondence: gabor.kovacs@meduniwien.ac.at; trojanow@upenn.edu
[1]Institute of Neurology, Medical University of Vienna, AKH 4J, Währinger Gürtel 18-20, 1097 Vienna, Austria
[2]Center for Neurodegenerative Disease Research (CNDR), Institute on Aging and Department of Pathology & Laboratory Medicine, Perelman School of Medicine (PSOM) at the University of Pennsylvania, HUP Maloney 3rd Floor, 36th and Spruce Street, Philadelphia, PA 19104 - 4283, USA
Full list of author information is available at the end of the article

further astroglial tau pathologies such as thorn-shaped astrocytes (TSA) and granular/fuzzy astrocytes (GFA) has been emphasized and the term, aging-related tau astrogliopathy (ARTAG) has been defined [31]. In ARTAG these morphologies appear in subependymal, subpial, perivascular, white matter (WM), and grey matter (GM) locations. In a recent study, we suggested a conceptual link between GM ARTAG and astroglial tau pathologies seen in primary FTLD-tauopathies [35]. In particular, GFA-like morphologies seen in primary FTLD-tauopathies can represent an early maturation phase of astroglial tau pathology [35], analogously to the concept of pretangles and neurofibrillary tangles [3]. These aspects support the notion that astrocytes might have an early role in primary FTLD-tauopathies as recognized also for example in CBD [40]. In addition, the distribution patterns and morphology of ARTAG shows overlap with chronic traumatic encephalopathy (CTE) [35, 41, 44].

The concept of cell-to-cell propagation of neurodegeneration-related proteins was a significant step in our understanding of NDDs [18]. In the human brain this is supported by the hierarchical or stereotypical involvement of anatomical regions, defined as stages or phases [9]. However, these focus only on neuronal (tau, α-synuclein, TDP-43) or extracellular (Aβ) protein pathologies. Hence, protein astrogliopathies have not been considered in these approaches. Here we report distribution patterns of ARTAG and primary-FTLD-tauopathy related astroglial tau pathologies and address the question whether sequential stages can be recognized.

## Material and methods

### Case cohort

This study includes 687 individuals from the collection of brains from longitudinally followed subjects in the Center Neurodegenerative Disease Research (CNDR) Brain Bank at the University of Pennsylvania, Philadelphia, PA (Table 1) [2, 55]. Cases were grouped as followed: CBD ($n = 40$), PSP ($n = 97$), PiD ($n = 22$), only PART ($n = 70$), only Alzheimer disease (AD) pathology ($n = 243$), and other disorders ($n = 215$) including multiple system atrophy ($n = 34$), Lewy body disorders ($n = 120$), and amyotrophic lateral sclerosis ($n = 61$). This pooled cohort of AD plus PART plus other disorders ($n = 528$) is termed here as non-FTLD-tauopathy group. Thus for better overview we did not include PART or the presence of AGD in the group of primary FTLD-tauopathies.

### Immunohistochemistry and evaluation of tau pathologies

Formalin fixed, paraffin-embedded tissue blocks from the investigated cases were evaluated. Immunostaining for tau was performed with anti-tau PHF-1 (Ser396/Ser404, 1:2000; Gift of Peter Davies). The Vectashield ABC detection kit, peroxidase/DAB, rabbit/mouse/rat (BA1000/BA2000/BA4001, 1:1000; Vector Laboratories) was used for the visualization of antibody reaction.

Following the consensus recommendations [31] we evaluated the presence (yes/no) of grey and white matter, subependymal and subpial ARTAG types in the 1) hippocampus pyramidal layers, dentate gyrus, inferior temporal gyrus, and amygdala: together representing medial temporal lobe (MTL) structures; 2) the middle frontal gyrus, anterior cingulate, inferior parietal gyrus, superior temporal gyrus and occipital cortex: together representing lobar structures; 3) the caudate-putamen, globus pallidus, thalamus, and basal forebrain: together representing subcortical structures; 4) the midbrain tegmentum, substantia nigra, locus coeruleus, pontine base, tegmentum and base of the medulla oblongata: together representing brainstem structures. Subependymal (inferior, anterior and posterior horns of the lateral ventricle, 3rd ventricle and aqueduct at different brainstem levels) locations were also evaluated. In all regions, we evaluated primary FTLD-tauopathy-related astroglial tau pathology as well. In addition, we documented the presence of neuronal and oligodendroglial tau pathology and grains.

For the subpial and WM ARTAG we stratified the regions into three groups: brainstem, basal brain regions (combination of basal forebrain and amygdala region) and lobar. For lobar regions we performed a

**Table 1** Demographic data of cases examined in this study

| | n | | Mean age | | Age range | | Men | | Women | |
|---|---|---|---|---|---|---|---|---|---|---|
| Disease group | All | ARTAG | All | ARTAG | All | ARTAG | All | ARTAG | All | ARTAG |
| CBD | 41 | 40 | 66.7 | 66.7 | 44–86 | 44–86 | 16 | 16 | 25 | 24 |
| PSP | 97 | 96 | 75.6 | 75.7 | 48–96 | 48–96 | 62 | 62 | 35 | 34 |
| PID | 22 | 17 | 67.1 | 66.7 | 31–84 | 31–84 | 13 | 11 | 9 | 6 |
| PART | 70 | 41 | 75.4 | 79.2 | 55–101 | 57–101 | 33 | 20 | 37 | 21 |
| AD | 243 | 152 | 80.5 | 82.3 | 60–98 | 60–98 | 107 | 71 | 136 | 81 |
| PART/AD/Other | 528 | 302 | 77.3 | 80.1 | 53–101 | 55–101 | 289 | 173 | 239 | 129 |

separate analysis for frontal, temporal, parietal and occipital lobes. For subependymal ARTAG we distinguished three regions: brainstem (aqueduct), 3rd ventricle and midline of the lateral ventricle together, and the inferior horn of the lateral ventricle. For GM ARTAG and primary FTLD-tauopathy related astroglial tau pathologies, we first stratified as brainstem, subcortical (basal ganglia), MTL and lobar. Next, we performed a detailed comparison of nine regions (frontal, parietal, temporal, occipital, amygdala, striatum, substantia nigra, pons and medulla oblongata tegmentum). In the same regions we evaluated the tau pathologies using a semiquantitative score (none, mild, moderate, severe); the median of these in each region was used to generate heatmaps [21, 35].

### Conceptual approach and statistical analysis

Our approach contains 5 steps: 1) We select cases showing a specific type of ARTAG; then 2) describe patterns of involvements of different anatomical regions; followed by 3) comparison of different anatomical regions to calculate conditional probabilities, which region might precede another one; complemented by 4) logistic regression to correct for influencing factors; and finally 5) evaluating clusters of cases showing different patterns of ARTAG involvement.

We applied conditional probability analysis as reported recently for the staging of TDP-43 pathology in AD [27]. Accordingly, we compared two regions in all combinations for discordance (one affected while the other not and vice versa). The null hypothesis was that region *A* being positive while region *B* being negative and the region *A* being negative and region *B* being positive is equally likely, thus *A* and *B* region is affected at the same time (i.e., being in the same stage). McNemar's test was used to assess the evidence against the null hypothesis. We used $p < 0.01$ to determine whether we can reject the null hypothesis. We generated a matrix for different ARTAG types involving various anatomical regions where each cell in the matrix corresponds to a conditional probability that one region is involved before another one. Conditional probability was calculated using crosstab function of SPSS.

If the conditional probability for one region is significantly higher than for the other region then we interpret that that this region is most likely affected before the other. However, this is interpreted analogously to the measurement of observer agreement for categorical data [36, 38]. Binary logistic regression models were additionally used to generate odds ratios (OR) and 95% confidence intervals (CI), where the presence of each ARTAG types in specific anatomical regions were the dependent variables, and age, sex and, as additional test, Braak stage of neurofibrillary degeneration, shown to influence the presence of ARTAG [35] were the independent variables. In case the OR > 1 with a significant *p* value we interpret this as high likelihood that two regions are affected together. In case OR < 1 with a significant p value we interpret this as low likelihood that the two regions are affected together, eventually meaning that they are affected independently from each other. For details on the methodological approach see Additional file 1.

We performed the statistical evaluation in six diagnostic groups (see case cohort). We report results for primary FTLD-tauopathies (PSP, CBD, Pick disease) and, in case there were no differences, the pooled cases of non-FTLD-tauopathies (where we included PART, AD and other disorders). We mention AD or PART cases separately only if a particular pattern is seen. We applied a significance level of 0.01 for McNemar's test and 0.05 for logistic regression with multiple independent variables. We chose a lower significance level than the traditional 0.05 for McNemar's test in order to reduce the likelihood of false positive findings. We provide the detailed tables of conditional probabilities and OR in the Additional file 2, Additional file 3 and Additional file 4 and here provide the combined interpretation and proposed sequential models.

In addition, we performed a hierarchical cluster analysis using the nearest neighbour approach to evaluate how cases within disease groups cluster together based on the 1) the patterns of primary FTLD-tauopathy related astroglial tau pathologies; 2) GM ARTAG with astroglial tau pathologies; and 3) subpial, WM and GM ARTAG in three major regions (lobar, subcortical/amygdala and brainstem. SPSS Statistics Version 24 was used for statistical analysis.

## Results

### Demographic summary of cases

Demographic data are summarized in Table 1. In sum 455 showed some type of ARTAG (Table 2). GM (68%) and subpial (58%) ARTAG were the most frequent, WM ARTAG was seen in 55% and subependymal in 22%. ARTAG was highly frequent in primary FTLD-tauopathies.

### Morphology of astrocytic tau immunoreactivity

TSAs are seen in subpial, subependymal, perivascular and WM locations in all disease groups. In CBD, in subpial and perivascular location the end-feet astroglial processes are densely stained with a stubby appearance, while the cell body less (Additional file 1: Figure S1a and b); this is reminiscent of the lack of the cell body staining in astrocytic plaques. The morphology of tau immunoreactive astrocytes varies in the WM in PSP and CBD and do not always show typical TSA morphology. In the GM TSAs are less frequently seen. When present, their distribution shows a close relation to adjacent WM, such as seen in deep cortical

**Table 2** Distribution of ARTAG types in different disease groups

| Disease | | ARTAG n | ARTAG % | SP n | SP % | SE n | SE % | WM n | WM % | GM n | GM % |
|---|---|---|---|---|---|---|---|---|---|---|---|
| All cases | no | 232 | 33.8 | 192 | 42 | 357 | 78 | 203 | 45 | 145 | 32 |
| | yes | 455 | 66.2 | 263 | 58 | 98 | 22 | 252 | 55 | 310 | 68 |
| | Sum | 687 | 100.0 | 455 | 100.0 | 455 | 100.0 | 455 | 100.0 | 455 | 100.0 |
| PART | no | 29 | 41.4 | 16 | 39.0 | 32 | 78.0 | 25 | 61.0 | 10 | 24.4 |
| | yes | 41 | 58.6 | 25 | 61.0 | 9 | 22.0 | 16 | 39.0 | 31 | 75.6 |
| | Sum | 70 | 100.0 | 41 | 100.0 | 41 | 100.0 | 41 | 100.0 | 41 | 100.0 |
| AD | no | 91 | 37.4 | 59 | 38.8 | 119 | 78.3 | 39 | 25.7 | 88 | 57.9 |
| | yes | 152 | 62.6 | 93 | 61.2 | 33 | 21.7 | 113 | 74.3 | 64 | 42.1 |
| | Sum | 243 | 100.0 | 152 | 100.0 | 152 | 100.0 | 152 | 100.0 | 152 | 100.0 |
| AD/PART/other | no | 226 | 42.8 | 123 | 40.7 | 236 | 78.1 | 115 | 38.1 | 140 | 46.4 |
| | yes | 302 | 57.2 | 179 | 59.3 | 66 | 21.9 | 187 | 61.9 | 162 | 53.6 |
| | Sum | 528 | 100.0 | 302 | 100.0 | 302 | 100.0 | 302 | 100.0 | 302 | 100.0 |
| CBD | no | 0 | 0.0 | 7 | 17.5 | 29 | 72.5 | 19 | 47.5 | 1 | 2.5 |
| | yes | 40 | 100.0 | 33 | 82.5 | 11 | 27.5 | 21 | 52.5 | 39 | 97.5 |
| | Sum | 40 | 100.0 | 40 | 100.0 | 40 | 100.0 | 40 | 100.0 | 40 | 100.0 |
| PSP | no | 1 | 1.0 | 48 | 50.0 | 76 | 79.2 | 54 | 56.3 | 2 | 2.1 |
| | yes | 96 | 99.0 | 48 | 50.0 | 20 | 20.8 | 42 | 43.8 | 94 | 97.9 |
| | Sum | 97 | 100.0 | 96 | 100.0 | 96 | 100.0 | 96 | 100.0 | 96 | 100.0 |
| PiD | no | 5 | 22.7 | 14 | 82.4 | 16 | 94.1 | 15 | 88.2 | 2 | 11.8 |
| | yes | 17 | 77.3 | 3 | 17.6 | 1 | 5.9 | 2 | 11.8 | 15 | 88.2 |
| | Sum | 22 | 100.0 | 17 | 100.0 | 17 | 100.0 | 17 | 100.0 | 17 | 100.0 |

*Abbreviations*: *SP* subpial, *SE* subependymal, *WM* white matter, *GM* grey matter

layers, amygdala, hippocampus dentate gyrus, nucleus accumbens bordering the frontobasal WM, or in the inferior olives. This looks like as TSAs creep into the GM from the WM (Additional file 1: Figure S1c and d). Similarly, in PSP (Additional file 1: Figure S1e-g) and CBD (Additional file 1: Figure S1 h-k) cases where neuronal tau pathology is mild or lacking the astrocytic tau pathology predominates in the deeper layers together with tau positive astrocytes in the WM.

The predominant morphology of GM ARTAG is GFA. In cortical areas these are not specifically accumulating in the depth of the sulci. Importantly, in all primary FTLD-tauopathies various astrocytic morphologies can be recognized in the GM close to each other reminiscent of a maturation process. This includes astrocytes with fine granular tau immunoreactivity in astrocytic processes reminiscent of GFAs followed by its more coarser accumulations either in a perinuclear location or remaining in distal segments of the astrocytic arborisation (Fig. 1 and Additional file 1: Figure S2). In CBD cases astrocytic plaques clearly predominate the astroglial tau pathology in the GM. Detection of GFA-like morphology requires meticulous search due to the dense neuronal, thread and astrocytic plaque pathology (Additional file 1: Figure S3). GFA-like morphology is better seen in PSP cases together with tufted astrocytes. In PiD the GM is predominated by ramified astrocytes or by GFA-like, and additional globular-like astroglial tau immunoreacitvities. The latter two morphologies are seen particularly in areas with less or lack of neuronal tau pathology (e.g. in the occipital cortex).

#### Spatial features of subpial ARTAG

First we evaluated the frequency and constellations of subpial ARTAG in three major regions in cases showing subpial ARTAG: basal brain areas (amygdala and basal forebrain together), lobar and brainstem (any location for both) in different case-cohorts. In cases showing subpial ARTAG the highest frequency was observed in basal brain areas except for CBD and PiD (data not shown) where the lobar location was more frequent (Fig. 2a and Additional file 2: Table S1).

In the pooled cohort of non-FTLD-tauopathy cases, basal brain regions frequently showed ARTAG alone followed by combinations either with lobar or brainstem ARTAG or both (Fig. 2a). A few cases only showed either pure lobar or pure brainstem subpial ARTAG. Conditional probability with McNemar's test supported the

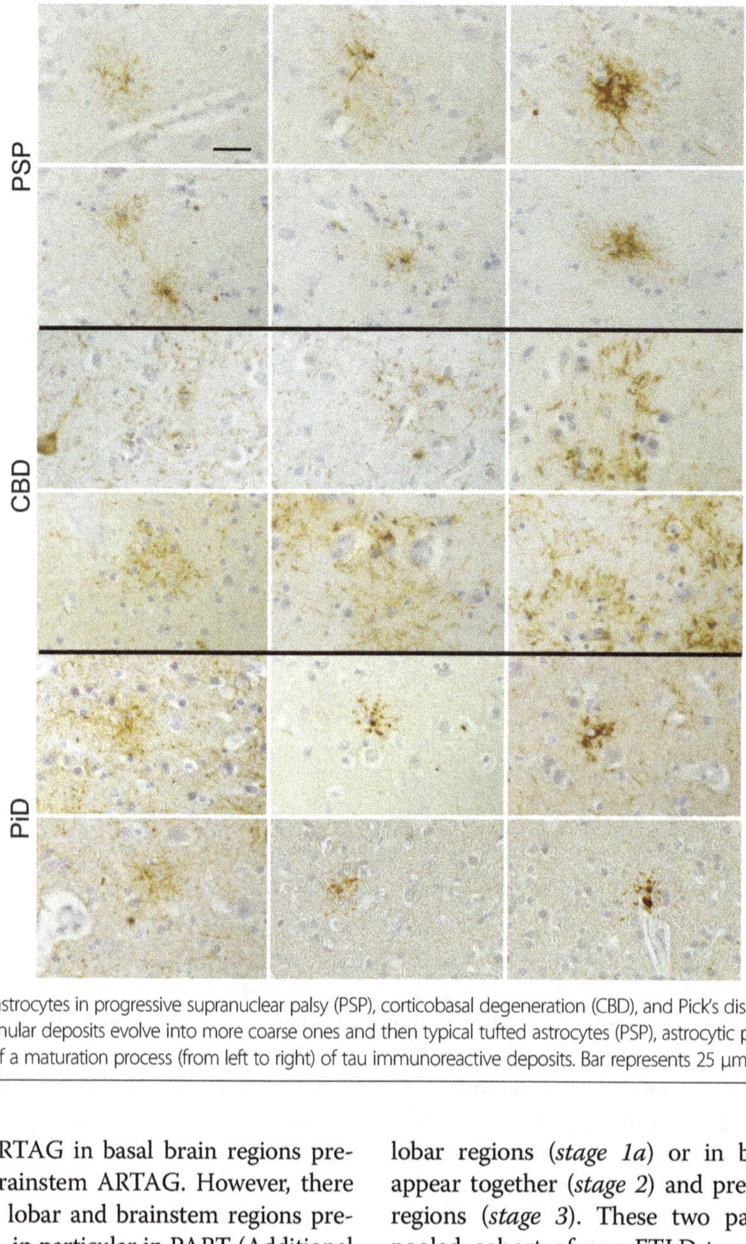


**Fig. 1** Tau immunoreactive astrocytes in progressive supranuclear palsy (PSP), corticobasal degeneration (CBD), and Pick's disease (PiD). Note the variety of morphologies where fine granular deposits evolve into more coarse ones and then typical tufted astrocytes (PSP), astrocytic plaques (CBD), and ramified astrocytes (PiD) reminiscent of a maturation process (from left to right) of tau immunoreactive deposits. Bar represents 25 μm for all images

concept that subpial ARTAG in basal brain regions precedes either lobar or brainstem ARTAG. However, there are several cases where lobar and brainstem regions precede basal brain regions, in particular in PART (Additional file 2: Table S1). Neither lobar or brainstem precedes the other, rather they are present with high likelihood together. Of note, in CBD the involvement of the brainstem always follow the presence of subpial ARTAG in lobar or basal brain regions (Additional file 2: Table S1). The number of cases with subpial ARTAG in the PiD group is too low to draw conclusions.

In summary, for subpial ARTAG, three patterns can be recognized. The first (Fig. 2b) is exemplified by the fact that basal brain regions show subpial ARTAG (*stage 1*). This is followed by a bidirectional sequence rostrally (lobar, *stage 2a*) or caudally (brainstem, *stage 2b*), which two, however, are usually affected together (*stage 3*). A second pattern (Fig. 2c) is when subpial ARTAG is only in lobar regions (*stage 1a*) or in brainstem (*stage 1b*) or appear together (*stage 2*) and precede that in basal brain regions (*stage 3*). These two patterns are seen in the pooled cohort of non-FTLD-tauopathies. The third pattern (Fig. 2d) is exemplified by CBD, where subpial tau immunoreactivity of astrocytic end-feet in lobar areas is the predominant pathology independently of subpial ARTAG in basal brain regions (together representing *stage 1*) and both are followed by the involvement of the brainstem, representing *stage 2*. PSP cases show overlapping features of these patterns. Heatmap of severity scores in the cohort of non-FTLD tauopathies reveals also a MTL to temporal and frontal lobe to parietal to occipital lobe and parallel also to the brainstem (Fig. 3a).

Next we were interested whether lobar subpial ARTAG shows a sequential involvement pattern (Additional file 2: Table S2). In non-FTLD-tauopathy cases there was no difference between frontal, parietal, and temporal lobes

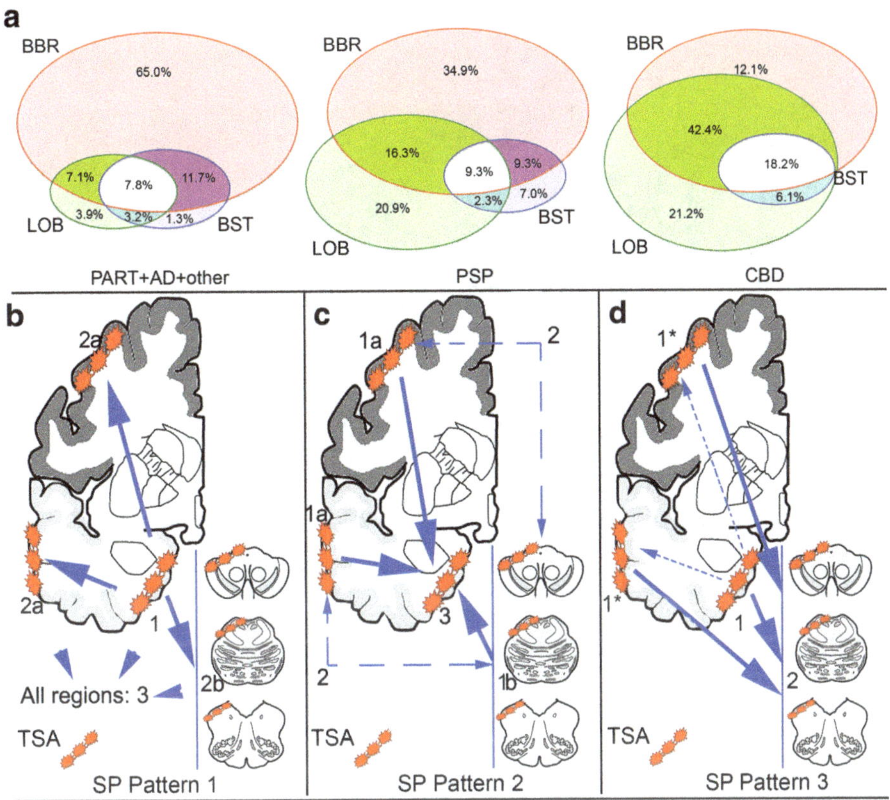


**Fig. 2** Frequencies and distribution patterns of subpial ARTAG. Frequency of subpial ARTAG in different regions (basal brain regions, BBR; lobar regions, LOB; and brainstem regions, BST) in a pooled cohort of non-FTLD-tauopathies (PART+AD+other), PSP, and CBD (**a**). Note the differences in concomitant involvement of regions. The sequential stages of subpial (SP) ARTAG in the pooled cohort of non-FTLD-tauopathies comprise pattern 1 (**b**) when basal brain regions show subpial ARTAG first (*stage 1*) followed by a bidirectional sequence rostrally (lobar) and caudally (brainstem), which two are affected rarely separately (*stages 2a or b*) and more frequently together (*stage 3*); pattern 2 (**c**) when subpial ARTAG in lobar regions or in brainstem appear first (*stage 1a or b*; two-headed dashed arrows indicate that we do not know which precedes the other); when affected together is *stage 2* and finally when additionally basal brain regions are involved is *stage 3*; and pattern 3 (**d**) as exemplified by CBD, where subpial tau immunoreactivity of astrocytic feet is the predominant pathology independently of subpial ARTAG in basal brain regions (together representing *stage 1*) and both are followed by the involvement of the brainstem, representing *stage 2*. The pathogenesis of subpial astrocyte feet tau immunoreactivity in CBD is most likely different from subpial lobar ARTAG (thus indicated with an asterisk), therefore this sequence could be termed as "masked" bidirectional. This means that the typical subpial TSAs in CBD follow the subpial ARTAG in the basal brain regions (indicated by dashed arrows) are masked by the predominant end-feet tau immunoreactivity

regarding which precedes the other, however, they all are affected before the occipital lobe. In CBD it seems that subpial glial end-feet tau immunoreactivity and TSAs is more likely to appear in the parietal and frontal lobes than the temporal and all precede the occipital lobe. In PSP, the frontal lobe shows significantly higher conditional probability values when compared to other lobes.

## Spatial features of subependymal ARTAG

The frequency of subependymal ARTAG was the highest in the MTL followed by subcortical and brainstem regions in all disease groups (Additional file 2: Table S3). Conditional probability analysis revealed significant results in the pooled cohort of non-FTLD-tauopathy cases and in PSP. A higher conditional probability is seen that the MTL is affected alone. Presence of subependymal ARTAG in subcortical regions seems to be independent from the MTL or brainstem. Subependymal ARTAG in the MTL usually precedes the involvement of the brainstem aqueduct. In summary, a clear sequential pattern cannot be defined.

## Spatial features of white matter ARTAG

First we evaluated the frequency and constellations in three major regions in cases showing WM ARTAG. The highest frequency was seen in the MTL (Additional file 2: Table S4). We observe different WM ARTAG patterns for AD, CBD, PART and PSP (Fig. 4a). The pooled cohort of all non-FTLD-tauopathy cases showed combined patterns as seen for AD and PART. Interestingly, in AD cases the presence of lobar WM ARTAG without other regions involved is high (20.8%). In the pooled cohort,

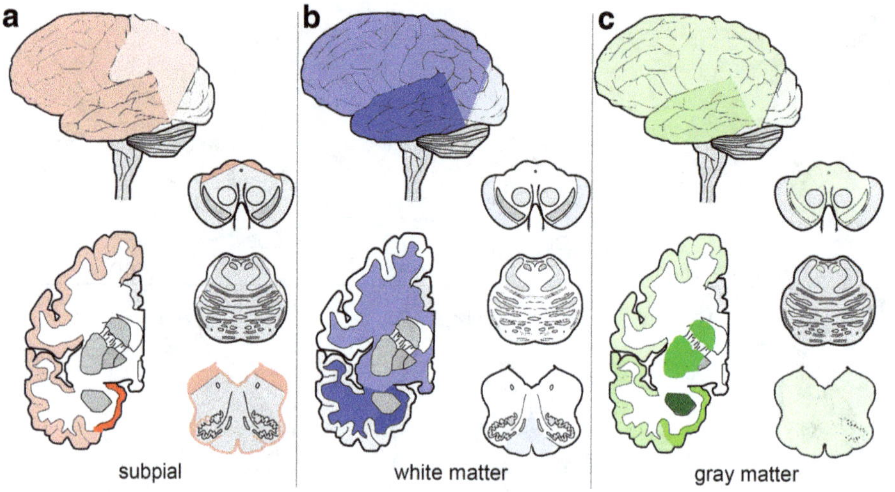


**Fig. 3** Heatmap of severity scores of subpial (**a**), white matter (**b**) and grey matter (**c**) ARTAG in the cohort of non-FTLD tauopathies. The more dark colours reflect higher severity scores

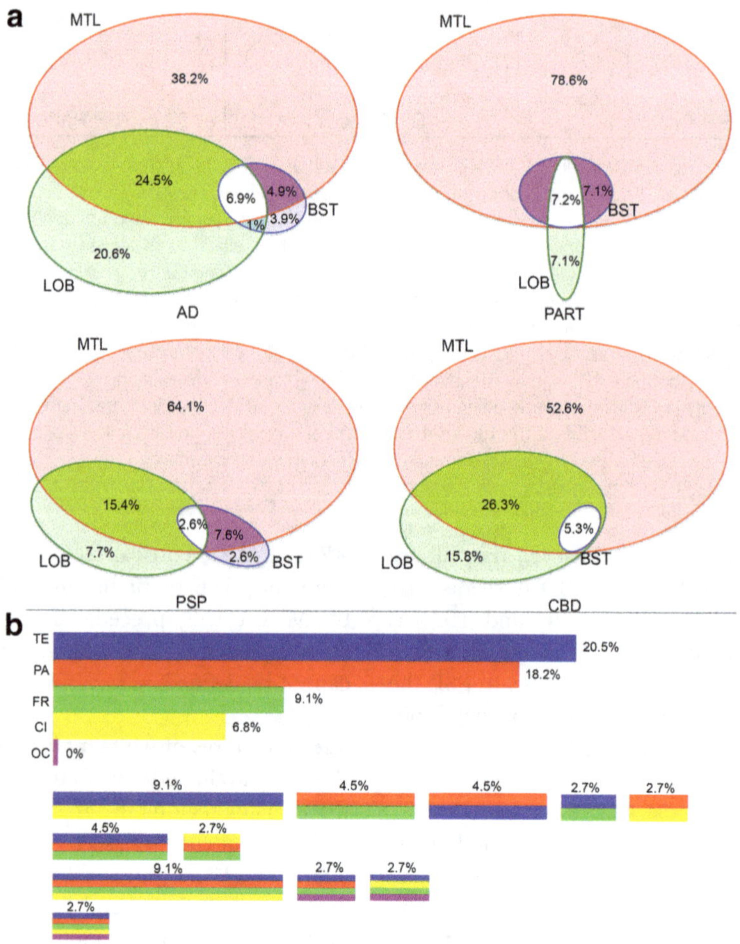


**Fig. 4** Frequency of white matter ARTAG in three major regions (**a**; medial temporal lobe, MTL; lobar regions, LOB; and brainstem regions, BST) in AD, PART, PSP, and CBD and its combinations in five lobar areas (**b**) in AD. Note the differences in concomitant involvement of regions. TE: temporal, PA: parietal, FR: frontal, CI: cingular, OC: occipital

the MTL shows higher conditional probability values when compared to lobar regions and brainstem, and lobar higher as brainstem (fair conditional probability). Logistic regression indicates, however, that WM ARTAG in lobar regions and MTL seems to be independent from each other. This is supported by moderate conditional probability values that lobar involvement precedes the MTL. Accordingly, two patterns of sequential distribution need to be distinguished. In the majority of cases WM ARTAG appears first in basal brain regions (Pattern 1, *stage 1*) followed by lobar regions (Pattern 1, *stage 2a*) or brainstem (Pattern 1, *stage 2b*) and then all regions are involved (*Stage 3*) (Fig. 5a). However, a further pathogenesis is suggested where lobar WM seems to be independent from basal brain region. In this case lobar involvement (Pattern 2, *stage 1*) is followed by the involvement of the basal brain regions (*stage 2a*) or occasionally the brainstem (*stage 2b*) and then all regions are involved (stage 3) (Fig. 5b). Evaluating severity scores and heatmaps reveals a MTL to temporal lobe to frontal-parietal to occipital and parallel to brainstem distribution (Fig. 3b).

Next we were interested in whether lobar WM ARTAG shows a sequential involvement pattern or not. We focused only on AD cases, since these show a high frequency of lobar WM ARTAG thereby rendering this analysis feasible. Briefly, lobar WM ARTAG is usually present in frontal, parietal, or temporal lobe usually in combination of these (Fig. 4b). Thus none of these seem to precede the other, however, in any constellation of frontal/parietal/temporal WM ARTAG this precedes the presence in the occipital lobe (Additional file 2: Table S5).

## Spatial features of grey matter ARTAG

First we evaluated the frequency and constellations of GM ARTAG in four major regions: MTL, lobar (pooled of frontal, parietal, temporal, and occipital lobes), subcortical (basal ganglia) and brainstem (any location) in different case-cohorts. We observed different patterns (Fig. 6 and Additional file 2: Table S6).

Non-FTLD-tauopathy cases are characterized by the predominant involvement of the MTL. A subset of cases shows pure involvement of subcortical areas or combined involvement of regions as seen in primary FTLD-tauopathies (Fig. 6). In comparisons, the MTL shows higher conditional probability then subcortical and brainstem regions then vice versa (Additional file 2: Table S6). The latter two shows fair (lobar) and moderate (brainstem) conditional probability values when compared to the MTL. Logistic regression reveals that these two regions show low ORs when compared to the MTL involvement. This suggests that there are situations when these are not affected together with the MTL. Subcortical seems to precede the involvement of the brainstem but not lobar areas reflected by a fair conditional probabilities. Higher ORs suggest that these regions are usually affected together (Additional file 2: Table S6).

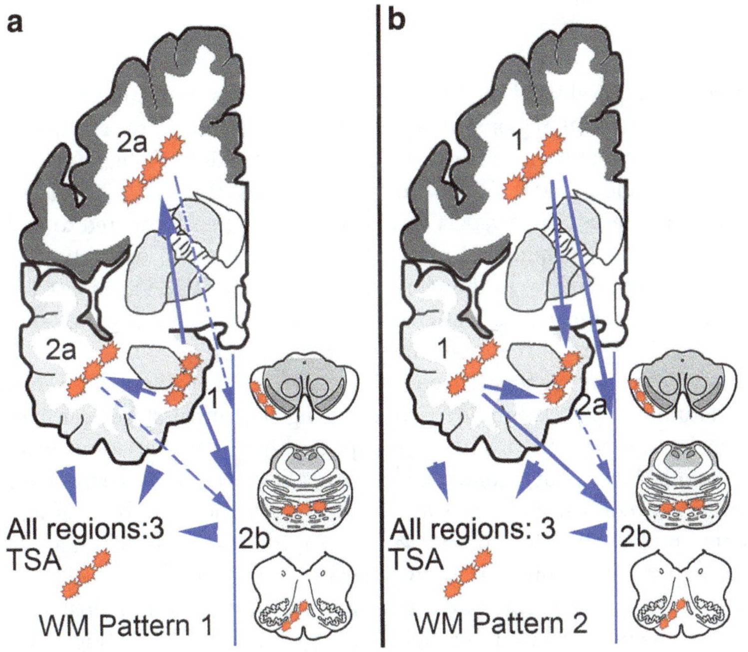


**Fig. 5** Sequential distribution patterns of white matter ARTAG in the pooled cohort of non-FTLD-tauopathies. Pattern 1 (**a**) is characterized by the appearance of white matter ARTAG in basal brain regions (*stage 1*) followed by lobar regions (*stage 2a*) or eventually brainstem (*stage 2b*) before involving all regions (*stage 3*). In Pattern 2 (**b**) lobar involvement (*stage 1*) is followed by the involvement of the basal brain regions or the brainstem (*stages 2 a or b*, respectively), before involving all regions (*stage 3*)

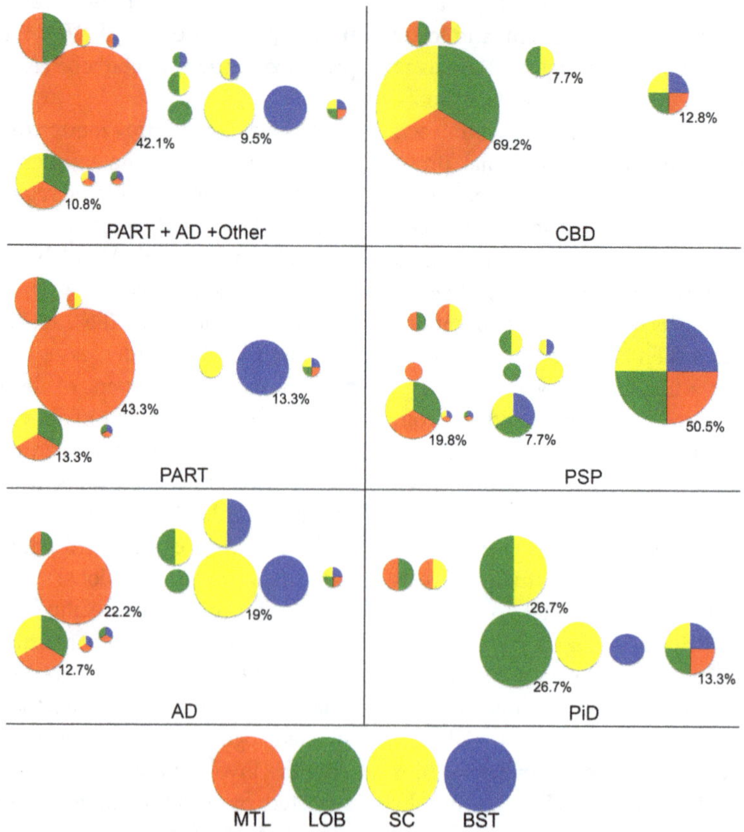


**Fig. 6** Frequency of combinations of grey matter ARTAG in different regions (medial temporal lobe, MTL; lobar regions, LOB; subcortical, SC; and brainstem regions, BST) in the pooled cohort of PART, AD and other non-FTLD tauopathies, AD, PART, PSP, Pick disease, and CBD. Note the differences and overlaps in concomitant involvement of regions. Only the three highest percentage values are shown in lower right corners for better overview. The size of the bubbles represent their frequency

To fine-tune the interpretation we evaluated the frontal, parietal, temporal, and occipital cortical regions, amygdala, striatum, substantia nigra, pons, and medulla oblongata for GM ARTAG (Additional file 3: Table S1). In the cohort of all non-FTLD-tauopathy cases the amygdala and striatum precede with fair (0.21–0.40) conditional probability cortical regions and brainstem regions. In the separated group of AD cases, for the comparisons with the striatum the conditional probabilities are in the moderate range (0.51–0.60). This is supported by higher frequency of involvement of the striatum in AD cases with GM ARTAG. The frontal, parietal and temporal cortical areas precede the occipital but with low (poor) conditional probability value. Comparison of cortical and brainstem regions show low conditional probability values but these are higher for the cortical regions. The amygdala shows fair conditional probability values when compared to brainstem areas. Logistic regression corrected for age, gender and Braak stages of neurofibrillary degenerations for this cohort of non-FTLD-tauopathy cases reveals that cortical areas are affected together with high (> 10) ORs. Importantly, high ORs are seen in the comparison of cortical areas and striatum but not with the amygdala. Brainstem areas are affected when amygdala already shows GM ARTAG (high ORs) and variably when the striatum (ORs: 0.85–1.12) is affected. Brainstem areas show high ORs when compared to each other (Additional file 3: Table S2). Finally, evaluating severity scores and heatmaps reveals a MTL and striatum to temporal lobe to frontal-parietal to occipital and parallel to brainstem distribution (Fig. 3c).

Based on these findings, a dualistic model with the following sequential stages can be proposed: GFAs first appear either in the striatum or in the amygdala (Pattern 1 or 2, Stage 1). The striatal pathway (Pattern 1, *stage 1*) proceeds either towards the amygdala (*stage 2a*), cortex (*stage 2b*), or rarely to brainstem (*stage 2c*) followed by *stage 3a* (striatum + amygdala + cortex) or *stage 3b* (striatum + amygdala + brainstem) and eventually involving all regions (*stage 4*) (Fig. 7a). Note that there is no *stage 3c* since the constellation of striatum+ cortex + brainstem has not been seen in this series (Fig. 6). If we exclude cases where amygdala GM ARTAG is present this sequence patterns remains very clear

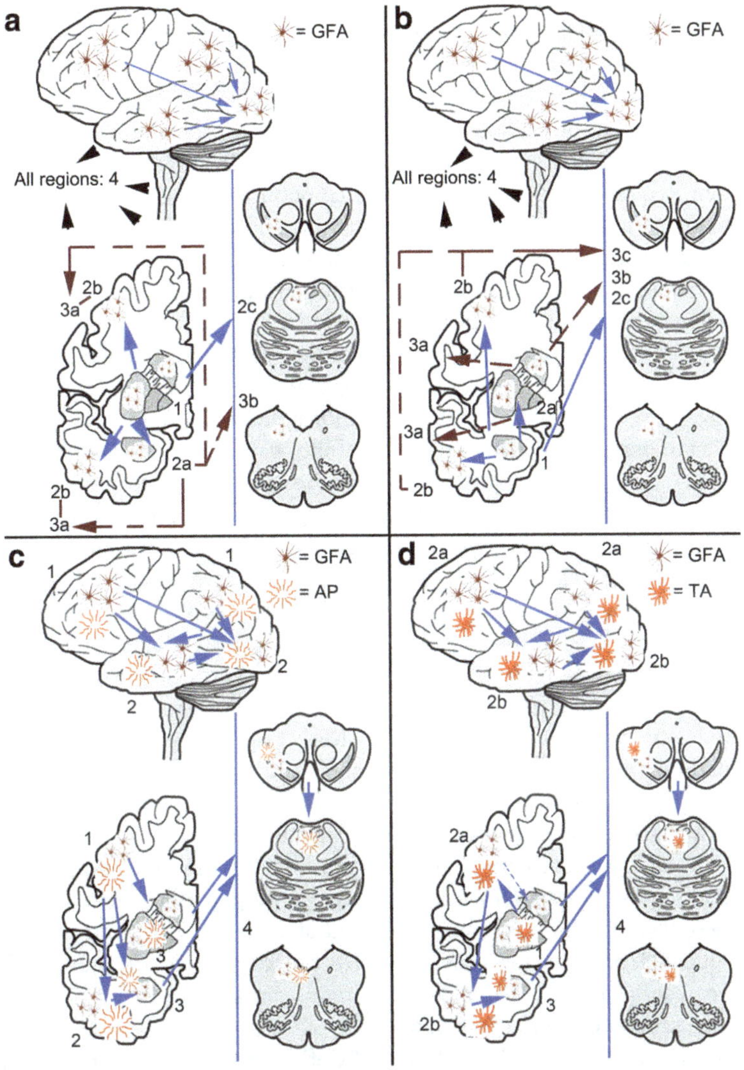


**Fig. 7** Sequential distribution patterns of astroglial tau pathology in the grey matter. In non-FTLD-tauopathies Patterns 1 and 2 are recognized. The distribution of grey matter ARTAG (granular-fuzzy astrocytes, GFA) shows Pattern 1 (**a**) characterized by the early involvement of the striatum (*stage 1*) followed by the amygdala (*stage 2a*), or cortex (here occipital is the latest to be involved) (*stage 2b*), or the brainstem (*stage 2c*); then a further region (striatum + amygdala + cortex, *stage 3a*; or striatum + amygdala + brainstem, *stage 3b*) followed by the involvement of all regions (*stage 4*). In pattern 2 (**b**) the amygdala (*stage 1*) precedes the involvement of the striatum (*stage 2a*) or the cortex (*stage 2b*), or the brainstem (*stage 2c*); then a further region (striatum + amygdala + cortex, *stage 3a*; or striatum + amygdala + brainstem, *stage 3b*; or amygdala + cortex + brainstem, *stage 3c*) followed by the involvement of all regions (*stage 4*). In CBD (**c**) the distribution of astrocytic plaques (AP) and grey matter ARTAG begins in the frontal (including premotor) and parietal cortex (*stage 1*) followed by temporal and occipital cortex (*stage 2*), paralelly moving into subcortical areas including either or both the striatum and the amygdala (*stage 3*) followed by the brainstem (*stage 4*) including the substantia nigra followed by pons and medulla oblongata. Regarding tufted astrocytes (TA) and grey matter ARTAG in PSP (**d**), a striatum (*stage 1*) to cortical (frontal-parietal to temporal to occipital) areas (*stage 2 and b, respectively*) to amygdala (*stage 3*) and to brainstem (*stage 4*), including the substantia nigra followed by pons and medulla oblongata, sequence can be recognized

(Additional file 3: Table S3), however, cortical regions show significantly higher, albeit poor conditional probability values when compared to brainstem regions. In pattern 2 the amygdala (*stage 1*) precedes the involvement of the striatum (*stage 2a*), the cortex (*stage 2b*) or very rarely the brainstem (*stage 2c*). This is followed by three combinations of *stage 3* (*a*: amygdala + striatum + cortex; *b*: amygdala + striatum + brainstem; *c*: amygdala +cortex + brainstem), and eventually followed by the involvement of all regions (*stage 4*) (Fig. 7b). This pattern is seen in cases where the striatum is not involved (Additional file 3: Table S4); here the conditional probability values are not significantly higher in cortical regions when compared to brainstem regions. There are only a few cases where a few GFAs can be noted alone in the brainstem or in the cortex.

Presence of GFA-like morphologies reveals different sequences in primary tauopathies. CBD is characterized by a fronto-parietal to temporal to occipital and to amygdala and to brainstem sequence represented by substantial to high (almost perfect) conditional probability values (Additional file 3: Table S1). However, there is a striatum to amygdala and brainstem sequence, which precedes cortical areas. PSP shows similar trends but the parietal cortex is less frequently an early affected cortical area and striatum is affected mostly before cortex. In contrast, in PiD GFA-like morphology is less frequent and therefore these sequential patterns cannot be recognized so markedly.

#### Spatial features of astrocytic tau immunoreactivity in primary FTLD-tauopathies

We also evaluated classical astrocytic plaques in CBD, tufted astrocytes in PSP, and ramified astrocytes in PiD, which presented overlapping patterns with GM ARTAG in the same cohorts (Additional file 3: Tables S1 and S5).

Astrocytic plaques in CBD in the frontal, parietal and temporal regions show high conditional probabilities in comparisons with other, subcortical and brainstem, regions. Occipital shows moderate conditional probability values except for the comparison with the striatum where this is zero and the striatum shows a high value (0.95). The amygdala and striatum clearly precedes brainstem regions. Comparison of the striatum and amygdala show high values for both indicating that sequential involvement cannot be clearly defined for these two regions. It is important to recognize combined sequential patterns for GFA-like morphologies and mature astroglial tau pathologies. A four-staged sequence can be proposed: frontal (including premotor) and parietal cortex (*stage 1*) is followed by temporal and occipital cortex (*stage 2*) parallel moving into subcortical areas including either or both the striatum and the amygdala (*stage 3*) followed by the brainstem (*stage 4*) including the substantia nigra followed by pons and medulla oblongata (Fig. 7c). It cannot be defined whether the striatum or the amygdala is the first to be affected by ARTAG after the cortex, although GFAs seem to be earlier in the striatum then the amygdala (conditional probability 0.96 versus 0.50) (Additional file 3: Table S1). This is supported by heatmap evaluation as reported in our recent study [35]. In summary, the astroglial tau pathology in CBD follows a cortical (frontal-parietal- to temporal-occipital) to subcortical, and to brainstem pathway.

Regarding tufted astrocytes and GM ARTAG in PSP, the striatum shows high conditional probabilities in comparisons with other regions including the amygdala. Cortical regions and amygdala shows moderate to high values in comparison with brainstem regions. Frontal and parietal shows significantly higher conditional probabilities when compared to temporal, occipital and amygdala. Between the latter three we do find significant differences for tufted astrocytes but for GFA-type morphologies cortical regions show significantly higher conditional probability values than the amygdala. Therefore, a striatum (*stage 1*) to cortical (frontal-parietal to temporal to occipital) areas (*stage 2 a and b, respectively*) to amygdala (*stage 3*) and to brainstem (*stage 4*), including the substantia nigra followed by pons and medulla oblongata, sequence can be recognized (Fig. 7d). This is supported by heatmap-analysis as reported in our recent study [35]. Of note, however, GFA-like morphologies may appear in some cases in cortical areas before the striatum indicated by moderate to substantial conditional probability values (Additional file 3: Table S1). In summary, PSP can be described predominantly as a subcortical-cortical pattern, however, an alternative pattern is to be considered, when the involvement of the cortex parallels, or eventually precedes, the striatum.

Finally, in contrast to the lack of sequential patterns for GFA-like morphologies, ramified astrocytes in PiD appear in frontal cortex before other lobar regions and the amygdala. However, the involvement of the striatum does not clearly sequentially follow the lobar regions and may be an initiating site for astroglial tau pathologies as well since it shows fair to moderate conditional probabilities in comparisons with other regions. GM ARTAG shows similar patterns but non-significant $p$ values. In summary, an overlapping pattern with PSP can be suspected either initiated in the cortex or in the striatum followed then by the other one of these and by the amygdala and brainstem areas.

#### Relation of tau pathological variables in different anatomical regions

To be able to interpret the spatial features in the whole brain we need to understand whether the presence of one type of ARTAG has any effect on the appearance of a further type of ARTAG. In other words we aimed to evaluate whether one type of ARTAG precedes any other type of ARTAG in the same anatomical region. We evaluated three representative anatomical regions: amygdala as a hotspot for all ARTAG types [35], frontal cortex, and mesencephalon with substantia nigra. The frequencies of ARTAG types showed different patterns in these regions (Fig. 8a and Additional file 3: Table S6).

Briefly, in the amygdala, subpial, WM, and perivascular appear together and precede the presence of subependymal ARTAG. GM ARTAG is independent from these and shows moderate conditional probability (0.59) when compared to the presence of grains as vice versa (0.009) (Fig. 8b). This phenomenon is not seen for further comparisons of ARTAG types with the presence of grains. In the frontal area conditional probability is significant only for the

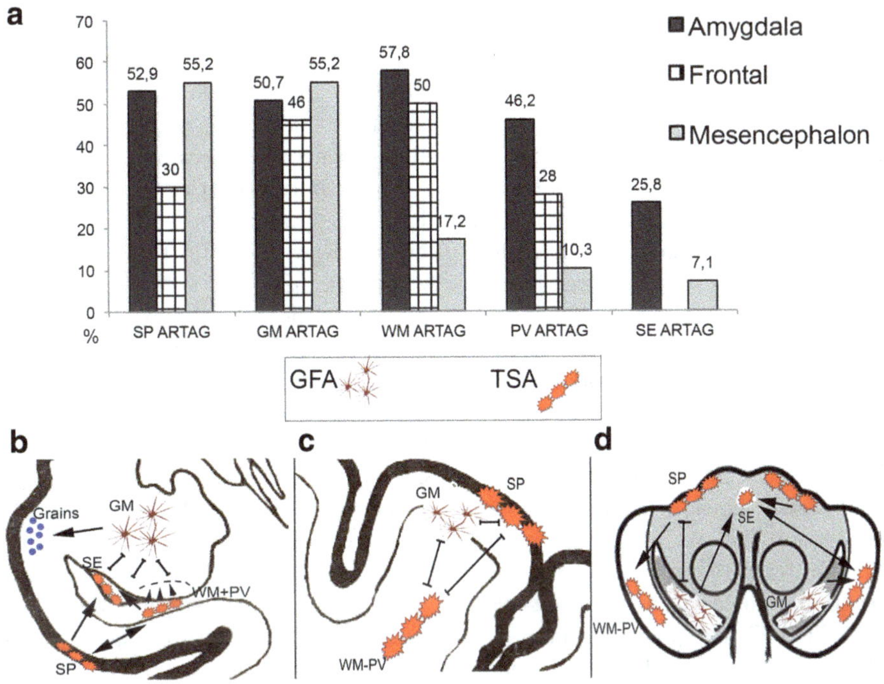


**Fig. 8** Frequency (**a**) and sequential distribution patterns of different ARTAG types in the amygdala region (**b**), frontal cortex (**c**) and mesencephalon (**d**) in pooled cases where any ARTAG type was seen. Arrows and small arrowheads indicate the proposed direction of the sequential distribution, two-headed arrows indicate concomitant, and lines the independent presence of different ARTAG types (SP: subpial, GM: grey matter, WM: white matter, PV: perivascular, SE: subependymal)

comparison of WM and perivascular ARTAG (0.36 versus 0.08). Logistic regression test reveals that the presence of WM ARTAG showed significant OR with perivascular ARTAG (6.08), indicating that they are strongly associated. The OR values are significant, but lower than 1, when compared to GM (OR: 0.06), subpial (OR: 0.16) ARTAG, indicating that they are most likely independent from WM ARTAG. Subpial and GM ARTAG show fair to moderate conditional probability values when compared (Fig. 8c) and non-significant OR value (< 1). In the mesencephalon, due to the low case numbers with ARTAG the multiple regression models did not reveal significant effects; however, in univariate regression model perivascular and WM ARTAG shows significant OR (15.3) OR values. Conditional probability analysis reveals moderate to substantial conditional probability values for GM ARTAG in the substantia nigra and subpial ARTAG when compared to subependymal, WM and perivascular ARTAG. Subpial ARTAG and GM ARTAG both show high conditional probability values (0.92) in their comparison in harmony with the very low OR in logistic regression test (Fig. 8d). WM and perivascular ARTAG shows significantly high OR value.

Finally, we were interested how many cases show primary-FTLD-tauopathy related astroglial tau pathology or GFAs without any neuronal tau pathology in the same region. Interestingly, cortical areas in primary FTLD-tauopathy cases not infrequently show astroglial tau depositions (Table 3). In the pooled cohort of other disease 0.2–1.5% of all examined cases show GFAs in any region without neuronal tau pathology (Table 3).

### Hierarchical cluster analysis

First we evaluated clustering of cases based on the presence of primary FTLD-tauopathy-related astroglial tau pathologies (i.e., tufted astrocytes, ramified astrocytes and astrocytic plaques) in three major anatomical regions

**Table 3** Percent of cases in different disease groups where astroglial tau pathology was seen without neuronal tau pathology

| | PSP | | CBD | | PiD | | All other | |
|---|---|---|---|---|---|---|---|---|
| | TA | GFA | AP | GFA | RA | GFA | TA | GFA |
| Frontal | 1.1 | 5.2 | 2.6 | 2.5 | 0 | 0 | 0.2 | 1 |
| Parietal | 7.7 | 11 | 0 | 0 | 0 | 5 | 0 | 1.4 |
| Temporal | 4.3 | 3.1 | 2.5 | 2.4 | 0 | 0 | 0 | 0.6 |
| Occipital | 26.2 | 32.9 | 2.6 | 7.3 | 5.3 | 26.3 | 0 | 0.3 |
| Amygdala | 0 | 0 | 0 | 0 | 0 | 0 | 0 | 0.2 |
| Dentate gyrus[a] | 0 | 2.2 | 0 | 0 | 0 | 0 | 0 | 1.4 |
| Striatum | 0 | 0 | 0 | 0 | 0 | 0 | 0.4 | 1.5 |
| Substantia nigra | 0 | 0 | 0 | 0 | 0 | 4.8 | 0 | 0.6 |

*TA* tufted astrocyte, *AP* astrocytic plaque, *RA* ramified astrocyte, *GFA* granular/fuzzy astrocyte
[a]Note that in the dentate gyrus the morphology resembles thorn-shaped astrocytes

(pooled lobar, subcortical and brainstem areas). Two major clusters are seen in primary tauopathies (Additional file 4: Figure S1); when all three regions or less show astrocytic tau pathology. In contrast to CBD, in PSP and PiD two further clusters are seen based on the presence of astrocytic tau pathology in two major regions (lobar and subcortical) or only in one these. In the pooled cohort on non-FTLD-tauopathies these types of astroglial tau pathologies are seen very rarely: cluster and pattern analysis and the morphology (i.e. tufted astrocytes) is reminiscent of PSP cases.

Next we added the presence of GM ARTAG in these three major anatomical regions to the cluster analysis (Additional file 4: Figure S2). In CBD and PiD this approach did not present more major clusters but more sub-clusters. In PSP GM ARTAG was usually present together with tufted astrocytes, however, there are several cases with individual constellations leading to several smaller groups. Importantly, there are PSP and PiD cases where the characteristic neuronal tau pathology is associated only with GM ARTAG (i.e., preceding immature form of astroglial tau pathologies). In the pooled cohort of non-primary FTLD-tauopathies, two major clusters are seen (presence or lack of tufted astrocytes). The majority of cases lack these astroglial tau pathologies and present small groups of cases with different constellations of GM ARTAG (see above).

Finally, we analysed cases with any type of ARTAG. Cases with GM ARTAG present a major cluster, which can be separated from those with additional WM and/or subpial ARTAG in various anatomical constellations leading to several smaller clusters consisting of a few cases (Additional file 4: Figure S3).

## Discussion

### General conceptual considerations

There are three fundamental aspects of neuropathological evaluation of neurodegenerative conditions [29]. First, clinical symptoms are thought to be associated with neuronal dysfunction and deposition of pathologically altered proteins in compartments of neurons. Second, these neurodegeneration-related proteins follow a hierarchical involvement of brain regions, which includes the likely cell-to-cell spreading of these proteins. Third, neuropathological examination of the human brain reveals changes in pathology distribution at different times in the course of a neurodegenerative disease. Together these concepts led to the development of staging strategies to describe the sequential involvement of brain regions with the aim of understanding the clinical progression [5, 7, 8, 10, 11, 21, 27, 47, 54] and defining the pre-clinical stage of diseases, which can be translated for clinical practice as in vivo biomarkers become available [14]. On the neuropathological level this means that even a few neurons showing immunoreactivity for a certain neurodegeneration-protein can be interpreted as an earliest stage of disease and not disregarded as a non-specific finding. These concepts, however, are based on a neuron-centric view of neurodegenerative diseases, in particular that stages are considered to follow neuronal networks.

The importance of astrocytes in neurodegeneration is increasingly recognized [15, 33, 57]. To evaluate astrocytes, however, a distinct conceptual approach is needed. Astrocytic networks are being recognized; furthermore, astrocytes show a complex spectrum of functions, which are associated with neurons as well as brain barriers [15, 33, 57]. The concept of protein astrogliopathies is mostly implemented for the diagnostic classification of tauopathies [33]. Astrocytic morphologies such as astrocytic plaques and tufted astrocytes should be considered as a dynamic process. Accordingly, PSP, CBD, and PiD are characterized by well-defined morphologies; however, these are the end stage of cytopathological maturation when protein pre-aggregates ripe into larger aggregates and finally form dense protein accumulations in certain segments of the astrocytes (Fig. 1). The first step of fine granular accumulation in astrocytic processes is followed by the transportation to distal or proximal segments of the astrocytic cytoskeleton and then by formation of aggregates that become argyrophilic and/or ubiquitinated [20, 33, 35, 48]. This interpretation provides a conceptual link between GFAs of ARTAG and primary FTLD-tauopathy-related astrocytic morphologies [33, 35].

Here we attempted to evaluate the patterns of ARTAG types. As expected the relative purity of neuron-based staging systems cannot be reproduced. As a limitation of our study we did not evaluate whole hemispheric sections and some of ARTAG types might have been missed in certain anatomical regions. However, analysis of patterns allows us to identify principles to appreciate better the heterogeneity of ARTAG in diverse NDD and pave the way to improved understanding of pathogenesis. First of all, our study supports the notion that the pathogenesis of GFA in the GM must be distinguished from TSAs in the subpial, subependymal, WM and perivascular locations [35]. Second, we show here that there is a regional difference in the interplay between ARTAG types represented by TSAs, e.g. subpial, WM and subependymal. This is exemplified by the observation that WM ARTAG is independent from the development of subpial ARTAG in lobar regions whereas strongly associates with that in basal brain areas and brainstem (see Fig. 8). Therefore, the interpretation of the sequential distribution of ARTAG types needs to consider further and local pathological variables. We applied several levels of evaluation to propose sequential patterns; our observations argue against an exclusive path for hierarchical involvement for any ARTAG type. This suggests distinct pathogenic events initiating ARTAG at specific locations, which then show sequential involvement of further anatomical areas.

### Sequential patterns of subpial, subependymal and white matter ARTAG

The distribution patterns of these three ARTAG types show considerable overlap. In addition, perivascular ARTAG is prominently associated with WM ARTAG and therefore not evaluated separately. Based on our observations, stages cannot be defined for subependymal ARTAG. It seems that in most cases subependymal ARTAG follows the development of subpial ARTAG suggesting that the pathogenic event, inducing subependymal ARTAG, needs to be more prominent or requires longer duration than in the situation when only subpial ARTAG develops. As discussed already, the aetiology of subpial ARTAG might be associated with dysfunction of the brain barriers [35, 41]. This is strongly supported by the prominent astroglial expression of connexin-43 and aquaporin-4 correlating with ARTAG [37]. Importantly, acute perivascular cellular uptake of blood-borne proteins is prominent in astrocytes and neurons, but not microglia in experimental concussion suggesting brain barrier disruption as a feature of concussion [25].

One pattern of subpial ARTAG seems to be initiated in basal regions proceeding towards the convexity of the brain (lobar areas) or dorsolateral parts of the brainstem. A second pattern, however, most likely begins in the convexity of the brain paralleled by the brainstem involvement but preceding the basal brain regions. Two aspects need to be considered for the interpretation: a pathogenesis related to the circulation of the CSF or local mechanical factors. During the circulation of the CSF from the lateral ventricles it enters the aqueduct and then the cerebellomedullary cistern at the brainstem level (i.e. via the foramen of Magendie and foramina of Luschka). The fluid then circulates in the subarachnoid space and reaches the basal areas before proceeding to the convexity. During the pulsatile flow of the CSF, the vascular expansion following cardiac systole occurs first at the base of the brain reversing then the flow of cisternal CSF superimposed by a circadian or diurnal rhythm [1]. Thus, subpial ARTAG might reflect the consequences of a "traffic jam" of CSF-flow at basal brain regions associated with the disturbance of CSF-brain barriers and with or without qualitative changes in the CSF. In this model the brainstem and the convexity develops ARTAG only later since the flow of the CSF may be less disrupted in these locations. A similar pattern of WM ARTAG mirrors this, in particular that in the initiating site of the amygdala, subpial and WM ARTAG strongly associates with each other. Interestingly WM tracts are important for oedema fluid movement and clearance [1]. Of particular note is the progression of WM ARTAG towards the occipital lobe from other lobar areas, which is reminiscent of the progression of NFT pathology in AD as suggested by the Braak stages [5]. Indeed, lobar WM ARTAG is frequent in AD [35], moreover, the possible role of cerebral arteries and the pulsatile CSF flow in the spreading of NFT degeneration has been also proposed based on other meticulous observations [45].

The existence of a second pattern of subpial and WM ARTAG raises the possibility of further pathogenic events such as a history of repeated mild traumatic brain injury (TBI) or a single severe TBI, where diffuse axonal injury across the WM is thought to be an important pathological feature [24]. Regarding subpial ARTAG, the early appearance of TSAs in the convexity of the brain and lateral parts of the brainstem raises the possibility of local mechanical compression. This would be analogous to the development of TSAs in the spinal cord in cervical spondylosis [50]. Subpial TSAs are frequent in CTE [44]. Blast injury has been also reported to be associated with tau positive astrocytes mainly in the frontal and parietal cortices [51]. It must be noted that in our series ARTAG was frequently not associated with the characteristic constellation of concomitant NFT pathology and ARTAG in the depth of the sulci as suggested for CTE [43]. However, our observations on two major patterns of subpial and WM ARTAG support the notion that the development of ARTAG and CTE type pathology shares common pathogenesis. In summary, it could be theorised that the basal region-to-convexity pattern is initiated by a disturbance in CSF circulation, while the convexity-to-basal brain region pattern might be initiated by, or associated with, mechanical perturbations of the brain such as occurs with mild TBI. The proposed spreading sequence of subpial and WM ARTAG could then most likely be linked to mild TBI and to alterations of the pulsatile flow of the CSF and interstitial fluid over the lifespan. As for TBI and CTE, the relative "dose", such as the frequency and severity of injury [23], associated with these pathologies is yet unknown.

Importantly, subpial astroglial tau pathology is different in CBD, in particular in lobar areas, i.e., the convexity of the brain, where the morphology of subpial TSAs is different in CBD. These are mostly the astrocytic feet immunostained and less the cell body as in typical TSAs, although a few TSAs can be recognized as well. Lobar subpial TSA always associates with tau pathology in the GM and WM contrasting non-FTLD tauopathies where lobar subpial ARTAG can be present alone. The pathogenesis of subpial astrocyte feet tau immunoreactivity in CBD is most likely different from subpial lobar ARTAG. Therefore the sequence (i.e., involvement of the convexity and basal brain region in *stage 1*) identified in CBD could be termed as "masked" bidirectional. This means that the basal brain regions-to-convexity and bidirectional to brainstem sequence seen in non-FTLD-tauopathies with the typical subpial TSA morphologies representing typical subpial ARTAG are masked by the predominant end-feet tau immunoreactivity.

**Sequential patterns of grey matter ARTAG**

Interpretation of the observations on astrocytic tau pathology requires an approach on two conceptual levels. First, at a cellular level the recognition of maturation phases of tau accumulation is important. Second, on the anatomical level, the relationship of astrocytic tau pathology to neuronal tau pathologies varies between anatomical regions. The most important finding of our study is that for GFAs in non-FTLD-tauopathies we can recognize a striatal and amygdala pathway each proceeding to cortical areas and brainstem. The striatal pattern is clearly reminiscent of the combined pattern of tufted astrocytes and GFAs seen in PSP. We are aware of the description of so called equivocal tufted astrocytes in pallido-nigro-luysian-atrophy showing different morphology and distribution [59], however, in our study we evaluated PSP cases with unequivocal tufted astrocytes. In our cohort the non-FTLD-tauopathy group included a wide range of neurodegenerative conditions, including PART cases. In PSP, as well as CBD and PiD, we have found a dissociation of the density of neuronal and astroglial tau pathologies [35]. There are also reports on the appearance of astroglial tau pathology in areas lacking neuronal tau pathology [21, 40]. Ling et al. [40] and Josephs et al. [26], by examining CBD and PSP cases, respectively, speculated that neuronal pathology is abundant in end-stage disease and therefore gradually overtake astroglial tau pathology. All together these support the notion that cases with concomitant early features of primary FTLD-tauopathies might be more frequent than previously assumed [35]. Even more, some of the cases with prominent GM ARTAG without prominent features of other disorders can be associated with clinical symptoms [34].

An interesting observation of our study is the high conditional probability that GFAs precede grains in the amygdala. Indeed GFAs are consistent finding in AGD [4, 16, 56]. We propose that cases with GFAs in the amygdala and without characteristic grains could be interpreted as pre-AGD pathologies. Interestingly, we observed this phenomenon in psychiatric conditions [35] and on the other hand psychiatric symptoms are not unusual in AGD [28]. In CBD tau pathology in the amygdala is probably mild in very early disease stages in the absence of secondary pathology [40], and eventually develops more when grain pathology, either as feature of CBD [53], or as additional AGD, is also present.

Importantly, we observed cases, which showed astroglial tau deposits with the lack of neuronal tau pathology in the same region. The question is whether astroglial tau pathology might precede neuronal tau pathology? We hypothesize that astroglia either phagocytizes pathological tau derived from the endings of projecting neurons or we observe local astroglial upregulation of tau as a response to a yet unidentified event. Alternatively, a reservoir of phosphorylated tau might be continuously released upon lysis of the axons as seen for example in TBI, where axons continue to degenerate for years after injury, a process that includes accumulations of phospho-Tau [24]. In some areas this might be again linked to CSF-brain barrier dysfunction, reflected by increased connexin-43 and aquaporin-4 expression in GM ARTAG-bearing astrocytes [37], supported also by observations that tufted astrocytes as well as astrocytic plaques tend to be positioned in close proximity to blood vessels [49]. Astrocytes do have phagocytic receptors and have been show to internalize or engulf pathological alpha-synuclein and most likely play a role in clearance and their degradation [12, 30, 39, 42, 46]. However, for tau this is not yet clearly defined. Experimental studies in tau transgenic mouse model of astrocytic tau pathologies suggest that this contributes to glial degeneration [19], and as a consequence of astrocytic tau pathology neuronal degeneration can be detected in the absence of neuronal tau inclusions [17]. Pattern analysis

| Subpial ARTAG | | | |
|---|---|---|---|
| **Pattern 1** | | | |
| BBR | Lobar | Brainstem | **Stage** |
| + | - | - | 1 |
| + | + | - | 2a |
| + | - | + | 2b |
| + | + | + | 3 |
| **Pattern 2** | | | |
| BBR | Lobar | Brainstem | **Stage** |
| - | + | - | 1a |
| - | - | + | 1b |
| - | + | + | 2 |
| + | + | + | 3 |
| **White matter ARTAG** | | | |
| **Pattern 1** | | | |
| BBR | Lobar | Brainstem | **Stage** |
| + | - | - | 1 |
| + | + | - | 2a |
| + | - | + | 2b |
| + | + | + | 3 |
| **Pattern 2** | | | |
| BBR | Lobar | Brainstem | **Stage** |
| - | + | - | 1 |
| + | + | - | 2a |
| - | + | + | 2b |
| + | + | + | 3 |

**Fig. 9** Staging scheme for subpial and white matter ARTAG

[35] indicates that neuronal tau is usually present locally where astroglial is seen or in projection areas. Some studies suggest dysfunction of pathological tau-harbouring protoplasmic astrocytes associated with neuronal dysfunction [48, 52]. This could help to better understand the relevance of astroglial tau pathology e.g. in the amygdala even without prominent tau pathology.

#### Implications for staging astroglial tau pathologies

Clear staging systems for PSP, CBD and PiD, such as for NFT pathology in AD [5] or Lewy bodies in Parkinson disease [6], are lacking. However, there are several studies indicating sequential distribution of pathologies [21, 58]. The wide spectrum of clinical presentations and pathological heterogeneity [22, 28] associated with these disorders hamper the development of uniform staging protocols. What lessons can be learned from our study? First, that the striatum, amygdala and cortex (mostly frontal-parietal) can be an initiating site to develop astroglial tau pathology. This can be a pure finding indicating a pathogenic event in these locations or combined (i.e. secondary) to the presence of neuronal tau pathology (i.e. in the form of pretangles) in the same region or in areas projecting to these regions (i.e., substantia nigra projecting to striatum or subcortical projecting to cortex). In later stages of the disease neuronal tau pathology increases in these locations. As a further aspect some types of tauopathies characterized by different tau strains may differ in the predominance of neuronal tau pathology, exemplified by PSP cases with prominent brainstem neuronal tau pathology with relative lower density of astroglial tau in other regions or the predominance of astroglial tau pathology in unusual locations such as the hippocampus [32]. Most likely strain specific staging systems should be considered and not unifying for all CBD or PSP cases. In this respect it is extremely important to recognize cases with low amount of GM ARTAG in certain areas theoretically representing pre-stages of one of the strains of primary FTLD-tauopathies.

For the practising neuropathologists an approach to the staging is summarized in Figs. 9 and 10. For subpial, WM, and GM ARTAG the final stages of different patterns are similar, thus the initiating pattern cannot be defined (i.e. only the stage number). Similarly, for GM

**Grey matter ARTAG**

**Pattern 1**

| Striatum | Amygdala | Cortex | Brainstem | **Stage** |
|---|---|---|---|---|
| + | - | - | - | 1 |
| + | + | - | - | 2a |
| + | - | + | - | 2b |
| + | - | - | + | 2c |
| + | + | + | - | 3a |
| + | + | - | + | 3b |
| + | + | + | + | 4 |

**Pattern 2**

| Striatum | Amygdala | Cortex | Brainstem | **Stage** |
|---|---|---|---|---|
| - | + | - | - | 1 |
| + | + | - | - | 2a |
| - | + | + | - | 2b |
| - | + | - | + | 2c |
| + | + | + | - | 3a |
| + | + | - | + | 3b |
| - | + | + | + | 3c |
| + | + | + | + | 4 |

**Grey matter ARTAG + other astroglial tau pathology**

**CBD**

| FR-PA Cortex | TE-OC Cortex | Striatum | Amygdala | Brainstem | **Stage** |
|---|---|---|---|---|---|
| + | - | - | - | - | 1 |
| + | + | - | - | - | 2 |
| + | + | + | + | - | 3 |
| + | + | + | + | + | 4 |

**PSP**

| FR-PA Cortex | TE-OC Cortex | Striatum | Amygdala | Brainstem | **Stage** |
|---|---|---|---|---|---|
| - | - | + | - | - | 1 |
| + | - | + | - | - | 2a |
| + | + | + | - | - | 2b |
| + | + | + | + | - | 3 |
| + | + | + | + | + | 4 |

**Fig. 10** Staging scheme for grey matter ARTAG and for all astroglial tau pathologies in corticobasal degeneration (CBD) and progressive supranuclear palsy (PSP). FR: frontal, PA: parietal, TE: temporal, OC: occipital cortex

ARTAG the initiating site cannot be defined when *stages 3a* or *3b* or 4 are seen. For primary FTLD-tauopathy related tau-astrogliopathies (combination of GFAs, tufted astrocytes or astrocytic plaques) the sequential stages can be better recognized (Fig. 10).

## Conclusions

Do the observations on subpial, subependymal and WM ARTAG have urgent therapeutic consequences? This remains to be seen since ARTAG was only defined clearly very recently and there is a need for more clinicopathological studies of ARTAG. This notwithstanding, the observations reported here reflect the various impacts the human brain undergoes during life, which may have effects on the physiological functioning of brain barriers. Developing in vivo markers for these ARTAG types or dysfunction of the CSF-brain barrier will help to understand their role in the pathogenesis of neurodegenerative conditions and eventually lead to better stratification of patients for therapies. For example therapies that require effective functioning of these barriers might be less advantageous for those individuals with prominent ARTAG. For GM ARTAG we show different patterns suggestive of complex relationships with other pathological alterations and eventually spreading mechanisms of astroglial tau pathologies. It will also be important to determine if there is glial cell-to-cell spread of ARTAG or spread of tau pathology between neurons and glia. The overlap of distribution patterns of GM ARTAG in diverse disorders and astroglial tau pathologies of primary-FTLD tauopathies supports the concept of common initiating events and pathogenesis.

## Additional files

**Additional file 1:** Summary of the statistical method and morphology of astroglial tau pathologies. (PDF 2229 kb)

**Additional file 2:** Pairwise conditional probability matrix and odds ratios of different ARTAG types. (PDF 876 kb)

**Additional file 3:** Pairwise conditional probability matrix and odds ratios of grey matter ARTAG and primary FTLD-tauopathy associated astroglial tau immunoreactivities. (PDF 437 kb)

**Additional file 4:** Hierarchical cluster analysis of astroglial tau pathologies in different disorders. (PDF 1463 kb)

**Acknowledgements**

The authors would like to thank the many patients who made this research possible.

**Funding**

Funding from the National Institutes of Health (AG10124, AG17586, R01NS094003, and R01NS038104) supported this study.

**Authors' contributions**

GGK designed the study, performed experiments, analyzed the data, and drafted the manuscript. JLR, EBL, DHS, TS contributed to the design of the study and the preparation of the histological slides. EBL, and JQT performed neuropathology workup. SXX and GGK conceptualized and performed the statistical analysis. VL and JQT participated in the study's design, data interpretation, and manuscript preparation. All were involved in critical review of the manuscript. All authors read and approved the final manuscript.

**Competing interests**

The authors declare that they have no competing interests.

**Author details**

[1]Institute of Neurology, Medical University of Vienna, AKH 4J, Währinger Gürtel 18-20, 1097 Vienna, Austria. [2]Center for Neurodegenerative Disease Research (CNDR), Institute on Aging and Department of Pathology & Laboratory Medicine, Perelman School of Medicine (PSOM) at the University of Pennsylvania, HUP Maloney 3rd Floor, 36th and Spruce Street, Philadelphia, PA 19104 - 4283, USA. [3]Perelman School of Medicine (PSOM) at the University of Pennsylvania, Philadelphia, PA, USA. [4]Department of Neurosurgery, Center for Brain Injury and Repair, the Perelman School of Medicine (PSOM) at the University of Pennsylvania, Philadelphia, PA, USA.

**References**

1. Abbott NJ, Pizzo ME, Preston JE, Janigro D, Thorne RG (2018) The role of brain barriers in fluid movement in the CNS: is there a 'glymphatic' system? Acta Neuropathol 135:387–407. https://doi.org/10.1007/s00401-018-1812-4
2. Arnold SE, Toledo JB, Appleby DH, Xie SX, Wang LS, Baek Y, Wolk DA, Lee EB, Miller BL, al LVM (2013) Comparative survey of the topographical distribution of signature molecular lesions in major neurodegenerative diseases. J Comp Neurol 521:4339–4355. https://doi.org/10.1002/cne.23430
3. Bancher C, Brunner C, Lassmann H, Budka H, Jellinger K, Wiche G, Seitelberger F, Grundke-Iqbal I, Iqbal K, Wisniewski HM (1989) Accumulation of abnormally phosphorylated tau precedes the formation of neurofibrillary tangles in Alzheimer's disease. Brain Res 477:90–99
4. Botez G, Probst A, Ipsen S, Tolnay M (1999) Astrocytes expressing hyperphosphorylated tau protein without glial fibrillary tangles in argyrophilic grain disease. Acta Neuropathol 98:251–256
5. Braak H, Braak E (1991) Neuropathological stageing of Alzheimer-related changes. Acta Neuropathol 82:239–259
6. Braak H, Del Tredici K, Rub U, de Vos RA, Jansen Steur EN, Braak E (2003) Staging of brain pathology related to sporadic Parkinson's disease. Neurobiol Aging 24:197–211
7. Brettschneider J, Arai K, Del Tredici K, Toledo JB, Robinson JL, Lee EB, Kuwabara S, Shibuya K, Irwin DJ, al FL (2014, 128) TDP-43 pathology and neuronal loss in amyotrophic lateral sclerosis spinal cord. Acta Neuropathol: 423–437. https://doi.org/10.1007/s00401-014-1299-6
8. Brettschneider J, Del Tredici K, Irwin DJ, Grossman M, Robinson JL, Toledo JB, Fang L, Van Deerlin VM, Ludolph AC, al LVM (2014) Sequential distribution of pTDP-43 pathology in behavioral variant frontotemporal dementia (bvFTD). Acta Neuropathol 127:423–439. https://doi.org/10.1007/s00401-013-1238-y
9. Brettschneider J, Del Tredici K, Lee VM, Trojanowski JQ (2015) Spreading of pathology in neurodegenerative diseases: a focus on human studies. Nat Rev Neurosci 16:109–120. https://doi.org/10.1038/nrn3887
10. Brettschneider J, Del Tredici K, Toledo JB, Robinson JL, Irwin DJ, Grossman M, Suh E, Van Deerlin VM, Wood EM, al BY (2013) Stages of pTDP-43 pathology in myotrophic lateral sclerosis. Ann Neurol 74:20–38. https://doi.org/10.1002/ana.23937
11. Brettschneider J, Irwin DJ, Boluda S, Byrne MD, Fang L, Lee EB, Robinson JL, Suh E, Van Deerlin VM, al TJB (2017) Progression of alpha-synuclein pathology in multiple system atrophy of the cerebellar type. Neuropathol Appl Neurobiol 43:315–329. https://doi.org/10.1111/nan.12362
12. Cavaliere F, Cerf L, Dehay B, Ramos-Gonzalez P, De Giorgi F, Bourdenx M, Bessede A, Obeso JA, Matute C, al IF (2017) In vitro alpha-synuclein

neurotoxicity and spreading among neurons and astrocytes using Lewy body extracts from Parkinson disease brains. Neurobiol Dis 103:101–112. https://doi.org/10.1016/j.nbd.2017.04.011

13. Crary JF, Trojanowski JQ, Schneider JA, Abisambra JF, Abner EL, Alafuzoff I, Arnold SE, Attems J, Beach TG, al BEH (2014, 128) Primary age-related tauopathy (PART): a common pathology associated with human aging. Acta Neuropathol:755–766. https://doi.org/10.1007/s00401-014-1349-0
14. Dubois B (2018) The emergence of a new conceptual framework for Alzheimer's disease. J Alzheimers Dis 62:1059–1066. https://doi.org/10.3233/JAD-170536
15. Ferrer I (2017) Diversity of astroglial responses across human neurodegenerative disorders and brain aging. Brain Pathol 27:645–674. https://doi.org/10.1111/bpa.12538
16. Ferrer I, Santpere G, van Leeuwen FW (2008) Argyrophilic grain disease. Brain 131:1416–1432. https://doi.org/10.1093/brain/awm305
17. Forman MS, Lal D, Zhang B, Dabir DV, Swanson E, Lee VM, Trojanowski JQ (2005) Transgenic mouse model of tau pathology in astrocytes leading to nervous system degeneration. J Neurosci 25:3539–3550. https://doi.org/10.1523/JNEUROSCI.0081-05.2005
18. Guo JL, Lee VM (2014) Cell-to-cell transmission of pathogenic proteins in neurodegenerative diseases. Nat Med 20:130–138. https://doi.org/10.1038/nm.3457
19. Higuchi M, Ishihara T, Zhang B, Hong M, Andreadis A, Trojanowski J, Lee VM (2002) Transgenic mouse model of tauopathies with glial pathology and nervous system degeneration. Neuron 35:433–446
20. Ikeda C, Yokota O, Nagao S, Ishizu H, Oshima E, Hasegawa M, Okahisa Y, Terada S, Yamada N (2016) The relationship between development of neuronal and astrocytic tau pathologies in subcortical nuclei and progression of Argyrophilic grain disease. Brain Pathol 26:488–505. https://doi.org/10.1111/bpa.12319
21. Irwin DJ, Brettschneider J, McMillan CT, Cooper F, Olm C, Arnold SE, Van Deerlin VM, Seeley WW, Miller BL, al LEB (2016) Deep clinical and neuropathological phenotyping of Pick disease. Ann Neurol 79:272–287. https://doi.org/10.1002/ana.24559
22. Irwin DJ, Cairns NJ, Grossman M, McMillan CT, Lee EB, Van Deerlin VM, Lee VM, Trojanowski JQ (2015) Frontotemporal lobar degeneration: defining phenotypic diversity through personalized medicine. Acta Neuropathol 129: 469–491. https://doi.org/10.1007/s00401-014-1380-1
23. Johnson VE, Stewart W, Arena JD, Smith DH (2017) Traumatic brain injury as a trigger of neurodegeneration. Adv Neurobiol 15:383–400. https://doi.org/10.1007/978-3-319-57193-5_15
24. Johnson VE, Stewart W, Smith DH (2013) Axonal pathology in traumatic brain injury. Exp Neurol 246:35–43. https://doi.org/10.1016/j.expneurol.2012.01.013
25. Johnson VE, Weber MT, Xiao R, Cullen DK, Meaney DF, Stewart W, Smith DH (2018) Mechanical disruption of the blood-brain barrier following experimental concussion. Acta Neuropathol. https://doi.org/10.1007/s00401-018-1824-0
26. Josephs KA, Mandrekar JN, Dickson DW (2006) The relationship between histopathological features of progressive supranuclear palsy and disease duration. Parkinsonism Relat Disord 12:109–112. https://doi.org/10.1016/j.parkreldis.2005.08.007
27. Josephs KA, Murray ME, Whitwell JL, Tosakulwong N, Weigand SD, Petrucelli L, Liesinger AM, Petersen RC, Parisi JE, Dickson DW (2016) Updated TDP-43 in Alzheimer's disease staging scheme. Acta Neuropathol 131:571–585. https://doi.org/10.1007/s00401-016-1537-1
28. Kovacs GG (2015) Invited review: neuropathology of tauopathies: principles and practice. Neuropathol Appl Neurobiol 41:3–23. https://doi.org/10.1111/nan.12208
29. Kovacs GG (2016) Molecular pathological classification of neurodegenerative diseases: turning towards precision medicine. Int J Mol Sci 17. https://doi.org/10.3390/ijms17020189
30. Kovacs GG, Breydo L, Green R, Kis V, Puska G, Lorincz P, Perju-Dumbrava L, Giera R, Pirker W, Lutz M et al (2014) Intracellular processing of disease-associated alpha-synuclein in the human brain suggests prion-like cell-to-cell spread. Neurobiol Dis 69:76–92. https://doi.org/10.1016/j.nbd.2014.05.020
31. Kovacs GG, Ferrer I, Grinberg LT, Alafuzoff I, Attems J, Budka H, Cairns NJ, Crary JF, Duyckaerts C, al GB (2016) Aging-related tau astrogliopathy (ARTAG): harmonized evaluation strategy. Acta Neuropathol 131:87–102. https://doi.org/10.1007/s00401-015-1509-x
32. Kovacs GG, Kwong LK, Grossman M, Irwin DJ, Lee EB, Robinson JL, Suh E, Van Deerlin VM, Lee VM, Trojanowski JQ (2018) Tauopathy with hippocampal 4-repeat tau immunoreactive spherical inclusions: a report of three cases. Brain Pathol 28: 274–283 doi https://doi.org/10.1111/bpa.12482
33. Kovacs GG, Lee VM, Trojanowski JQ (2017) Protein astrogliopathies in human neurodegenerative diseases and aging. Brain Pathol 27:675–690. https://doi.org/10.1111/bpa.12536
34. Kovacs GG, Molnar K, Laszlo L, Strobel T, Botond G, Honigschnabl S, Reiner-Concin A, Palkovits M, Fischer P, Budka H (2011) A peculiar constellation of tau pathology defines a subset of dementia in the elderly. Acta Neuropathol 122:205–222. https://doi.org/10.1007/s00401-011-0819-x
35. Kovacs GG, Robinson JL, Xie SX, Lee EB, Grossman M, Wolk DA, Irwin DJ, Weintraub D, Kim CF, al ST (2017) Evaluating the patterns of aging-related tau Astrogliopathy unravels novel insights into brain aging and neurodegenerative diseases. J Neuropathol Exp Neurol 76:270–288. https://doi.org/10.1093/jnen/nlx00
36. Kovacs GG, Xie SX, Lee EB, Robinson JL, Caswell C, Irwin DJ, Toledo JB, Attems J, Bencze J, al BKF (2017) Multisite assessment of aging-related tau astrogliopathy (ARTAG). J Neuropathol Exp Neurol 76:605–619. https://doi.org/10.1093/jnen/nlx041
37. Kovacs GG, Yousef A, Kaindl S, Lee VM, Trojanowski JQ (2017) Connexin-43 and aquaporin-4 are markers of ageing-related tau astrogliopathy (ARTAG)-related astroglial response. Neuropathol Appl Neurobiol. https://doi.org/10.1111/nan.12427
38. Landis JR, Koch GG (1977) The measurement of observer agreement for categorical data. Biometrics 33:159–174
39. Lindstrom V, Gustafsson G, Sanders LH, Howlett EH, Sigvardson J, Kasrayan A, Ingelsson M, Bergstrom J, Erlandsson A (2017) Extensive uptake of alpha-synuclein oligomers in astrocytes results in sustained intracellular deposits and mitochondrial damage. Mol Cell Neurosci 82:143–156. https://doi.org/10.1016/j.mcn.2017.04.009
40. Ling H, Kovacs GG, Vonsattel JP, Davey K, Mok KY, Hardy J, Morris HR, Warner TT, Holton JL, Revesz T (2016) Astrogliopathy predominates the earliest stage of corticobasal degeneration pathology. Brain 139:3237–3252. https://doi.org/10.1093/brain/aww256
41. Liu AK, Goldfinger MH, Questari HE, Pearce RK, Gentleman SM (2016) ARTAG in the basal forebrain: widening the constellation of astrocytic tau pathology. Acta Neuropathol Commun 4:59. https://doi.org/10.1186/s40478-016-0330-7
42. Loria F, Vargas JY, Bousset L, Syan S, Salles A, Melki R, Zurzolo C (2017) Alpha-Synuclein transfer between neurons and astrocytes indicates that astrocytes play a role in degradation rather than in spreading. Acta Neuropathol 134:789–808. https://doi.org/10.1007/s00401-017-1746-2
43. McKee AC, Cairns NJ, Dickson DW, Folkerth RD, Keene CD, Litvan I, Perl DP, Stein TD, Vonsattel JP, al SW (2016) The first NINDS/NIBIB consensus meeting to define neuropathological criteria for the diagnosis of chronic traumatic encephalopathy. Acta Neuropathol 131:75–86. https://doi.org/10.1007/s00401-015-1515-z
44. McKee AC, Stein TD, Kiernan PT, Alvarez VE (2015) The neuropathology of chronic traumatic encephalopathy. Brain Pathol 25:350–364. https://doi.org/10.1111/bpa.12248
45. Papp MI, Kovacs T (2013) Progression of Alzheimer-type neurofibrillary tangles is related to the proximodistal segments of the hemispheric arteries. Curr Alzheimer Res 10:818–828
46. Puska G, Lutz MI, Molnar K, Regelsberger G, Ricken G, Pirker W, Laszlo L, Kovacs GG (2018) Lysosomal response in relation to alpha-synuclein pathology differs between Parkinson's disease and multiple system atrophy. Neurobiol Dis 114:140–152. https://doi.org/10.1016/j.nbd.2018.02.019
47. Saito Y, Ruberu NN, Sawabe M, Arai T, Tanaka N, Kakuta Y, Yamanouchi H, Murayama S (2004) Staging of argyrophilic grains: an age-associated tauopathy. J Neuropathol Exp Neurol 63:911–918
48. Santpere G, Ferrer I (2009) Delineation of early changes in cases with progressive supranuclear palsy-like pathology. Astrocytes in striatum are primary targets of tau phosphorylation and GFAP oxidation. Brain Pathol 19: 177–187. https://doi.org/10.1111/j.1750-3639.2008.00173.x
49. Shibuya K, Yagishita S, Nakamura A, Uchihara T (2011) Perivascular orientation of astrocytic plaques and tuft-shaped astrocytes. Brain Res 1404: 50–54. https://doi.org/10.1016/j.brainres.2011.06.014
50. Shimizu H, Kakita A, Takahashi H (2008) Spinal cord tau pathology in cervical spondylotic myelopathy. Acta Neuropathol 115:185–192. https://doi.org/10.1007/s00401-007-0321-7
51. Shively SB, Horkayne-Szakaly I, Jones RV, Kelly JP, Armstrong RC, Perl DP (2016) Characterisation of interface astroglial scarring in the human brain after blast exposure: a post-mortem case series. Lancet Neurol 15:944–953. https://doi.org/10.1016/S1474-4422(16)30057-6
52. Song YJ, Halliday GM, Holton JL, Lashley T, O'Sullivan SS, McCann H, Lees AJ, Ozawa T, Williams DR, al LPJ (2009) Degeneration in different parkinsonian syndromes relates to astrocyte type and astrocyte protein expression. J Neuropathol Exp Neurol 68:1073–1083. https://doi.org/10.1097/NEN.0b013e3181b66f1b
53. Tatsumi S, Mimuro M, Iwasaki Y, Takahashi R, Kakita A, Takahashi H, Yoshida M (2014) Argyrophilic grains are reliable disease-specific features of corticobasal

degeneration. J Neuropathol Exp Neurol 73:30–38. https://doi.org/10.1097/NEN.0000000000000022
54. Thal DR, Rub U, Orantes M, Braak H (2002) Phases of a beta-deposition in the human brain and its relevance for the development of AD. Neurology 58:1791–1800
55. Toledo JB, Van Deerlin VM, Lee EB, Suh E, Baek Y, Robinson JL, Xie SX, McBride J, Wood EM, al ST (2014) A platform for discovery: The University of Pennsylvania Integrated Neurodegenerative Disease Biobank. Alzheimers Dement 10:477–484 e471. https://doi.org/10.1016/j.jalz.2013.06.003
56. Tolnay M, Clavaguera F (2004) Argyrophilic grain disease: a late-onset dementia with distinctive features among tauopathies. Neuropathology 24: 269–283
57. Verkhratsky A, Zorec R, Parpura V (2017) Stratification of astrocytes in healthy and diseased brain. Brain Pathol 27:629–644. https://doi.org/10.1111/bpa.12537
58. Williams DR, Holton JL, Strand C, Pittman A, de Silva R, Lees AJ, Revesz T (2007) Pathological tau burden and distribution distinguishes progressive supranuclear palsy-parkinsonism from Richardson's syndrome. Brain 130: 1566–1576. https://doi.org/10.1093/brain/awm104
59. Yokoyama Y, Toyoshima Y, Shiga A, Tada M, Kitamura H, Hasegawa K, Onodera O, Ikeuchi T, Someya T, al NM (2016) Pathological and Clinical Spectrum of Progressive Supranuclear Palsy: With Special Reference to Astrocytic Tau Pathology. Brain Pathol 26:155–166. https://doi.org/10.1111/bpa.12265

12

# CD74 regulates complexity of tumor cell HLA class II peptidome in brain metastasis and is a positive prognostic marker for patient survival

P. S. Zeiner[1,2†], J. Zinke[1†], D. J. Kowalewski[3,4], S. Bernatz[1], J. Tichy[2], M. W. Ronellenfitsch[2], F. Thorsen[5], A. Berger[6], M. T. Forster[7], A. Muller[8], J. P. Steinbach[2,9], R. Beschorner[10], J. Wischhusen[11], H. M. Kvasnicka[12], K. H. Plate[1,9], S. Stefanović[3], B. Weide[13], M. Mittelbronn[1,9,14,15,16,17] and P. N. Harter[1,9*]

**Abstract**

Despite multidisciplinary local and systemic therapeutic approaches, the prognosis for most patients with brain metastases is still dismal. The role of adaptive and innate anti-tumor response including the Human Leukocyte Antigen (HLA) machinery of antigen presentation is still unclear. We present data on the HLA class II-chaperone molecule CD74 in brain metastases and its impact on the HLA peptidome complexity.

We analyzed CD74 and HLA class II expression on tumor cells in a subset of 236 human brain metastases, primary tumors and peripheral metastases of different entities in association with clinical data including overall survival. Additionally, we assessed whole DNA methylome profiles including CD74 promoter methylation and differential methylation in 21 brain metastases. We analyzed the effects of a siRNA mediated CD74 knockdown on HLA-expression and HLA peptidome composition in a brain metastatic melanoma cell line.

We observed that CD74 expression on tumor cells is a strong positive prognostic marker in brain metastasis patients and positively associated with tumor-infiltrating T-lymphocytes (TILs). Whole DNA methylome analysis suggested that CD74 tumor cell expression might be regulated epigenetically via CD74 promoter methylation. $CD74^{high}$ and $TIL^{high}$ tumors displayed a differential DNA methylation pattern with highest enrichment scores for antigen processing and presentation. Furthermore, CD74 knockdown in vitro lead to a reduction of HLA class II peptidome complexity, while HLA class I peptidome remained unaffected.

In summary, our results demonstrate that a functional HLA class II processing machinery in brain metastatic tumor cells, reflected by a high expression of CD74 and a complex tumor cell HLA peptidome, seems to be crucial for better patient prognosis.

**Keywords:** CD74, HLA class II, Brain metastasis, HLA peptidome, Tumor infiltrating lymphocytes

* Correspondence: patrick.harter@kgu.de
†Equal contributors
1Edinger Institute (Institute of Neurology), Goethe-University, Heinrich-Hoffmann-Str. 7, D-60528 Frankfurt am Main, Germany
9German Cancer Research Center DKFZ Heidelberg, Germany and German Cancer Consortium DKTK partner site, Frankfurt/Mainz, Germany
Full list of author information is available at the end of the article

## Introduction

Brain metastases (BM) are the most frequent brain tumors in humans. Despite multimodal therapies including radio-chemotherapy, neurosurgery and/or stereotactic irradiation patient survival is still poor, often not exceeding 6–12 months [3, 43]. During the last years clinical trials focusing on modulation of the immune response (mostly by targeting immune checkpoints) have shown promising results in peripheral tumors of different cancer entities [13, 37, 55]. Unfortunately, knowledge about treatment response in BM is still poor. Recently, Frenard and colleagues showed that ipilimumab treatment (CTLA-4-dependent checkpoint-inhibitor) failed to prevent metastases formation in the per se immune privileged environment of the brain in patients suffering from metastatic melanoma [12] despite a potentially enhanced systemic immune response. Nevertheless, it has recently been shown that the PD-1 antibodies nivolumab and pembrolizumab might have significant activity in BM patients, indicating a potential tumor control function in BM of melanoma patients [34]. Interestingly, it has been described that the mutational load of metastatic melanomas predicts a better response to CTLA-4 blockade [41]. Likewise, hypermutated tumors with DNA mismatch-repair gene defects respond significantly better to PD-1 blockade as compared to tumors without DNA mismatch-repair gene defects and lower mutational load [25]. Even across different tumor entities, the response to immunotherapy is associated with mutational load as presented in humans via human leukocyte antigen (HLA) molecules [2]. This indicates that the mutational landscape presented via HLA molecules might be crucial for an adequate immune and thus therapy response.

Antigens are presented either via HLA class I or class II molecules. Tumor cell-derived (neo)-antigens are presented by the ubiquitously expressed HLA class I molecules, although recent data demonstrates murine mutant epitopes also on major histocompatibility complex (MHC) class II molecules [22]. HLA class II presentation is usually found on antigen presenting cells such as dendritic cells, macrophages and microglial cells. The expression of HLA class II molecules is not exclusively restricted to immune cells, HLA class II molecules have been described on cancer cells already several decades ago [8, 24, 48] and the loss of heterozygosity in HLA does correlate with tumor immune escape [29]. Further, HLA class II-dependent help from CD4-positive TILs might significantly support anti-tumor immune response [1] (the term TILs will be used throughout the manuscript describing the population of tumor infiltrating T-lymphocytes mainly consisting of CD3-, CD4- and CD8-positive cells). However, the clinical relevance of HLA class II expression on cancer cells might depend on the cancer type. Whereas e.g. in colorectal cancer HLA class II expression has been described to be associated with a favorable clinical outcome [23, 31, 40], HLA class II expression on e.g. melanomas or sarcomas has been linked with poor clinical outcome [30, 46]. Still there is the question whether the mere amount of HLA class II molecules on cancer cells is mediating these effects or weather modulations of the antigen processing and assembly machinery are resulting in differential presentation of immunogenic antigens on the cell surface.

CD74, also known as invariant chain (li) is essential for assembly and stabilization during HLA class II antigen presentation. HLA class II molecules are synthesized in the endoplasmic reticulum (ER) where they assemble with CD74, the latter being involved in proper folding and stabilization of HLA class II molecules. CD74 also facilitates the export of HLA class II complexes from the ER to lysosomal compartments where antigens are loaded and CD74 becomes proteolytically degraded by cathepsins leaving the CLIP peptide in the HLA class II binding groove. Although CD74 has recently been shown to be involved in cross-presentation on HLA class I molecules, the main function seem to be the chaperoning during HLA class II antigen presentation [4, 52]. CD74 itself is upregulated in a variety of peripheral (e.g. melanoma: [47], lung cancer: [28]) and especially hematopoietic neoplasms [6, 7]. Several studies in peripheral tumors suggest pro-neoplastic effects of CD74 [9, 20, 27] or even show a negative association of CD74 expression with overall survival in vivo [33]. On the contrary other studies observed controversial CD74 effects with prolonged overall survival and an association with HLA class II expression [11, 54]. The exact mechanisms how CD74 might functionally influence neoplastic behavior remain multifaceted including the function as a receptor for macrophage migration inhibitory factor (MIF) [26] and a predominant expression on non-neoplastic antigen-presenting cells of the microenvironment in some tumor entities [26].

Here we analyze expression profiles and clinical relevance of the major assembly and stabilization molecule CD74 in a large cohort of BM patients. Furthermore, we analyzed the consequences of CD74 expression on the HLA peptidome of a brain metastatic cancer cell line.

## Material and methods

### Patient tissue and tissue microarrays (TMAs)

Data analyses was performed on paraffin embedded tissue samples which were processed to tissue micro arrays (TMAs) (deriving from the UCT tumor bank, Goethe-University, Frankfurt am Main, Germany, member of the German Cancer Consortium (DKTK), Heidelberg, Germany and German Cancer Research Center (DKFZ), Heidelberg, Germany or from the local biobank "Blut-und Gewebebank zur Erforschung des malignen Melanoms" Department of Dermatology,

University Hospital Tuebingen, Tuebingen, Germany). Written consent was obtained from each patient. The study protocol was endorsed by the local ethical committee (Goethe-University Medical School/UCT Frankfurt GS-04/09, SNO-08-2015). In total, we investigated 236 embedded tissue samples including BM of: melanoma ($n$ =96), non small cell lung cancer (NSCLC, $n$ =56), breast carcinoma ($n$ = 31), renal cell carcinoma (RCC, $n$ =18), small cell lung cancer (SCLC $n$ =8), colon carcinoma ($n$ = 10), carcinomas which were not otherwise specified (carcinoma NOS $n$ =8) and specimens of rare tumors summarized as others ($n$ = 9). Histopathology of BM was performed by board certified neuropathologists (KHP, MM and PNH). Histopathology of primary tumors and peripheral metastases was performed by a board certified pathologist (HMK). Further clinical data is shown in Additional file 1: Figure S1.

**Immunohistochemistry (IHC) and immunofluorescence (IF)**

For immunohistochemical and immunofluorescent analyses of TMAs, whole mount sections and paraffin embedded cell pellets (of melanoma cell lines H1_DL2 (human brain seeking cell line deriving from melanoma BM) [45, 53], SK-MEL-2 (human skin metastatic melanoma), SK-MEL-28, UACC-257 (both human melanoma), the breast cancer cell lines MDA-MB-231 and JIMT-1 (both brain seeking clones of human pleural metastatic breast cancer) and the lung adenocarcinoma cell line PC14-PE6 (brain seeking clone of human lung adenocarcinoma)) the following antibodies were used: anti-CD3 (Dako A0452, dilution for IHC 1:500), anti-CD4 (Roche #790–4423, clone SP35, undiluted), anti-CD8 (Dako, clone C8/144B, dilution for IHC 1:100), anti-CD74 (Abcam, ab9514, dilution for IHC/IF 1:100/1:200), anti-Ki67 (Dako M7240, dilution for IHC 1:200) anti-HLA class II (Dako M0775, dilution for IHC/IF 1:1000 detecting HLA-DP, DQ, and DR) and anti-panCK (Dako, clone MNF116, dilution for IHC/IF 1:1000). TMA tissue blocks were cut in slices of 3 μm thickness using a microtome (Leica Microsystems, Nussloch GmbH, Nussloch, Germany) and placed onto SuperFrost slides (Thermo Scientific, Dreieich, Germany). IHC was performed according to standardized protocols using the Discovery XT automated immunostaining system (Ventana Medical Systems, München, Germany). IHC stainings were analyzed using a light microscope (BX41, Olympus, Hamburg, Germany). IF stainings were performed as described previously [57] and were evaluated using the Eclipse 80i fluorescent microscope (Nikon Eclipse 80i, Nikon, Japan).

**Statistical analyses of tissue micro array data**

Quantification of CD4-positive TILs was performed on all BM with regard to positive lymphocytic cells related to all cells, while the amount of CD3-, CD8- and PD-1-positive TILs has already been calculated and described [16]. CD74- and HLA class II- (both intracellular and membrane-associated) positive tumor cells related to the total cell number were calculated using a semi quantitative IHC H-score ("histo" score) ranging from 0 to 300. Each staining intensity level (1 = weak, 2 = moderate, 3 = strong) and the percentage of positively stained cells in these particular levels (1, 2 or 3) were determined in the whole tissue sample. The staining intensity levels were then multiplied with the frequency of positively stained cells (in %). Finally, these scores per level were put together, ending up with a final score ranging from 0 to 300. PD-L1 expression on tumor cells has already been described [16]. CD74 expression in tumor cells was compared to clinical parameters such as, overall survival, Karnofsky Performance Status (KPS) or in case of melanoma the Graded Prognostic Assessment (GPA) score. If not otherwise stated, $p$-values are indicated including their 95% confidence intervals ($^{*}p < 0.05$; $^{**}p < 0.01$; $^{***}p < 0.0001$). A significance level of alpha =0.05 was selected. Statistical analyses were performed using JMP 11.0 software (SAS, Cary, NC, USA). Graphics were prepared using GraphPad Prism 6 software (GraphPad Software, Inc., La Jolla, CA, USA).

**CD74 siRNA knockdown**

The melanoma brain metastasis cell line H1 which shows a tropism for the brain was grown in DMEM GlutaMax (Invitrogen) supplemented with 10% Fetal Bovine Serum (FBS Superior, Biochrome) and 1% Penicillin-Streptomycin (P/S, Sigma-Aldrich) at 37 °C and 5% CO2. Cells were seeded directly into the transfection mix consisting of DMEM (without FBS and P/S) and siRNA pools against human CD74 (NCBI gene ID: 972, sp972_5) in a final concentration of 6 nM for 96 h according to the manufacturer's protocol. Unspecific (control siPools) served as a control condition (siTOOLs Biotech GmbH, Munich, Germany) [15]. LipofectamineTM 2000 (Invitrogen, Darmstadt, Germany) was used as a transfection reagent (5 μL in a six-well format, 30 μL in a 10-cm-format or T-175 flasks). To generate cyto pellets $2 \times 10^6$ cells were seeded in a 10 cm petri dish applying a total volume of 10 ml/dish including transfection reagent, siRNA pools and DMEM. For extraction of RNA for qRT-PCR and RNA microarray as well as protein for immunoblotting $3 \times 10^5$ cells/well of a 6-well plate in a total volume of 2 ml/well were seeded. These experiments were performed in triplicates. For peptidome analysis $8 \times 10^6$ cells were seeded in T-175 cell culture flasks in a final volume of 15 ml (11xT-175 flasks per condition: siRNA pools against human CD74 versus unspecific control siPools, including each an additional flask for validation with immunoblotting as well as qRT-PCR).

**Quantitative-RealTime-PCR (qRT-PCR)**

Total RNA was extracted according to the manufacturer's protocol of the RNeasy Mini Kit (Qiagen, Hilden, Germany) from several metastatic cancer cell lines (melanoma cell lines: H1_DL2, SK-MEL-2, SK-MEL-28, UACC-257, breast cancer cell lines: MDA-MB-231, Jimt-1 and the lung adenocarcinoma cell line PC14-PE6) as well as the H1 cell line after CD74 knockdown with siRNA pools. The concentration of total RNA was determined photometrically with the NanoDrop™ 2000 spectral photometer (Thermo Scientific, Dreieich, Germany). Reverse transcription of 1 µg of RNA into complementary DNA (cDNA) was performed according to the manufacturer's protocol of the RevertAidTM H Minus First Strand cDNA synthesis Kit (Thermo Scientific, Dreieich, Germany) using random hexamer primers. To digest template RNA after cDNA synthesis 1 µl of Ribonuclease H was added and incubated for 30 min at 37 °C. The quantitative polymerase chain reaction (qPCR) reactions were prepared in a final volume of 20 µ using SYBR green master mix (Thermo Fisher Scientific, Waltham, MA, USA) on a MyiQ Single Color Real-Time PCR Detection System (BIO-RAD, Hercules, CA, USA). CD74_551 (fw 5'-CCCGGAGAACCTGAGACACCT-3', rv 5'-CCAAGGAGTGCCTGCTCATT-3') and the internal standard control RPLP0 (fw 5'-GAGTCCTGGCC TTGTCTGTGG-3', rv 5'-TCCGACTCTTCCTTGGCT TCA-3') were designed as described previously [57]. Analyses were performed in triplicates. ΔCT and ΔΔCT values were determined.

**TaqMan® Array human antigen processing and presentation by MHCS**

On the gene signature plate TaqMan® Array Human Antigen Processing and Presentation by MHCS (Fisher Scientific, Schwerte, Germany) 44 genes related to antigen processing and presentation as well as 4 endogenous control genes were tested in duplicates per condition according to the manufacturer's protocol using the TaqMan® Gene Expression Master Mix (Fisher Scientific, Schwerte, Germany) on a MyiQ Single Color Real-Time PCR Detection System (BIO-RAD, Hercules, CA, USA). The aforementioned array was performed in the brain seeking melanoma metastasis cell line H1 after CD74 knockdown with siRNA pools. Unspecific control siPools (negative pools) served as a control condition. ΔCT and ΔΔCT values were determined.

**RNA microarray**

RNA microarray analyses were performed using the brain seeking melanoma brain metastasis cell line H1 after CD74 knockdown with siRNA pools (see above). Unspecific control siPools (negative pools) served as control. Analyses were performed in triplicates. The comprehensive RNA microarray using the HumanHT-12 v4 Expression BeadChip Kit was completed at the Genomics and Proteomics Core Facility at the German Cancer Research Center, Heidelberg, Germany (DKFZ). Major transcripts of HLA class II components were analyzed for confirmation of TaqMan® data.

**Immunoblot analysis**

Protein lysates of H1 cells after CD74 knockdown with siRNA pools were generated as described previously [18]. Unspecific control siPools (neg. pools) served as a control condition. Protein concentration was determined by using the Pierce® BCA Protein Assay Kit (Thermo Scientific, Dreieich, Germany) according to the manufacturer's instructions. Electrophoretic separation of denatured proteins was performed on 15% SDS-polyacrylamide-gels using the Bio-Rad (Bio-Rad, München, Germany) electrophoresis system, followed by immunoblotting and immunodetection as described previously [57]. The following antibodies were used: anti-CD74 (Abcam, ab9514, dilution for WB 1:50), as a loading control anti-Lamin B1 (Abcam, ab16048, dilution for WB 1:4500). Immunoblots were developed with the Odyssey Fc (LI-COR, Lincoln, NE, USA). For quantitative analysis of immunoblots a densitometry approach was used as previously described with normalization of CD74 signal to Lamin B1 signal [18].

**Flow cytometry (FACS)**

Membranous CD74 (anti-CD74, abcam, ab9514, dilution for FACS 1:50) expression of the brain seeking melanoma metastasis cell line H1 and the melanoma cell line SKMEL-28 was tested by FACS (FACSCanto-II flow cytometer (BD Bioscience)) against the positive control Raji as described previously [57]. HLA class II (anti-HLA-DR, Biolegend, clone L243, dilution for FACS 1:100) cell surface expression was assessed in H1 cells after CD74 knockdown with siRNA pools, unspecific control siPools (negative pools) serving as control treatment condition. An anti-mouse IgG1 antibody (Dako, Hamburg, Germany) was used as an isotype control for CD74 stainings and an anti-mouse IgG2a antibody (Dako, Hamburg, Germany) for HLA class II stainings respectively. Data were analyzed by Flow Jo software (TreeStar, Ashland, OR, USA).

**Whole DNA methylome analyses and CD74 promoter methylation status**

CD74 promoter associated CpGs were analyzed in 21 NSCLC BM using the EPIC 850 k whole methylome Chip (Illumina, San Diego, USA) following standard protocols for tissue and DNA processing. Hybridization was performed as indicated by the manufacturer. Data were preprocessed using Illumina Genome Studio, further analysis was performed using JMP 11.0 (SAS, Cary, NC, USA). Mean beta-values were compared between CD74 high ($n = 11$) and low ($n = 10$) expressors as assessed in IHC (median H-Score 20). The following target promoter associated CpG sites were analyzed: cg01601628, cg11619961, cg11915469, cg13362637, cg14484145, cg165 91228, cg18664712, cg19928046, cg19966212, cg229755 68, cg24548564, cg26129545. Whole methylome analysis was performed using Partek Genomic Suite software (Partek Incorborated, St. Louis, Missouri, USA). We hypothetically stratified both CD74$^{high}$ and TIL$^{high}$ tumors versus tumors not showing these features. Differential methylation was performed using M-values after functional normalization. CpGs were regarded as differentially methylated with an unadjusted $p$-value of $p < 0.0001$. Differentially methylated CpGs were further processed with Partek Gene Ontology (GO) enrichment analysis.

#### HLA peptidome analysis by mass spectrometry

HLA class I and class II molecules were isolated from $5 \times 10^7$ CD74siRNA treated and mock treated H1 cells using standard immunoaffinity purification as described previously [21]. We independently transfected nine replicates each of control and siRNA knockdown condition (nine T175 flasks each). Due to the large amounts of cells which are necessary for sufficiently deep HLA peptidome analysis, we pooled all cells for each condition. Mass spectrometry was performed in 5 technical replicates for each condition to allow for statistical evaluation of label-free quantitation data. The pan-HLA class I-specific mAb W6/32 was utilized for isolation of class I molecules. A 1:1 mixture of the pan-HLA class II-specific mAb Tü-39 and the HLA-DR-specific mAB L243 was utilized for the isolation of HLA class II.

Label-free relative quantitation (LFQ) of the HLA peptidome composition was performed by LC-MS analysis of HLA class II ligand extracts from treated and control cells in five technical replicates. Peptide samples were separated by nanoflow high-performance liquid chromatography (RSLCnano, Thermo Fisher Scientific) using a 50 μm × 25 cm PepMap C18 column (Thermo Fisher Scientific) and a linear gradient ranging from 2.4% to 32.0% acetonitrile over the course of 90 min. Eluting peptides were analyzed in an online-coupled Orbitrap Fusion Lumos mass spectrometer (Thermo Fisher Scientific) in data dependent acquisition mode using collision-induced dissociation fragmentation. MS2 spectra for 2+ and 3+ precursors of 400–650 m/z were acquired at 30 k resolution with AGC target values of 70,000 and maximum injection times of 150 ms. Normalized collision energy was set to 35%, dynamic exclusion was set to 7 s. On column peptide amounts for the 5 LFQ replicates were adjusted based on initial dose-finding LC-MS analysis.

Database search was performed using SequestHT node of ProteomeDiscoverer 1.4.1.14 (Thermo Fisher Scientific) to search against the human proteome as comprised in the Swiss-Prot database (version of September 27th 2013, 20,279 reviewed protein sequences contained) without enzymatic restriction. Precursor mass tolerance was set to 5 ppm, fragment mass tolerance to 0.02 Da. Oxidized methionine was allowed as a dynamic modification. The false discovery rate (FDR) was estimated using Percolator [19] and limited to 1%. Peptide lengths were to 8–25 amino acids.

Relative quantification of HLA ligands was performed based on the peak area of the corresponding precursor MS1 extracted ion chromatogram. Imputation of missing values, 2-tier normalization for technical variability in MS signal intensity and calculation of fold-change and $p$-values (heteroskedastic t-test using Benjamini-Hochberg correction) for differential peptide presentation was performed using an in-house R script.

The mass spectrometry proteomics data have been deposited to the ProteomeXchange Consortium via the PRIDE [51] partner repository with the dataset identifier PXD008937.

### Results

#### CD74 is expressed by tumor cells in BM and is associated with a better overall survival in vivo.

In a first step, we assessed protein expression profiles of CD74 in BM from distinct primary tumor entities. CD74 was expressed by tumor cells (Fig. 1a, b) and by myeloid cells such as tumor associated microglia and macrophages (TAMs) as previously shown by our group in primary brain tumors [57]. We solely analyzed CD74 expression in tumor cells not in TAMs. CD74 tumor cell expression was heterogeneous among all investigated entities (Fig. 1a-c) with highest expression levels in BM of RCC and NSCLC (mean H-Score of 133.9 and 73.2) respectively. We detected lowest levels in SCLC (mean H-Score of 16.2). Despite the strong variation of mean values, we found high and low expressors in all investigated entities (Fig. 1c, median H-Score 20). Most interestingly, high CD74 expression on tumor cells was associated with prolonged patient overall survival after BM surgery in the total cohort as well as in our largest subcohorts of BM deriving from NSCLC and melanoma (Fig. 1d). Interestingly, CD74 expression in tumor cells was not associated with clinical parameters such as Karnofsky Performance Status (KPS) or in case of melanoma the Graded Prognostic Assessment (GPA) Score (Additional file 1: Figure S1). Furthermore, non-cerebral, peripheral melanoma metastases (skin metastases) did not show a significant survival benefit (Additional file 2: Figure S2a). In peripheral melanoma skin metastases, we did not find a significant difference in CD74 expression between tumor stage III and tumor stage IV patients (Additional file 2: Figure S2b). Furthermore, we had the opportunity to analyze primary tumors ($n = 10$), peripheral

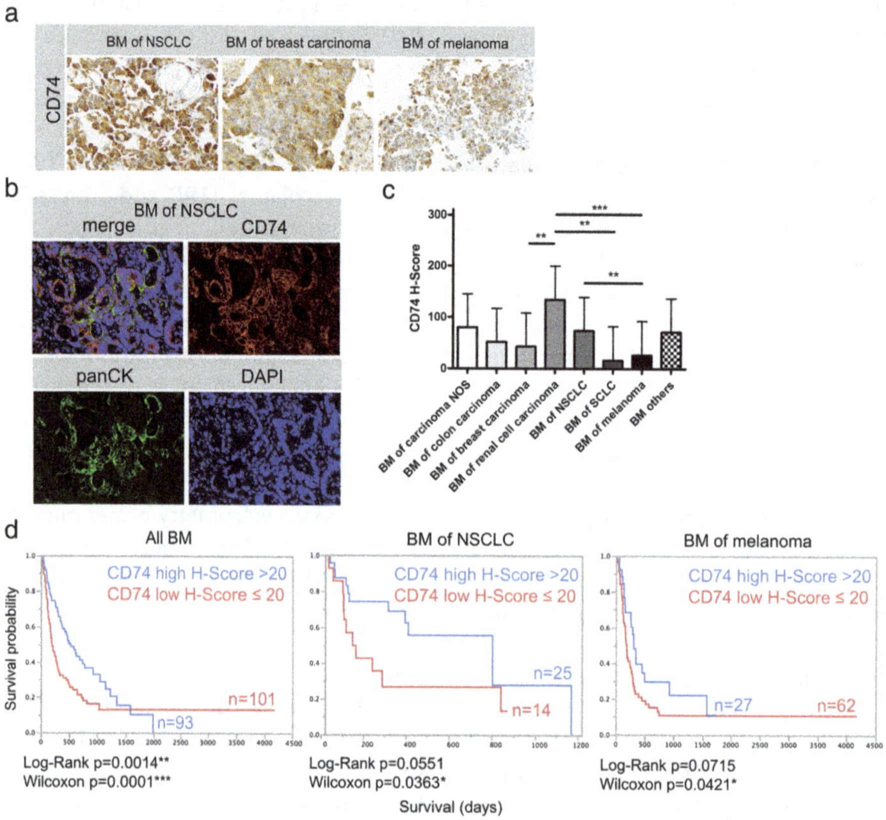


**Fig. 1** CD74 expression in human brain metastases. **a** Immunohistochemical staining against CD74 in three examples of BM from NSCLC, breast carcinoma and melanoma. **b** Example for CD74 and panCK showing co-expression in a NSCLC BM. **c** H-Score mean values and standard error of the mean (SEM) of all investigated BM entities (mean CD74 H-Score values: carcinoma NOS 79.4 ($n = 8$); colon carcinoma 51.4 ($n = 10$); breast carcinoma 42.5 ($n = 31$); RCC 133.9 ($n = 18$); NSCLC 73.2 ($n = 56$); SCLC 16.3 ($n = 8$); melanoma 26.5 ($n = 96$); others 71.1 ($n = 9$)). **d** Kaplan-Meier Survival analyses in the total BM cohort and in the subcohorts of NSCLC and melanoma after median split (median H-Score 20) according to CD74 expression

metastases ($n = 4$) as well as BM ($n = 56$) of NSCLC patients. We did not observe any significant differences between these different stages of disease with regard to CD74 expression (Additional file 2: Figure S2c). Matched-pair analysis of CD74 expression in primary tumors and BM did not reveal a clear trend (Additional file 2: Figure S2d).

### CD74 expression in BM is associated with immune cell infiltration

As CD74 is a HLA class II chaperone molecule which guides and stabilizes assembly as well as influences the intracellular transport of HLA class II molecules, we next investigated whether CD74 expression is associated with HLA class II expression profiles. Despite heterogeneous expression patterns of CD74 and HLA class II in individual cases (Fig. 2a, b), H-Score values strongly correlated between CD74 and HLA class II in our total cohort of BM (Spearman's ρ 0.5440, $p < 0.0001$; Fig. 2c). More than half of the investigated BM showing high CD74 expression also showed high HLA class II values (Fig. 2c). However, CD74 low expressors did not necessarily show low expression levels for HLA class II expression. Interestingly, HLA class II expression alone showed no significant association with overall survival (Additional file 3: Figure S3a). Moreover, HLA class II expression was significantly reduced in BM as compared to their primary tumors ($p < 0.002$, Additional file 3: Figure S3b), which might indicate that the mere amount of HLA class II molecules is not the crucial step for a functional immune response in BM.

We recently found that the mere amount of TILs (CD3-positive and CD8-positive lymphocytes as well as subsets of these cells) is not associated with patient survival [16]. In the total cohort of BM as well as in the subcohort of melanoma BM the positive prognostic marker CD74 on tumor cells is nevertheless significantly associated with increased numbers of TILs (including CD3-, CD4- and CD8-positive TILs) (Fig. 2d, e). In the cohort of NSCLC BM, $CD74^{high}$ expressors also showed a trend towards increased CD3- and CD8-positive TILs, while we did not observe significant differences with regard to CD4-positive cells.

Current therapeutic strategies focus on targeting the immune checkpoint axis PD-1 and PD-L1. Although the

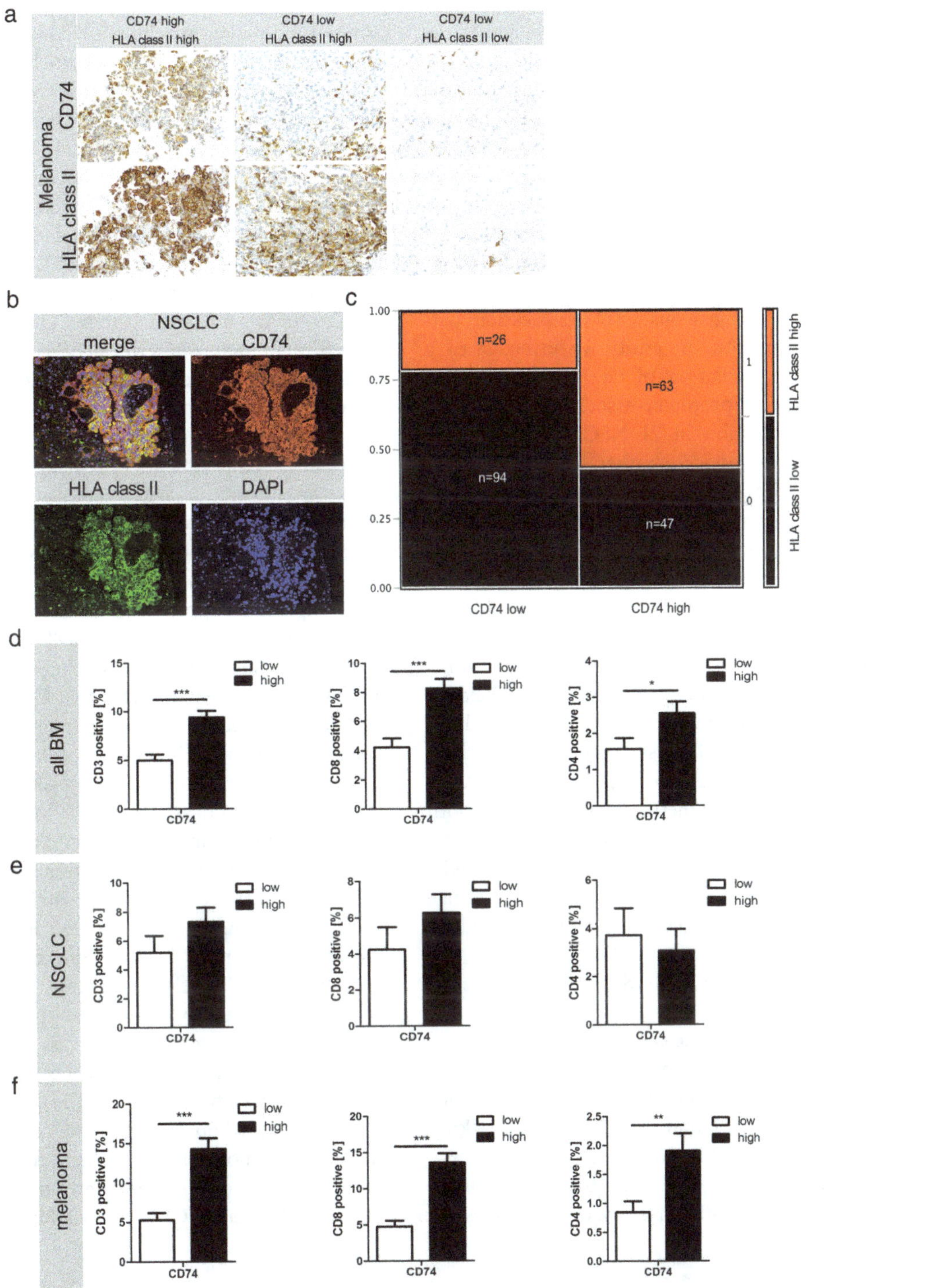


**Fig. 2** CD74 association with HLA class II and TILs. **a** Immunohistochemical staining against HLA class II members and CD74 revealing a heterogeneous expression pattern in tumor cells of BM from melanoma. CD74 positive myeloid cells were excluded from further analysis. **b** Immunofluorescent doublestaining indicating an overlap of CD74 and HLA class II in the majority of tumors. **c** Contingency table showing, that more than 50% of CD74 high tumors also showed high levels of HLA class II. **d**, **e** and (**f**) illustrating the association between CD74 expression and TILs in different BM entities

expression of these molecules is not prognostic for BM [16] and e.g. resected NSCLC [49], we investigated the association of PD-1/CD8 positive TILs as well as PD-L1 positive tumor cells with CD74 in BM. We only found a weak significant positive correlation between PD-L1 and CD74 in BM from melanoma (Table 1).

### CD74$^{high}$ and TIL$^{high}$ tumors show a differential methylation pattern in which genes associated with antigen processing and presentation are enriched among differentially methylated CpGs

To further assess heterogeneous CD74 expression patterns among the same tumor entity we investigated a potential epigenetic regulation of CD74 expression in BM. We investigated promoter-associated CpGs for hypo- or hypermethylation in 21 NSCLC BM. As expected, mean beta-values were rather low, as CD74 is strongly expressed by TAMs as previously shown [49]. Nevertheless, we detected significantly reduced beta-values in CD74$^{high}$ versus CD74$^{low}$ protein expressors (Fig. 3a), indicating a potential epigenetic regulation of CD74 expression in tumor cells from BM. We further asked whether there might be a differential methylation pattern between BM with a potential highly functional immune response, which we hypothetically defined as CD74$^{high}$ and TIL$^{high}$ tumors (CD74 TIL high) and tumors not showing both of these features (CD74 TIL low). Differential methylation analyses revealed 74 CpG sites being differentially methylated between both groups (Fig. 3b). Gene ontology enrichment analysis of differentially methylated CpGs of NSCLC BM showed a strong enrichment for processes of immune response and especially for antigen processing and presentation (Fig. 3c, d) (differentially methylated CpG sites are shown in Additional file 4: Table S1).

### CD74 is expressed in metastatic cell lines of different entities without showing a relevant surface expression

We assessed CD74 expression levels in tumor cell lines from different entities (H1 and H1_DL2 (brain seeking cell line from melanoma BM), SKMEL-2 (skin metastatic melanoma), SKMEL-28, UACC-257 (both melanoma), MDA-MB-231, Jimt1 (both brain seeking clones of pleural metastatic breast cancer), PC-14 (brain seeking clone of lung adenocarcinoma)). We were able to detect CD74 expression by immunocytochemistry notably in H1_DL2, SKMEL-2 and SKMEL-28, mildly in UACC-257 and MDA-MB-231 but not significantly present in Jimt1 and PC-14 (Fig. 4a) cells. H1 cells yielded similar results as H1_DL2 (data not shown). qRT-PCR showed highest RNA levels for H1_DL2 melanoma cells (Fig. 4b). Besides its role as an assembly and stabilization molecule during HLA class II processing, CD74 has also been described as a MIF receptor, acting on the cell membrane [26]. To further analyze whether CD74 was expressed on the cell membrane we performed FACS analysis of brain seeking human BM cell lines. Interestingly, we did not detect CD74 cell surface expression in unfixed H1 melanoma cells indicating a functional restriction to mainly intracellular compartments (Fig. 4c).

### CD74 knock-down may influence HLA class II-mediated antigen presentation by reducing the complexity of the HLA class II peptidome

CD74 expression appeared to be restricted to intracellular compartments of H1 brain seeking melanoma cells. CD74 expression is further associated with the presence of TILs. We thus hypothesized that CD74 may contribute to antigen processing and presentation in BM. We hence asked whether an siRNA-mediated knockdown of CD74 would affect the HLA class II processing machinery.

CD74 siRNA knockdown in H1 brain metastatic cells (Fig. 5a-d) did not influence HLA class II expression on protein level (Fig. 5a), transcriptional level (as assessed by TaqMan® array designed for the detection of the human antigen processing and presentation machinery by HLAs (Fig. 5f) corroborated by RNA-microarray (Fig. 5g)) nor did it influence HLA class II expression on the tumor cell surface as assessed by FACS analysis (Fig. 5e). Interestingly, none of the crucial HLA class I and II processing factors showed a significant regulation upon CD74 knockdown on transcriptional level (Fig. 5f).

As CD74 knockdown did neither alter the amount of HLA class II molecules nor affect central regulators of the HLA class I and II family on transcriptional level, we assessed whether a CD74 knockdown directly affects

**Table 1** Association between CD74 expression, PD-L1 expression and PD1/CD8-positive TILs in BM

| | PD1/CD8 all | PD1/CD8 NSCLC | PD1/CD8 melanoma | PD-L1 all | PD-L1 NSCLC | PD-L1 melanoma |
|---|---|---|---|---|---|---|
| CD74 all | ρ=0.0251<br>$p = 0.7184$ | | | ρ=0.0900<br>$p = 0.1815$ | | |
| CD74 NSCLC | | ρ=0.0190<br>$p = 0.8980$ | | | ρ=0.0793<br>$p = 0.5613$ | |
| CD74 melanoma | | | ρ=0.3947<br>$p = 0.5108$ | | | ρ=0.2912<br>$p = 0.0072$ |

Correlation analyses (Spearmen's ρ and corresponding *p*-values) between CD74 expression, PD-L1 and PD1/CD8-positive TILs in the total cohort of BM, melanoma BM and BM from NSCLC

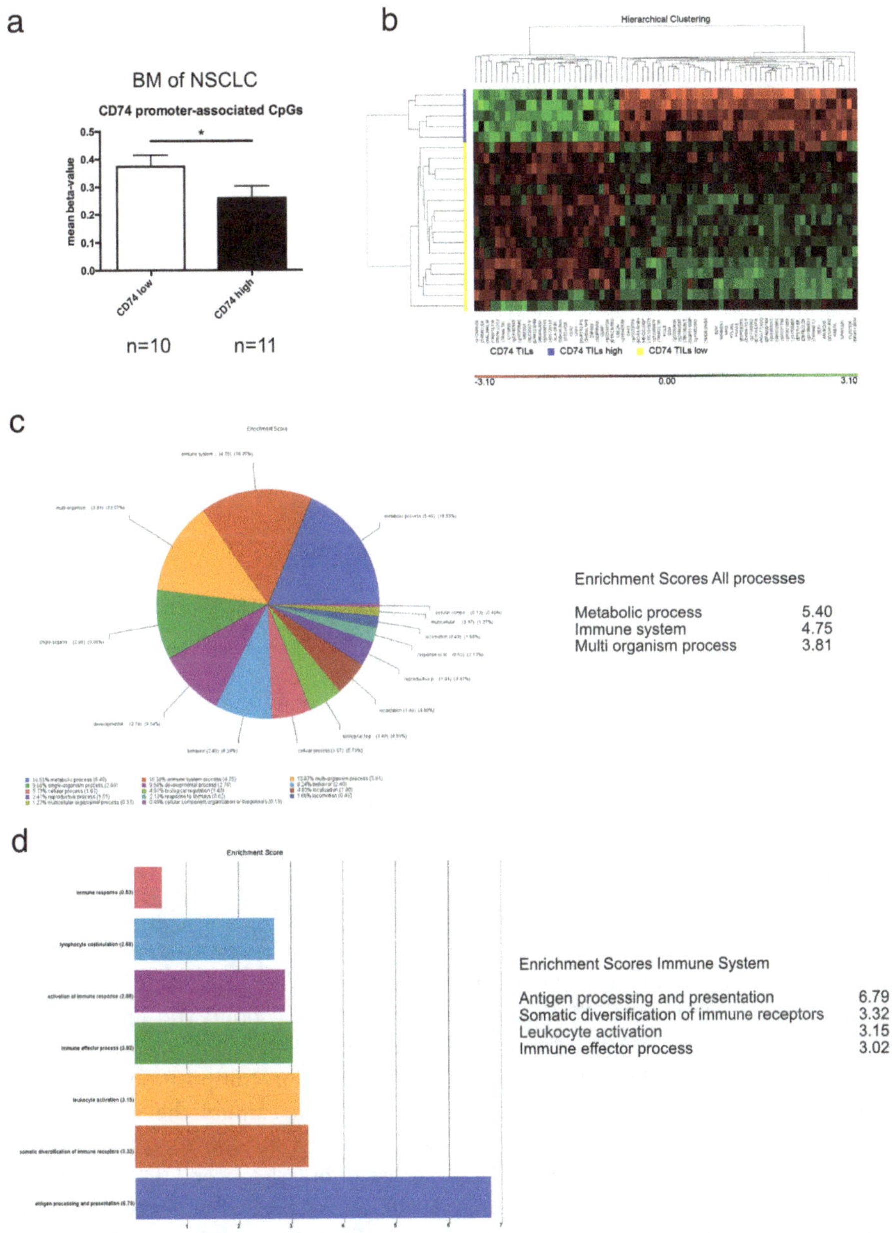


**Fig. 3** CD74 promoter methylation and whole DNA methylation patterns in NSCLC BM. **a** Mean beta-values of promoter-associated CpGs in 21 BM from NSCLC. CD74 low expressors are associated with significantly increased mean beta-values. **b** Differentially methylated CpGs of 21 BM from NSCLC, stratified by the combinatory parameters CD74 high + TILs high (CD74 TILs high, $n = 5$, blue) versus tumors not showing these combined features (CD74 TILs low, $n = 16$, yellow). Hierarchical cluster analysis showing 74 differentially methylated CpGs (M-values are shown, unadjusted $p$-value < 0.0001, Additional file 4: Table S1). **c** Gene ontology enrichment analysis of biological processes, (**d**) gene ontology enrichment analysis of Immune System processes

antigen presentation by altering the HLA class II peptidome composition. Label-free quantitation mass spectrometry of the HLA peptidome of H1 brain metastatic tumor cells suggests that the overall amount of class II peptides - approximated by the summed signal intensity of all peptide identifications – does not substantially differ between control and CD74 knockdown condition (Fig. 6a). The number of unique class II peptide identifications on the other hand was reduced by 47% in CD74 siRNA treated H1 cells compared to control indicating a reduced complexity of the class II peptidome (Fig. 6b), whereas HLA class I peptidome composition was not affected (data not shown). Volcano plot analysis of differential source protein presentation in the class II peptidome (Fig. 6c) revealed 52/781 (6.7%) source proteins to be significantly overrepresented (≥2 average

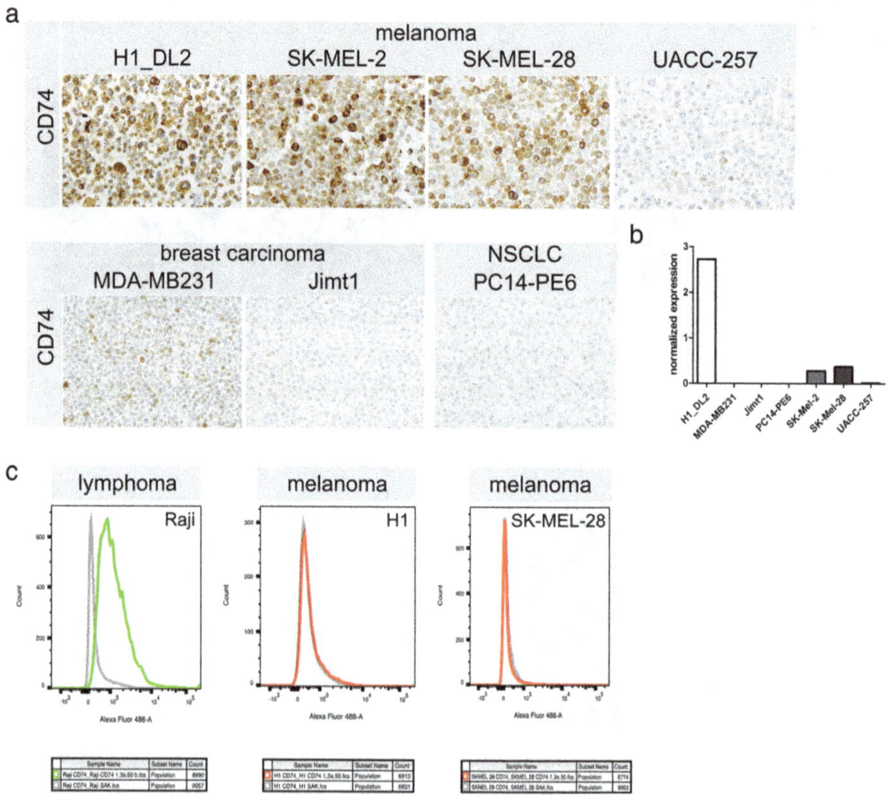


**Fig. 4** CD74 expression in vitro using brain seeking BM cell lines. **a** Immunocytochemistry against CD74 in different brain seeking human BM cell lines. **b** Normalized results of CD74 transcript expression using qPCR. H1 and H1_DL2 cell line showed similar results, both on protein and transcript level (data not shown). **c** FACS analyses of unfixed cell lines. Positive control cell line Raji showing CD74 expression on the cell surface, while H1 and SK-MEL-28 cell lines don't show CD74 on the cell surface

fold-change in LFQ signal intensity of corresponding class II peptides, avg. $p$-value≤0.01) on CD74 siRNA treated H1 cells, whereas 101/781 (12.9%) showed down-modulation. Functional Annotation Clustering revealed molecules of cell signaling pathways, of the lysosomal and of the ribosomal compartment as main down-regulated HLA class II ligands upon CD74 knockdown (Fig. 6d). Interestingly, most upregulated ligands upon CD74 knockdown were found in the group of ribosomal proteins as well as rRNA binding molecules, where to date relatively few neoantigens have been found [14].

## Discussion and conclusions

BM are the most frequent CNS tumors and constitute a fatal disease, which is often accompanied with a short disease interval and high patients' disability. Still, therapeutic strategies are limited and include whole brain radiotherapy (WBRT), stereotactic irradiation (SI), surgery, chemotherapy (CTX) or a combination of different approaches.

In recent years immunomodulatory therapeutic strategies mainly targeting immune checkpoints led to a considerable improvement of patient survival and quality of life and have therefore been rapidly approved for therapy in different cancer entities [38]. These drugs re-invigorate an exhausted lymphocytic immune response against the tumor cells. Thus, a successful response strongly depends on the cellular composition of the microenvironment. In peripheral tumors the composition of lymphocytic infiltration is a well accepted prognostic marker and in case of breast cancer TILs have already reached the status of an established biomarker [17]. In CNS tumors and especially BM the relevance of the mere amount of TILs is however still controversial and might not be a sufficient prognostic tool [5, 16].

In the present study, we showed that CD74 expression in tumor cells, a major assembly and stabilization molecule of the HLA class II machinery, is a strong prognostic factor for BM patients. In contrast to peripheral metastases we observed this prognostic value in the cohort of all investigated BM and in the subcohorts of NSCLC and melanoma BM. This indicates a specific role for CD74 functionality in the microenvironment of BM. Interestingly, CD74 expression has been described to be prognostic in particular subcohorts of peripheral tumors such as basal like and triple negative breast cancer, but not in the total investigated cohort in these studies [11, 54]

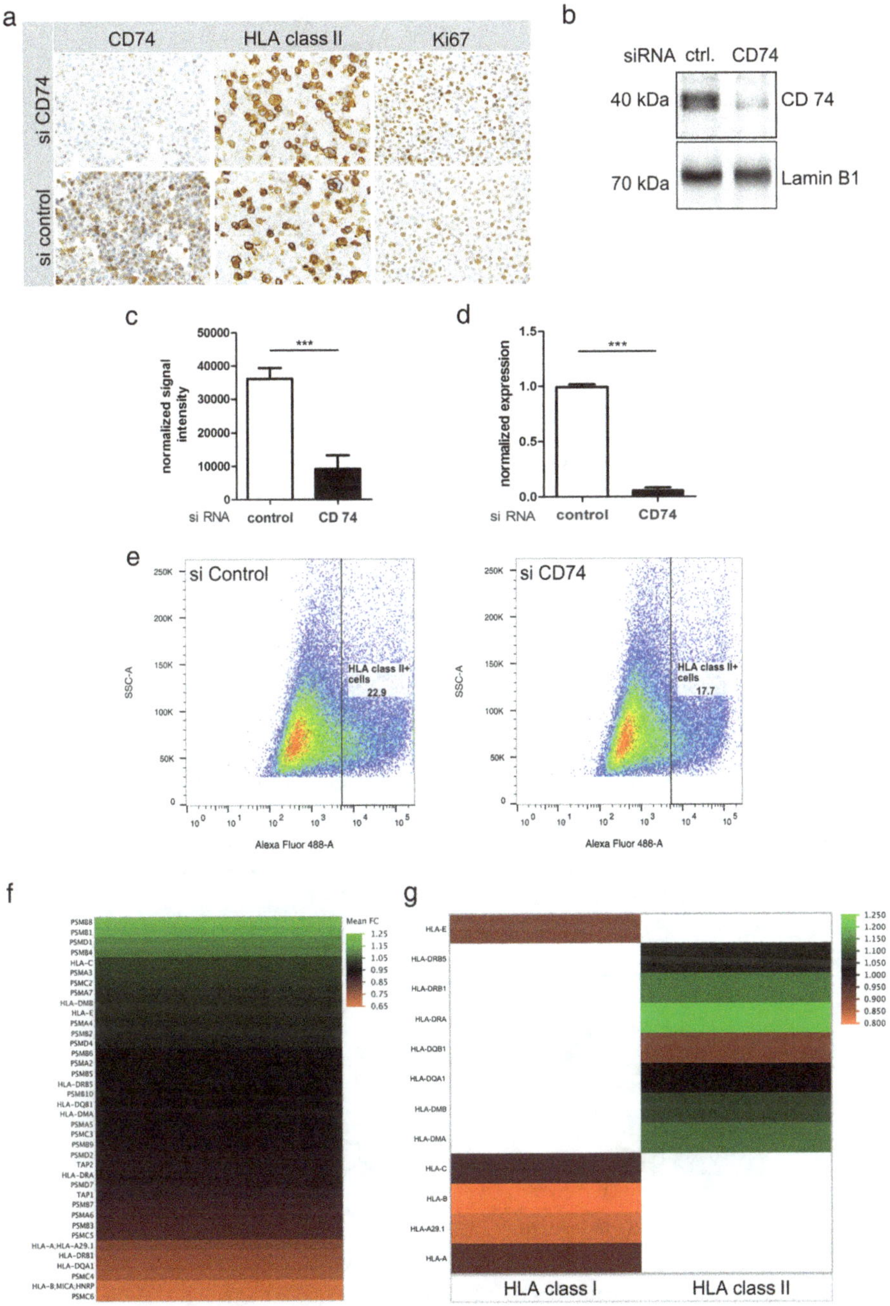


**Fig. 5** The influence of CD74 siRNA mediated knockdown on HLA class I and II machinery in H1 brain metastatic melanoma cells. **a** Immunocytochemistry of H1 melanoma cells against CD74, HLA class II molecules and Ki67. **b + c** Western blot analysis of siRNA-mediated CD74 knock-down versus siRNA-control with (**c**) protein quantification normalized against Lamin B1. **d** qRT-PCR analysis of siRNA-mediated CD74 knock-down versus control. **e** FACS analyses against HLA class II molecules on H1 melanoma cells. Differential transcript expression of H1 siRNA CD74 versus control siRNA (**f**, **g**). **f** TaqMan® array focusing on the transcriptome of the human antigen processing and presentation machinery by HLAs, (**g**) excerpt of micro-array data with regard to HLA class I and II transcripts

indicating, that there might be a more global genetic or epigenetic regulatory event. In line with the heterogeneous CD74 expression levels among the same tumor entity, we found CD74 promoter methylation to be associated with low CD74 protein expression in NSCLC BM, indicating an epigenetic regulatory event in these tumors. Rather low apparent levels of promoter methylation in these tumors can be explained by CD74 expression not being restricted to tumor cells. Instead CD74 is a major member of the HLA class II machinery which is highly expressed by antigen presenting cells such as TAMs [57]. A total CD74 promoter methylation in tumor tissue is therefore most

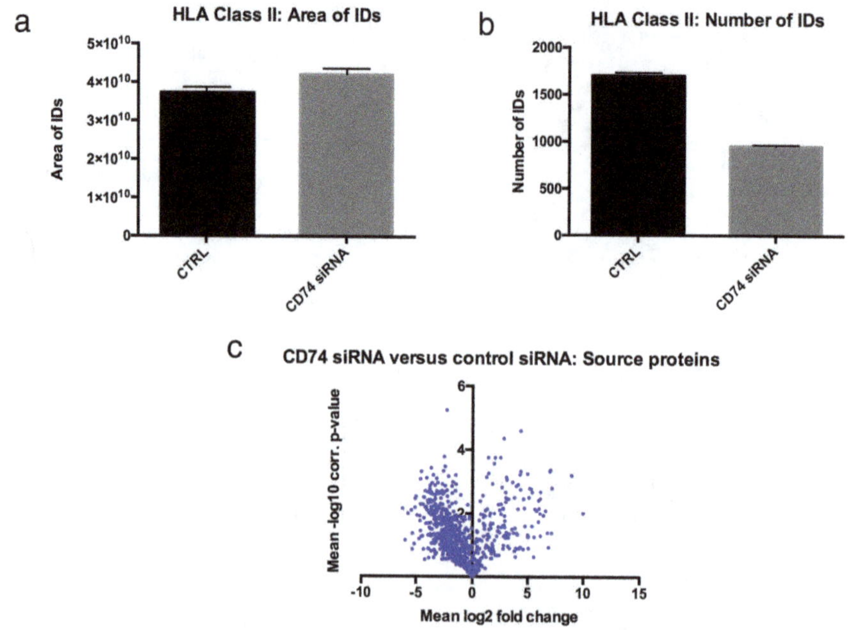


d

| DAVID Functional Annotation Clustering HLA class II peptidome | | | | |
|---|---|---|---|---|
| Annotation Cluster | Downregulated ligands | ES | Upregulated ligands | ES |
| 1 | Cell signaling | 10.2* | Ribosome/Translation | 12.3* |
| 2 | Lysosome | 8.5* | Ribosomal ribonucleic acid (rRNA) binding | 3.3* |
| 3 | Ribosome/Translation | 4.8* | Endoplasmic reticulum | 2.1* |
| 4 | Cell adhesion | 4.4* | mRNA processing | 1.6 |
| 5 | Endoplasmic reticulum/Protein processing | 4.3* | Neurodegeneration | 1.3 |

Abbreviations: ES = Enrichment Score, * ES > 2.0

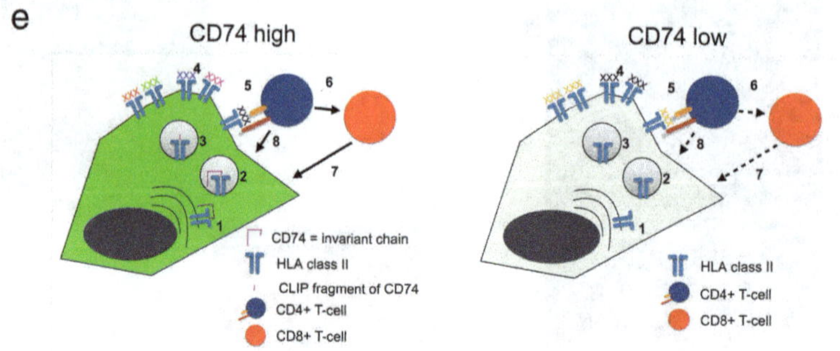


**Fig. 6** Effects of siRNA mediated CD74 knockdown on the HLA class II peptidome of H1 brain metastatic melanoma cells. **a** Summed MS1 intensities and (**b**) Number of identifications of HLA class II ligands in label-free quantitation mass spectrometry (error bars represent standard error of the mean (SEM). **c** Volcano plot of differentially presented source proteins in CD74 knockdown vs control (**d**) DAVID Functional Annotation Clustering of differentially represented HLA class II source proteins. **e** Schematic illustration of CD74 functions (left) and consequences of CD74 knockdown/downregulation (right) in brain metastatic tumor cells. 1: HLA class II and invariant chain complex in the endoplasmic reticulum and Golgi apparatus, 2: HLA class II compartment, 3: Processing of invariant chain by proteases, CLIP fragment remains and is exchanged for an antigenic peptide, 4: Complex antigens are expressed on the tumor cell surface when CD74 is highly expressed, 5: Tumor cell - CD4-positive lymphocyte interaction, 6: Recruitment of CD8-positive T-cells, 7: direct lysis by CD8 or 8: CD4-positive cells. Dotted lines illustrate impaired tumor cell – lymphocyte interactions. XXX denote HLA class II ligands. Multiple colors of ligands denote high peptidome complexity

unlikely. Interestingly, CD74 and HLA class II expression have been shown to be reactivated upon treatment of ovarian cancer cells with histone deacetylase and DNA methyltransferase inhibitors, which in turn lead to a reduced tumor growth in an experimental in vivo model [50]. The underlying mechanisms of this favorable reactivation of HLA class II members as well as downstream effects still remain unclear. Epigenetic regulation of the HLA class II machinery by class II transactivator protein (CIITA) has been described in various cancer cell lines. Methylation of CIITA promoter IV seems to reduce interferone-gamma-inducible HLA-DR expression on cancer cells [36, 44, 56]. Moreover, about 3% of the HLA ligandome was recently found to be detectable both on HLA class I and II. Processing of such peptides detected on both class I and class II was proposed to require the cellular class II presentation machinery [32], implicating that a loss of CD74 expression could also affect presentation of neoantigens on HLA class I.

In our current study, we found CD74 tumor cell expression to be associated with the frequency of TILs. Nevertheless the mere amount of TILs and subsets (including PD-1-positive TILs) has not been prognostic for BM patients in one of our previous studies [16]. Unlike CD74 expression, the mere HLA class II expression was also not prognostic in our investigated BM cohorts (Additional file 2: Figure S2), although (similar to CD74) HLA class II expression is considered as a potential prognostic factor for some peripheral cancer entities like ovarian cancer or triple negative and basal like breast cancer in the aforementioned studies [11, 54]. Interestingly, we found a significantly reduced expression of HLA class II molecules in BM as compared to their primary tumors, raising the question whether the mere amount of HLA class II molecules on tumor cells might be limiting for a functional immune response in the microenvironment of BM. However, immune responses do not only depend on the available antigen-presenting molecules. Instead, the quality or complexity of the presented HLA peptidome is also crucial for an adequate immune response.

Our results suggest, that upon CD74 knockdown in a brain metastatic melanoma cell line the complexity of the HLA class II peptidome was strongly reduced, while the mere amount of HLA class II molecules did not appear to vary between knockdown and control condition, nor did we observe significant changes of HLA class I and II transcripts upon CD74 knockdown. This suggests that CD74 directly influences the diversity of the HLA class II peptidome on tumor cells. The prognostic significance of CD74 hence suggests that the complexity of the HLA class II peptidome might be critical for a functional HLA class II dependent immune response in BM. However, while the search for tumor-specific antigens has prompted thorough investigations of the HLA class I peptidome, the HLA class II peptidome of cancer cells has only been explored in much lesser detail, which may be due to the old and grossly oversimplified concept that endogenous antigens are presented on HLA class I while HLA class II would mainly present exogenous antigens. Nevertheless, previous studies already identified HLA class II dependent cancer-specific phosphopeptides which could become targets for immunotherapy. Likewise, a recent study identified cancer specific antigens on HLA class I and II molecules even in low mutated tumors such as ovarian carcinomas [10, 39]. In fact, only about 20% of antigens presented on HLA class II seem to derive from exogenous sources incorporated by endocytosis, while the remainder consists of endogenous proteins from plasma, lysosomal or endosomal membraneous compartments, and to a minor extent also from the cytoplasm, nucleus and golgi apparatus [42]. Interestingly, upon CD74 knockdown in melanoma brain metastatic cells we observed a significantly decreased presentation of HLA class II source proteins belonging to cell signaling pathways and the lysosomal compartment, while ribosomal sources were upregulated. Whether these downregulated peptides are the crucial peptides responsible for an anti-tumor response in CD74 high expressing tumors remains an open question which should be addressed in future studies.

Since different cancer entities show different biological behavior especially with regard to CD74 expression and its function, there is no universal answer whether CD74 is mainly associated with aggressiveness or positive prognosis. Here we could demonstrate that BM with high CD74 expression show a better clinical course. Although we investigated a fair number of samples (especially in our largest subgroup of melanoma BM patients), our patient cohorts are still limited especially regarding subgroups of other cancer entities. Thus, results of survival analyses of subgroups should be confirmed in larger subcohorts of future studies. Furthermore, we show that this expression might be epigenetically regulated via CD74 promoter methylation at least in BM deriving from NSCLC. Additional studies in other BM entities would be reasonable and a potential association of a differential whole DNA methylation pattern with a functional immune response should be target of future studies. On a functional level we showed that CD74 regulates tumor cell HLA class II immune peptidome complexity, which may be a central immunological event for a clinically relevant HLA class II restricted anti-tumor response in BM. To answer this question properly, the exact role of CD74 in tumor cells for functional immune responses including the impact on the function of different effector cell subsets like TILs and NK-cells has to be addressed in detail in additional studies. HLA class II peptidome analyses in patient samples of $CD74^{high}$ versus $CD74^{low}$ expressors are likewise highly relevant and unfortunately a technical limitation of the current study. Moreover, given that recent studies point out the importance of an unimpaired antigen-processing machinery for a successful immunotherapy response [35] CD74 in cancer cells should also be explored as a putative predictive marker for immunotherapies.

## Additional files

**Additional file 1: Figure S1.** Clinical data of the different BM cohorts and association of CD74 expression with clinical parameters. Correlation analyses were performed using Spearmen's correlation analyses (Spearmen's ρ and corresponding *p*-values are depicted). (JPEG 1333 kb)

**Additional file 2: Figure S2.** CD74 expression in different stages of melanoma (a, b) and NSCLC (c). Matched-pairs analysis of primary tumors and BM (different primary tumor entities) (d). (JPEG 1243 kb)

**Additional file 3: Figure S3.** (a) HLA class II dependent Kaplan-Meier survival analyses in the total BM cohort as well as in the two largest subcohorts of NSCLC and melanoma. (b) Matched-pairs analysis of primary tumors and BM (different primary tumor entities). (JPEG 2138 kb)

**Additional file 4: Table S1.** Table showing differentially methylated CpGs between BM of NSCLC with a highly functional immune response, defined as $CD74^{high}$ and $TIL^{high}$ tumors (CD74 TIL high) and tumors not showing both of these features (CD74 TIL low). (CSV 1 kb)

**Acknowledgments**
MM would like to thank the Luxembourg National Research Fond (FNR) for the support (FNR PEARL P16/BM/11192868 grant).

**Authors' contributions**

PSZ performed in vitro as well as in vivo experiments using cell culture and paraffin-embedded tissue, analyzed data, wrote the manuscript and was involved in the study design and conception. JZ performed in vitro as well as in vivo experiments using cell lines and paraffin-embedded tissue, analyzed data, wrote the manuscript and was involved in the study design and conception. DJK carried out HLA peptidome analyses, wrote the manuscript and was involved in the study design. SB performed in vivo analyses on tissue microarrays. JT and MWR provided clinical data and performed image analyses. FT and AB performed cell line characterizations. MTF provided tissue and clinical data. AM performed bioinformatic analyses. JPS provided and analyzed clinical data. RB analyzed tissue specimens and provided clinical data. JW wrote the manuscript and was involved in study design and conception. HMK analyzed tissue specimens and provided clinical data. KHP analyzed tissue specimens, provided equipment and wrote the manuscript. SS provided equipment and analyzed HLA peptidome data. BW provided clinical data, performed human data analyses and was involved in study design and conception. MM analyzed human data, wrote the manuscript and was involved in study design and conception. PNH supervised and conceived the study, performed in vivo and in vitro analyses and wrote the manuscript. All authors read and approved the final manuscript.

**Competing interests**

The authors declare that they have no conflict of interest.

**Author details**
[1]Edinger Institute (Institute of Neurology), Goethe-University, Heinrich-Hoffmann-Str. 7, D-60528 Frankfurt am Main, Germany. [2]Dr. Senckenberg Institute of Neurooncology, Goethe-University, Frankfurt am Main, Germany. [3]Department of Immunology, Institute for Cell Biology, University of Tuebingen, Tuebingen, Germany. [4]Immatics Biotechnologies GmbH, Tübingen, Germany. [5]Department of Biomedicine, The Kristian Gerhard Jebsen Brain Tumour Research Center and The Molecular Imaging Center, University of Bergen, Bergen, Norway. [6]Institute for Virology, Goethe-University, Frankfurt am Main, Germany. [7]Department of Neurosurgery, Goethe-University, Frankfurt am Main, Germany. [8]Department of Oncology, Luxembourg Institute of Health, Luxembourg, Luxembourg. [9]German Cancer Research Center DKFZ Heidelberg, Germany and German Cancer Consortium DKTK partner site, Frankfurt/Mainz, Germany. [10]Department of Pathology and Neuropathology, University of Tuebingen, Tuebingen, Germany. [11]Department of Gynecology, University of Wuerzburg, Wuerzburg, Germany. [12]Goethe-University, Dr. Senckenberg Institute for Pathology, Frankfurt am Main, Germany. [13]Department of Dermatology, University of Tuebingen, Tuebingen, Germany. [14]Luxembourg Centre of Neuropathology (LCNP), 3555 Dudelange, Luxembourg. [15]Laboratoire National de Santé, Department of Pathology, 3555 Dudelange, Luxembourg. [16]Luxembourg Centre for Systems Biomedicine (LCSB), University of Luxembourg, 4361 Esch-sur-Alzette, Luxembourg. [17]NORLUX Neuro-Oncology Laboratory, Department of Oncology, Luxembourg Institute of Health (L.I.H.), 1526 Luxembourg, Luxembourg.

**References**

1. Ahrends T, Spanjaard A, Pilzecker B, Bąbała N, Bovens A, Xiao Y, Jacobs H, Borst J (2017) CD4+T cell help confers a cytotoxic T cell effector program including Coinhibitory receptor downregulation and increased tissue invasiveness. Immunity 47:848–861.e5. https://doi.org/10.1016/j.immuni.2017.10.009
2. Alexandrov LB, Nik-Zainal S, Wedge DC, Aparicio SAJR, Behjati S, Biankin AV, Bignell GR, Bolli N, Borg A, Børresen-Dale AL, Boyault S, Burkhardt B, Butler AP, Caldas C, Davies HR, Desmedt C, Eils R, Eyfjörd JE, Foekens JA, Greaves M, Hosoda F, Hutter B, Ilicic T, Imbeaud S, Imielinsk M, Jäger N, Jones DTW, Jonas D, Knappskog S, Koo M, Lakhani SR, López-Otín C, Martin S, Munshi NC, Nakamura H, Northcott PA, Pajic M, Papaemmanuil E, Paradiso A, Pearson JV, Puente XS, Raine K, Ramakrishna M, Richardson AL, Richter J, Rosenstiel P, Schlesner M, Schumacher TN, Span PN, Teague JW, Totoki Y, Tutt ANJ, Valdés-Mas R, Van Buuren MM, van 't Veer L, Vincent-Salomon A, Waddell N, Yates LR, Zucman-Rossi J, Andrew Futreal P, McDermott U, Lichter P, Meyerson M, Grimmond SM, Siebert R, Campo E, Shibata T, Pfister SM, Campbell PJ, Stratton MR (2013) Signatures of mutational processes in human cancer. Nature 500:415–421. https://doi.org/10.1038/nature12477
3. Barnholtz-Sloan JS, Sloan AE, Davis FG, Vigneau FD, Lai P, Sawaya RE (2004) Incidence proportions of brain metastases in patients diagnosed (1973 to 2001) in the metropolitan Detroit cancer surveillance system. J Clin Oncol 22:2865–2872. https://doi.org/10.1200/JCO.2004.12.149
4. Basha G, Omilusik K, Chavez-Steenbock A, Reinicke AT, Lack N, Choi KB, Jefferies WA (2012) A CD74-dependent MHC class I endolysosomal cross-presentation pathway. Nat Immunol 13:237–245. https://doi.org/10.1038/ni.2225
5. Berghoff AS, Ricken G, Widhalm G, Rajky O, Dieckmann K, Birner P, Bartsch R, Höller C, Preusser M (2015) Tumour-infiltrating lymphocytes and expression of programmed death ligand 1 (PD-L1) in melanoma brain metastases. Histopathology 66:289–299. https://doi.org/10.1111/his.12537
6. Burton JD, Ely S, Reddy PK, Stein R, Gold DV, Cardillo TM, Goldenberg DM (2004) CD74 is expressed by multiple myeloma and is a promising target for therapy. Clin Cancer Res 10:6606–6611. https://doi.org/10.1158/1078-0432.CCR-04-0182
7. Chamuleau MED, Souwer Y, Van Ham SM, Zevenbergen A, Westers TM, Berkhof J, Meijer CJ, Van De Loosdrecht AA, Ossenkoppele GJ (2004) Class II-associated invariant chain peptide expression on myeloid leukemic blasts predicts poor clinical outcome. Cancer Res 64:5546–5550. https://doi.org/10.1158/0008-5472.CAN-04-1350
8. Concha A, Ruiz-Cabello F, Cabrera T, Nogales F, Collado A, Garrido F (1995) Different patterns of HLA-DR antigen expression in normal epithelium, hyperplastic and neoplastic malignant lesions of the breast. Int J Immunogenet 22:299–310. https://doi.org/10.1111/j.1744-313X.1995.tb00246.x
9. Cuthbert RJ, Wilson JM, Scott N, Coletta PL, Hull MA (2009) Differential CD74 (major histocompatibility complex class II invariant chain) expression in mouse and human intestinal adenomas. Eur J Cancer 45:1654–1663. https://doi.org/10.1016/j.ejca.2009.02.005
10. Depontieu FR, Qian J, Zarling AL, McMiller TL, Salay TM, Norris A, English AM, Shabanowitz J, Engelhard VH, Hunt DF, Topalian SL (2009) Identification of tumor-associated, MHC class II-restricted phosphopeptides as targets for immunotherapy. Proc Natl Acad Sci U S A 106:12073–12078. https://doi.org/10.1073/pnas.0903852106

11. Forero A, Li Y, Chen D, Grizzle WE, Updike KL, Merz ND, Downs-Kelly E, Burwell TC, Vaklavas C, Buchsbaum DJ, Myers RM, LoBuglio AF, Varley KE (2016) Expression of the MHC class II pathway in triple-negative breast cancer tumor cells is associated with a good prognosis and infiltrating lymphocytes. Cancer Immunol Res:1–11. https://doi.org/10.1158/2326-6066.CIR-15-0243
12. Frenard C, Peuvrel L, Jean MS, Brocard A, Knol AC, Nguyen JM, Khammari A, Quereux G, Dreno B (2016) Development of brain metastases in patients with metastatic melanoma while receiving ipilimumab. J Neuro-Oncol 126: 355–360. https://doi.org/10.1007/s11060-015-1977-9
13. Gettinger SN, Horn L, Gandhi L, Spigel DR, Antonia SJ, Rizvi NA, Powderly JD, Heist RS, Carvajal RD, Jackman DM, Sequist LV, Smith DC, Leming P, Carbone DP, Pinder-Schenck MC, Topalian SL, Hodi FS, Sosman JA, Sznol M, McDermott DF, Pardoll DM, Sankar V, Ahlers CM, Salvati M, Wigginton JM, Hellmann MD, Kollia GD, Gupta AK, Brahmer JR (2015) Overall survival and long-term safety of nivolumab (anti-programmed death 1 antibody, BMS-936558, ONO-4538) in patients with previously treated advanced non-small-cell lung cancer. J Clin Oncol 33:2004–2012. https://doi.org/10.1200/JCO.2014.58.3708
14. Goudarzi KM, Lindström MS (2016) Role of ribosomal protein mutations in tumor development (review). Int J Oncol 48:1313–1324. https://doi.org/10.3892/ijo.2016.3387
15. Hannus M, Beitzinger M, Engelmann JC, Weickert MT, Spang R, Hannus S, Meister G (2014) SiPools: highly complex but accurately defined siRNA pools eliminate off-target effects. Nucleic Acids Res 42:8049–8061. https://doi.org/10.1093/nar/gku480
16. Harter PN, Bernatz S, Scholz A, Zeiner PS, Zinke J, Kiyose M, Blasel S, Beschorner R, Senft C, Bender B, Ronellenfitsch MW, Wikman H, Glatzel M, Meinhardt M, Juratli TA, Steinbach JP, Plate KH, Wischhusen J, Weide B, Mittelbronn M (2015) Distribution and prognostic relevance of tumor-infiltrating lymphocytes (TILs) and PD-1/PD-L1 immune checkpoints in human brain metastases. Oncotarget 6:40836–40849. https://doi.org/10.18632/oncotarget.5696
17. Hendry S, Salgado R, Gevaert T, Russell PA, John T, Thapa B, Christie M, van de Vijver K, Estrada MV, Gonzalez-Ericsson PI, Sanders M, Solomon B, Solinas C, Van den Eynden GGGM, Allory Y, Preusser M, Hainfellner J, Pruneri G, Vingiani A, Demaria S, Symmans F, Nuciforo P, Comerma L, Thompson EA, Lakhani S, Kim S-R, Schnitt S, Colpaert C, Sotiriou C, Scherer SJ, Ignatiadis M, Badve S, Pierce RH, Viale G, Sirtaine N, Penault-Llorca F, Sugie T, Fineberg S, Paik S, Srinivasan A, Richardson A, Wang Y, Chmielik E, Brock J, Johnson DB, Balko J, Wienert S, Bossuyt V, Michiels S, Ternes N, Burchardi N, Luen SJ, Savas P, Klauschen F, Watson PH, Nelson BH, Criscitiello C, O'Toole S, Larsimont D, de Wind R, Curigliano G, André F, Lacroix-Triki M, van de Vijver M, Rojo F, Floris G, Bedri S, Sparano J, Rimm D, Nielsen T, Kos Z, Hewitt S, Singh B, Farshid G, Loibl S, Allison KH, Tung N, Adams S, Willard-Gallo K, Horlings HM, Gandhi L, Moreira A, Hirsch F, Dieci MV, Urbanowicz M, Brcic I, Korski K, Gaire F, Koeppen H, Lo A, Giltnane J, Rebelatto MC, Steele KE, Zha J, Emancipator K, Juco JW, Denkert C, Reis-Filho J, Loi S, Fox SB (2017) Assessing tumor-infiltrating lymphocytes in solid tumors: a practical review for pathologists and proposal for a standardized method from the international Immuno-oncology biomarkers working group: part 2: TILs in melanoma, gastrointestinal tract carcinomas, non-small cell lung carcinoma and mesothelioma, endometrial and ovarian carcinomas, squamous cell carcinoma of the head and neck, genitourinary carcinomas, and primary brain tumors. Adv Anat Pathol doi. https://doi.org/10.1097/PAP.0000000000000161
18. Ilina EI, Armento A, Sanchez LG, Reichlmeir M, Braun Y, Penski C, Capper D, Sahm F, Jennewein L, Harter PN, Zukunft S, Fleming I, Schulte D, Le F, Behrends C, Ronellenfitsch MW, Naumann U, Mittelbronn M (2017) Effects of soluble CPE on glioma cell migration are associated with mTOR activation and enhanced glucose flux. Oncotarget. https://doi.org/10.18632/oncotarget.18747
19. Käll L, Canterbury JD, Weston J, Noble WS, MacCoss MJ (2007) Semi-supervised learning for peptide identification from shotgun proteomics datasets. Nat Methods 4:923–925. https://doi.org/10.1038/nmeth1113
20. Koide N, Yamada T, Shibata R, Mori T, Fukuma M, Yamazaki K, Aiura K, Shimazu M, Hirohashi S, Nimura Y, Sakamoto M (2006) Establishment of perineural invasion models and analysis of gene expression revealed an invariant chain (CD74) as a possible molecule involved in perineural invasion in pancreatic cancer. Clin Cancer Res 12:2419–2426. https://doi.org/10.1158/1078-0432.CCR-05-1852
21. Kowalewski DJ, Stefanović S (2013) Biochemical large-scale identification of MHC class I ligands. Methods Mol Biol 960:145–157. https://doi.org/10.1007/978-1-62703-218-6_12
22. Kreiter S, Vormehr M, van de Roemer N, Diken M, Löwer M, Diekmann J, Boegel S, Schrörs B, Vascotto F, Castle JC, Tadmor AD, Schoenberger SP, Huber C, Türeci Ö, Sahin U (2015) Mutant MHC class II epitopes drive therapeutic immune responses to cancer. Nature 520:692–696. https://doi.org/10.1038/nature14426
23. Kunihiro M, Tanaka S, Haruma K, Yoshihara M, Sumii K, Kajiyama G, Shimamoto F (1998) Combined expression of HLA-DR antigen and proliferating cell nuclear antigen correlate with colorectal cancer prognosis. Oncology 55:326–333. https://doi.org/10.1159/000011870
24. Lazzaro B, Anderson AE, Kajdacsy-Balla A, Hessner MJ (2001) Antigenic characterization of medullary carcinoma of the breast: HLA-DR expression in lymph node positive cases. Appl Immunohistochem Mol Morphol 9:234–241
25. Le DT, Uram JN, Wang H, Bartlett BR, Kemberling H, Eyring AD, Skora AD, Luber BS, Azad NS, Laheru D, Biedrzycki B, Donehower RC, Zaheer A, Fisher GA, Crocenzi TS, Lee JJ, Duffy SM, Goldberg RM, de la Chapelle A, Koshiji M, Bhaijee F, Huebner T, Hruban RH, Wood LD, Cuka N, Pardoll DM, Papadopoulos N, Kinzler KW, Zhou S, Cornish TC, Taube JM, Anders RA, Eshleman JR, Vogelstein B, Diaz LA (2015) PD-1 blockade in tumors with mismatch-repair deficiency. N Engl J Med 372:2509–2520. https://doi.org/10.1056/NEJMoa1500596
26. Leng L, Metz CN, Fang Y, Xu J, Donnelly S, Baugh J, Delohery T, Chen Y, Mitchell RA, Bucala R (2003) MIF signal transduction initiated by binding to CD74. J Exp Med 197:1467–1476. https://doi.org/10.1084/jem.20030286
27. Maharshak N, Cohen S, Lantner F, Hart G, Leng L, Bucala R, Shachar I (2010) CD74 is a survival receptor on colon epithelial cells. World J Gastroenterol 16:3258–2366. https://doi.org/10.3748/wjg.v16.i26.3258
28. McClelland M, Zhao L, Carskadon S, Arenberg D (2009) Expression of CD74, the receptor for macrophage migration inhibitory factor, in non-small cell lung cancer. Am J Pathol 174:638–646. https://doi.org/10.2353/ajpath.2009.080463
29. McGranahan N, Rosenthal R, Hiley CT, Rowan AJ, Watkins TBK, Wilson GA, Birkbak NJ, Veeriah S, Van Loo P, Herrero J, Swanton C (2017) Allele-specific HLA loss and immune escape in lung cancer evolution. Cell. https://doi.org/10.1016/j.cell.2017.10.001
30. Moretti S, Pinzi C, Berti E, Spallanzani A, Chiarugi A, Boddi V, Reali UM, Giannotti B (1997) In situ expression of transforming growth factor beta is associated with melanoma progression and correlates with Ki67, HLA-DR and beta 3 integrin expression. Melanoma Res 7:313–321
31. Morita M, Tanaka K, Kawanishi H, Tsuji M, Ookusa T, Takada H, Okamura A, Hioki K (1995) Immunohistochemically demonstrated expression of HLA-DR antigen in colorectal adenocarcinomas and its relation to clinicopathological features. J Surg Oncol 59:233–238. https://doi.org/10.1002/jso.2930590407
32. Müller M, Gfeller D, Coukos G, Bassani-Sternberg M (2017) "Hotspots" of antigen presentation revealed by human leukocyte antigen ligandomics for neoantigen prioritization. Front Immunol. https://doi.org/10.3389/fimmu.2017.01367
33. Nagata S, Jin YF, Yoshizato K, Tomoeda M, Song M, Iizuka N, Kitamura M, Takahashi H, Eguchi H, Ohigashi H, Ishikawa O, Tomita Y (2009) CD74 is a novel prognostic factor for patients with pancreatic cancer receiving multimodal therapy. Ann Surg Oncol 16:2531–2538. https://doi.org/10.1245/s10434-009-0532-3
34. Parakh S, Park JJ, Mendis S, Rai R, Xu W, Lo S, Drummond M, Rowe C, Wong A, Mcarthur G, Haydon A, Andrews MC, Cebon J, Guminski A, Kefford RF, Long GV, Menzies AM, Klein O, Carlino MS (2017) Efficacy of anti-PD-1 therapy in patients with melanoma brain metastases. Br J Cancer 116:1558–1563. https://doi.org/10.1038/bjc.2017.142
35. Patel SJ, Sanjana NE, Kishton RJ, Eidizadeh A, Vodnala SK, Cam M, Gartner JJ, Jia L, Steinberg SM, Yamamoto TN, Merchant AS, Mehta GU, Chichura A, Shalem O, Tran E, Eil R, Sukumar M, Guijarro EP, Day CP, Robbins P, Feldman S, Merlino G, Zhang F, Restifo NP (2017) Identification of essential genes for cancer immunotherapy. Nature. https://doi.org/10.1038/nature23477
36. Reith W, LeibundGut-Landmann S, Waldburger JM (2005) Regulation of MHC class II gene expression by the class II transactivator. Nat Rev Immunol 5:793–806. https://doi.org/10.1038/nri1708
37. Robert C, Schachter J, Long GV, Arance A, Grob JJ, Mortier L, Daud A, Carlino MS, McNeil C, Lotem M, Larkin J, Lorigan P, Neyns B, Blank CU, Hamid O, Mateus C, Shapira-Frommer R, Kosh M, Zhou H, Ibrahim N, Ebbinghaus S, Ribas A (2015) Pembrolizumab versus Ipilimumab in Advanced Melanoma. N Engl J Med 372:150419053123009. https://doi.org/10.1056/NEJMoa1503093
38. Rotte A, Jin JY, Lemaire V (2017) Mechanistic overview of immune checkpoints to support the rational design of their combinations in cancer immunotherapy. Ann Oncol:1–13. https://doi.org/10.1093/annonc/mdx686

39. Schuster H, Peper JK, Bösmüller HC, Röhle K, Backert L, Bilich T, Ney B, Löffler MW, Kowalewski DJ, Trautwein N, Rabsteyn A, Engler T, Braun S, Haen SP, Walz JS, Schmid-Horch B, Brucker SY, Wallwiener D, Kohlbacher O, Fend F, Rammensee H-G, Stefanović S, Staebler A, Wagner P (2017) The immunopeptidomic landscape of ovarian carcinomas. Proc Natl Acad Sci 201707658. https://doi.org/10.1073/pnas.1707658114
40. Sconocchia G, Eppenberger-Castori S, Zlobec I, Karamitopoulou E, Arriga R, Coppola A, Caratelli S, Spagnoli GC, Lauro D, Lugli A, Han J, Iezzi G, Ferrone C, Ferlosio A, Tornillo L, Droeser R, Rossi P, Attanasio A, Ferrone S, Terracciano L (2014) HLA class II antigen expression in colorectal carcinoma tumors as a favorable prognostic marker. Neoplasia 16:31–42. https://doi.org/10.1593/neo.131568
41. Snyder A, Makarov V, Merghoub T, Yuan J, Zaretsky JM, Desrichard A, Walsh LA, Postow MA, Wong P, Ho TS, Hollmann TJ, Bruggeman C, Kannan K, Li Y, Elipenahli C, Liu C, Harbison CT, Wang L, Ribas A, Wolchok JD, Chan TA (2014) Genetic basis for clinical response to CTLA-4 blockade in melanoma. N Engl J Med:2189–2199. https://doi.org/10.1056/NEJMoa1406498
42. Sofron A, Ritz D, Neri D, Fugmann T (2016) High-resolution analysis of the murine MHC class II immunopeptidome. Eur J Immunol 46:319–328. https://doi.org/10.1002/eji.201545930
43. Sperduto PW, Kased N, Roberge D, Xu Z, Shanley R, Luo X, Sneed PK, Chao ST, Weil RJ, Suh J, Bhatt A, Jensen AW, Brown PD, Shih HA, Kirkpatrick J, Gaspar LE, Fiveash JB, Chiang V, Knisely JPS, Sperduto CM, Lin N, Mehta M (2012) Summary report on the graded prognostic assessment: an accurate and facile diagnosis-specific tool to estimate survival for patients with brain metastases. J Clin Oncol 30:419–425. https://doi.org/10.1200/JCO.2011.38.0527
44. Steimle V, Siegrist C, Mottet A, Lisowska-Grospierre B, Mach B (1994) Regulation of MHC class II expression by interferon-gamma mediated by the transactivator gene CIITA. Science (80- ) 265:106–109. https://doi.org/10.1126/science.8016643
45. Sundstrom T, Daphu I, Wendelbo I, Hodneland E, Lundervold A, Immervoll H, Skaftnesmo KO, Babic M, Jendelova P, Sykova E, Lund-Johansen M, Bjerkvig R, Thorsen F (2013) Automated tracking of nanoparticle-labeled melanoma cells improves the predictive power of a brain metastasis model. Cancer Res 73:2445–2456. https://doi.org/10.1158/0008-5472.CAN-12-3514
46. Swanson PE, Wick MR (1990) HLA-DR (Ia-like) reactivity in tumors of bone and soft tissue: an immunohistochemical comparison of monoclonal antibodies LN3 and LK8D3 in routinely processed specimens. Mod Pathol 3:113–119
47. Tanese K, Hashimoto Y, Berkova Z, Wang Y, Samaniego F, Lee JE, Ekmekcioglu S, Grimm EA (2015) Cell surface CD74–MIF interactions drive melanoma survival in response to interferon-γ. J Invest Dermatol. https://doi.org/10.1038/jid.2015.259
48. Taramelli D, Fossati G, Mazzocchi A, Parmiani G, Delia D, Ferrone S (1986) Classes i and ii hla and melanoma-associated antigen expression and modulation on melanoma cells isolated from primary and metastatic lesions. Cancer Res 46:433–439
49. Tsao MS, Le Teuff G, Shepherd FA, Landais C, Hainaut P, Filipits M, Pirker R, Le Chevalier T, Graziano S, Kratze R, Soria JC, Pignon JP, Seymour L, Brambilla E (2017) PD-L1 protein expression assessed by immunohistochemistry is neither prognostic nor predictive of benefit from adjuvant chemotherapy in resected non-small cell lung cancer. Ann Oncol 28:882–889. https://doi.org/10.1093/annonc/mdx003
50. Turner TB, Meza-Perez S, Londoño A, Katre A, Peabody JE, Smith HJ, Forero A, Norian LA, Straughn JM, Buchsbaum DJ, Randall TD, Arend RC (2017) Epigenetic modifiers upregulate MHC II and impede ovarian cancer tumor growth. Oncotarget 8:44159–44170. https://doi.org/10.18632/oncotarget.17395
51. Vizcaíno JA, Csordas A, Del-Toro N, Dianes JA, Griss J, Lavidas I, Mayer G, Perez-Riverol Y, Reisinger F, Ternent T, Xu QW, Wang R, Hermjakob H (2016) 2016 update of the PRIDE database and its related tools. Nucleic Acids Res 44:D447–D456. https://doi.org/10.1093/nar/gkv1145
52. Wälchli S, Kumari S, Fallang LE, Sand KMK, Yang W, Landsverk OJB, Bakke O, Olweus J, Gregers TF (2014) Invariant chain as a vehicle to load antigenic peptides on human MHC class I for cytotoxic T-cell activation. Eur J Immunol 44:774–784. https://doi.org/10.1002/eji.201343671
53. Wang J, Daphu I, Pedersen PH, Miletic H, Hovland R, Mørk S, Bjerkvig R, Tiron C, McCormack E, Micklem D, Lorens JB, Immervoll H, Thorsen F (2011) A novel brain metastases model developed in immunodeficient rats closely mimics the growth of metastatic brain tumours in patients. Neuropathol Appl Neurobiol 37:189–205. https://doi.org/10.1111/j.1365-2990.2010.01119.x
54. Wang ZQ, Milne K, Webb JR, Watson PH (2017) CD74 and intratumoral immune response in breast cancer. Oncotarget. https://doi.org/10.18632/oncotarget.8610
55. Wolchok JD, Kluger H, Callahan MK, Postow MA, Rizvi NA, Lesokhin AM, Segal NH, Ariyan CE, Gordon R-A, Reed K, Burke MM, Caldwell A, Kronenberg SA, Agunwamba BU, Zhang X, Lowy I, Inzunza HD, Feely W, Horak CE, Hong Q, Korman AJ, Wigginton JM, Gupta A, Sznol M (2013) Nivolumab plus ipilimumab in advanced melanoma. N Engl J Med 369:122–133. https://doi.org/10.1056/NEJMoa1302369
56. Wright KL, Ting JPY (2006) Epigenetic regulation of MHC-II and CIITA genes. Trends Immunol 27:405–412. https://doi.org/10.1016/j.it.2006.07.007
57. Zeiner PS, Preusse C, Blank AE, Zachskorn C, Baumgarten P, Caspary L, Braczynski AK, Weissenberger J, Bratzke H, Reiß S, Pennartz S, Winkelmann R, Senft C, Plate KH, Wischhusen J, Stenzel W, Harter PN, Mittelbronn M (2015) MIF receptor CD74 is restricted to microglia/macrophages, associated with a M1-polarized immune milieu and prolonged patient survival in gliomas. Brain Pathol 25:491–504. https://doi.org/10.1111/bpa.12194

# Type 2 diabetes impairs odour detection, olfactory memory and olfactory neuroplasticity; effects partly reversed by the DPP-4 inhibitor Linagliptin

Grazyna Lietzau[1,3*], William Davidsson[1], Claes-Göran Östenson[2], Fausto Chiazza[1], David Nathanson[1], Hiranya Pintana[1], Josefin Skogsberg[4], Thomas Klein[5], Thomas Nyström[1], Vladimer Darsalia[1*] and Cesare Patrone[1*]

**Abstract**

Recent data suggest that olfactory deficits could represent an early marker and a pathogenic mechanism at the basis of cognitive decline in type 2 diabetes (T2D). However, research is needed to further characterize olfactory deficits in diabetes, their relation to cognitive decline and underlying mechanisms.

The aim of this study was to determine whether T2D impairs odour detection, olfactory memory as well as neuroplasticity in two major brain areas responsible for olfaction and odour coding: the main olfactory bulb (MOB) and the piriform cortex (PC), respectively. Dipeptidyl peptidase-4 inhibitors (DPP-4i) are clinically used T2D drugs exerting also beneficial effects in the brain. Therefore, we aimed to determine whether DPP-4i could reverse the potentially detrimental effects of T2D on the olfactory system.

Non-diabetic Wistar and T2D Goto-Kakizaki rats, untreated or treated for 16 weeks with the DPP-4i linagliptin, were employed. Odour detection and olfactory memory were assessed by using the block, the habituation-dishabituation and the buried pellet tests. We assessed neuroplasticity in the MOB by quantifying adult neurogenesis and GABAergic inhibitory interneurons positive for calbindin, parvalbumin and carletinin. In the PC, neuroplasticity was assessed by quantifying the same populations of interneurons and a newly identified form of olfactory neuroplasticity mediated by post-mitotic doublecortin (DCX) + immature neurons.

We show that T2D dramatically reduced odour detection and olfactory memory. Moreover, T2D decreased neurogenesis in the MOB, impaired the differentiation of DCX+ immature neurons in the PC and altered GABAergic interneurons protein expression in both olfactory areas. DPP-4i did not improve odour detection and olfactory memory. However, it normalized T2D-induced effects on neuroplasticity.

The results provide new knowledge on the detrimental effects of T2D on the olfactory system. This knowledge could constitute essentials for understanding the interplay between T2D and cognitive decline and for designing effective preventive therapies.

**Keywords:** Diabetes, DPP-4 inhibitors, Goto-Kakizaki rats, Olfaction, Neuroplasticity, Piriform cortex

* Correspondence: grazyna.lietzau@ki.se; vladimer.darsalia@ki.se; cesare.patrone@ki.se
[1]Department of Clinical Science and Education, Södersjukhuset, Internal Medicine, Karolinska Institutet, Stockholm, Sweden
Full list of author information is available at the end of the article

## Introduction

Cognitive decline, dementia and Alzheimer's disease (AD) are often preceded by olfactory deficits [reviewed in [18, 20]]. Interestingly, some studies show that type 2 diabetic (T2D) patients present olfactory impairments such as elevated odour detection threshold [39], reduced odour-identification ability [26, 51, 68], and increased risk of anosmia [9]. Since there is also a strong association between T2D and different forms of cognitive decline and dementia, including AD [6, 14, 40, 42, 90], olfactory dysfunction in T2D could represent an early indicator and perhaps even one of the pathogenic mechanisms at the base of future cognitive impairment. A few recent studies support this hypothesis [82, 91]. However, other studies could not detect olfactory deficits in diabetes [2, 9, 71] and these discrepancies call for further investigation. Moreover, the potential impairment of cognitive functions related to olfaction (e.g *olfactory memory*) needs to be studied in T2D, since the disruption of these functions in non-diabetics has been associated with aging and cognitive decline [12, 13, 50, 75, 85, 92].

The mechanisms at the basis of impaired olfaction in T2D have been poorly investigated, although some interesting studies have been performed in animal models of obesity/pre-diabetes. Livingston et al. have shown that obese, insulin-resistant rats have a decreased level of tyrosine-phosphorylated proteins in the main olfactory bulb (MOB) and piriform cortex (PC) [57] which are the two brain areas responsible for olfaction [67] and odour coding [5, 25], respectively. Furthermore, insulin binding in the MOB of these rats is decreased [4].

The brain's ability to reorganize neural circuits in order to adapt to the environmental changes is called *neuroplasticity*. Olfaction requires *neuroplasticity* for both detecting and coding new odours and GABAergic inhibitory interneurons play an important role in this context [36]. Interestingly, the vulnerability of GABAergic inhibitory interneurons in the olfactory system has been associated with AD [79]. The potential effects of T2D on the interneuron-mediated *neuroplasticity* in the olfactory system have been investigated only in one study showing that calbindin (CB) + interneurons are affected by T2D [56].

Olfactory *neuroplasticity* is also regulated by adult neurogenesis in the MOB. This process occurs during the adult life and starts in the subventricular zone (SVZ) bordering the lateral ventricle. In the SVZ, neural stem cells (NSCs) produce undifferentiated and proliferative doublecortin (DCX) + neuroblasts that migrate towards the MOB where they differentiate mainly into interneurons playing an important role in the *neuroplasticity* of the MOB [31, 81]. While the detrimental effects of T2D on the NSCs in the SVZ have been recently shown [3, 49, 59, 60], it remains to be determined whether neurogenesis in the MOB is affected by T2D.

Another form of *neuroplasticity* in the olfactory system is represented by DCX+ immature neurons in the PC. In contrast to DCX+ cells in the MOB (see above), these cells are post-mitotic, non-proliferative immature neurons of embryonic origin. The pool of these cells decreases during aging due to continuous differentiation into mature neurons following new olfactory learning demands [41, 66]. Whether T2D affects these cells is unknown.

Recent studies suggest that olfactory deficits, in addition to their potential role as biomarkers, could also play an important role in the pathogenesis of AD [18, 21]. If so, the normalization of olfactory deficits in T2D could have a therapeutic preventive role against cognitive decline. Dipeptidyl peptidase-4 inhibitors (DPP-4i) are a growing class of clinically used T2D drugs [19, 83] that have also shown beneficial effects in the CNS of animal models of AD [15, 22, 45–47, 77] and in T2D patients with AD [37], even independently from glycemic regulation [27, 70]. Whether some of these beneficial effects occur via the normalization of impaired olfaction is unknown.

In this study, we addressed some of these issues in a lean and spontaneous model of T2D: the Goto Kakizaki (GK) rat [69]. Specifically, we investigated whether T2D impairs *odour detection* and *olfactory memory*. To determine whether T2D impairs the *neuroplasticity* in the olfactory system, we investigated whether GABAergic inhibitory interneurons and adult neurogenesis in the MOB as well as GABAergic interneurons and the immature DCX+ neurons in the PC are affected by T2D. Finally, we determined whether a chronic treatment with DPP-4i could reverse the identified factors affected by T2D.

## Materials and methods

### Animals and the T2D model

Rats were housed in 12-h light/dark cycle with free access to food and water. All experiments were conducted in accordance with the Guide for the Care and Use of Laboratory Animals published by U.S. National Institute of Health and approved by the regional ethics committee for animal experimentation (ethical permits granted by Stockholm's Djurförsöksetiska Nämnd: S7–13 and N43/16).

As experimental model of T2D, the GK rat was used. This non-obese strain originates from selective breeding of Wistar rats and becomes spontaneously hyperglycemic during early adulthood [69]. The GK rats develop deficiency in insulin secretion and peripheral insulin/leptin resistance [73].

### Experimental design

In total, sixty five 4–7-months-old male GK rats and age-matched, non-diabetic Wistar rats were used in 2 studies:

*Study 1*: To determine the effect of T2D on *odour detection*, *olfactory memory* and *neuroplasticity*-related markers, we used T2D GK rats ($n = 9$) and Wistar rats ($n = 11$) as non-diabetic controls. The experimental design is summarized in Fig. 1a.

*Study 2*: To determine the potential effect of chronic DPP4i on the olfactory system, T2D GK rats ($n = 23$) were treated with linagliptin (mixed in the standard rodent chow at 83 mg/kg, estimated daily intake at ≈5–8 mg/kg/bw) for 16 weeks. Control GK rats ($n = 22$) received the chow of the same composition, but without the drug. *Odour detection, olfactory memory* and *neuroplasticity*-related markers were determined as in Study 1. The rationale for the dose of 5–8 mg/kg/bw and the duration of the treatment were to strongly and chronically inhibit DPP-4 activity. We employed middle-aged rats rather than old rats in the view to test the preventive potential of Linagliptin to decrease olfactory impairment. The experimental design is summarized in Fig. 1b.

#### Body weight and glycemic level

Blood glucose levels (after 6 h of fasting; LifeScan glucometer, US) and body weight were measured in all animals. As previously published by us and others [33, 56, 73], results showed lower body weight (363.4 ± 9.3 vs. 503.4 ± 13.1, $p < 0.0001$) as well as increased hyperglycemia (11.8 ± 0.6 vs. 4.7 ± 0.2, $p < 0.0001$) in GK rats compared to Wistar controls (Additional file 1: Figure S1 A and B, respectively).

#### Dipeptidyl peptidase 4 (DPP-4) activity and glucagon-like peptide-1 (GLP-1) levels

In order to verify the bioactivity of linagliptin, plasma DPP-4 activity and total active GLP-1 levels were determined by enzyme immunoassay (EIA) and by the GLP-1 assay kit (Meso Scale discovery, Gaithersburg, MD, USA).

#### Olfactory assays

To assess the odour detection ability and the olfactory memory, the block test, the habituation-dishabituation test, and the buried pellet test were used [52]. The detailed description of the olfactory testing procedures and analyzed parameters are provided in the Additional file 1.

#### Immunohistochemistry

For immunohistochemistry (IHC): the rats were deeply anesthetized with sodium pentobarbital and transcardially perfused with saline followed by 4% paraformaldehyde (PFA). Brains were post-fixed overnight in 4% PFA and placed in 20% sucrose solution until they sank. Brains were cut into 40 μm-thick coronal sections (apart from the olfactory bulb, which was cut in sagittal plane) using Leica SM2010 R sliding microtome (Leica, Germany).

The following primary antibodies were used: rabbit polyclonal against parvalbumin (PV) (1:1500, Abcam, UK), rabbit polyclonal against calbindin (CB) (1:400, Abcam, UK), rabbit monoclonal against calretinin (CR) (1:300,

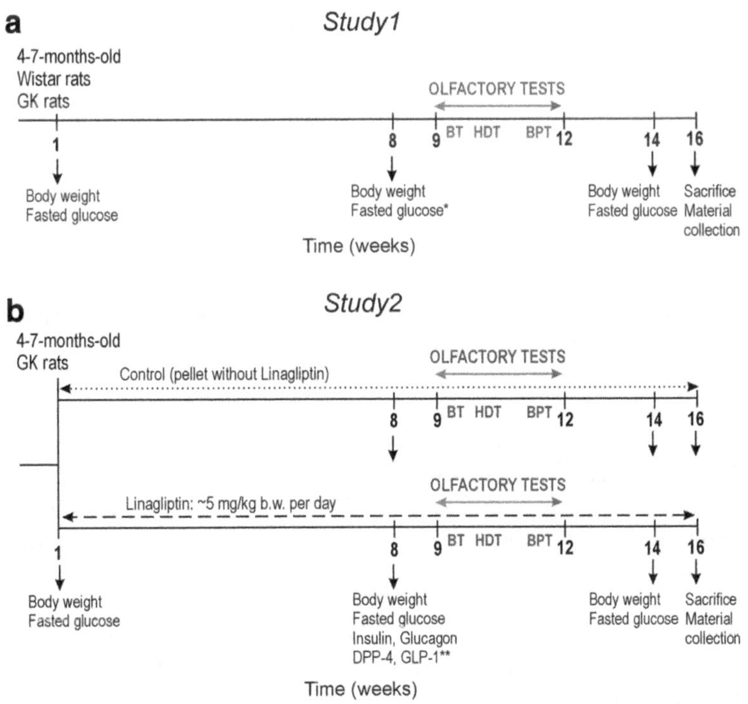


**Fig. 1** Experimental timeline of studies. Abbreviations: BT – block test, BPT – buried pellet test, DPP-4 – dipeptidyl peptidase 4, GK rat – Goto-Kakizaki rat, GLP-1 – glucagon-like peptide-1, HDT – habituation-dishabituation test. *Data presented in Additional file 1: Figure S1, **data presented in Additional file 1: Figure S3

Vector Laboratories, US), goat polyclonal against doublecortin (DCX) (1:300, SantaCruz Biotechnology, US), mouse monoclonal against neuronal nuclei marker (NeuN) (1:300, Merck Millipore, US). Antigen retrieval was performed in 1 mM EDTA, pH 8.0 (for PV, CB and CR) in 70 °C for 35 min. After cooling, free-floating sections were incubated with primary antibodies overnight at 4°C in PBS containing 5% of natural horse serum (NHS) and 0.25% Triton-X100. Then, primary antibodies were detected by either fluorescent dye-conjugated [Alexa Fluor488 (DCX), Alexa Fluor594 (NeuN) (both 1:200, Life Technologies, US)] or biotin-conjugated secondary antibodies (1:200, Vector Laboratories, Sweden). The sections were incubated with the secondary antibodies for 2 h at RT in PBS containing 5% NHS and 0.25% Triton-X100. For chromogenic visualization, avidin-biotin complex (ABC kit, Vector Laboratories, Sweden) and diaminobenzidine (DAB; Sigma-Aldrich, US) were used.

To evaluate the density of projecting neurons in the mitral cell layer of the MOB, Nissl staining was performed.

#### Quantitative analyses of IHC

The PV-, CB-, CR-, DCX/NeuN- positive cells were quantified using a computerized stereology toolbox equipped with Visiopharm v. 4.2.1.0 software for digital image analysis (NewCast, Denmark), connected to Olympus BX51 epifluorescent/light microscope (Olympus, Japan). Positive cells were counted on three coronal sections *per* animal located in 0.24, – 1.80 and – 3.36 mm distance to Bregma (PC) and two representative sagittal sections *per* animal (MOB). Accessory olfactory bulb was excluded from all assessments. The cell density per 1 $mm^2$ was determined. Due to low number of DCX+ cells *per* section in PC and their characteristic localization (mostly in II layer), total number of DCX+ and DCX/NeuN+ cells in PC was estimated on sections located between – 1.20 and – 3.48 mm in relation to Bregma. Measurements of the mean cell volume (in $\mu m^3$) of CB+ cells were made, using nucleator technique [28], by Visiopharm software. To assess the extent of interneuronal connectivity of CB+ cells, neuronal arborization (number of neurites/branching) was quantified [38]. Neuronal arborization was evaluated as showed in Additional file 1: Figure S2. Due to lack of visible neurites in CB+ cells in the MOB and negative preliminary results regarding differences in the mean volume of these interneurons, we present only the results of the arborisation/volume measurements for CB+ cells in the PC.

#### Western blot

The PC and the MOB were dissected and snap frozen for further analyses. The tissue was homogenized in RIPA lysis buffer containing protease inhibitory cocktail (Sigma-Aldrich) on ice for 30 min. Total protein concentration was determined by Lowry assay (Bio-Rad Laboratories, US). Samples containing 4 μg/μl total protein were mixed with LDS sample buffer (Novex, Life Technologies, US) and incubated in 95 °C for 5 min. After electrophoresis on Bolt 4–12% Bis-TrisPlus gel (ThermoFisher Scientific, US), proteins were transferred on nitrocellulose membrane (iBlot 2 Dry Blotting System, 25 V for 6 min, ThermoFisher, US). Immuno-detection was performed with antibodies against: 1) PV (1:500, polyclonal, rabbit, Abcam, US), 2) CB (1:100 polyclonal, rabbit antibody, Abcam), 3) CR (1:1000, monoclonal, rabbit, Abcam, US), and 4) β-actin (1:450, monoclonal, mouse, SantaCruz Biotechnology). Secondary antibodies used: bovine anti-rabbit (1:10,000; SantaCruz Biotechnology) and goat anti-mouse (1:5000; SantaCruz Biotechnology, US) were conjugated with horseradish peroxidase (HRP). Immuno-reactive bands were developed using ECL substrate for HRP (GE Healthcare, Sweden) and documented with a GelDoc chemiluminescent system (Bio-Rad Laboratories, US). Normalization against β-actin was performed.

#### Statistics

To analyze the data from behavioral experiments, nonparametric tests (Mann-Whitney *U*-test, Wilcoxon Signed Rank test) were employed to account for heterogeneity of variance. Additionally, for analyses of the behavioral data one-way and two-way ANOVA followed by appropriate post-hoc tests were applied (see Figure legends for detailed information). Cell density and relative protein content were compared using unpaired two-tailed *t* test. Multiple *t*-tests were applied to compare neuronal arborization. The statistical analyses were performed using GraphPad Prism 7 (USA). All data are presented as means ±S.E.M. and differences between the groups were considered significant when *p*-values were less than 0.05 ($^{*,\Delta}p < 0.05$; $^{**,\Delta\Delta}p < 0.01$, $^{***}p < 0.001$, $^{****}p < 0.0001$).

## Results

### Odour detection and olfactory memory in T2D rats

#### *T2D rats have deficits in odour detection ability and olfactory memory*

To assess the potential impairment of *odour detection* in T2D rats with confirmed hyperglycemia (see Materials and methods), we measured the mean sniffing time for various odours and the time to find a fragrant object. The results show that GK rats, compared to non-diabetic controls, spent less time sniffing new odours in the block test (8.5 ± 2.2 vs. 19.66 ± 5.1 s., $p = 0.04$, Fig. 2a) and the habituation-dishabituation test (odour 1 = vanilla: 1.9 ± 0.7 vs. 17.6 ± 2.5 s., $p < 0.0001$; odour 2 = lemon: 8.6 ± 1.6 vs. 16.8 ± 2.9 s., $p = 0.01$, Fig. 2b). GK rats also needed much more time to find the fragrant object in the buried pellet test (181.2 ± 26.1 vs. 20.3 ± 2.3 s., $p = 0.0003$, Fig. 2c).

To assess *olfactory memory*, we repeatedly measured the mean sniffing time for the same odour (the habituation-

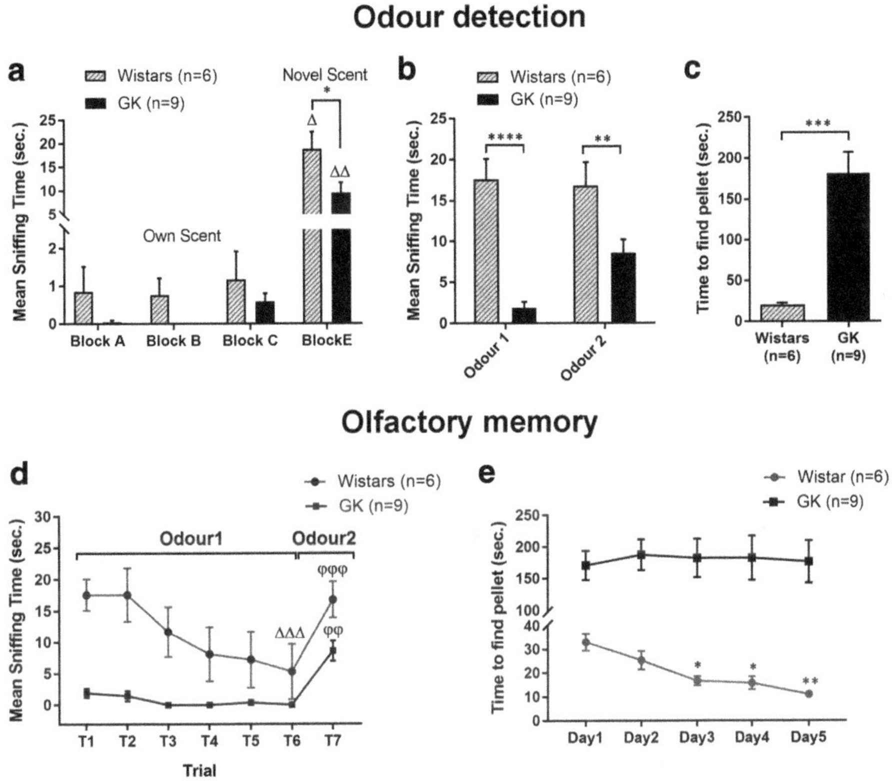


**Fig. 2** Diabetic rats show deficits in odour detection and olfactory memory. **a** Mean sniffing time of wooden blocks covered with a scent of the tested rat (blocks *A-C*) and unknown rat (block *E*) in the block test. *comparison of time spent sniffing block E between non-diabetic Wistar and T2D GK rats done by the Mann-Whitney *U*-test; $^{\Delta}$comparison of time spent sniffing block E with other blocks done by the Wilcoxon Signed Rank test. **b** Mean sniffing time of the scented cartridge covered with vanilla (odour 1) and lemon (odour 2) in the habituation-dishabituation test. Two-way ANOVA followed by Sidak's multiple comparisons test. **c** Mean time to find pellet in the buried pellet test. Mann-Whitney *U*-test. **d** Mean sniffing time of the scented cartridge (vanilla/lemon) during 7 trials of the habituation-dishabituation test. Habituation was determined as significant difference in sniffing time between the first and last presentation of the same odour. $^{\Delta}$comparision of sniffing time of odour 1 between T1 and T6. Dishabituation was determined as significant difference between the last presentation of an odour and the first presentation of an alternative odour. $^{\varphi}$comparision of sniffing time between T6 (odour 1) and T7 (odour 2). Repeated measures One-way ANOVA followed by Bonferroni's test. **e** Mean time to find pellet in buried pellet test performed during 5 consecutive days. Repeated measures One-way ANOVA with Greenhouse-Geisser correction followed by Bonferoni's multiple comparisons test. The data are means ±S.E.M., $^{*,\Delta}p < 0.05$, $^{**,\Delta\Delta,\varphi\varphi}p < 0.01$, $^{***,\Delta\Delta\Delta,\varphi\varphi\varphi}p < 0.001$, $^{****}p < 0.0001$

dishabituation test) and the time to find the fragrant object (the buried pellet test). The results show that during consecutive trials, GK rats did not improve neither sniffing time (ie. they did not habituate) nor time to find the fragrant object (Fig. 2d and e, respectively) in comparison to Wistar rats. However, both strains discriminate between odour 1 and 2. (Fig. 2d). No differences in time to approach the scented object (Additional file 1: Figure S3A and B) or in movement activity (Additional file 1: Figure S3 C and D) were detected between GK and Wistar rats in both olfactory tests.

Overall, these results indicate that T2D is associated with to a dramatic reduction in *odour detection* and *olfactory memory*.

### The effect of T2D on neuroplasticity in the MOB and PC

#### *T2D affects CB+ interneurons in the MOB*

We did not observe major structural changes in the MOB of GK and Wistar rats (e.g. by quantifying the mitral cells; data not shown). However, when we quantified CB+ interneurons in the MOB, the results show a trend, albeit not statistically significant, towards a decrease in the density of CB+ interneurons in diabetic compared with control rats ($p = 0.09$; Fig. 3a-c). Moreover, results show 18% decrease in CB expression in the MOB of GK rats versus Wistars by Western blot analysis ($p = 0.04$; Fig. 3d-e). Difference in neither the cell density nor expression of other interneuronal markers (i.e. PV and CR) between GK and Wistar rats was found (data not shown).

#### *T2D reduces neurogenesis in the MOB*

Adult neurogenesis in the MOB was assessed by counting DCX+ neuroblasts in this brain area. The results showed a dramatic reduction (over 50% decrease) in the density of DCX+ immature neurons in the MOB

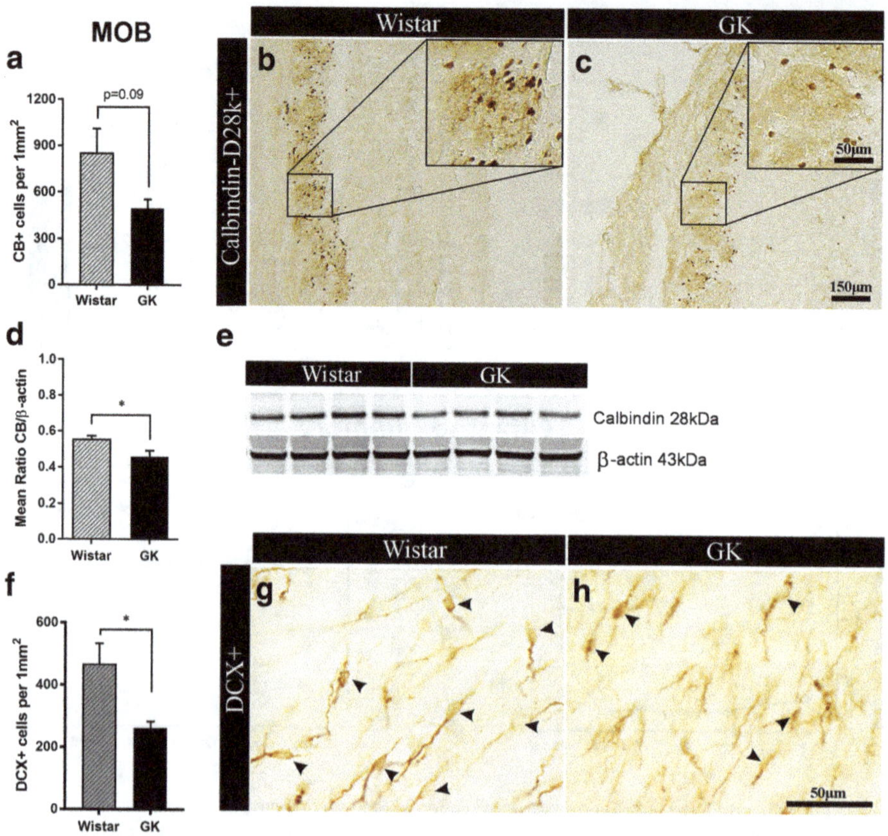


**Fig. 3** Diabetes affects calbindin+ interneurons and impairs adult neurogenesis in the olfactory bulb. **a** Density of CB+ interneurons. **b-c** representative microphotographs of CB+ staining in the MOB of non-diabetic Wistar versus T2D GK rats ($n = 5$–$6$). **d** Relative level of CB expression normalized against beta-actin and, **e** representative bands showing CB expression level in the MOB of non-diabetic vs. T2D rats ($n = 4$), (Western blot). **f** Density of immature DCX+ neurons and, **g-h** representative microphotographs of DCX+ staining in the MOB of Wistar vs. GK rats ($n = 7$) (black arrows indicate DCX+ cells). Two-tailed, unpaired *t*-test. The data are means ±S.E.M., * $p < 0.05$

of GK compared with Wistar rats (261.7 ± 20.3 vs. 468.5 ± 65.9 cell/mm$^2$, $p = 0.02$, Fig. 3f-h) indicating that MOB adult neurogenesis is severely impaired by T2D.

### *T2D impairs PV+ interneurons in the PC*

In our previous study, we showed vulnerability of GABAergic CB+ interneurons in the PC of GK rats during aging [56]. In the present study, we investigated the potential effect of T2D on PV+ and CR+ interneurons in the PC. We did not observe any significant difference in the density of PV+ interneurons between T2D and control rats (Fig. 4a-c). Results showed, however, 17% decrease in the expression of PV in the PC of diabetic compared with non-diabetic rats ($p = 0.046$; Fig. 4d, e), by Western blot analysis. No difference in either density of CR+ cells, or expression of this protein between GK and Wistars was recorded (data not shown). In summary, these results indicate that T2D affects PV+ interneurons in the PC.

### *T2D impairs the neuronal differentiation of DCX+ immature neurons in the PC*

To assess the *neuroplasticity* related to adaptation to new odours, we quantified post-mitotic DCX+ immature neurons in the PC of 6 months-old T2D GK and non-diabetic rats. The results show that the total number of DCX+ cells was significantly higher (168% increase) in GK versus Wistar rats (39.2 ± 8.8 vs. 14.6 ± 3.4 cells; Fig. 4f-h). To determine whether the increase of DCX+ cells in GK rats corresponded to a decrease in neuronal differentiation, we double-stained DCX+ cells with the mature neuronal marker NeuN which is acquired by these cells during the differentiation process. Interestingly, the results show 52% increase in DCX/NeuN+ cells in the PC of the middle-aged T2D GK rats versus non-diabetic control rats (38.5 ± 4.7 vs. 25.3 ± 3.6 cells, $p = 0.049$; Fig. 4i-o). Overall, the results indicate an impairment of the differentiation rate of DCX+ cells (and thus of this form of *neuroplasticity*) in the PC of T2D rats.

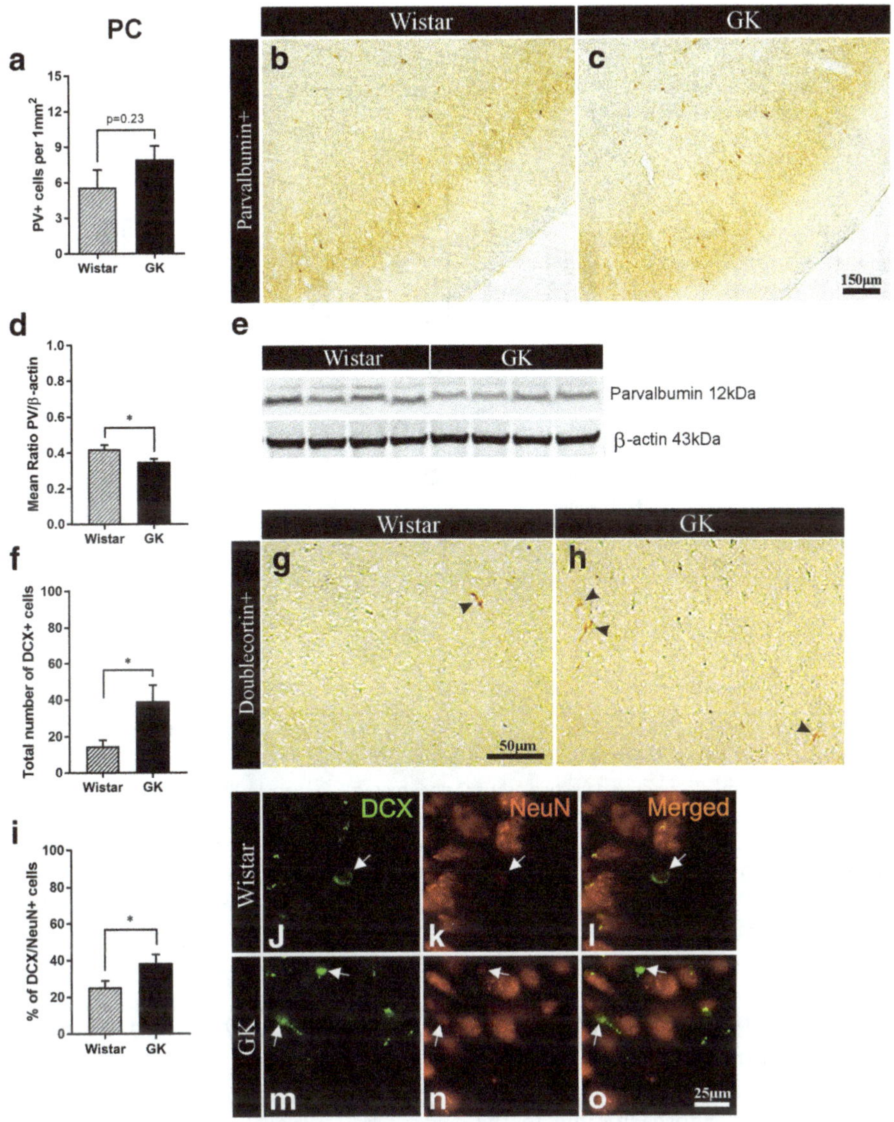

**Fig. 4** Diabetes decreases parvalbumin expression and impairs neuroblast differentiation in the piriform cortex. **a** Density of PV+ interneurons and, **b-c** representative microphotographs of PV+ staining in the PC of non-diabetic Wistar versus T2D GK rats ($n = 7$). **d** Relative level of PV normalized against beta-actin and, **e** representative bands showing PV expression level in the PC of non-diabetic vs. T2D rats ($n = 4$) (Western blot). **f** Total number and, **g-h** representative microphotographs of post-mitotic immature DCX+ neurons of embryonic origin in the PC of middle-aged Wistar vs. GK rats. **i** Percent of "differentiating" DCX/NeuN+ neurons and, **j-o** representative microphotographs of double-stained DCX/NeuN+ neurons (white arrows) in the PC of Wistar vs. GK rats ($n = 7–9$). Two-tailed, unpaired *t*-test. The data are means ±S.E.M., * $p < 0.05$

### Odour detection and olfactory memory in GK rats treated with the DPP-4i linagliptin

Chronic linagliptin treatment led to a 55% reduction in peripheral DPP-4 activity (45.2 ± 2.3 vs. 100.0 ± 5.5% of control, $p < 0.0001$; Additional file 1: Figure S4A) and to increase active GLP-1 levels (0.66 ± 0.1 vs. 0.04 ± 0.002 pg/ml, $p < 0.0001$; Additional file 1: Figure S4B) versus the untreated controls. These results demonstrate the bioactivity of linagliptin. However, the chronic linagliptin treatment did not affect the glucagon and insulin concentrations, body weight, and glycemic levels (Additional file 1: Figure S4C-F). One possibility to explain these results is that linagliptin was less efficient in reducing DPP-4 activity (55% reduction in our study vs. more than 80% reduction in the previous studies [16, 17]).

#### *Chronic DPP-4 inhibition does not improve odour detection and olfactory memory in T2D rats*

Chronic treatment of GK rats with linagliptin for 16 weeks did not improve *odour detection* (Fig. 5a and b) and did not shorten the time to uncover the food (Fig. 5c). Similarly, the results showed no difference in the *olfactory memory*

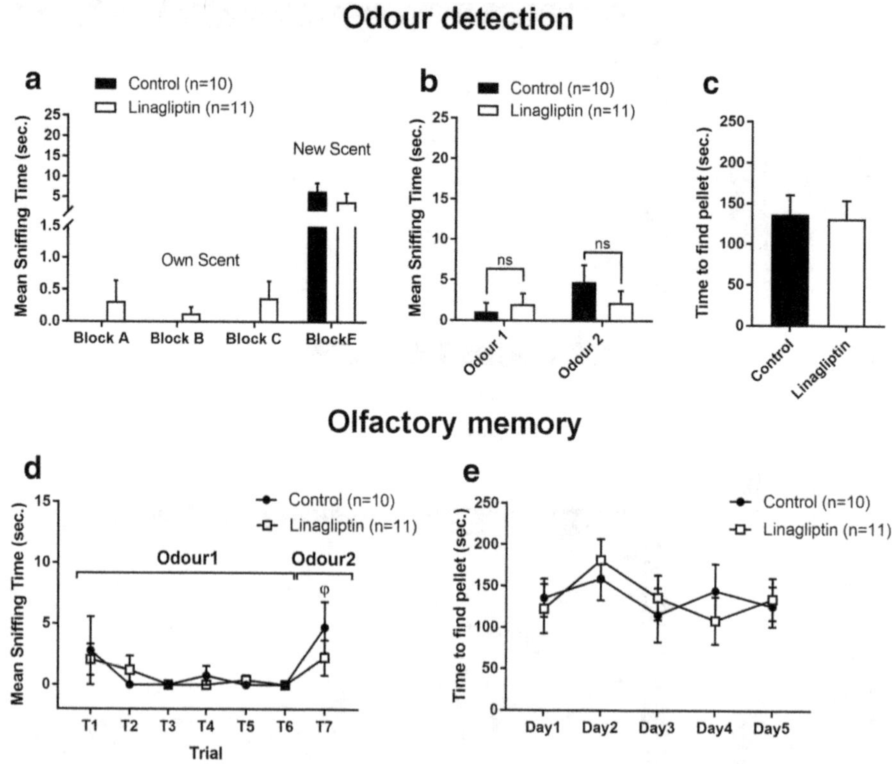


**Fig. 5** Chronic DPP-4 inhibition does not affect odour detection and olfactory memory in diabetic rats. **a** Mean sniffing time of wooden blocks covered with a scent of the tested rat (block *A-C*) and unknown rat (block *E*) in the block test. **b** Mean sniffing time of the scented cartridge covered with vanilla and lemon odour in the habituation dishabituation test. **c** Mean time to find pellet in the buried pellet test. **d** Mean sniffing time of the scented cartridge (vanilla/lemon) during 7 trials of the habituation dishabituation test. **e** Mean time to find pellet in the buried pellet test performed during 5 consecutive days. For comparisons between linagliptin-treated and untreated GK rats in this Study 2, the same statistical tests were performed as in Study 1 (see Fig. 2). The data are expressed as means ±S.E.M., $^{\varphi}p < 0.05$

between linagliptin and control-treated GK rats (Fig. 5d and e). Interestingly, while untreated GK rats discriminated between the odours, linagliptin-treated rats did not. No significant difference in the approach time to the fragrant object as well as the movement activity between the linagliptin-treated and control GK rats was recorded (data not shown).

## The effect of chronic DPP-4 inhibition on neuroplasticity in the MOB and PC of T2D rat

### *Chronic DPP-4 inhibition normalizes CB+ interneurons in the MOB of T2D rats*

In the MOB, no significant difference in the density of CB+ interneurons was observed in untreated versus linagliptin-treated GK rats (Fig. 6a-c). However, the results show 22% increase ($p = 0.002$; Fig. 6d and e) in CB expression in the MOB after chronic treatment with linagliptin compared to the control group. No significant differences in neither cell density nor expression of PV- and CR-positive interneurons were observed (data not shown). These results suggest that DPP-4i can normalize the T2D-induced down-regulation of CB in the MOB (see Fig. 3d).

### *Chronic DPP-4 inhibition has no effect on adult neurogenesis in the MOB of T2D rats*

No difference in the density of DCX+ cells was observed in the MOB of linagliptin-treated versus control rats (data not shown) indicating no effect of this drug on adult neurogenesis in the MOB.

### *DPP-4 inhibition normalizes CB+ interneurons in the PC of T2D rats*

In the PC, the results showed over 40% increase in the number of CB+ interneurons after chronic linagliptin treatment compared to the control group (1849 ± 124 versus 1278 ± 86 cells, $p = 0.002$) (Fig. 7a-c) suggesting a significant role of DPP-4i in the regulation of *neuroplasticity* driven by these cells in the PC. The results showed no difference between control and linagliptin-treated group in neither the density of both PV- and CR+ interneurons nor the expression of these interneuronal markers (data not shown).

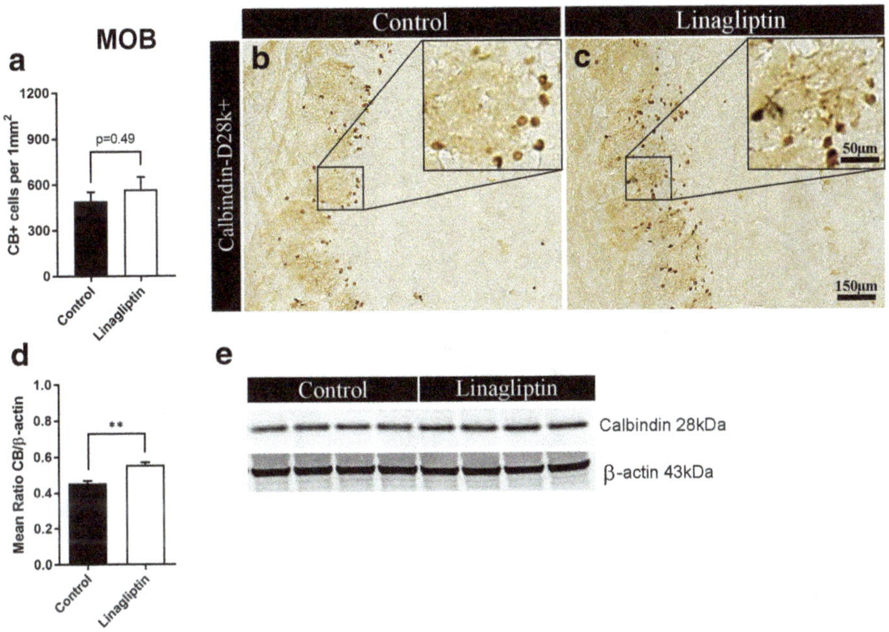


**Fig. 6** Chronic DPP-4 inhibition increases calbindin expression in the olfactory bulb of diabetic rats. **a** Density of CB+ interneurons and, **b-c** representative microphotographs of CB+ staining in the MOB of control vs. linagliptin-treated GK rats ($n = 6$). **d** Relative level of CB normalized against beta-actin and, **e** representative bands showing CB expression level in the MOB of control vs. linagliptin-treated GK rats ($n = 4$), (Western blot). Two-tailed, unpaired *t*-test. The data are means ±S.E.M., ** $p < 0.01$

### *DPP-4 inhibition exerts neurotrophic effects on CB+ interneurons in the PC of T2D rats*

Interestingly, the average soma volume of CB+ interneurons in the PC of the linagliptin-treated GK rats was 14% larger compared to the untreated rats (1567 ± 56 versus 1373 ± 49 μm$^3$, $p = 0.02$; Fig. 7d-f). Moreover, the results show differences in the neuronal arborization of the CB+ interneurons in the PC after chronic treatment with linagliptin. Specifically, the number of neuronal branches per cell (see Material and Methods for the quantification procedures) was significantly increased in the PC of the linagliptin-treated animals compared to control group (level 3: 1.67 ± 0.17 vs. 1.05 ± 0.2, $p = 0.03$; level 4: 0.45 ± 0.06 vs. 0.16 ± 0.05, $p = 0.002$; level 5: 0.11 ± 0.02 vs. 0.04 ± 0.02, $p = 0.02$; Fig. 7g-i). Overall, these morphometric changes indicate a neurotrophic effect mediated by linagliptin on CB+ interneurons suggesting that DPP-4i regulate the *neuroplasticity* driven by CB+ interneurons in the PC.

### *DPP-4 inhibition promotes neuronal differentiation in the PC of T2D rats*

Sixteen weeks of DPP-4 inhibition resulted in no significant difference in the number of DCX+ neurons in the PC of GK rats compared with control rats (Fig. 7j). However, when looking at the rate of their differentiation into mature neurons, linagliptin induced a strong 36%-decrease in DCX/NeuN double-stained neurons versus the control (24.5 ± 2.6 vs. 38.5 ± 4.7, $p = 0.03$; Fig. 7k). These results indicate that DPP-4 inhibition promotes the neuronal differentiation of these cells.

## Discussion

The primary aim of this study was to investigate the potential effects of T2D on *odour detection* and *olfactory memory*. Secondly, we determined whether important neuronal populations regulating the *neuroplasticity* in the two major brain areas involved in smelling and odour coding (the MOB and the PC) were affected by T2D. We show that T2D dramatically decreases *odour detection* and *olfactory memory*. These functional effects correlated with the decrease in CB expression and adult neurogenesis in the MOB. Moreover, T2D decreased PV expression and impaired the differentiation of DCX+ immature neurons in the PC. The third aim of the study was to determine whether a therapy mediated by DPP-4i could counteract the identified T2D effects on the olfactory system. While a chronic treatment with DPP-4i could not improve *odour detection* and *olfactory memory*, PV regulation in the PC and adult neurogenesis in the MOB, this pharmacological treatment could normalize CB+ interneurons in the MOB and PC. In addition, DPP-4i could exert neurotrophic effects on CB+ interneurons and promoted neuronal differentiation of immature DCX+ neurons in the PC.

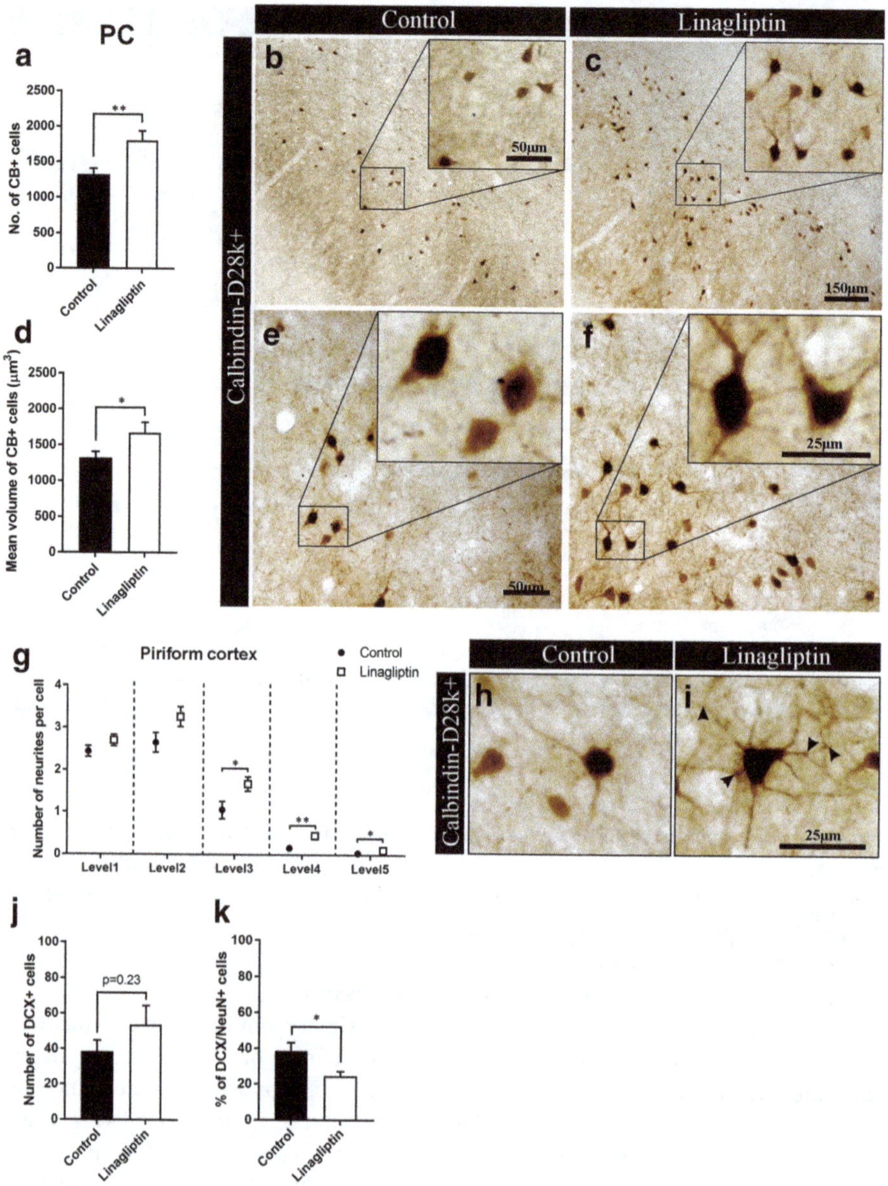


**Fig. 7** Chronic DPP-4 inhibition increases the number, the mean volume, and the arborization of calbindin+ interneurons and it promotes neuroblast differentiation in the piriform cortex of diabetic rats. **a** Density of CB+ interneurons and, **b-c** representative microphotographs of CB+ staining in the PC of control vs. linagliptin-treated GK rats ($n = 9$). **d** Mean volume and, **e-f** illustrating microphotographs of CB+ interneurons in the PC of control vs. linagliptin-treated GK rats. **g** Neuronal arborization and, **h-i** illustrating microphotographs of CB+ interneurons in the PC of the compared groups ($n = 9$). **j** Total number of DCX+ immature neurons and, **k** percent of double-stained DCX/NeuN+ "differentiating" neurons ($n = 8$). Two-tailed, unpaired *t*-test. The data are means ±S.E.M., * $p < 0.05$, ** $p < 0.01$

### The effects of T2D on *odour detection, olfactory memory* and *olfactory neuroplasticity*

The relation between diabetes and olfactory deficits was shown for the first time already in the 60's [39]. Since then a few other clinical studies have reported that diabetes could negatively impact olfactory functions [26, 51, 68]. However, a great limitation of these studies was the low number of patients. Moreover, discrepancies in the results of these studies, also in relation to differences between T1D and T2D [2, 9, 71], need to be clarified in order to undoubtedly prove the deleterious effects of T2D on the olfactory system. Importantly, the association between olfactory dysfunction in T2D with cognitive decline and dementia (including AD) has been suggested by a few clinical studies [82, 91]. However, the findings need to be further confirmed by employing additional and more reliable olfactory tests, since the ones used so far vary greatly in terms of sensitivity and reliability, as well as in the power to separate sensory and cognitive components of the olfactory functions. This is an important factor as suggested by a recent study by Markopoulou and colleagues who showed that individuals with olfactory dysfunction had poor inter-test consistency among the sets of odours identified incorrectly in successive replicate tests, even before severe olfactory dysfunction appeared [61]. Another important aspect, to prove the potential association of olfactory deficits in T2D with cognitive decline, is that olfactory parameters directly related to cognition, such as *olfactory memory* [12, 13, 24, 50, 75, 92] have, to the best of our knowledge, not been previously investigated.

In the attempt to address experimentally some of these questions, we employed a lean and spontaneous animal model of T2D, the GK rat. We used this model to rule out obesity-related factors. Furthermore, GK rats have recently been shown to present CNS complications and impaired mechanisms at the basis of cognition and memory [10, 33, 54–56, 62–65, 73]. Using three different functional tests, we show that T2D impairs *odour detection*. We also provide, for the first time, experimental evidence that *olfactory memory* is strongly impaired in T2D. Interestingly, recent works showed that hyperlipidemic and fructose-based diets disrupt odour-related learning [48, 74, 87]. These findings could be relevant for the understanding of the interplay between T2D and cognitive decline/dementia and they call for new clinical studies aimed at determining whether *olfactory memory* is impaired in T2D patients and, if so, whether this impairment correlates with the incidence of cognitive decline and dementia.

In the attempt to identify some of the pathophysiological mechanisms at the basis of impaired *odour detection* and *olfactory memory* in T2D, we investigated specific populations of neuronal cells involved in the regulation of the *neuroplasticity* of the MOB and the PC. We found decreased expression of CB (and a strong trend toward a decrease in the density of CB+ interneurons) in the MOB of GK rats. Interestingly, the vulnerability of CB+ interneurons in the AD brain has been known since the late 80's [32, 34]. More recently, it has been suggested to represent a pathogenic mechanism at the basis of AD development [1, 43]. Importantly, decreased CB+ interneurons in the MOB of an AD mouse model has been recently shown [80]. To our knowledge, this is the first report showing that CB is decreased by T2D in the MOB. Although speculative, this data suggest that this decrease could represent an early step in the development of cognitive decline in T2D.

Adult neurogenesis in the MOB is an important cellular process at the basis of olfactory functions and olfaction-related *neuroplasticity* [31, 81]. NSC proliferation and survival in the SVZ (where NSCs are generated) are impaired by T2D [3, 49, 59, 60]. However, NSC proliferation and survival are only the initial steps of adult neurogenesis and thus cannot not fully depict the effect of T2D on this process. Immature neuroblasts derived from NSCs migrate from the SVZ to the MOB and it is here where they differentiate into neurons, i.e. the ultimate result of adult neurogenesis. Therefore, investigation of the potential effects of T2D on neurogenesis requires assessment of the neurogenesis process specifically within the MOB. Impairment of the MOB's neurogenesis has been shown in one elegant study by Wakabayashi and colleagues with STZ-induced T1D [89]. However, MOB neurogenesis in T2D has not been previously investigated. Our results are in line with the results by Wakabayashi in T1D and they show a dramatic decrease in the number of DCX+ neuroblasts in the MOB of GK rats. Interestingly, deficits in adult neurogenesis in the MOB may mediate premature cognitive decline in AD [29]. This suggests that the impairment of this process in T2D could also represent an early pathogenic mechanism at the basis of cognitive decline in diabetics.

The next step in our study was to investigate potential changes induced by T2D in the PC, which is critical for odour coding [5]. The PC receives direct synaptic input from the MOB via the lateral olfactory tract and it is connected to higher brain centers such as the entorhinal cortex. Interestingly, the disruption of this region mediates early olfactory deficits in AD [53]. In the PC, the role of interneurons is fundamental for the synaptic inhibition after olfactory stimulation by a range of different odours [72, 93]. When investigating the potential effects of T2D on interneurons in the PC, we found that the expression of PV was decreased in GK rats. Importantly, PV+ interneurons play a crucial role in the regulation of cognition [11] and their dysfunction has been suggested to be a key mechanism in AD's development [88]. Furthermore, PV+ interneurons are particularly vulnerable to AD in humans [8] and PV expression is lower in AD patients versus healthy controls [35]. Finally, a recent study by Saiz-Sanchez et al. showed that PV+ interneurons in the PC are up-regulated in the AD human brain [78]. Although electrophysiology experiments are needed to well characterize the functional role of PV+ interneurons in the PC, our data support the hypothesis that PV dysregulation in T2D could be linked to impaired *odour detection* and *olfactory memory*. This could represent an early pathogenic process at the basis of cognitive decline in T2D. These findings in the PC are supported by our recent work showing that impairment of PV+ interneurons in the hippocampus of T2D rats correlates with decreased gamma oscillations [55] which is an important mechanism at the basis of cognition.

The number of DCX+ immature neurons in the PC decreases along the course of life due to continuous differentiation into mature neurons. This pool of post-mitotic cells is generated prenatally [76] and, therefore, they are not derived from adult neurogenesis [66]. The knowledge at the basis of this process is largely unknown. However, it is believed that DCX+ cells represent a newly identified form of olfactory *neuroplasticity* in relation to olfactory learning and adaptation to new olfactory stimuli [7, 41, 84, 86]. Our results show that T2D dramatically reduces this process suggesting, for the first time, a potential negative effect of T2D on the adaptation to new odours. Whether the impairment of this form of *neuroplasticity* can be related to cognitive decline in T2D remains to be investigated.

#### The effects of DPP-4i on *odour detection, olfactory memory* and olfactory *neuroplasticity* in T2D

In addition to be used clinically for the regulation of glycemia in T2D, DPP-4i mediate neurotrophic, neurogenic and neuroprotective effects in the brain, also independently of glycemia regulation [27, 70]. We investigated the potential efficacy of a chronic treatment with the DPP-4i linagliptin to counteract the identified functional and structural deficits induced by T2D on the olfactory system. We used linagliptin because the drug showed positive effects in animal models of neurodegenerative diseases [44] and cerebral stroke [16, 17].

Furthermore, glucose normalization was not obtained in GK rats (see Results), which allowed us to focus on potential glucose independent effects of the drug.

We show that linagliptin normalize some of the T2D-dysregulated *neuroplasticity* parameters (i.e. CB+ interneurons in the MOB and PC and immature DCX+ neurons in the PC). However, this treatment improved neither *odour detection* nor *olfactory memory* in T2D GK rats. Furthermore, linaglipin-treated rats showed impaired odour discrimination. One possibility to explain the lack of behavioral efficacy is that the employed olfactory tests in this study are not sensitive enough to detect pharmacologically-mediated improvements. New studies employing highly sensitive olfactometers could be useful in this respect as Thiebaud et al. have recently shown by studying the effects of a hyperlipidemic diet on olfaction in the mouse [87]. Another potential explanation is that the T2D-induced impairment in *odour detection* and *olfactory memory* is mainly driven by hyperglycemia (which is well known to have detrimental effects on the brain [58]), while *neuroplasticity* changes are glycemia-independent. In support of this hypothesis is the fact that Linagliptin was ineffective in the regulation of glycemia in the GK rat, as also recently shown [30]. If this is the case, the GK rat might not be the best model to study the effects of DPP-4i on *odour detection* nor *olfactory memory* and this is a weakness of our study. However, this aspect could also be a strength of this study allowing for the identification of glycemic-independent effects (on *neuroplasticity)* of T2D on the olfactory system. Additional studies investigating *odour detection* and *olfactory memory* in other T2D models, where DPP-4i efficiently regulate glycemia, will answer this question. Finally, another potential reason to explain the lack of effect of linagliptin on *odour detection* and *olfactory memory* is that low DPP-4 activity has been associated with inflammation of the nasal mucosa [23]. Although speculative, this effect could have masked a potential beneficial action of linagliptin on *odour detection* and/or *olfactory memory* and this is, in our sense, the most likely interpretation.

Despite the need to answer these questions by new studies, our results indicate that a chronic therapy mediated by DPP-4i can normalize the effect of T2D on CB+ interneurons in both the MOB and the PC by also inducing morphological and neurotrophic changes. This effect is potentially very interesting in relation to the established importance of these interneurons in AD progression [1, 32, 34, 43, 80]. Therefore, our results may suggest the preventive potential of DPP-4i to counteract these detrimental processes in the CNS. We also provided evidence that DPP-4i strongly (50%) decreases the number of DCX/NeuN double positive cells in the PC of GK rats. This indicates enhanced differentiation of immature DCX+ neurons into mature neurons and likely an improved capacity for adaptation to new smells. These results provide the first experimental evidence for the effect of DPP-4i on this newly identified form of *neuroplasticity* in the PC. Whether the improvement of this form of *neuroplasticity* can be associated with improved cognition in T2D remains to be investigated.

### Conclusions

In conclusion, the results of our study prove the detrimental effects of diabetes on *odour detection* in a lean model of T2D. Importantly, this study gains new knowledge about the detrimental impact of T2D on *olfactory memory* providing a strong rationale for testing this parameter in future clinical studies, e.g. as an early predictor for cognitive decline in T2D. We also show, for the first time, how T2D affects *neuroplasticity* in both the MOB and the PC by identifying the impairment of specific cellular mechanisms. These mechanisms could turn out to be key for understanding not only how T2D impairs olfaction but also the interplay between impaired olfaction in T2D and cognitive decline and dementia. While we could not demonstrate the efficacy of DPP-4i to improve *odour detection* and *olfactory memory*, our results show that linagliptin could improve cellular parameters related to the *neuroplasticity* in the olfactory system that were impaired by T2D. This provides new knowledge on the mechanisms at the basis of the beneficial effects of DPP-4 inhibitors in the T2D brain that could be exploited to design preventive therapies to treat cognitive decline in diabetes.

**Acknowledgments**
We thank Dr. Fuad Bahram (Södersjukhuset) for technical assistance and Dr. Hans Pettersson for advice on statistical analyses. We also express our gratitude to KI medical students Ioni Appelberg and Timo Oosterveld for performing part of the IHC experiments and analyzing the data.
Work in our laboratories is supported by The Swedish Heart-Lung Foundation, Diabetesfonden, Konung Gustaf V:s och Drotttning Victorias Frimurarestiftelse, the NovoNordisk foundation, EFSD, Åhlén Stiftelse, Stohnes Stiftelse, O. E. och Edla Johanssons Stiftelse, Magnus Bergvalls Stiftelse, STROKE Riksförbundet, Tornspiran stiftelse, Gamla Tjänarinnor Stiftelse, Syskonen Svensson Stiftelse and by the regional agreement on medical training and clinical research (ALF) between Stockholm County Council and the Karolinska Institutet (KI).

**Authors' contributions**
GL conceived and designed the study, performed behavioral and great part of immunohistochemistry studies, supervised Western blot studies, acquired and processed images and figures, performed statistical analyses, contributed to discussion and wrote the manuscript. WD performed some of the Western blot and immunohistochemistry studies. CGÖ provided the GK rat, contributed to discussion and edited the manuscript. FC & HP performed some of the immunohistochemistry studies and helped with the immunohistochemistry experiments. DN provided some resources and contributed to discussion. JS & TK provided the resources to perform the study, supervised GLP-1 quantification and DPP-4 activity studies, contributed to discussion and edited the manuscript. TN provided expertise and resources, contributed to discussion and edited the manuscript. VD conceived and designed the study and performed the glycemic tests, contributed to discussion and edited the manuscript. CP conceived, designed, and coordinated the study, contributed to discussion and wrote the manuscript. All authors read and approved the final manuscript.

**Competing interests**
Work in our laboratory is supported by Boehringer Ingelheim Pharma GmbH & Co. Thomas Klein and Josefin Skogsberg are employees of Boehringer Ingelheim AB, Sweden and Boehringer Ingelheim Pharma GmbH & Co, respectiviely. Thomas Nyström has received unrestricted grants from AstraZenca and consultancy fees from Boehringer Ingelheim, Eli Lilly, Novo Nordisk, Merck and Sanofi-Aventis.

**Author details**
[1]Department of Clinical Science and Education, Södersjukhuset, Internal Medicine, Karolinska Institutet, Stockholm, Sweden. [2]Department of Molecular Medicine and Surgery, Karolinska Institutet, Stockholm, Sweden. [3]Department of Anatomy and Neurobiology, Medical University of Gdansk, Gdansk, Poland. [4]Boehringer Ingelheim AB, Stockholm, Sweden. [5]Boehringer Ingelheim Pharma GmbH & Co. KG, Biberach, Germany.

**References**
1. Ahmadian SS, Rezvanian A, Peterson M, Weintraub S, Bigio EH, Mesulam MM, Geula C (2015) Loss of calbindin-D28K is associated with the full range of tangle pathology within basal forebrain cholinergic neurons in Alzheimer's disease. Neurobiol Aging 36:3163–3170. https://doi.org/10.1016/j.neurobiolaging.2015.09.001
2. Altundag A, Ay SA, Hira S, Salihoglu M, Baskoy K, Deniz F, Tekeli H, Kurt O, Yonem A, Hummel T (2017) Olfactory and gustatory functions in patients with non-complicated type 1 diabetes mellitus. Eur Arch Otorhinolaryngol 274:2621–2627. https://doi.org/10.1007/s00405-017-4497-8
3. Bachor TP, Karbanova J, Buttner E, Bermudez V, Marquioni-Ramella M, Carmeliet P, Corbeil D, Suburo AM (2017) Early ciliary and prominin-1 dysfunctions precede neurogenesis impairment in a mouse model of type 2 diabetes. Neurobiol Dis 108:13–28. https://doi.org/10.1016/j.nbd.2017.07.010
4. Baskin DG, Stein LJ, Ikeda H, Woods SC, Figlewicz DP, Porte D, Jr., Greenwood MR, Dorsa DM (1985) Genetically obese Zucker rats have abnormally low brain insulin content. Life Sci 36: 627–633
5. Bekkers JM, Suzuki N (2013) Neurons and circuits for odor processing in the piriform cortex. Trends Neurosci 36:429–438. https://doi.org/10.1016/j.tins.2013.04.005
6. Biessels GJ, Reagan LP (2015) Hippocampal insulin resistance and cognitive dysfunction. Nat Rev Neurosci 16:660–671. https://doi.org/10.1038/nrn4019
7. Bonfanti L, Olive S, Poulain DA, Theodosis DT (1992) Mapping of the distribution of polysialylated neural cell adhesion molecule throughout the central nervous system of the adult rat: an immunohistochemical study. Neuroscience 49:419–436
8. Brady DR, Mufson EJ (1997) Parvalbumin-immunoreactive neurons in the hippocampal formation of Alzheimer's diseased brain. Neuroscience 80: 1113–1125
9. Bramerson A, Johansson L, Ek L, Nordin S, Bende M (2004) Prevalence of olfactory dysfunction: the skovde population-based study. Laryngoscope 114:733–737. https://doi.org/10.1097/00005537-200404000-00026
10. Candeias E, Sebastiao I, Cardoso S, Carvalho C, Santos MS, Oliveira CR, Moreira PI, Duarte AI (2017) Brain GLP-1/IGF-1 signaling and autophagy mediate Exendin-4 protection against apoptosis in type 2 diabetic rats. Mol Neurobiol. https://doi.org/10.1007/s12035-017-0622-3
11. Cardin JA, Carlen M, Meletis K, Knoblich U, Zhang F, Deisseroth K, Tsai LH, Moore CI (2009) Driving fast-spiking cells induces gamma rhythm and controls sensory responses. Nature 459:663–667. https://doi.org/10.1038/nature08002
12. Cassano T, Romano A, Macheda T, Colangeli R, Cimmino CS, Petrella A, LaFerla FM, Cuomo V, Gaetani S (2011) Olfactory memory is impaired in a triple transgenic model of Alzheimer disease. Behav Brain Res 224:408–412. https://doi.org/10.1016/j.bbr.2011.06.029
13. Coronas-Samano G, Baker KL, Tan WJ, Ivanova AV, Verhagen JV (2016) Fus1 KO mouse as a model of oxidative stress-mediated sporadic Alzheimer's disease: circadian disruption and long-term spatial and olfactory memory impairments. Front Aging Neurosci 8:268. https://doi.org/10.3389/fnagi.2016.00268
14. Cukierman T, Gerstein HC, Williamson JD (2005) Cognitive decline and dementia in diabetes–systematic overview of prospective observational studies. Diabetologia 48:2460–2469. https://doi.org/10.1007/s00125-005-0023-4
15. D'Amico M, Di Filippo C, Marfella R, Abbatecola AM, Ferraraccio F, Rossi F, Paolisso G (2010) Long-term inhibition of dipeptidyl peptidase-4 in Alzheimer's prone mice. Exp Gerontol 45:202–207. https://doi.org/10.1016/j.exger.2009.12.004
16. Darsalia V, Larsson M, Lietzau G, Nathanson D, Nystrom T, Klein T, Patrone C (2016) Gliptins-mediated neuroprotection against stroke requires chronic pre-treatment and is glucagon-like peptide-1 receptor independent. Diabetes Obes Metab. https://doi.org/10.1111/dom.12641
17. Darsalia V, Ortsater H, Olverling A, Darlof E, Wolbert P, Nystrom T, Klein T, Sjoholm A, Patrone C (2013) The DPP-4 inhibitor linagliptin counteracts stroke in the normal and diabetic mouse brain: a comparison with glimepiride. Diabetes 62:1289–1296. https://doi.org/10.2337/db12-0988
18. Daulatzai MA (2015) Olfactory dysfunction: its early temporal relationship and neural correlates in the pathogenesis of Alzheimer's disease. J Neural Transm (Vienna) 122:1475–1497. https://doi.org/10.1007/s00702-015-1404-6
19. Deacon CF, Holst JJ (2013) Dipeptidyl peptidase-4 inhibitors for the treatment of type 2 diabetes: comparison, efficacy and safety. Expert Opin Pharmacother 14:2047–2058. https://doi.org/10.1517/14656566.2013.824966
20. Doty RL (2017) Olfactory dysfunction in neurodegenerative diseases: is there a common pathological substrate? Lancet Neurol 16:478–488. https://doi.org/10.1016/S1474-4422(17)30123-0
21. Franks KH, Chuah MI, King AE, Vickers JC (2015) Connectivity of pathology: the olfactory system as a model for network-driven mechanisms of Alzheimer's disease pathogenesis. Front Aging Neurosci 7:234. https://doi.org/10.3389/fnagi.2015.00234
22. Gault VA, Lennox R, Flatt PR (2015) Sitagliptin, a dipeptidyl peptidase-4 inhibitor, improves recognition memory, oxidative stress and hippocampal neurogenesis and upregulates key genes involved in cognitive decline. Diabetes Obes Metab. https://doi.org/10.1111/dom.12432
23. Giger R, Nicoucar K, Kurt AM, Grouzman E, Lacroix JS (2000) Study of the enzyme peptidyl peptidase IV in nasal mucosa. Schweiz Med Wochenschr Suppl 125:99S–101S

24. Gilbert PE, Murphy C (2004) The effect of the ApoE epsilon4 allele on recognition memory for olfactory and visual stimuli in patients with pathologically confirmed Alzheimer's disease, probable Alzheimer's disease, and healthy elderly controls. J Clin Exp Neuropsychol 26:779–794. https://doi.org/10.1080/13803390490509439
25. Gottfried JA (2010) Central mechanisms of odour object perception. Nat Rev Neurosci 11:628–641. https://doi.org/10.1038/nrn2883
26. Gouveri E, Katotomichelakis M, Gouveris H, Danielides V, Maltezos E, Papanas N (2014) Olfactory dysfunction in type 2 diabetes mellitus: an additional manifestation of microvascular disease? Angiology 65:869–876. https://doi.org/10.1177/0003319714520956
27. Groeneveld ON, Kappelle LJ, Biessels GJ (2016) Potentials of incretin-based therapies in dementia and stroke in type 2 diabetes mellitus. J Diabetes Invest 7:5–16. https://doi.org/10.1111/jdi.12420
28. Gundersen HJ, Bagger P, Bendtsen TF, Evans SM, Korbo L, Marcussen N, Moller A, Nielsen K, Nyengaard JR, Pakkenberg B et al (1988) The new stereological tools: disector, fractionator, nucleator and point sampled intercepts and their use in pathological research and diagnosis. APMIS 96:857–881
29. Hamilton LK, Aumont A, Julien C, Vadnais A, Calon F, Fernandes KJ (2010) Widespread deficits in adult neurogenesis precede plaque and tangle formation in the 3xTg mouse model of Alzheimer's disease. Eur J Neurosci 32:905–920. https://doi.org/10.1111/j.1460-9568.2010.07379.x
30. Hardigan T, Yasir A, Abdelsaid M, Coucha M, El-Shaffey S, Li W, Johnson MH, Ergul A (2016) Linagliptin treatment improves cerebrovascular function and remodeling and restores reduced cerebral perfusion in type 2 diabetes. Am J Physiol Regul Integr Comp Physiol 311:R466–R477. https://doi.org/10.1152/ajpregu.00057.2016
31. Hardy D, Saghatelyan A (2017) Different forms of structural plasticity in the adult olfactory bulb. Neurogenesis (Austin) 4:e1301850. https://doi.org/10.1080/23262133.2017.1301850
32. Hof PR, Morrison JH (1991) Neocortical neuronal subpopulations labeled by a monoclonal antibody to calbindin exhibit differential vulnerability in Alzheimer's disease. Exp Neurol 111:293–301
33. Hussain S, Mansouri S, Sjoholm A, Patrone C, Darsalia V (2014) Evidence for cortical neuronal loss in male type 2 diabetic Goto-Kakizaki rats. JAD. https://doi.org/10.3233/JAD-131958
34. Ichimiya Y, Emson PC, Mountjoy CQ, Lawson DE, Heizmann CW (1988) Loss of calbindin-28K immunoreactive neurones from the cortex in Alzheimer-type dementia. Brain Res 475:156–159
35. Inaguma Y, Shinohara H, Inagaki T, Kato K (1992) Immunoreactive parvalbumin concentrations in parahippocampal gyrus decrease in patients with Alzheimer's disease. J Neurol Sci 110:57–61
36. Isaacson JS (2010) Odor representations in mammalian cortical circuits. Curr Opin Neurobiol 20:328–331. https://doi.org/10.1016/j.conb.2010.02.004
37. Isik AT, Soysal P, Yay A, Usarel C (2017) The effects of sitagliptin, a DPP-4 inhibitor, on cognitive functions in elderly diabetic patients with or without Alzheimer's disease. Diabetes Res Clin Pract 123:192–198. https://doi.org/10.1016/j.diabres.2016.12.010
38. Jan YN, Jan LY (2010) Branching out: mechanisms of dendritic arborization. Nat Rev Neurosci 11:316–328. https://doi.org/10.1038/nrn2836
39. Jorgensen MB, Buch NH (1961) Studies on the sense of smell and taste in diabetics. Acta Otolaryngol 53:539–545
40. Kalaria RN (2009) Neurodegenerative disease: diabetes, microvascular pathology and Alzheimer disease. Nature reviews. Neurology 5:305–306. https://doi.org/10.1038/nrneurol.2009.72
41. Klempin F, Kronenberg G, Cheung G, Kettenmann H, Kempermann G (2011) Properties of doublecortin-(DCX)-expressing cells in the piriform cortex compared to the neurogenic dentate gyrus of adult mice. PLoS One 6: e25760. https://doi.org/10.1371/journal.pone.0025760
42. Kodl CT, Seaquist ER (2008) Cognitive dysfunction and diabetes mellitus. Endocr Rev 29:494–511. https://doi.org/10.1210/er.2007-0034
43. Kook SY, Jeong H, Kang MJ, Park R, Shin HJ, Han SH, Son SM, Song H, Baik SH, Moon M et al (2014) Crucial role of calbindin-D28k in the pathogenesis of Alzheimer's disease mouse model. Cell Death Differ 21:1575–1587. https://doi.org/10.1038/cdd.2014.67
44. Kornelius E, Lin CL, Chang HH, Li HH, Huang WN, Yang YS, Lu YL, Peng CH, Huang CN (2015) DPP-4 inhibitor Linagliptin attenuates Abeta-induced cytotoxicity through activation of AMPK in neuronal cells. CNS Neurosci Ther 21:549–557. https://doi.org/10.1111/cns.12404
45. Kosaraju J, Gali CC, Khatwal RB, Dubala A, Chinni S, Holsinger RM, Madhunapantula VS, Muthureddy Nataraj SK, Basavan D (2013) Saxagliptin: a dipeptidyl peptidase-4 inhibitor ameliorates streptozotocin induced Alzheimer's disease. Neuropharmacology 72:291–300. https://doi.org/10.1016/j.neuropharm.2013.04.008
46. Kosaraju J, Holsinger RM, Guo L, Tam KY (2016) Linagliptin, a dipeptidyl Peptidase-4 inhibitor, mitigates cognitive deficits and pathology in the 3xTg-AD mouse model of Alzheimer's disease. Mol Neurobio. https://doi.org/10.1007/s12035-016-0125-7
47. Kosaraju J, Madhunapantula SV, Chinni S, Khatwal RB, Dubala A, Muthureddy Nataraj SK, Basavan D (2014) Dipeptidyl peptidase-4 inhibition by Pterocarpus Marsupium and Eugenia Jambolana ameliorates streptozotocin induced Alzheimer's disease. Behav Brain Res 267:55–65. https://doi.org/10.1016/j.bbr.2014.03.026
48. Lacroix MC, Caillol M, Durieux D, Monnerie R, Grebert D, Pellerin L, Repond C, Tolle V, Zizzari P, Baly C (2015) Long-lasting metabolic imbalance related to obesity alters olfactory tissue homeostasis and impairs olfactory-driven behaviors. Chem Senses 40:537–556. https://doi.org/10.1093/chemse/bjv039
49. Lang BT, Yan Y, Dempsey RJ, Vemuganti R (2009) Impaired neurogenesis in adult type-2 diabetic rats. Brain Res 1258:25–33. https://doi.org/10.1016/j.brainres.2008.12.026
50. Larsson M, Hedner M, Papenberg G, Seubert J, Backman L, Laukka EJ (2016) Olfactory memory in the old and very old: relations to episodic and semantic memory and APOE genotype. Neurobiol Aging 38:118–126. https://doi.org/10.1016/j.neurobiolaging.2015.11.012
51. Le Floch JP, Le Lievre G, Labroue M, Paul M, Peynegre R, Perlemuter L (1993) Smell dysfunction and related factors in diabetic patients. Diabetes Care 16:934–937
52. Lehmkuhl AM, Dirr ER, Fleming SM (2014) Olfactory assays for mouse models of neurodegenerative disease. JOVE:e51804. https://doi.org/10.3791/51804
53. Li W, Howard JD, Gottfried JA (2010) Disruption of odour quality coding in piriform cortex mediates olfactory deficits in Alzheimer's disease. Brain J Neurol 133:2714–2726. https://doi.org/10.1093/brain/awq209
54. Li XH, Xin X, Wang Y, Wu JZ, Jin ZD, Ma LN, Nie CJ, Xiao X, Hu Y, Jin MW (2013) Pentamethylquercetin protects against diabetes-related cognitive deficits in diabetic Goto-Kakizaki rats. JAD 34:755–767. https://doi.org/10.3233/JAD-122017
55. Lietzau G, Darsalia V, Pintana H, Ostenson CG, Nystrom T, Fisahn A, Patrone C (2017) Type 2 diabetes alters hippocampal gamma oscillations: a potential mechanism behind impaired cognition. Psychoneuroendocrinology 82:46–50. https://doi.org/10.1016/j.psyneuen.2017.04.012
56. Lietzau G, Nystrom T, Ostenson CG, Darsalia V, Patrone C (2016) Type 2 diabetes-induced neuronal pathology in the piriform cortex of the rat is reversed by the GLP-1 receptor agonist Exendin-4. Oncotarget. https://doi.org/10.18632/oncotarget.6823
57. Livingston JN, Unger JW, Moxley RT, Moss A (1993) Phosphotyrosine-containing proteins in the CNS of obese Zucker rats are decreased in the absence of changes in the insulin receptor. Neuroendocrinology 57:481–488
58. Luitse MJ, Biessels GJ, Rutten GE, Kappelle LJ (2012) Diabetes, hyperglycaemia, and acute ischaemic stroke. Lancet Neurol 11:261–271. https://doi.org/10.1016/S1474-4422(12)70005-4
59. Mansouri S, Barde S, Ortsater H, Eweida M, Darsalia V, Langel U, Sjoholm A, Hokfelt T, Patrone C (2013) GalR3 activation promotes adult neural stem cell survival in response to a diabetic milieu. J Neurochem 127:209–220. https://doi.org/10.1111/jnc.12396
60. Mansouri S, Ortsater H, Pintor Gallego O, Darsalia V, Sjoholm A, Patrone C (2011) Pituitary adenylate cyclase-activating polypeptide counteracts the impaired adult neural stem cell viability induced by palmitate. J Neurosci Res. https://doi.org/10.1002/jnr.22803
61. Markopoulou K, Chase BA, Robowski P, Strongosky A, Narozanska E, Sitek EJ, Berdynski M, Barcikowska M, Baker MC, Rademakers Ret al (2016) Assessment of olfactory function in MAPT-associated neurodegenerative disease reveals odor-identification irreproducibility as a non-disease-specific, general characteristic of olfactory dysfunction. PLoS One 11: e0165112 https://doi.org/10.1371/journal.pone.0165112
62. Matsunaga Y, Negishi T, Hatakeyama A, Kawagoe Y, Sawano E, Tashiro T (2016) Impairment of synaptic development in the hippocampus of diabetic Goto-Kakizaki rats. Int J Dev Neurosci 53:58–67. https://doi.org/10.1016/j.ijdevneu.2016.07.004
63. Moreira PI, Santos MS, Moreno AM, Seica R, Oliveira CR (2003) Increased vulnerability of brain mitochondria in diabetic (Goto-Kakizaki) rats with aging and amyloid-beta exposure. Diabetes 52:1449–1456
64. Moreira T, Malec E, Ostenson CG, Efendic S, Liljequist S (2007) Diabetic type II Goto-Kakizaki rats show progressively decreasing exploratory activity and

learning impairments in fixed and progressive ratios of a lever-press task. Behav Brain Res 180:28–41. https://doi.org/10.1016/j.bbr.2007.02.034
65. Murakawa Y, Zhang W, Pierson CR, Brismar T, Ostenson CG, Efendic S, Sima AA (2002) Impaired glucose tolerance and insulinopenia in the GK-rat causes peripheral neuropathy. Diabetes Metab Res Rev 18:473–483. https://doi.org/10.1002/dmrr.326
66. Nacher J, Bonfanti L (2015) New neurons from old beliefs in the adult piriform cortex? A commentary on: occurrence of new neurons in the piriform cortex. Front Neuroanat 9:62. https://doi.org/10.3389/fnana.2015.00062
67. Nagayama S, Homma R, Imamura F (2014) Neuronal organization of olfactory bulb circuits. Front Neural Circuits 8:98. https://doi.org/10.3389/fncir.2014.00098
68. Naka A, Riedl M, Luger A, Hummel T, Mueller CA (2010) Clinical significance of smell and taste disorders in patients with diabetes mellitus. Eur Arch Otorhinolaryngol 267:547–550. https://doi.org/10.1007/s00405-009-1123-4
69. Ostenson CG, Efendic S (2007) Islet gene expression and function in type 2 diabetes; studies in the Goto-Kakizaki rat and humans. Diabetes Obes Metab 9(Suppl 2):180–186. https://doi.org/10.1111/j.1463-1326.2007.00787.x
70. Patrone C, Eriksson O, Lindholm D (2014) Diabetes drugs and neurological disorders: new views and therapeutic possibilities. Lancet Diabetes Endocrinol 2:256–262. https://doi.org/10.1016/S2213-8587(13)70125-6
71. Patterson DS, Turner P, Smart JV (1966) Smell threshold in diabetes mellitus. Nature 209:625
72. Poo C, Isaacson JS (2009) Odor representations in olfactory cortex: "sparse" coding, global inhibition, and oscillations. Neuron 62:850–861. https://doi.org/10.1016/j.neuron.2009.05.022
73. Portha B, Giroix MH, Tourrel-Cuzin C, Le-Stunff H, Movassat J (2012) The GK rat: a prototype for the study of non-overweight type 2 diabetes. Methods Mol Biol 933:125–159. https://doi.org/10.1007/978-1-62703-068-7_9
74. Riviere S, Soubeyre V, Jarriault D, Molinas A, Leger-Charnay E, Desmoulins L, Grebert D, Meunier N, Grosmaitre X (2016) High fructose diet inducing diabetes rapidly impacts olfactory epithelium and behavior in mice. Sci Rep 6:34011. https://doi.org/10.1038/srep34011
75. Roman FS, Alescio-Lautier B, Soumireu-Mourat B (1996) Age-related learning and memory deficits in odor-reward association in rats. Neurobiol Aging 17:31–40
76. Rubio A, Belles M, Belenguer G, Vidueira S, Farinas I, Nacher J (2016) Characterization and isolation of immature neurons of the adult mouse piriform cortex. Dev Neurobiol 76:748–763. https://doi.org/10.1002/dneu.22357
77. Sa-Nguanmoo P, Tanajak P, Kerdphoo S, Jaiwongkam T, Pratchayasakul W, Chattipakorn N, Chattipakorn SC (2017) SGLT2-inhibitor and DPP-4 inhibitor improve brain function via attenuating mitochondrial dysfunction, insulin resistance, inflammation, and apoptosis in HFD-induced obese rats. Toxicol Appl Pharmacol 333:43–50. https://doi.org/10.1016/j.taap.2017.08.005
78. Saiz-Sanchez D, De la Rosa-Prieto C, Ubeda-Banon I, Martinez-Marcos A (2015) Interneurons, tau and amyloid-beta in the piriform cortex in Alzheimer's disease. Brain Struct Funct 220:2011–2025. https://doi.org/10.1007/s00429-014-0771-3
79. Saiz-Sanchez D, Flores-Cuadrado A, Ubeda-Banon I, de la Rosa-Prieto C, Martinez-Marcos A (2016) Interneurons in the human olfactory system in Alzheimer's disease. Exp Neurol 276:13–21. https://doi.org/10.1016/j.expneurol.2015.11.009
80. Saiz-Sanchez D, Ubeda-Banon I, De la Rosa-Prieto C, Martinez-Marcos A (2012) Differential expression of interneuron populations and correlation with amyloid-beta deposition in the olfactory cortex of an AbetaPP/PS1 transgenic mouse model of Alzheimer's disease. JAD 31:113–129. https://doi.org/10.3233/JAD-2012-111889
81. Sakamoto M, Kageyama R, Imayoshi I (2014) The functional significance of newly born neurons integrated into olfactory bulb circuits. Front Neurosci 8:121. https://doi.org/10.3389/fnins.2014.00121
82. Sanke H, Mita T, Yoshii H, Yokota A, Yamashiro K, Ingaki N, Onuma T, Someya Y, Komiya K, Tamura Y et al (2014) Relationship between olfactory dysfunction and cognitive impairment in elderly patients with type 2 diabetes mellitus. Diabetes Res Clin Pract 106:465–473. https://doi.org/10.1016/j.diabres.2014.09.039
83. Scheen AJ (2015) A review of gliptins for 2014. Expert Opin Pharmacother 16:43–62. https://doi.org/10.1517/14656566.2015.978289
84. Seki T, Arai Y (1991) Expression of highly polysialylated NCAM in the neocortex and piriform cortex of the developing and the adult rat. Anat Embryol (Berl) 184:395–401
85. Seubert J, Laukka EJ, Rizzuto D, Hummel T, Fratiglioni L, Backman L, Larsson M (2017) Prevalence and correlates of olfactory dysfunction in old age: a population-based study. The journals of gerontology series a, biological sciences and medical. Sciences 72:1072–1079. https://doi.org/10.1093/gerona/glx054
86. Shapiro LA, Ng KL, Kinyamu R, Whitaker-Azmitia P, Geisert EE, Blurton-Jones M, Zhou QY, Ribak CE (2007) Origin, migration and fate of newly generated neurons in the adult rodent piriform cortex. Brain Struct Funct 212:133–148. https://doi.org/10.1007/s00429-007-0151-3
87. Thiebaud N, Johnson MC, Butler JL, Bell GA, Ferguson KL, Fadool AR, Fadool JC, Gale AM, Gale DS, Fadool DA (2014) Hyperlipidemic diet causes loss of olfactory sensory neurons, reduces olfactory discrimination, and disrupts odor-reversal learning. J Neurosci 34:6970–6984. https://doi.org/10.1523/JNEUROSCI.3366-13.2014
88. Verret L, Mann EO, Hang GB, Barth AM, Cobos I, Ho K, Devidze N, Masliah E, Kreitzer AC, Mody let al (2012) Inhibitory interneuron deficit links altered network activity and cognitive dysfunction in Alzheimer model. Cell 149: 708–721 Doi https://doi.org/10.1016/j.cell.2012.02.046
89. Wakabayashi T, Hidaka R, Fujimaki S, Asashima M, Kuwabara T (2016) Diabetes impairs Wnt3 protein-induced neurogenesis in olfactory bulbs via glutamate transporter 1 inhibition. J Biol Chem 291:15196–15211. https://doi.org/10.1074/jbc.M115.672857
90. Xu W, Caracciolo B, Wang HX, Winblad B, Backman L, Qiu C, Fratiglioni L (2010) Accelerated progression from mild cognitive impairment to dementia in people with diabetes. Diabetes 59:2928–2935. https://doi.org/10.2337/db10-0539
91. Xu ZP, Yang SL, Zhao S, Zheng CH, Li HH, Zhang Y, Huang RX, Li MZ, Gao Y, Zhang SJet al (2016) Biomarkers for early diagnostic of mild cognitive impairment in Type-2 diabetes patients: a multicentre, retrospective, nested case-control study. EBioMedicine 5: 105–113 https://doi.org/10.1016/j.ebiom.2016.02.014
92. Young JW, Sharkey J, Finlayson K (2009) Progressive impairment in olfactory working memory in a mouse model of mild cognitive impairment. Neurobiol Aging 30:1430–1443. https://doi.org/10.1016/j.neurobiolaging.2007.11.018
93. Zhan C, Luo M (2010) Diverse patterns of odor representation by neurons in the anterior piriform cortex of awake mice. J Neurosci 30:16662–16672. https://doi.org/10.1523/JNEUROSCI.4400-10.2010

14

# Exosomes taken up by neurons hijack the endosomal pathway to spread to interconnected neurons

Juan Carlos Polanco[1], Chuanzhou Li[1], Nela Durisic[2], Robert Sullivan[2] and Jürgen Götz[1*]

**Abstract**

In Alzheimer disease and related disorders, the microtubule-associated protein tau aggregates and forms cytoplasmic lesions that impair neuronal physiology at many levels. In addition to affecting the host neuron, tau aggregates also spread to neighboring, recipient cells where the misfolded tau aggregates, in a manner similar to prions, actively corrupt the proper folding of soluble tau, and thereby impair cellular functions. One vehicle for the transmission of tau aggregates are secretory nanovesicles known as exosomes. Here, we established a simple model of a neuronal circuit using a microfluidics culture system in which hippocampal neurons A and B were seeded into chambers 1 and 2, respectively, extending axons via microgrooves in both directions and thereby interconnecting. This system served to establish two models to track exosome spreading. In the first model, we labeled the exosomal membrane by coupling tetraspanin CD9 with either a green or red fluorescent tag. This allowed us to reveal that interconnected neurons exchange exosomes only when their axons extend in close proximity. In the second model, we added exosomes isolated from the brains of tau transgenic rTg4510 mice (i.e. exogenous, neuron A-derived) to neurons in chamber 1 (neuron B) interconnected with neuron C in chamber 2. This allowed us to demonstrate that a substantial fraction of the exogenous exosomes were internalized by neuron B and passed then on to neuron C. This transportation from neuron B to C was achieved by a mechanism that is consistent with the hijacking of secretory endosomes by the exogenous exosomes, as revealed by confocal, super-resolution and electron microscopy. Together, these findings suggest that fusion events involving the endogenous endosomal secretory machinery increase the pathogenic potential and the radius of action of pathogenic cargoes carried by exogenous exosomes.

**Keywords:** Alzheimer, Tau, Spreading, Exosomes, Endosomes, Protein aggregates, Organelle fusion, Axonal transport

## Introduction

Alzheimer disease (AD), the most common form of aging dementia, is characterized by problems with memory, thinking and behavior [50]. These clinical features are strongly associated with the accumulation of two types of insoluble protein deposits in the AD brain, which are composed of either the amyloid-β (Aβ) peptide or the microtubule-associated protein tau and impair neuronal function at many levels [5, 32, 44, 50]. The Aβ deposits are referred to as amyloid plaques and are found in the interstitial space of the brain, whereas the lesions composed of aggregated tau, known as neurofibrillary tangles (NFTs), are intraneuronal [5, 32, 44, 50]. Tau pathology progresses through well-defined stereotyped stages, which appears to be initiated in the locus coeruleus and slowly spreads via the entorhinal cortex and hippocampus to the neocortex [12, 13]; however the role of the locus coeruleus is controversial [4]. This pattern of tau spreading led to the suggestion that AD progression occurs by neuron-to-neuron transmission involving trans-synaptic transport of seeds of tau aggregation from affected to anatomically interconnected recipient neurons [12, 13]. It has since been established that the intercellular transfer of misfolded forms of tau known as "seeds" contributes to the progression of AD, with tau seeds acting in a manner similar to prions, triggering the robust conversion of soluble tau into insoluble large filamentous aggregates and NFTs [14, 30, 50].

* Correspondence: j.goetz@uq.edu.au
[1]Clem Jones Centre for Ageing Dementia Research (CJCADR), Queensland Brain Institute (QBI), The University of Queensland, Brisbane, QLD 4072, Australia
Full list of author information is available at the end of the article

Several modes of neuron-to-neuron transfer of tau seeds have been described, including via extracellular vesicles such as exosomes [22, 51, 66], trans-synaptically mediated transfer of tau aggregates between interconnected neurons [15, 23], tunneling nanotubes [61] or the uptake of free-floating tau aggregates and fibrils [30, 35]. In vitro evidence suggests that reducing the pool of extracellular tau seeds, irrespective of whether these are moving freely or are transported by exosomes or any other mechanism of inter-neuronal transfer, results in an in vivo reduction of tau pathology by maintaining the level of extracellular tau seeds below a pathological concentration threshold [5, 15, 29, 30, 36, 51, 61]. Our research focuses on exosomes, membranous secreted nanovesicles 30–150 nm in size, that are produced in late endosomes by the inward budding of the endosomal membrane, which is progressively pinched off to generate and accumulate intraluminal nanovesicles [11, 38, 45]. The late endosome, loaded with intraluminal nanovesicles, then gradually develops into large multivesicular bodies (MVBs). These MVBs can fuse with the plasma membrane to release the intraluminal nanovesicles into the extracellular environment, and once secreted these free nanovesicles are termed "exosomes" [11, 38, 45].

A number of studies have shown that exosomes can transport Aβ and derivatives of the amyloid precursor protein (APP) from which Aβ originates [48, 52, 58]. They also contain phosphorylated tau as demonstrated for exosomes that have been isolated from the blood and cerebrospinal fluid of AD patients [26, 55]. Furthermore, immuno-electron microscopy of AD brain tissue has revealed that human Aβ plaques are enriched in exosomal proteins [52]. Mouse models of AD have been instrumental in demonstrating that exosome reduction in vivo is associated with a lower Aβ plaque load in the brain [20, 21]. Similarly, depletion of microglia and inhibition of exosome synthesis has been found to halt tau propagation in the brains of tauopathy mouse models [3]. Taken together, these studies support the notion that reducing exosome secretion results in reduced Aβ plaque formation and tau propagation. Related to this, we have demonstrated that tau seeds are contained within exosomes isolated from the brains of tauopathy mice, that they have a distinct phosphorylation pattern, and that only exosomes derived from cells undergoing tau aggregation are able to seed and corrupt soluble tau in recipient cells, a phenomenon that occurs in a threshold-dependent manner [6, 51].

An important question in the field is how the seeds are taken up and handled by recipient cells. Here, neuron-to-neuron transmission of exosomes emerges as an important pathomechanism for the progression of AD. Such a mechanism implies that a neuron generates exosomes in endosomes, an organelle which is more abundant in the soma than in axons [65], after which the mature MVBs undergo anterograde transport along the axons until they fuse with the plasma membrane to release the exosome at the synapse of an interconnected cell. Evidence for such a trans-synaptic mechanism has been provided by studies in *Drosophila* which investigated exosomes carrying Wnt signals at the neuromuscular junction [41, 42]. In our study, we used simple microfluidics circuit systems to demonstrate that exosomes are not only being exchanged between interconnected neurons A and B, but that a recipient neuron C can receive exosomes that have either been generated by an interconnected neuron B or are passed on via this interconnected neuron after processing of 'exogenous' exosomes that have been internalized from neuron A. This 'longer-distance action' of exosomes appears to be linked to the hijacking of secretory endosomes present in neuron B of this simple circuit. We discuss how such fusion events potentially increase the pathogenic potential and the radius of action of pathogenic cargoes carried by exogenous exosomes.

## Materials and methods

### Mouse strains and collection of brain tissue

C57BL/6 mice were used at embryonic day 17 (E17) to isolate hippocampal neurons for tissue culture experiments. rTg4510 mice expressing human four-repeat tau with the P301L mutation linked to hereditary tauopathy [56] were used at 4–6 months of age for exosome isolation. Animal experimentation was approved by the Animal Ethics Committee of the University of Queensland (approval number QBI/412/14/NHMRC).

### Isolation and purification of brain exosomes

Exosomes were isolated from the interstitial space of mouse brains using a previously established protocol [48, 51]. In brief, each brain was dissected and gently chopped before being incubated in 7 ml of 0.2% *w/v* Collagenase type III (LS004182, Worthington) in serum-free Hibernate-A medium (A12475-01, Life Technologies) for 30 min at 37 °C. The dissociation reaction was stopped with 14 ml of ice-cold Hibernate-A containing 1× Complete protease inhibitor cocktail (Roche), 50 mM NaF and 200 nM $Na_3VO_4$. The tissue was then gently dissociated with a 10 ml pipette, keeping the cells intact during pipetting them up and down, followed by a series of differential 4 °C centrifugations at 300 g for 10 min, 2000 g for 10 min and 10,000 g for 30 min to sequentially discard the pellet containing cells, membranes, and nanodebris, respectively. The supernatant from the final centrifugation step was passed through a 0.22 µm syringe filter (Millex-GP, Millipore) and centrifuged at 120,000 g for 70 min at 4 °C to pellet the exosomes. The pellet containing the exosomes was then washed with 5 ml phosphate-buffered saline (PBS, 17-516Q, Lonza), after which the pellets from five mouse brains per genotype (25 ml) were pooled. This preparation was centrifuged at 120,000 g for 70 min at 4 °C to obtain a pellet that was resuspended in 2 ml of 0.95 M sucrose in 20 mM HEPES (15630–080, Life Technologies), then purified using a sucrose step gradient column (six 2 ml steps at 2.0, 1.65, 1.3, 0.95, 0.6 and 0.25 M sucrose from bottom to top). The sucrose gradient was centrifuged at 200,000 g for 16 h at 4 °C. The exosome-containing fraction 3 (0.95 M; ρ = 1.12 g/ml sucrose) was collected together with the interphase and resuspended in 6 ml ice-cold PBS, followed by a 120,000 g centrifugation for 70 min at 4 °C. Finally, the sucrose-purified exosome pellet was resuspended in 100 μl PBS containing 1× Complete protease inhibitor cocktail (Roche). A 10 μl aliquot of exosomes in PBS was homogenized with 10 μl of 2× RIPA buffer (300 mM NaCl, 100 mM Tris-HCl pH 7.4, 0.50% (*w*/*v*) sodium deoxycholate, 0.2% (*v*/*v*) Nonidet P-40) to determine the protein content with a Micro BCA™ Protein Assay Kit (23,235, Thermo-Fisher).

#### Fluorescence labeling of exosome membranes

To track exogenous exosomes isolated from mouse brains, we labeled their membranes with an appropriate fluorescent stain that stably incorporates a fluorescent dye with long aliphatic tails into the exosome membrane. In our study, the fluorescent membrane probes CellVue® Claret Far-Red Fluorescent Membrane Linker (Sigma), PKH67 Green Fluorescent Membrane Linker (Sigma) and FM™ 1–43FX Fixable Membrane Stain (Thermo-Fisher) were used to separately label sucrose-purified exosomes according to the manufacturer's instructions. The labeling reaction was stopped with 6 ml of 2% bovine serum albumin, followed by ultra-centrifugation at 100,000 g for 70 min, washing with PBS and another round of ultra-centrifugation, followed by resuspension of the fluorescently labeled exosomes in PBS.

#### Primary neuronal culture and microfluidic devices

Hippocampal neurons were isolated by standard methods using C57BL/6 mice sacrificed at E17 and grown in culture chamber microfluidic devices (Xona Microfluidics) placed on 24 × 60 mm coverslips (#1,5 Menzel-Glaser) that had been coated with poly-D-lysine (PDL), to form a non-plasma bond with the device. 60,000–80,000 neurons were plated per chamber using Neurobasal medium (21,103,049, Thermo-Fisher) supplemented with 5% fetal bovine serum (FBS; Hyclone), 2% B27 (17,504,044, Thermo-Fisher), 1 mM GlutaMAX (35,050,061, Thermo-Fisher) and 50 U/ml penicillin/streptomycin (15,070,063, Thermo-Fisher). The medium was changed to serum-free Neurobasal medium minus phenol red (12,348,017, Thermo-Fisher), supplemented with 28 nM 2-mercaptoethanol (21,985,023, Thermo-Fisher) 24 h post-seeding, and half of the medium was changed twice a week. A hydrostatic pressure gradient that prevents diffusion between culture chamber (Ch) 1 and Ch2 was established by adding twice the volume of culture medium to Ch2. To perform electron microscopy, the microfluidic devices were placed on plastic culture dishes coated with PDL. All cultures were maintained at 37 °C and 5% $CO_2$ for up to 12 days. Neurons grown in the microfluidic devices were analyzed at 8–12 days in vitro (DIV8–12).

#### Plasmids, virus preparation and electroporations

CD9 is a tetraspanin that is expressed on plasma, endosomal and exosomal membranes [2, 8, 64]. To label and track exosomes, dispersed primary hippocampal neurons were transfected with the plasmids mCherry-CD9–10 (Addgene # 55013) and Dendra2-CD9–10 (Addgene #57705), kind gifts from Dr. Michael Davidson to Addgene. For transfection, $4 \times 10^6$ neurons were electroporated with 4 μg plasmid DNA using a Nucleofector™ 2b device and the Amaxa Basic Primary Neurons Nucleofector® Kit (VPI-1003, Lonza). After electroporation, the neurons were resuspended in FBS-containing Neurobasal plating medium, centrifuged for 5 min at 100 g and then resuspended in Neurobasal plating medium to obtain a concentration of 8000 neurons per μl before seeding the neurons in the chambers of the microfluidic device. To detect endosomes, neurons were also transduced with a commercial baculovirus expressing the late endosomal marker LAMP1 (lysosomal-associated membrane protein 1) tagged with RFP (Thermo, C10597). After 48 h they were fixed in paraformaldehyde and imaged.

#### Confocal microscopy and image analysis

Fluorescence images at a 63× magnification were obtained with a Zeiss LSM 710 inverted laser scanning confocal microscope using a 1-2× optical zoom. For fluorescent particle quantification of endosomes, 4–10 non-overlapping confocal images at a 63× magnification were analyzed per sample using the open source ImageJ software (version 1.51r, Wayne Rasband, National Institutes of Health, Bethesda). The acquisition parameters remained invariable for all images. The fluorescence signal was adjusted by image segmentation applying a 'Triangle' threshold to specifically detect endosomal fluorescent particles in the green (Dendra2-CD9) and red (mCherry-CD9) channels. The thresholded binary images with particles were processed to reduce noise using the Image-J 'Despeckle' plugin, followed by the 'Watershed' filter to separate overlapping particles in the binary images. Particles were quantified in the segmented images with the 'Analyze Particles' ImageJ plugin using the parameter size 0.2–10 squared microns (μm [2]) and circularity 0.1–1 (value of 1 indicating a perfect circle). Occasionally, fluorescent detection of CD9 in the plasma membrane generated fragments of neurites that were included as endosomal particles by ImageJ. Those inconsistencies were manually curated and excluded from the analysis using the ROI Manager. Then, the 'Image Calculator' plugin was used to multiply the segmented binary images from the green and red channels in order to quantify the number of endosomal particles that had both colors.

### Super-resolution microscopy

Super-resolution microscopy was performed as a combination of Photo-Activated Localization Microscopy (PALM) using the fluorescent protein Dendra2 as the label for CD9 and direct Stochastic Optical Reconstruction Microscopy (dSTORM) using CellVue Claret. All super-resolution experiments were performed on an Elyra STORM/SIM microscope (Carl Zeiss, GmbH) equipped with a 100× oil-immersion objective, a focus lock system, an EMCCD Andor iXon Ultra 897 camera (Andor Technologies) and a super-resolution multiband dichroic and emission filter set (405/488/561/635-A-000,m Semrock). Neurons were imaged in highly inclined illumination mode at 20 kHz. Zen 2012 SP2 (black) software (Carl Zeiss, GmbH) was used for image reconstruction and channel alignment in the dual color experiments.

### Electron microscopy and DAB photoconversion

Exosomes labeled with FM™1-43FX Fixable Membrane Stain (Thermo-Fisher) were added to primary hippocampal neurons grown in chamber 1 of microfluidic devices bound to 6 cm plastic culture dishes (Falcon, 353,002). 24 h after exosome uptake, the cultures were briefly washed 3× for 5 min with PBS to remove cellular debris and non-internalized exosomes, fixed with 4% paraformaldehyde (Sigma, 15,827) in PBS for 20 min, and again washed in PBS 3× for 5 min. The cultures were then incubated in 100 mM ammonium chloride solution (Sigma, 213,330) for 20 min, after which they were washed in PBS. Fixed cultures were incubated in 1.5 mg/ml diaminobenzidine (DAB, Sigma D5637) in PBS for 30 min at 4 °C. DAB forms a stable, insoluble precipitate that has a dark appearance and can be easily distinguished by electron microscopy [33, 34]. We therefore photoconverted the FM™ 1-43FX stain into a DAB precipitate using a light box equipped with four 24-watt lamps (Atiaquaristik), two lamps at 420–460 nm and two at 400–500 nm, refrigerated with a cooling fan to prevent heating of the samples. Fluorescence bleaching and complete DAB photoconversion were confirmed by direct visualization using an axioscope (Zeiss).

For electron microscopy, samples were processed using protocols of the Biowave Pro+ (Pelco) microwave tissue processor maintaining the samples at room temperature. Biowave procedures included fixation in 2.5% glutaraldehyde (Proscitech, C003) in PBS for 3 min, osmication with 4% osmium (Proscitech, C010) and 3% potassium ferrocyanide (Sigma, P8131), and washing in $dH_2O$ 5× for 3 min, followed by incubation in 1% thiocarbohydrazide (Sigma, 88,535) for 20 min. After this, the samples were stained in 2% osmium tetroxide, washed in $dH_2O$ 5 × for 3 min and then stained in 1% uranyl acetate (Proscitech, C079) for 30 min. After 5 washes in $dH_2O$ for 3 min, the samples were stained in 20 mM lead aspartate (Proscitech, C151, Sigma, A9256) for 30 min at 60°C. Cultures were dehydrated through a graded series of ethanol followed by 100% acetone and then infiltrated into Epon resin (C038), followed by resin polymerization at 60 °C for 48 h. Resin-embedded samples were cut at 70 nm using a diamond knife (Diatome) and then collected onto 200 × mesh copper grids (Proscitech, GCu200) and imaged on a Hitachi HT7700 transmission electron microscope at 80 kV using an AXT 2Kx2K CMOS digital camera.

## Results

### Establishing neuronal circuits with microfluidic devices

We tested different neuronal cultures in microfluidic devices in order to identify an appropriate neuronal circuit to analyze exosome spreading and tracking. Neuronal cultures grown in the chambers of microfluidic devices are separated by thin microgrooves, which allows for fluidically isolating neuronal cell bodies (somata) from axons (but not dendrites), with axons extending into a connected chamber and thereby establishing synaptic connections [15, 16, 23, 62]. We first tested triple chamber devices (Ch1, Ch2, Ch3) seeded with neurons A, B and C, respectively, interconnected with microgrooves for axonal projections. However, we found that from 8 to 9 days in vitro (DIV8–9) onwards, axons from red neurons seeded in Ch1 grew into Ch3, thereby bypassing neuron B and establishing direct connections A-C, confounding our experimental design (Additional file 1: Figure S1). We therefore opted for the two models that are illustrated in Fig. 1.

(i) Model 1 (Fig. 1a) connects two neurons (A and B) that were individually labeled using a discriminating fluorescence marker (red or green). CD9 was used as a marker for plasma, endosomal and exosomal membranes. To label and track exosomes, dispersed primary hippocampal neurons were transfected with either mCherry-CD9–10 (red) or Dendra2-CD9–10

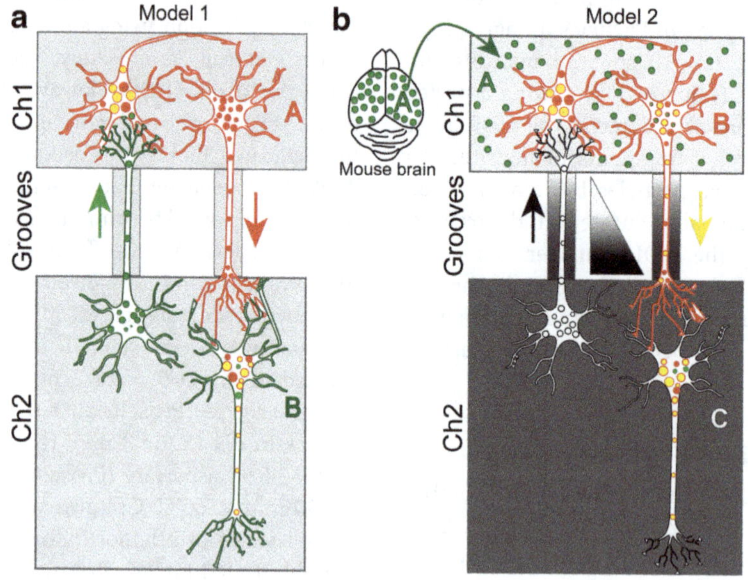


**Fig. 1** Schematic of experimental designs used to establish neuronal circuits using microfluidic devices. Neurons expressing the tetraspanin CD9 together with either a red or green fluorescent tag were used to track exosomal, endosomal and plasma membranes. **a** Model 1 of two differently colored neurons (A-red and B-green) seeded separately into the two chambers Ch1 and Ch2. Red axons extend from Ch1 to Ch2, but green axons can also project from Ch2 to Ch1. The potential combination of colors by transmission of exosomes is shown in yellow. **b** Model 2 of three interconnected neurons (A-green, B-red, C-no color) seeded into chambers Ch1 and Ch2. The exosomes from A (green) are internalized by B (red) and can potentially be anterogradely transported to C (no color). Combination of colors is shown in yellow. The gradient of the triangle depicts a hydrostatic pressure gradient that prevents diffusion from Ch1 to Ch2. Note that sizes of neurons and culture chambers are not shown at scale

(green) in chambers Ch1 and Ch2, respectively. The exchange of fluorescence in either direction can be detected with model system 1.

(ii) Model 2 (Fig. 1b) is a proxy for the connection of three neurons (A, B and C) exchanging exosomes and separated in Ch1 and Ch2. Instead of having an intact neuron A, we used brain-derived exosomes from rTg4510 mice [51, 56] labeled with a green fluorescent membrane dye (PKH67) that were added to neuron B (red, expressing mCherry-CD9) in Ch1, whereas the interconnected neuron C in Ch2 was a 'non-fluorescent' neuron. Diffusion from Ch1 to Ch2 of brain neuron A-derived exosomes was prevented by establishing a hydrostatic pressure gradient by adding twice the volume of culture medium to Ch2 (Fig. 1b).

### Interconnected neurons exchange exosomes

Exosomes are highly enriched in the protein superfamily termed tetraspanins, which organize plasma membrane microdomains [2]. The tetraspanins CD9, CD63, CD81 and CD151 have a broad tissue distribution [2]. They are abundant in various types of endocytic membranes, including exosome-generating MVBs [8], and have been widely used as exosomal markers because of their prevalence in exosomes and their role in exosome biogenesis, protein loading and sorting of cargoes into exosomes [64]. We used CD9 to mark exosomes, by fusing it with either Dendra-2 or mCherry to track the transmission of exosomes between interconnected hippocampal neurons. Cells were electroporated with each plasmid directly before plating and seeded separately into microfluidic chambers according to model 1 (red - > Ch1, green - > Ch2) (Fig. 1a).

As expected, fluorescence was detected that delineated the plasma membrane of hippocampal neurons (Fig. 2a). In addition, somatic punctae representing endosomes were visualized that displayed a much stronger signal (Fig. 2a). Interestingly, the red endosomal punctae in the cell bodies in Ch1 also exhibited a green fluorescence signal in those neurons that were in close proximity to, and possibly interconnected to, Dendra2-CD9-expressing and -projecting axons (Fig. 2 b-c). Importantly, we observed that the exchange in fluorescence was restricted to the endosomal punctae, given that axons with different colors running in parallel in opposite directions within the microgrooves did not exhibit double fluorescence (Fig. 2 d-f). Similarly, we found no evidence for a fluorescence exchange at the plasma membranes. The reverse was also true, in that green cell bodies (Fig. 2 g-i, Ch2) acquired red fluorescence when they were in close proximity to mCherry-CD9-positive axons (Fig. 2i). For endosome quantification, we used segmentation of fluorescence confocal images and determined the percentage of endosomal punctae having both

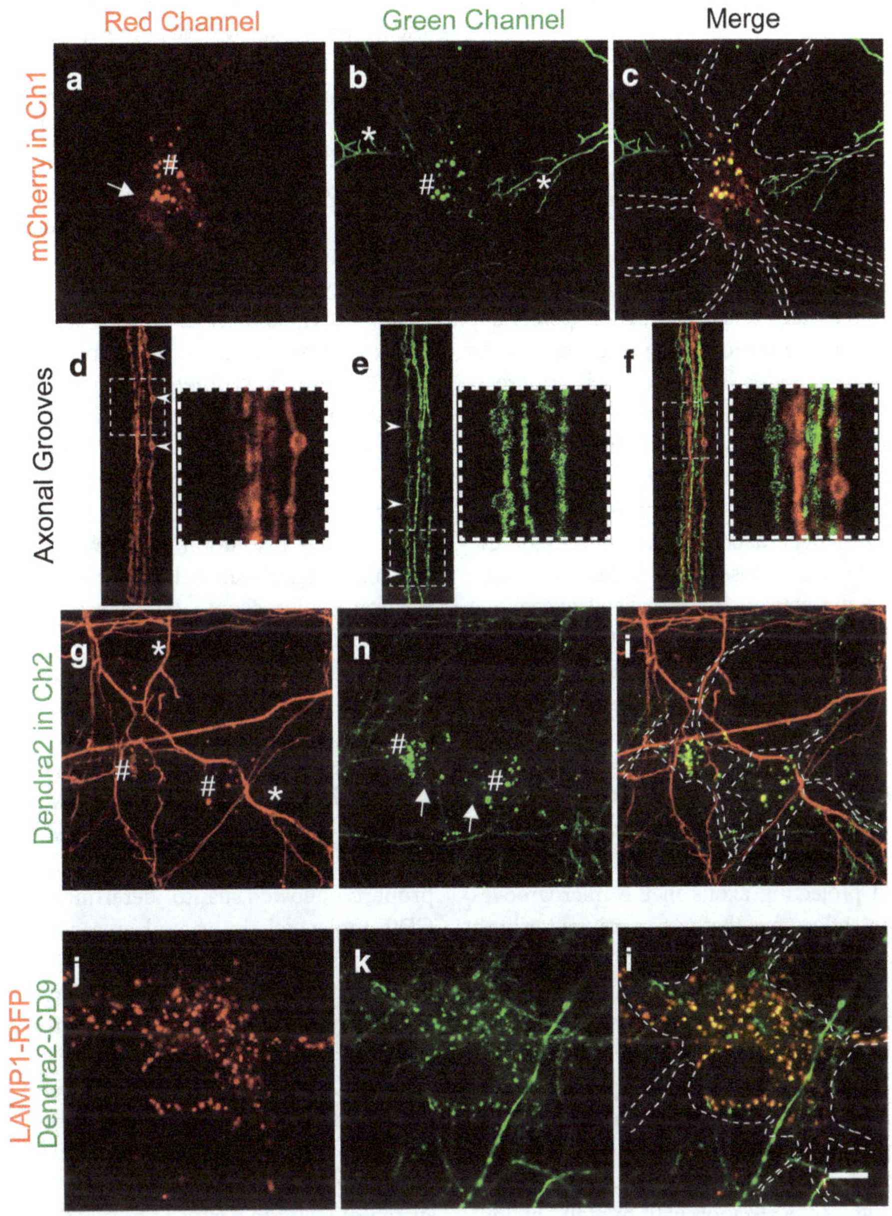


**Fig. 2** Transmission of exosomes between interconnected neurons. Culture performed according to Model 1, with neuron A being labeled with mCherry-CD9 (red) and neuron B labeled with Dendra2-CD9 (green). **a-c** Confocal images of mCherry-CD9-positive neurons in Ch1. The red channel (**a**) shows that CD9 is detected in the neuronal plasma membrane (**a**, white arrow) and is strongly present in endosomal somatic punctae (**a**, #). The green channel (**b**) reveals that Dendra2-positive axons (*) from Ch2 can reach mCherry-CD9-positive neurons in Ch1. Interestingly, red neurons only show green fluorescence in endosomal punctae when they are close to green axons (**b**, #). **d-f** Images of axonal grooves revealing that axons grow in both directions but never exchange fluorescence. White arrowheads indicate CD9-positive globular enlargements, which appear to be migrating endosomes based on single color fluorescence. The square (dashed lines) outlines a magnification of the axonal region (right square). **f** The magnification shows that the axonal endosomes are either green or red, but do not display both colors. This indicates that the fluorescence exchange found in the soma is post-synaptic. **g-i** Images of Ch2 containing Dendra2-CD9-expressing neurons. Similarly, Dendra2-expressing green endosomal punctae in Ch2 (**h**, #) show red fluorescence (**g**, #) when in proximity to red axons (**g**, *) projecting from Ch1. White arrows indicate the plasma membrane. **j-l** Colocalization of Dendra2-CD9-expressing endosomal punctae with the late endosome marker LAMP1 tagged with RFP (transduced with a baculovirus). Scale bar: 10 μm for all images

colors, which was 34.5% ± 5.8% (mean ± SEM, $n = 6$, 22 neurons), indicating a potential transfer of exosomes between neurons. Together, these results suggest a trans-synaptic transfer of exosomes that are generated by secretory endosomes. To confirm the endocytic origin of the visualized Dendra2-CD9-positive somatic punctae, we demonstrated colocalization with the late endosomal marker LAMP-1 (Fig. 2 j-l), a protein that remains on the limiting membrane of late endosomes during the formation of MVBs [49].

### A subset of exosomes are internalized and passed on to a third interconnected neuron

Having demonstrated the transfer of exosomes between two interconnected neurons, we sought to investigate whether all transferred exosomes find their final destination in the neurons that internalized them or whether some exosomes might have a somatic 'free pass' and be transferred to a third, interconnected neuron, thereby potentially increasing the pathogenic radius of action of exosomes. As outlined in Fig. 1b, a proxy for this situation is the treatment of neuron B in Ch1 with exosomes isolated from neuron A (rTg4510 brains) by labeling their membranes with the green fluorescent dye PKH67 (Fig. 1b, model 2). After internalization, exosomes would be processed neuron B, either by lysosomal degradation or by transfer of the exosomal content to the cytosol. We asked, however, whether a subset of the neuron B-internalized exogenous exosomes would be transported to neuron C in Ch2. To differentiate between the neurons in Ch1 and Ch2, only those in Ch1 were electroporated with mCherry-CD9 whereas those in Ch2 lacked fluorescence signal. As expected, PKH67-positive exogenous exosomes were internalized by the neurons in Ch1 and 67.0% ± 9.8% (mean ± SEM, $n = 6$, 41 neurons) of the endosomal particles contained both colors (Fig. 3 a-c). Interestingly, we also observed that the red projecting axons in the microgrooves contained migrating endosomes that were positive for both mCherry-CD9 and PKH67 (Fig. 3 d-f). Furthermore, neurons in Ch2 in close proximity to these red projecting axons exhibited somatic endosomal fluorescent punctae in which the two fluorescent signals colocalized (Fig. 3 g-i), with 40.3% ± 5.0% (mean ± SEM, n = 6, 18 neurons) of the endosomes containing both red and green fluorescence. In addition, an early pilot characterization of model 2 revealed that a subset of the exosomes isolated from rTg4510 mice added to Ch1 exhibited colocalization with human tau and, with only a fraction of the exosomes migrating into Ch2, an even smaller subset carried tau seeds as demonstrated with an antibody for human tau (Additional file 1: Figure S2). Together, these results support the notion that the endosomes containing internalized exogenous exosomes fuse with endogenous endosomes containing intraluminal nanovesicles, which are fated to be secreted as mCherry-CD9-positive exosomes, potentially contributing to the spreading of pathological human tau.

### Super-resolution microscopy supports fusion events between endosomes containing endogenous and exogenous exosomes

The results described in Fig. 3 revealed the presence of a number of fluorescent punctae moving along axons and presenting a signal from endogenous and exogenous membranes that we hypothesized to be derived from intraluminal nanovesicles (exosomes). However, the size of the punctae (0.5–1.5 μm approximately) visualized by confocal microscopy corresponded more with endosomes than exosomes (30–150 nm). We therefore turned to super-resolution microscopy in order to visualize discrete fluorescent particles inside the endosomes and better demonstrate the potential 'hijacking' of endogenous secretory endosomes.

We used stochastic super-resolution in which the fluorescence emission of a photoconvertible protein (Dendra2) or a synthetic organic fluorophore (CellVue Claret) can be sequentially activated in a semi-controlled manner to generate blinking of single fluorophores, thereby allowing for single molecule localization-based super-resolution imaging [9, 24, 53]. Using this technique, image resolution is achievable in the order of tens of nanometers, well below the diffraction limit of conventional microscopy. To analyze the endosomal punctae that contain colocalized endogenous and exogenous exosomes, we electroporated the neurons in Ch1 with Dendra2-CD9. In its native form Dendra2 is a fluorescent protein that emits green light. However, when illuminated at the low power level of 405 nm laser light, it is photoconverted to red fluorescence [31], and this 'blinking' generated by the color switch is used to determine the position of each individual fluorophore. This property allowed us to determine the localization of CD9 molecules in the plasma and endosomal membranes with a precision of 25 nm (Fig. 4 a-j).

Using the model 2 design (Fig. 1b), Dendra2-CD9-transfected neurons in Ch1 were treated with exosomes the membranes of which were labeled with CellVue Claret, a far-red dye with a chemical structure similar to that of other photo-switchable fluorescent probes [19, 59]. We used photoconversion of Dendra2 to locate endosomal membranes with a precision of 25 nm and the photoswitch of CellVue Claret to localize the membranes of exogenous exosomes with precision of 35 nm (Fig. 4 e-j).

Fig. 4a shows a representative conventional image of a dendrite the plasma membrane of which was labeled with Dendra2-CD9. Subsequent photoconversion and localization of single Dendra2 molecules produced a super-resolved image of the same dendrite (Fig. 4b). Previously obscured details including the plasma membrane of the dendrite can now be clearly resolved (Fig. 4b). Due to the limited localization precision of Dendra2, the neuronal plasma membrane appears as a 41 ± 4 nm thick dotted line as determined for the cross-section (yellow line in Fig. 4c, graphed in Fig. 4d). However, we were able to discriminate between the plasma membranes of axons and dendrites, and the endosomal particles located between them. Many endogenous endosomes in the neuronal soma,

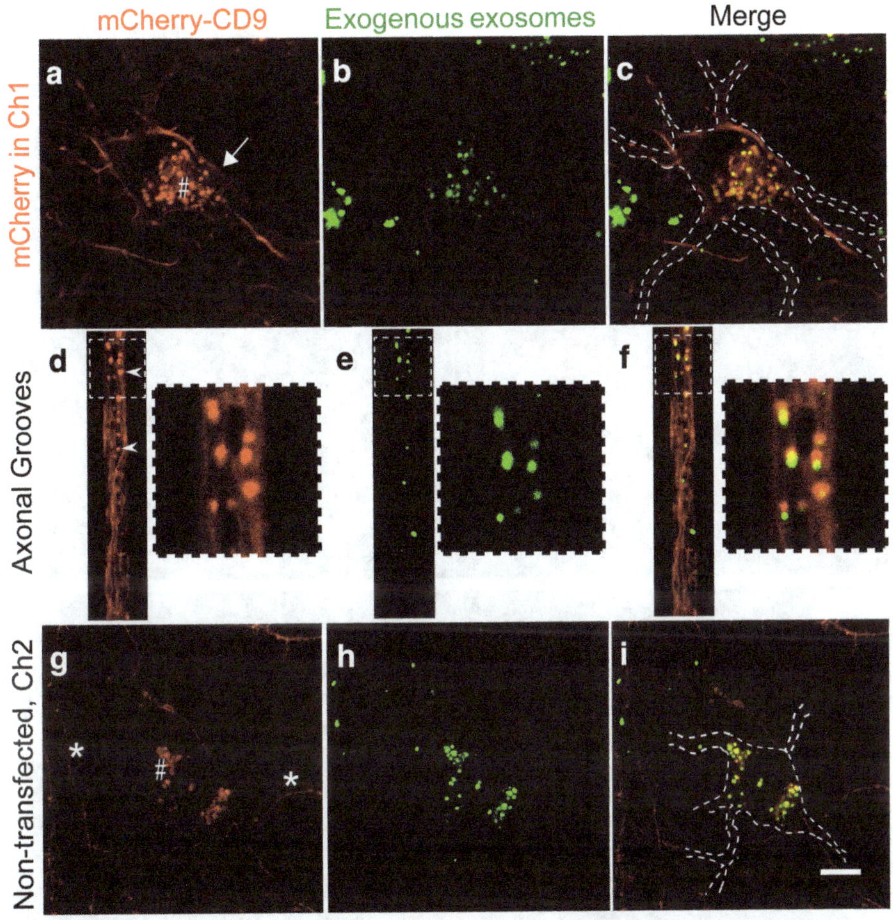


**Fig. 3** Neurons internalize exosomes but also share them with interconnected neurons. Culture performed according to Model 2, with neuron A-derived exosomes labeled with PKH67 (green), neuron B labeled with mCherry-CD9 (red) and neuron C being unlabeled (no color). **a-c** Confocal images in Ch1 containing mCherry-CD9-labeled neurons. The red channel (**a**) shows CD9 in the neuronal plasma membrane (**a**, white arrow) and a strong signal in endosomal somatic punctae (**a**, #). The green channel (**b**) reveals that PKH67-green is also detectable in somatic endosomal punctae where it colocalizes with endogenous somatic endosomes in red (**c**). **d-f** mCherry-CD9-labeled axons extending towards Ch2 and transporting red endosomal punctae (d, white arrowheads), which also carry green exogenous exosomes labeled with PKH67 (**e-f**). The square (dashed line) outlines a magnified axonal region. **f** Magnification showing that the axonal endosomes are labeled with both colors, meaning that they contain endogenous and exogenous cargoes. This implies that exogenous exosomes are axonally transported together with endogenous vesicles. **g-i** Hippocampal neurons in Ch2 that were not electroporated. These neurons only acquired red somatic endosomal punctae (**g**, #) when in proximity to red axons projecting from Ch1 (**g**, *). Endosomal punctae also show PKH67 green fluorescence (**h-i**), indicating post-synaptic acquisition of both exogenous and endogenous exosomes. Scale bar: 10 μm for all images

axons and dendrites in red colocalized with the exogenous exosomes labeled with CellVue Claret pseudocolored in green (Fig. 4 e-j). Fusion events between both types of endosomes were evident in endosomal particles located in axons (Fig. 4 e-g) as well as in the somata and dendrites (Fig. 4 h-j). This is consistent with the incorporation of exogenous exosomes into host neurons and their endosomes (green in Fig. 4 e-j). However, as our localization precision was only 35 nm, it did not allow us to visualize potential intraluminal nanovesicles as discrete particles, probably because these vesicles lie very close to one another inside endosomes. Instead, we observed an apparent uneven thickness of endosomal structures. For example, Fig. 4h and f shows the fusion between endogenous (red) and exogenous (green) particles. It is evident that the endogenous endosome is larger than the exogenously acquired exosome but potential internal nanovesicles (red) cannot be visualized.

### Electron microscopy reveals the hijacking of endogenous endosomes at a high resolution

Super-resolution images strongly support fusion events between endosomes containing either endogenous or exogenous intraluminal nanovesicles (exosomes). However, we were not able to visualize discrete intraluminal vesicles. Given that electron microscopy provides substantially higher resolution than super-resolution microscopy [25], we again adopted model 2 (Fig. 1b) and performed

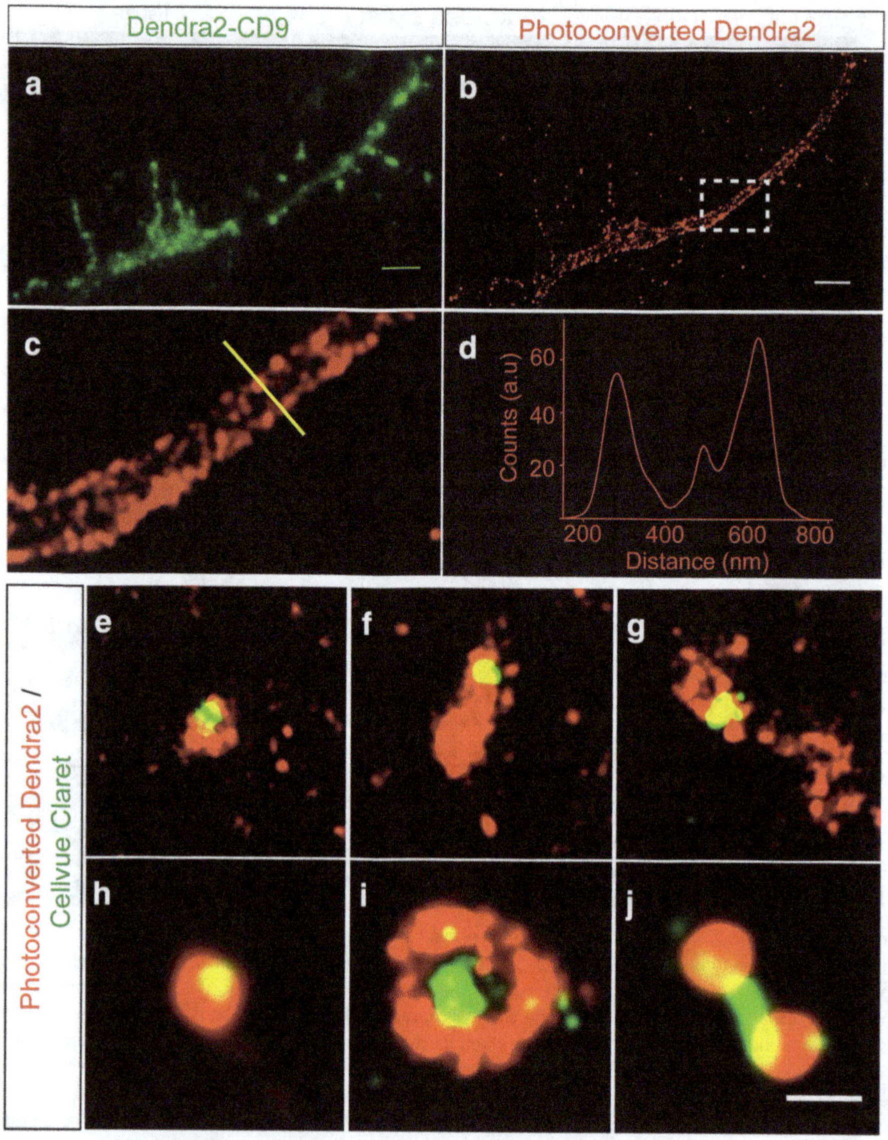


**Fig. 4** Super-resolution microscopy reveals that endosomes can carry both exogenous and endogenous exosomes. Culture performed according to Model 2, with neuron A-derived exosomes being labeled with the CellVue® Claret far-red fluorescent membrane dye (pseudocolored in green), neuron B labeled with Dendra2-CD9 (natively green but red when photoconverted) and neuron C containing no label (no color). **a** Conventional and (**b**) super-resolution images of a dendrite expressing Dendra2-labeled CD9. In the high-resolution image, structural features such as the plasma membrane become visible (scale bar 2 µm). **c** Magnification of the outlined rectangular region in (**b**). **d** Cross-section along the yellow line in (**c**) where the width of the dendrite and the thickness of the plasma membrane were measured. **e-j** Examples of colocalized endogenous endosomes and exogenous exosomes. **e**, **f** and **g**) showing events detected in axons. Panels h, i and j illustrate fusion events in soma and dendrites. In (**h**) and (**i**) exogenous exosomes are found close to the center of endosomal structures. Endosomal intraluminal nanovesicles cannot be resolved in red endosomal structures, but they contribute to the broader red fluorescence in the structure (ie: **f**, **h** and **i**). Scale bar 500 nm

electron microscopy after first labeling the membranes of exogenous exosomes with FM1–43FX. When specimens are fixed, this fluorescent probe oxidizes the substrate diaminobenzidine (DAB), thereby converting it into a precipitated and electron-dense reaction product [46]. Photooxidized DAB can therefore be used to track vesicles by electron microscopy and differentiate between endogenous and exogenous vesicles [27, 33, 34, 37]. We found that the majority of endosomes in the neuronal soma contained exogenous material, as evident by the DAB precipitate (Fig. 5a, black arrowheads), and that only a few endosomes were DAB-negative, indicative of an exclusively endogenous origin (Fig. 5a, white arrowheads). This is also shown in the high magnification images that reveal a mixture of DAB-positive (black arrowheads) and DAB-negative (black arrows) intraluminal nanovesicles (Fig. 5 b-c). Fig 5c supports the notion that more than one fusion/internalization event occurred for the imaged

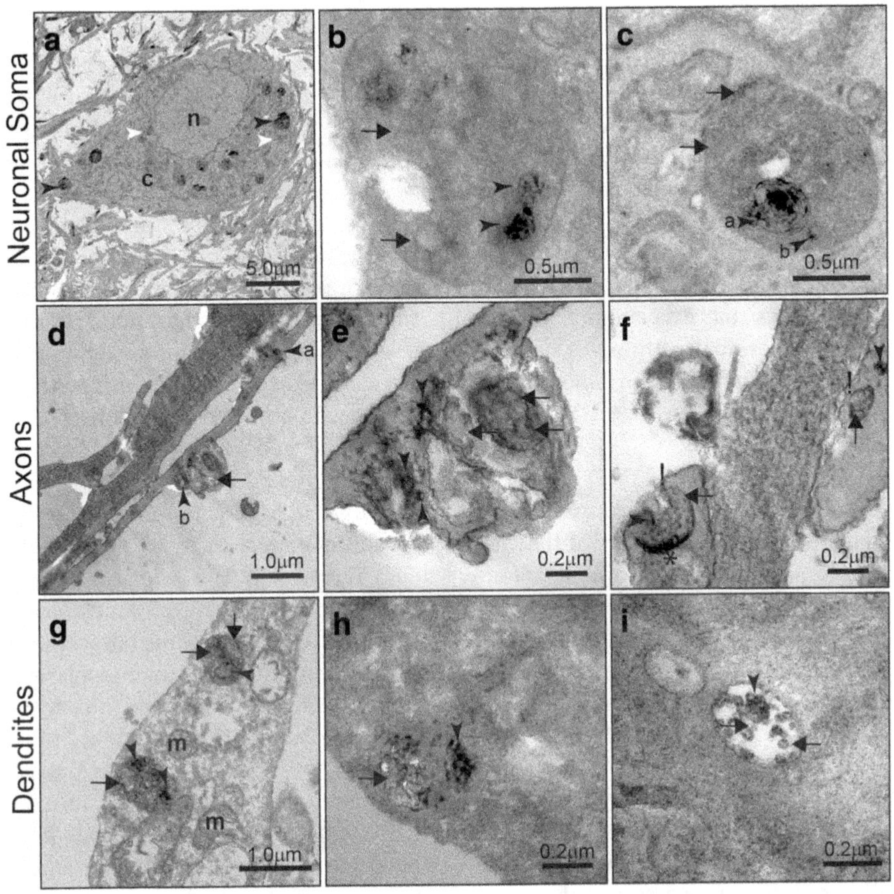


**Fig. 5** Hijacking of endogenous endosomes revealed by electron microscopy. Hippocampal neurons in microfluidic devices in Ch1 according to model 2 were treated with exosomes isolated from mouse brains and labeled with FM1–43FX, a fluorescent dye that reacts with diaminobenzidine (DAB) to form insoluble dark precipitates that are visualized by electron microscopy. **a** Electron microscopy image of a neuronal soma in Ch1, showing that the majority of endosomes contain DAB-positive exosomes of exogenous origin (black arrowheads). A few endosomes are DAB-negative (white arrowheads). **b** High magnification of endosomes located in the neuronal soma, showing a mixture of exogenous DAB-positive exosomes (black arrowheads) and endogenous DAB-negative intraluminal nanovesicles (black arrows). **c** Somatic endosome showing engulfment and fusion with a smaller endosome containing DAB-positive exosomes (black arrowhead "**a**"). An exogenous DAB-positive exosome can be seen close to the fused endosome (black arrowhead "**b**"). Endogenous DAB-negative intraluminal nanovesicles are also visualized (black arrows). **d-f** Endosomes found in axons. (d) Low magnification of axons transporting a small DAB-positive endosome (black arrowhead "**a**") and a large endosome in front of it (black arrowhead "**b**"). **e** High magnification of a large axonal endosome containing a mixture of DAB-positive (black arrowheads) and DAB-negative vesicles (black arrows). **f** Axonal termini showing endosome fusion with the plasma membrane (indicated with "!") during exosome release and potential residue of the back-fusion with the limiting membrane of the endosome (*). Exogenous DAB-positive (black arrowheads) and endogenous DAB-negative exosomes (black arrows). **g-i** Endosomes found in dendrites. **g** Low magnification of a dendrite demonstrating the presence of endosomes carrying both DAB-positive exosomes (black arrowheads) and DAB-negative intraluminal nanovesicles (black arrows). **h** and **i** High magnification of dendritic endosomes carrying DAB-positive exosomes less than 100 nm diameter (black arrowheads) together with DAB-negative vesicles of a similar size (black arrows). m, mitochondria; n, nucleus

endosomes (1.2 μm), as shown by the internalization of an endosome of approximately 400 nm containing smaller DAB-positive intraluminal nanovesicles (Fig. 5c, black arrowhead "a"). However, a DAB-positive intraluminal nanovesicle of less than 100 nm located outside "a" probably has been internalized during a separate fusion event (Fig. 5c, black arrowhead "b").

Interestingly, when axons were imaged (Fig. 5 d-f), we were able to observe small endosomes containing DAB-positive nanovesicles moving freely inside the axonal lumen (Fig. 5d, black arrowhead "a"). However, we also noted a large convoluted endosome which appeared to stretch the axonal lumen and membrane (Fig. 5d, black arrowhead "b"). High magnification images of this axonal endosome revealed a complex structure with a mixture of endogenous and exogenous intraluminal nanovesicles (Fig. 5e). It is worth noting that because FM1–43FX exosomes were only added to the cell bodies in Ch1, the endosomes carrying the DAB-positive material (Fig. 5 d-f) were quite likely moving anterogradely. Furthermore, the axonal termini showed fusion events with the plasma membrane in what appeared to be the secretion of exosomes (Fig. 5f). Dendrites contained a similar type of ultrastructure, exhibiting endosomes containing a mixture of exogenous DAB-positive nanovesicles and endogenous DAB-negative vesicles (Fig. 5 g-i). Together, the cumulative evidence of super-resolution and electron microscopy data strongly supports the notion that endosomes containing endogenous intraluminal nanovesicles fuse with endosomes loaded with internalized exogenous exosomes. The fact that these mixed endosomes move in dendrites and axons and are presumably secreted, suggests that exogenous exosomes can hijack the secretory endosomal pathway of neurons and be secreted in conjunction with exosomes of endogenous origin.

## Discussion

Our study supports the notion that exosomes are invasive, hijacking the endosomal secretory machinery of the cells that internalized them to achieve a longer distance of action and a potentially higher pathogenicity. Previous studies have established that early endosomes arise from primary endocytic vesicles which fuse with each other to form a larger endocytic structure [40]. It is likely that endocytic vesicles containing internalized exosomes fuse with endocytic vesicles containing different cargoes and that, during endosome maturation towards the generation of intraluminal nanovesicles, this results in a late endosome sheltering both endogenous vesicles and exosomes taken up from another cell. It can be assumed that most of the internalized exosomes are used by the cell itself, by either undergoing lysosomal degradation or recovery of some components via the trans-Golgi network [39, 57], or by the release of exosomal contents into the cytosol via back-fusion mechanisms [10, 63]. However, our data show that not all internalized exosomes are destined for destruction or recovery, as some are actually re-secreted together with endogenous exosomes.

The hijacking of endosomes is not unique to exosomes. For instance, some enveloped RNA viruses hijack MVBs in order to be released from infected cells [17]. DNA viruses, such as the herpes virus, hijack the exosomal pathway of their host to facilitate virion assembly, promote the export of host proteins involved in immune regulation, and transfer viral-derived molecules that can assume activity in recipient cells [54]. Even the bacterium *Chlamydia trachomatis* has the capacity to hijack intracellular trafficking and lipid transport pathways of the host cell in order to promote infection [47]. However, different from the mechanism that occurs with intracellular pathogens, the hijacking of endosomes as revealed in our study does not require genome replication as with viruses or bacteria.

Perhaps the hijacking mechanism most similar to that which we report is used by the proteinaceous lethal toxin known as anthrax which exploits MVBs. Anthrax toxins can persist in intraluminal nanovesicles for days, fully sheltered from proteolytic degradation in MVBs and can be delivered to the extracellular medium as exosomes [1]. It is tempting to speculate that the fusion of exogenous exosomes with endosomes destined to secrete intraluminal nanovesicles would equally shelter the exogenous exosomes from proteolytic degradation in the MVBs which could eventually be secreted together with de novo generated exosomes. An alternative mechanism could be that, given the endocytic origin of exosomes, these contain markers for secretion and drive a subpopulation of exosomes into the secretory pathway. Comparison with the internalization of microvesicles, which are not of endocytic origin [38, 45], might provide insight into this possibility.

Tau protein aggregation is a hallmark of AD and other neurodegenerative diseases collectively termed tauopathies. Tau accumulation in the brain hinders neuronal physiology at many levels, including axonal transport and synaptic transmission, mitochondrial and proteasomal functions, induction of endoplasmic reticulum stress and even nuclear effects on chromatin relaxation [28, 50]. It is assumed that the ability of exosomes to carry misfolded or aggregated proteins significantly enhances the progression of tauopathies in a manner similar to what has been reported for prions [6, 38, 50, 51]. However, it has been proposed that an increase in pathogenic exosomes could end up in traffic jams during endosome transport, which could cause a reduction of glutamate receptor recycling [60]. Traffic jams could increase the number of intraluminal nanovesicles in the MVBs, thereby increasing the number of released exosomes; or increase the content of exosomes with AD-associated proteins like tau or Aβ, leading to an accelerated spread of disease [60]. We observed that brain-derived exosomes are strongly internalized by neurons, resulting in a somata with high numbers of endosomes. Similarly, axons exhibited endosomes of varied sizes moving inside the axonal lumen, where sometimes massive endosomes were caught stretching the axonal membrane. We reasoned that huge endosomes, probably generated by the upregulated endosomal activity, are more difficult to transport along axons and might end up in traffic jams that could strongly affect neuronal physiology. Interestingly, synaptic activity increases the secretion of exosomes [18, 43], and hippocampal hyperactivity has been observed in patients with mild cognitive impairment [7], where the compounded action of both mechanisms might also generate endosomal traffic jams acting as upstream drivers of AD pathogenesis.

In this study, we demonstrated features of exosome spreading between interconnected neurons in agreement with what is expected of this type of vesicle of endocytic origin. However, we also provide evidence for a novel hijacking mechanism of endosomes by exogenous exosomes, which might result in a longer-distance action and therefore increase the pathogenic potential and the radius of action of the exosomes. These intriguing findings demonstrate that exosomes are more invasive that previously anticipated acting as amplifiers in the spread of pathogenic molecules in neurodegenerative diseases.

## Conclusion

Our study reveals an unusual intracellular trafficking of exosomes in that not all internalized exosomes are degraded or their constituents recovered by the cell. Instead, endosome hijacking leads to the generation of a persistent subpopulation of exosomes with a longer distance of action and potential pathogenicity.

### Abbreviations

Aβ: Amyloid-β; AD: Alzheimer disease; APP: Amyloid precursor protein; DAB: Diaminobenzidine; DIV: Days in vitro; E: Embryonic day; MVBs: Multivesicular bodies; NFTs: Neurofibrillary tangles

### Acknowledgements

This study was supported by the Estate of Dr. Clem Jones AO, as well as grants from the Australian Research Council (ARC) [DP160103812], the National Health and Medical Research Council of Australia [GNT1037746, GNT1127999], and the State Government of Queensland (DSITI, Department of Science, Information Technology and Innovation). Confocal and super-resolution microscopy were facilitated by the Queensland Brain Institute's Advanced Microscopy Facility, supported by the ARC LIEF grant (LE130100078). Electron microscopy was performed at the Australian Microscopy & Microanalysis Research Facility at the Centre for Microscopy and Microanalysis, the University of Queensland. We thank Linda Cumner, Tishila Palliyaguru, Trish Hitchcock and the animal care team for animal maintenance, and Rowan Tweedale and Esmi Zajaczkowski for critically reading the manuscript.

### Authors' contributions

All authors read and approved the final manuscript. (J.C.P.): conception and design of experiments, collection and/or assembly of data, data analysis and interpretation, and manuscript writing; (C.L., N.D., R.S.): collection and/or assembly of data, data analysis and interpretation, and manuscript writing; (J.G.): data analysis and interpretation, manuscript writing, financial support, and final approval of manuscript.

### Competing interests

The authors declare that they have no competing interests.

### Author details

[1]Clem Jones Centre for Ageing Dementia Research (CJCADR), Queensland Brain Institute (QBI), The University of Queensland, Brisbane, QLD 4072, Australia. [2]Queensland Brain Institute (QBI), The University of Queensland, Brisbane, QLD 4072, Australia.

### References

1. Abrami L, Brandi L, Moayeri M, Brown MJ, Krantz BA, Leppla SH et al (2013) Hijacking multivesicular bodies enables long-term and exosome-mediated long-distance action of anthrax toxin. Cell Rep 5:986–996. https://doi.org/10.1016/j.celrep.2013.10.019
2. Andreu Z, Yanez-Mo M (2014) Tetraspanins in extracellular vesicle formation and function. Front Immunol 5:442. https://doi.org/10.3389/fimmu.2014.00442
3. Asai H, Ikezu S, Tsunoda S, Medalla M, Luebke J, Haydar T et al (2015) Depletion of microglia and inhibition of exosome synthesis halt tau propagation. Nat Neurosci 18:1584–1593. https://doi.org/10.1038/nn.4132
4. Attems J, Thal DR, Jellinger KA (2012) The relationship between subcortical tau pathology and Alzheimer's disease. Biochem Soc Trans 40:711–715. https://doi.org/10.1042/BST20120034
5. Baker S, Gotz J (2016) A local insult of okadaic acid in wild-type mice induces tau phosphorylation and protein aggregation in anatomically distinct brain regions. Acta Neuropathol Commun 4:32. https://doi.org/10.1186/s40478-016-0300-0
6. Baker S, Polanco JC, Gotz J (2016) Extracellular vesicles containing P301L mutant tau accelerate pathological tau phosphorylation and oligomer formation but do not seed mature neurofibrillary tangles in ALZ17 mice. J Alzheimers Dis 54:1207–1217. https://doi.org/10.3233/JAD-160371
7. Bakker A, Krauss GL, Albert MS, Speck CL, Jones LR, Stark CE et al (2012) Reduction of hippocampal hyperactivity improves cognition in amnestic mild cognitive impairment. Neuron 74:467–474. https://doi.org/10.1016/j.neuron.2012.03.023
8. Berditchevski F, Odintsova E (2007) Tetraspanins as regulators of protein trafficking. Traffic 8:89–96. https://doi.org/10.1111/j.1600-0854.2006.00515.x
9. Betzig E, Patterson GH, Sougrat R, Lindwasser OW, Olenych S, Bonifacino JS et al (2006) Imaging intracellular fluorescent proteins at nanometer resolution. Science 313:1642–1645. https://doi.org/10.1126/science.1127344
10. Bissig C, Gruenberg J (2014) ALIX and the multivesicular endosome: ALIX in wonderland. Trends Cell Biol 24:19–25. https://doi.org/10.1016/j.tcb.2013.10.009
11. Boyiadzis M, Whiteside TL (2017) The emerging roles of tumor-derived exosomes in hematological malignancies. Leukemia 31:1259–1268. https://doi.org/10.1038/leu.2017.91
12. Braak H, Braak E (1995) Staging of Alzheimer's disease-related neurofibrillary changes. Neurobiol Aging 16:271–278 discussion 278-284
13. Braak H, Del Tredici K (2011) Alzheimer's pathogenesis: is there neuron-to-neuron propagation? Acta Neuropathol 121:589–595. https://doi.org/10.1007/s00401-011-0825-z
14. Brundin P, Melki R, Kopito R (2010) Prion-like transmission of protein aggregates in neurodegenerative diseases. Nat Rev Mol Cell Biol 11:301–307. https://doi.org/10.1038/nrm2873
15. Calafate S, Buist A, Miskiewicz K, Vijayan V, Daneels G, de Strooper B et al (2015) Synaptic contacts enhance cell-to-cell tau pathology propagation. Cell Rep 11:1176–1183. https://doi.org/10.1016/j.celrep.2015.04.043
16. Calafate S, Flavin W, Verstreken P, Moechars D (2016) Loss of Bin1 promotes the propagation of tau pathology. Cell Rep 17:931–940. https://doi.org/10.1016/j.celrep.2016.09.063
17. Calistri A, Salata C, Parolin C, Palu G (2009) Role of multivesicular bodies and their components in the egress of enveloped RNA viruses. Rev Med Virol 19:31–45. https://doi.org/10.1002/rmv.588
18. Chivet M, Javalet C, Laulagnier K, Blot B, Hemming FJ, Sadoul R (2014) Exosomes secreted by cortical neurons upon glutamatergic synapse activation specifically interact with neurons. J Extracell Vesicles 3:24722. https://doi.org/10.3402/jev.v3.24722
19. Dempsey GT, Vaughan JC, Chen KH, Bates M, Zhuang X (2011) Evaluation of fluorophores for optimal performance in localization-based super-resolution imaging. Nat Methods 8:1027–1036. https://doi.org/10.1038/nmeth.1768
20. Dinkins MB, Dasgupta S, Wang G, Zhu G, Bieberich E (2014) Exosome reduction in vivo is associated with lower amyloid plaque load in the 5XFAD mouse model of Alzheimer's disease. Neurobiol Aging 35:1792–1800. https://doi.org/10.1016/j.neurobiolaging.2014.02.012
21. Dinkins MB, Enasko J, Hernandez C, Wang G, Kong J, Helwa I et al (2016) Neutral Sphingomyelinase-2 deficiency ameliorates Alzheimer's disease pathology and improves cognition in the 5XFAD mouse. J Neurosci 36:8653–8667. https://doi.org/10.1523/JNEUROSCI.1429-16.2016

22. Dujardin S, Begard S, Caillierez R, Lachaud C, Delattre L, Carrier S et al (2014) Ectosomes: a new mechanism for non-exosomal secretion of tau protein. PLoS One 9:e100760. https://doi.org/10.1371/journal.pone.0100760
23. Dujardin S, Lecolle K, Caillierez R, Begard S, Zommer N, Lachaud C et al (2014) Neuron-to-neuron wild-type tau protein transfer through a trans-synaptic mechanism: relevance to sporadic tauopathies. Acta Neuropathol Commun 2:14. https://doi.org/10.1186/2051-5960-2-14
24. Durisic N, Laparra-Cuervo L, Sandoval-Alvarez A, Borbely JS, Lakadamyali M (2014) Single-molecule evaluation of fluorescent protein photoactivation efficiency using an in vivo nanotemplate. Nat Methods 11:156–162. https://doi.org/10.1038/nmeth.2784
25. Ehmann N, Sauer M, Kittel RJ (2015) Super-resolution microscopy of the synaptic active zone. Front Cell Neurosci 9:7. https://doi.org/10.3389/fncel.2015.00007
26. Fiandaca MS, Kapogiannis D, Mapstone M, Boxer A, Eitan E, Schwartz JB et al (2015) Identification of preclinical Alzheimer's disease by a profile of pathogenic proteins in neurally derived blood exosomes: a case-control study. Alzheimers Dement 11:600–607 e601. https://doi.org/10.1016/j.jalz.2014.06.008
27. Fomina AF, Deerinck TJ, Ellisman MH, Cahalan MD (2003) Regulation of membrane trafficking and subcellular organization of endocytic compartments revealed with FM1-43 in resting and activated human T cells. Exp Cell Res 291:150–166
28. Gerakis Y, Hetz C (2017) Emerging roles of ER stress in the etiology and pathogenesis of Alzheimer's disease. FEBS J: Doi https://doi.org/10.1111/febs.14332
29. Guo JL, Buist A, Soares A, Callaerts K, Calafate S, Stevenaert F et al (2016) The dynamics and turnover of tau aggregates in cultured cells: insights into therapies for Tauopathies. J Biol Chem 291:13175–13193. https://doi.org/10.1074/jbc.M115.712083
30. Guo JL, Lee VM (2014) Cell-to-cell transmission of pathogenic proteins in neurodegenerative diseases. Nat Med 20:130–138. https://doi.org/10.1038/nm.3457
31. Gurskaya NG, Verkhusha VV, Shcheglov AS, Staroverov DB, Chepurnykh TV, Fradkov AF et al (2006) Engineering of a monomeric green-to-red photoactivatable fluorescent protein induced by blue light. Nat Biotechnol 24:461–465. https://doi.org/10.1038/nbt1191
32. Hatch RJ, Wei Y, Xia D, Gotz J (2017) Hyperphosphorylated tau causes reduced hippocampal CA1 excitability by relocating the axon initial segment. Acta Neuropathol 133:717–730. https://doi.org/10.1007/s00401-017-1674-1
33. Henkel AW, Lubke J, Betz WJ (1996) FM1-43 dye ultrastructural localization in and release from frog motor nerve terminals. Proc Natl Acad Sci U S A 93:1918–1923
34. Henkel AW, Simpson LL, Ridge RM, Betz WJ (1996) Synaptic vesicle movements monitored by fluorescence recovery after photobleaching in nerve terminals stained with FM1-43. J Neurosci 16:3960–3967
35. Holmes BB, Diamond MI (2014) Prion-like properties of tau protein: the importance of extracellular tau as a therapeutic target. J Biol Chem 289: 19855–19861. https://doi.org/10.1074/jbc.R114.549295
36. Holmes BB, Furman JL, Mahan TE, Yamasaki TR, Mirbaha H, Eades WC et al (2014) Proteopathic tau seeding predicts tauopathy in vivo. Proc Natl Acad Sci U S A 111:E4376–E4385. https://doi.org/10.1073/pnas.1411649111
37. Hoshino A, Costa-Silva B, Shen TL, Rodrigues G, Hashimoto A, Tesic Mark M et al (2015) Tumour exosome integrins determine organotropic metastasis. Nature 527:329–335. https://doi.org/10.1038/nature15756
38. Howitt J, Hill AF (2016) Exosomes in the pathology of neurodegenerative diseases. J Biol Chem 291:26589–26597. https://doi.org/10.1074/jbc.R116.757955
39. Hu YB, Dammer EB, Ren RJ, Wang G (2015) The endosomal-lysosomal system: from acidification and cargo sorting to neurodegeneration. Transl Neurodegener 4:18. https://doi.org/10.1186/s40035-015-0041-1
40. Huotari J, Helenius A (2011) Endosome maturation. EMBO J 30:3481–3500. https://doi.org/10.1038/emboj.2011.286
41. Korkut C, Ataman B, Ramachandran P, Ashley J, Barria R, Gherbesi N et al (2009) Trans-synaptic transmission of vesicular Wnt signals through Evi/Wntless. Cell 139:393–404. https://doi.org/10.1016/j.cell.2009.07.051
42. Korkut C, Li Y, Koles K, Brewer C, Ashley J, Yoshihara M et al (2013) Regulation of postsynaptic retrograde signaling by presynaptic exosome release. Neuron 77:1039–1046. https://doi.org/10.1016/j.neuron.2013.01.013
43. Lachenal G, Pernet-Gallay K, Chivet M, Hemming FJ, Belly A, Bodon G et al (2011) Release of exosomes from differentiated neurons and its regulation by synaptic glutamatergic activity. Mol Cell Neurosci 46:409–418. https://doi.org/10.1016/j.mcn.2010.11.004
44. Li C, Gotz J (2017) Somatodendritic accumulation of tau in Alzheimer's disease is promoted by Fyn-mediated local protein translation. EMBO J 36: 3120–3138. https://doi.org/10.15252/embj.201797724
45. Mathivanan S, Ji H, Simpson RJ (2010) Exosomes: extracellular organelles important in intercellular communication. J Proteome 73:1907–1920. https://doi.org/10.1016/j.jprot.2010.06.006
46. Meisslitzer-Ruppitsch C, Rohrl C, Neumuller J, Pavelka M, Ellinger A (2009) Photooxidation technology for correlated light and electron microscopy. J Microsc 235:322–335. https://doi.org/10.1111/j.1365-2818.2009.03220.x
47. Paul B, Kim HS, Kerr MC, Huston WM, Teasdale RD, Collins BM (2017) Structural basis for the hijacking of endosomal sorting nexin proteins by chlamydia trachomatis. elife 6. https://doi.org/10.7554/eLife.22311
48. Perez-Gonzalez R, Gauthier SA, Kumar A, Levy E (2012) The exosome secretory pathway transports amyloid precursor protein carboxyl-terminal fragments from the cell into the brain extracellular space. J Biol Chem 287: 43108–43115. https://doi.org/10.1074/jbc.M112.404467
49. Piper RC, Katzmann DJ (2007) Biogenesis and function of multivesicular bodies. Annu Rev Cell Dev Biol 23:519–547. https://doi.org/10.1146/annurev.cellbio.23.090506.123319
50. Polanco JC, Li C, Bodea LG, Martinez-Marmol R, Meunier FA, Gotz J (2018) Amyloid-beta and tau complexity - towards improved biomarkers and targeted therapies. Nat Rev Neurol 14:22–39. https://doi.org/10.1038/nrneurol.2017.162
51. Polanco JC, Scicluna BJ, Hill AF, Gotz J (2016) Extracellular vesicles isolated from the brains of rTg4510 mice seed tau protein aggregation in a threshold-dependent manner. J Biol Chem 291:12445–12466. https://doi.org/10.1074/jbc.M115.709485
52. Rajendran L, Honsho M, Zahn TR, Keller P, Geiger KD, Verkade P et al (2006) Alzheimer's disease beta-amyloid peptides are released in association with exosomes. Proc Natl Acad Sci U S A 103:11172–11177. https://doi.org/10.1073/pnas.0603838103
53. Rust MJ, Bates M, Zhuang X (2006) Sub-diffraction-limit imaging by stochastic optical reconstruction microscopy (STORM). Nat Methods 3:793–795. https://doi.org/10.1038/nmeth929
54. Sadeghipour S, Mathias RA (2017) Herpesviruses hijack host exosomes for viral pathogenesis. Semin Cell Dev Biol 67:91–100. https://doi.org/10.1016/j.semcdb.2017.03.005
55. Saman S, Kim W, Raya M, Visnick Y, Miro S, Saman S et al (2012) Exosome-associated tau is secreted in tauopathy models and is selectively phosphorylated in cerebrospinal fluid in early Alzheimer disease. J Biol Chem 287:3842–3849. https://doi.org/10.1074/jbc.M111.277061
56. Santacruz K, Lewis J, Spires T, Paulson J, Kotilinek L, Ingelsson M et al (2005) Tau suppression in a neurodegenerative mouse model improves memory function. Science 309:476–481. https://doi.org/10.1126/science.1113694
57. Schulze H, Kolter T, Sandhoff K (2009) Principles of lysosomal membrane degradation: cellular topology and biochemistry of lysosomal lipid degradation. Biochim Biophys Acta 1793:674–683. https://doi.org/10.1016/j.bbamcr.2008.09.020
58. Sharples RA, Vella LJ, Nisbet RM, Naylor R, Perez K, Barnham KJ et al (2008) Inhibition of gamma-secretase causes increased secretion of amyloid precursor protein C-terminal fragments in association with exosomes. FASEB J 22:1469–1478. https://doi.org/10.1096/fj.07-9357com
59. Shim SH, Xia C, Zhong G, Babcock HP, Vaughan JC, Huang B et al (2012) Super-resolution fluorescence imaging of organelles in live cells with photoswitchable membrane probes. Proc Natl Acad Sci U S A 109:13978–13983. https://doi.org/10.1073/pnas.1201882109
60. Small SA, Simoes-Spassov S, Mayeux R, Petsko GA (2017) Endosomal traffic jams represent a pathogenic hub and therapeutic target in Alzheimer's disease. Trends Neurosci 40:592–602. https://doi.org/10.1016/j.tins.2017.08.003
61. Tardivel M, Begard S, Bousset L, Dujardin S, Coens A, Melki R et al (2016) Tunneling nanotube (TNT)-mediated neuron-to neuron transfer of pathological tau protein assemblies. Acta Neuropathol Commun 4:117. https://doi.org/10.1186/s40478-016-0386-4
62. Taylor AM, Blurton-Jones M, Rhee SW, Cribbs DH, Cotman CW, Jeon NL (2005) A microfluidic culture platform for CNS axonal injury, regeneration and transport. Nat Methods 2:599–605. https://doi.org/10.1038/nmeth777

63. Traub LM (2010) The reverse logic of multivesicular endosomes. EMBO Rep 11:79–81. https://doi.org/10.1038/embor.2009.281
64. Villarroya-Beltri C, Baixauli F, Gutierrez-Vazquez C, Sanchez-Madrid F, Mittelbrunn M (2014) Sorting it out: regulation of exosome loading. Semin Cancer Biol 28:3–13. https://doi.org/10.1016/j.semcancer.2014.04.009
65. Von Bartheld CS, Altick AL (2011) Multivesicular bodies in neurons: distribution, protein content, and trafficking functions. Prog Neurobiol 93: 313–340. https://doi.org/10.1016/j.pneurobio.2011.01.003
66. Wang Y, Balaji V, Kaniyappan S, Kruger L, Irsen S, Tepper K et al (2017) The release and trans-synaptic transmission of tau via exosomes. Mol Neurodegener 12:5. https://doi.org/10.1186/s13024-016-0143-y

# Transcription factors *Tp73*, *Cebpd*, *Pax6*, and *Spi1* rather than DNA methylation regulate chronic transcriptomics changes after experimental traumatic brain injury

Anssi Lipponen[1], Assam El-Osta[2,3], Antony Kaspi[2], Mark Ziemann[2], Ishant Khurana[2], Harikrishnan KN[2], Vicente Navarro-Ferrandis[1], Noora Puhakka[1], Jussi Paananen[4,5] and Asla Pitkänen[1*]

**Abstract**

Traumatic brain injury (TBI) induces a wide variety of cellular and molecular changes that can continue for days to weeks to months, leading to functional impairments. Currently, there are no pharmacotherapies in clinical use that favorably modify the post-TBI outcome, due in part to limited understanding of the mechanisms of TBI-induced pathologies. Our system biology analysis tested the hypothesis that chronic transcriptomics changes induced by TBI are controlled by altered DNA-methylation in gene promoter areas or by transcription factors. We performed genome-wide methyl binding domain (MBD)-sequencing (seq) and RNA-seq in perilesional, thalamic, and hippocampal tissue sampled at 3 months after TBI induced by lateral fluid percussion in adult male Sprague-Dawley rats. We investigated the regulated molecular networks and mechanisms underlying the chronic regulation, particularly DNA methylation and transcription factors. Finally, we identified compounds that modulate the transcriptomics changes and could be repurposed to improve recovery. Unexpectedly, DNA methylation was not a major regulator of chronic post-TBI transcriptomics changes. On the other hand, the transcription factors ***Cebpd***, ***Pax6***, ***Spi1***, and ***Tp73*** were upregulated at 3 months after TBI (False discovery rate $< 0.05$), which was validated using digital droplet polymerase chain reaction. Transcription regulatory network analysis revealed that these transcription factors regulate apoptosis, inflammation, and microglia, which are well-known contributors to secondary damage after TBI. Library of Integrated Network-based Cellular Signatures (LINCS) analysis identified 118 pharmacotherapies that regulate the expression of ***Cebpd***, ***Pax6***, ***Spi1***, and ***Tp73***. Of these, the antidepressant and/or antipsychotic compounds trimipramine, rolipramine, fluspirilene, and chlorpromazine, as well as the anti-cancer therapies pimasertib, tamoxifen, and vorinostat were strong regulators of the identified transcription factors, suggesting their potential to modulate the regulated transcriptomics networks to improve post-TBI recovery.

**Keywords:** DNA methylation, LINCS analysis, MBD-seq, Recovery, RNA-seq, Treatment

## Introduction

Every year, 2.5 million people in Europe and the USA sustain traumatic brain injury (TBI) [15, 28, 74]. TBI is a major cause of disability and death in patients younger than 45 years of age [65]. Despite a large number of preclinical and clinical studies, an effective pharmacotherapy to improve post-TBI outcome is still lacking [22, 25, 76]. This is due in part to the complexity of the secondary pathologies induced by TBI, including neurodegeneration, inflammation, oxidative stress, axonal and myelin injury, and vascular changes [64, 79, 80]. These pathologies progress in parallel and serial time windows over weeks to months in experimental models [7, 46, 91, 112] and humans [36, 49, 98]. As these observations suggest complex and long-lasting transcriptomics regulation, we propose that a network therapy rather than a

* Correspondence: asla.pitkanen@uef.fi
[1]Epilepsy Research Laboratory, A. I. Virtanen Institute for Molecular Sciences, University of Eastern Finland, PO Box 1627, FIN-70211 Kuopio, Finland
Full list of author information is available at the end of the article

monotherapy approach will be more effective for repair of the ongoing damage.

To date, a number of studies have investigated transcriptomics changes at a genome-wide scale at 24-48 h after TBI [14, 17, 38, 42, 47, 48, 59, 63, 78, 85, 97, 99, 104, 122, 123, 125, 128–130, 136]. Of these 19 genome-wide gene expression studies, 11 report dysregulation of transcription factors in the acute post-TBI phase [17, 48, 59, 78, 85, 97, 104, 123, 128–130]. Four hypothesis-driven analyses focusing on individual transcription factors report the dysregulation of *Jun* [133], *Cebpd* [105], *Runx1* [70], and *Olig2* [9] in the acute post-TBI phase. Most of the studies, however, analyzed only acute post-TBI time-points and a single brain area, typically the hippocampus or cortex. Further, very few studies have explored the mechanisms that regulate post-TBI gene expression, such as genome-wide DNA methylation [20, 39, 83].

We hypothesized that TBI results in chronic transcriptomics changes that are controlled by DNA-methylation changes in the gene promoter areas or by transcription factors. To test this, we induced TBI in rats by lateral fluid-percussion, and subjected the perilesional cortex, ipsilateral thalamus, and ipsilateral hippocampus to MBD-seq and RNA-seq. As bioinformatics analysis and laboratory validation indicated that transcription factors rather than DNA methylation regulate chronic transcriptomics changes, we further conducted LINCS analysis to identify compounds that regulate gene expression of these transcription factors and could therefore be repurposed to improve post-TBI outcome via transcription factor-mediated mechanisms.

## Materials and methods

### Animals

TBI was induced by lateral fluid-percussion injury (FPI) with an impact pressure of 3.30 ± 0.01 atm in 14 adult male Sprague-Dawley rats (330–370 g at the time of TBI or sham operation; Harlan, The Netherlands) as previously described [54, 81]. Eleven sham-operated animals served as experimental controls. At 3 months after TBI, the perilesional cortex, thalamus, and hippocampus were collected as described in Lipponen et al. [69]. Briefly, the rats were anesthetized with 5% isoflurane and decapitated. The brain was removed from the skull, flushed with 0.9% cold (4 °C) sodium chloride, and placed onto a slicing matrix on ice (#15007, Rodent Brain Matrix, Ted Pella, Inc., Redding, CA, USA). Two 2-mm-thick coronal slices were cut (between − 2.2 and − 6.2 from the bregma), from which the perilesional cortex, ipsilateral thalamus, and ipsilateral hippocampus (including dentate gyrus) were dissected on top of the light table under the magnifying glass. Brain tissue samples were snap-frozen in liquid nitrogen, and stored at -70 °C until RNA and DNA extraction.

All animal operations were approved by The Animal Ethics Committee of the Provincial Government of Southern Finland and carried out according to the guidelines of the European Community Council Directives 2010/63/EU.

### Preparation of MBD- and RNA-seq libraries and sequencing

#### *DNA and RNA extraction*

Brain tissue from five TBI and five sham-operated rats was used for methyl-binding domain sequencing (MBD-seq) and RNA-sequencing (RNA-seq). DNA and RNA were co-purified from the perilesional cortex, ipsilateral hippocampus, or ipsilateral thalamus using a DNeasy Blood&Tissue kit (#69504, Qiagen, Hilden, Germany). Quality control of the total RNA was performed using a MultiNA electrophoresis device (Shimazu, Kyoto, Japan).

#### *RNA-seq library and sequencing*

The mRNA library preparation and RNA-sequencing were performed as described in Lipponen et al. [69]. Briefly, mRNA was enriched using Dynabeads Oligo (dT)25 beads (#61002, Invitrogen, Carlsbad, CA, USA), and the sequencing libraries were compiled with the NEBNext mRNA Library Prep Reagent Set (#E6100S, New England Biolabs, Ipswich, MA, USA). Quality control of the sequencing libraries was performed with a MultiNA electrophoresis device (Shimazu, Kyoto, Japan). Sequencing of the mRNA libraries for the perilesional cortex and hippocampus was carried out with an Illumina Genome Analyzer IIx (San Diego, CA, USA), and for the thalamus using an Illumina HiSeq 2000 (San Diego, CA, USA). The Illumina Off-Line Basecaller v1.8 was used for base-calling. RNA-seq raw data can be downloaded from the NCBI Gene Expression Omnibus (GEO; series accession number GSE80174).

#### *MBD-seq library and sequencing*

For MBD-seq, 2 µg of DNA was fragmented by sonication, and the quality was controlled with a MultiNA electrophoresis device (Shimazu, Kyoto, Japan). Methylated DNA was enriched with a 2-M sodium chloride elution using MethylMiner™kit (Thermo Fischer Scientific, Waltham, MA, USA), and quantified using a Qubit fluorometer (Thermo FisherScientific, Waltham, MA, USA). The sequencing library was prepared from 5 ng of enriched methylated DNA using an NEB Next DNA library kit (#E6040S, New England Biolabs, Ipswich, MA, USA). Then, MBD-sequencing and base-calling for the perilesional cortex, hippocampus, and thalamus were carried out as described above. Raw MBD-seq data was saved to the NCBI Gene Expression Omnibus (GEO; series accession number GSE107837).

## Mapping of sequencing data, and identification of differentially methylated regions and differentially expressing genes

### *Methylation*

Quality control of the MBD-sequencing raw reads was performed using FastQC [3]. Sequencing raw reads were mapped to the Ensemble RN5 genome with Spliced Transcripts Alignment to a Reference (STAR) software (version 2.3.0e_r291) [24] with parameter alignIntronMax 1 to prohibit splicing and allow genomic mapping. The mapping percentages were 71.2 ± 4.0% for the perilesional cortex, 63.3 ± 3.2% for the ipsilateral hippocampus, and 71.3 ± 2.7% for the ipsilateral thalamus. Differentially-methylated gene promoters (5000 bp upstream and 200 bp downstream from the transcription start site), exons, and gene body area were identified with blocksStats function in the Repitools 1.21.1 R package [115] with R version 3.1.0. The adjusted *p*-value was calculated with a Benjamini–Hochberg false discovery rate (FDR). DNA methylation was considered significantly changed if the FDR was < 0.05.

### *Gene expression*

RNA-seq quality control, mapping, and identification of differentially expressed genes were previously described in detail (Lipponen et al. 2016) [69]. Shortly, quality control of the RNA-seq reads was performed using FastQC [3] and reads were aligned to the Ensemble RN5 genome with STAR software (version 2.3.0e_r291) [24]. Differentially expressed genes were identified with DEseq2 [72] R package (R version 3.1.0) and the Benjamini–Hochberg false discovery rate (FDR) was used to calculate the adjusted *p*-value. Gene expression was considered to be significantly differentially expressed when FDR < 0.05.

## Effect of DNA methylation in the promoter, exon, or gene body region on gene expression

### *Gene set enrichment analysis*

To analyze the effect of DNA methylation located in the gene promoter, exon, or gene body areas on gene expression, we performed Gene Set Enrichment Analysis (GSEA) [116]. First, we prepared ranked lists from the gene expression data in the perilesional cortex, hippocampus, and thalamus by ranking the genes in order according to the p-value of mRNA differential expression. Upregulated genes were assigned with a positive rank number and downregulated genes with a negative rank number. Then, we generated three gene sets (genes with differentially methylated promoters, exons, or gene body areas) from each of the three brain areas (perilesional cortex, hippocampus, thalamus). Enrichment of these sets within the ranked lists was studied using GSEA, and enrichment was considered significant when the FDR q-value was < 0.05.

### *Linear regression analysis*

To confirm the GSEA results, we analyzed the association of DNA methylation in the gene promoter, exon, and gene body areas on gene expression using two different linear regression models: (a) association of DNA methylation on gene expression, (b) association of TBI on gene expression via DNA methylation. Regression analysis was carried out with lm-function in R v3.1.0. Genes with average mRNA read number < 50 were filtered out from the analysis. Regression was considered significant when FDR < 0.05.

## Validation of gene promoter methylation and gene expression

Digital droplet polymerase chain reaction (ddPCR) and pyrosequencing were used to confirm the gene expression changes in the RNA-seq and the methylation changes in the MBD-seq, respectively, of the four top hits. Of the four top hits, ***Gpr12*** and ***Lrp1b*** were downregulated in the mRNA-seq and showed increased promoter methylation in the MBD-seq in the perilesional cortex, ***Ppid*** showed increased promoter methylation in the thalamus, and ***Wdr26*** showed increased promoter methylation in the hippocampus (Table 1).

**Table 1** Gene promoter methylation and gene expression of *Wdr26, Lrp1b, Ppid* and *Gpr12* in perilesional cortex, hippocampus and ipsilateral thalamus according MBD and RNA-seq

| | | *Wdr26* | *Lrp1b* | *Ppid* | *Gpr12* |
|---|---|---|---|---|---|
| Perilesional Cx | ***Gene expression*** | | | | |
| | log2FC | − 0.161 | **− 0.441** | − 0.222 | **− 0.531** |
| | FDR | 0.300607 | **0.022273** | 0.242403 | **0.000197** |
| | ***Methylation*** | | | | |
| | log2FC | 0.313 | **1.402** | 0.038 | **1.407** |
| | FDR | 1 | **0.01901** | 1 | **0.014662** |
| Hippocampus | ***Gene expression*** | | | | |
| | log2FC | −0.129 | −0.166 | −0.036 | 0.224 |
| | FDR | 0.999825 | 0.999825 | 0.999825 | 0.999825 |
| | ***Methylation*** | | | | |
| | log2FC | **2.660** | −0.602 | **1.930** | 0.179 |
| | FDR | **1.87E-14** | 1 | **1.4E-07** | 1 |
| Thalamus | ***Gene expression*** | | | | |
| | log2FC | 0.140 | −0.097 | −0.074 | **− 0.687** |
| | FDR | 0.721246 | 0.795279 | 0.873954 | **0.000388** |
| | ***Methylation*** | | | | |
| | log2FC | 0.241 | 0.159 | 0.059 | −0.014 |
| | FDR | 1 | 1 | 1 | 1 |

Abbreviations: *Cx* perilesional cortex, *FC* fold-change. ***Statistical significances:*** log2FC change and corresponding FDR (< 0.05) are shown in bolded font

*Extraction of RNA for ddPCR and DNA for pyrosequencing*

Brain tissue from nine TBI and six sham-operated animals was collected as described above. The animals belonged to the same cohort of injured rats used for the RNA-seq and MBD-seq analyses.

RNA and DNA were extracted simultaneously from the perilesional cortex, thalamus, or hippocampus using a *mir*Vana miRNA isolation kit (#AM1560, Life Technologies (Ambion) Carlsbad, CA, USA), QIAshredder (#79654, Qiagen), and AllPrep DNA/RNA Mini Kit (#80204, Qiagen) as previously described [90]. Briefly, to avoid clogging the spin columns, brain tissue was divided into 2–5 pieces (each ~ 10 mg) on dry ice. Each tissue piece was then placed into a 2-ml microcentrifuge tube together with one metal ball and 800 μl of Ambion Lysis/binding buffer, and homogenized with a TissueLyser (Qiagen) for 3 min (30 Hz). For further homogenization, the lysate was transferred to a QIAshedder spin column and centrifuged (16,000 g) for 2 min at 4 °C. Flow-through lysate was transferred back to the QIAshedder spin column and centrifuged again. For DNA extraction, lysate was transferred to a Qiagen All Prep DNA spin column and centrifuged (10,000 g) for 1 min at room temperature. The spin-column was washed and eluted according to the instructions provided in the AllPrep DNA/RNA Mini Kit for DNA extraction.

Flow-through from the All Prep DNA spin column was used for RNA extraction using a *mir*Vana miRNA isolation kit. Briefly, miRNA homogenate additive (70 μl) was added to the flow-through. The mixture was vigorously vortexed for 30 s and then incubated on ice for 10 min. Acid-phenol:chloroform (700 μl) was then added, mixed, and centrifuged (16,000 g) for 30 s. The aqueous upper phase was transferred to a new microcentrifuge tube. Five hundred microliters of water was added to the lower phase, mixed, and centrifuged (16,000 g) for 30 s. The upper aqueous phase was collected into the same tube as the aqueous phase from the previous extraction cycle. Then, 100% ethanol (625 μl) was added to the tube, mixed, and transferred to the *mir*Vana miRNA isolation spin column. Finally, RNA was washed and eluted from the spin column according to instructions provided with the *mir*Vana miRNA isolation kit. Finally, RNA extracted from each brain region was pooled.

*Pyrosequencing*

Percentage (ratio of methylated/nonmethylated DNA * 100) of DNA methylated cytosines at a given CpG site in the ***Ppid, Lrp1b,*** *or* ***Wrd26*** gene promoters, or at two CpG sites in the ***Gpr12*** promoter was measured with pyrosequencing using the PSQ 96MA 2.1 platform (Biotage AB, Uppsala, Sweden) in the Genome Center of the University of London (Additional file 1). The Mann-Whitney U test was used to assess the significance of the difference in the percentage of methylation between the TBI and sham-operated animals ($p < 0.05$ was considered statistically significant) (Table 2).

*ddPCR*

RNA quality was checked with a 2100 Bioanalyzer (Agilent, Santa Clara, CA, USA) and RNA 6000 Nano Kit (#5067–1511, Agilent). The RNA integrity number (RIN) was > 8.0 in all but one sample (RIN 7.8). Therefore, 50 ng of RNA from all 15 samples was translated to cDNA using an iScript Advanced cDNA synthesis kit (#172–5038, BioRad, Hercules, CA, USA). Gene expression of ***Ppid, Gpr12, Lrp1b,*** *and* ***Wrd26*** was validated by ddPCR using ***Actb*** as a reference gene. ddPCR was conducted using QX200 ddPCR EvaGreen Supermix solution (#186–4033, BioRad) and a PrimerPCR gene expression assay (Actb; #dRnoEG5146006, Gpr12; #dRnoEG5125945, Lrp1b; #dRnoEG5140109, Ppid; #dRnoEG5125166, Wdr26; #dRnoEG5145659, BioRad) according to the manufacturer's instructions. Droplets were generated and their fluorescence measured with a QX200 Droplet Digital PCR System (BioRad). Fluorescent droplets were classified as "positive" and "negative", and then the concentration of each gene (copy/μl) was calculated using QuantaSoft 1.7.4 (BioRad). Target gene concentrations were normalized according to the ***Actb*** reference gene, log2 fold-changes were calculated, and the significance in the difference in droplet counts between the TBI and sham-operated rats was assessed using the Mann-Whitney U test (Table 2).

**Identification of transcription factors that chronically regulate post-TBI transcriptomics**

***Transcription regulatory network of the perilesional cortex and ipsilateral thalamus***

To analyze the regulation of post-TBI transcriptomics by transcription factors in the perilesional cortex and ipsilateral thalamus, and to further visualize their target genes, we downloaded the transcription regulatory network (TRN) from the SignaLink 2.0 database [31, 60]. Then, RNA-seq data from both brain areas (fold-change and FDR between sham-operated experimental controls and TBI animals) was integrated with the SignaLink 2.0 TRN in Cytoscape 3.4 [108]. To visualize the regulated targets of each selected transcription factor, differentially expressed transcription factors in mRNA-seq (FDR < 0.05 and log2FC < − 1 or > 1) and their nearest downstream neighbors in the TRN were detached from the SignaLink 2.0 network. Further analysis focused on the four transcription factors that had the highest number of regulated target genes in TRN.

**Table 2** Validation of gene promoter methylation by pyrosequencing and gene expression by ddPCR in the perilesional cortex, thalamus and hippocampus. As negative controls, we also assessed the methylation and gene expression in the ipsilateral hippocampus and thalamus. *Wdr26, Lrp1b,* and *Ppid* genes had only one CpG site whereas *Gpr12* gene had two CpG sites

| | | *Wdr26* | *Lrp1b* | *Ppid* | *Gpr12* | |
|---|---|---|---|---|---|---|
| Perilesional Cx | ***Gene expression*** | | | | | |
| | Log2FC | **−0.94944** | − 0.17498 | **− 0.60015** | −0.37159 | |
| | p-value | **0.007592** | 0.7756 | **0.03596** | 0.3277 | |
| | ***Methylation*** | | | | | |
| | Average methylation (%) | 85.31 | 67.28 | 59.52 | CpG site1: 73.43 | CpG site2: 76.57 |
| | Difference TBI - sham (%) | 1.07 | −0.17 | 2.39 | CpG site1:0.43 | CpG site2:0.35 |
| | p-value | 0.1135 | 0.9546 | 0.3636 | CpG site1: 0.8639 | CpG site2: 1 |
| Hippocampus | ***Gene expression*** | | | | | |
| | Log2FC | −0.6746 | −0.6457 | −1.3397 | −0.3415 | |
| | p-value | 0.366 | 0.1375 | 0.366 | 0.366 | |
| | ***Methylation*** | | | | | |
| | Average methylation (%) | 87.22 | 59.92 | 57.25 | CpG site1: 69.06 | CpG site2: 73.48 |
| | Difference TBI - sham (%) | 1.10 | −2.73 | 2.65 | CpG site1: 1.70 | CpG site2: −0.59 |
| | p-value | 0.366 | 0.2343 | 0.366 | CpG site1: 0.5338 | CpG site2: 1 |
| Thalamus | ***Gene expression*** | | | | | |
| | Log2FC | −0.8936 | −0.4964 | −0.9309 | **−1.3735** | |
| | p-value | 0.181 | 0.3277 | 0.06633 | **0.001598** | |
| | ***Methylation*** | | | | | |
| | Average methylation (%) | 85.11 | 65.82 | 49.95 | CpG site1: 74.23 | CpG site2: 77.40 |
| | Difference TBI - sham (%) | 1.07 | −2.33 | 7.69 | CpG site1: −0.95 | CpG site2: −0.93 |
| | p-value | 0.1469 | 0.5287 | 0.3884 | CpG site1: 0.7756 | CpG site2: 0.1135 |

*Abbreviations: Cx* cortex, *FC* fold-change. ***Statistical significances:*** log2FC change and corresponding p-value (< 0.05) are shown in bolded font

### Validation of gene expression of the top four transcription factors

#### *ddPCR*

Digital droplet PCR of the four top transcription factors (***Cebpd, Pax6, Spi1,*** and ***Tp73***) using ***Actb*** as a reference gene was performed to confirm the change in the expression of transcription factors coding genes. Analysis was performed using the same RNA samples, cDNA synthesis method, and ddPCR EvaGreen Supermix solution as for the validation of MBD-seq data (see above). A PrimerPCR gene expression assay (Actb; #dRnoEG5146006, Cebpd; #dRnoEG5126239, Pax6; #dRnoEG5125771, Spi1; #dRnoEG5139059, Tp73; #dRnoEG5139860, BioRad) was performed according to the manufacturer's instructions. Droplets were generated and their fluorescence measured with the QX200 Droplet Digital PCR System. QuantaSoft 1.7.4 was used to classify droplets as "positive" and "negative", and to calculate the concentration of gene copies/µl as described earlier. Finally, the target gene concentration was normalized with the reference gene concentration, the log2 fold-change of the concentration was calculated, and the significance in the difference in concentrations between the TBI and sham-operated rats was assessed using the Mann-Whitney U test.

### Identification of compounds modifying the transcription factor gene expression with the LINCS database

#### *Compounds modifying transcription factors gene expression*

Next, we searched the LINCS database (http://data.lincscloud.org.s3.amazonaws.com/index.html) to identify compounds that modify the expression of the four top transcription factors revealed by the SignaLink 2.0 database analysis. An in-house–created R script was used to run LINCS through an application programming interface. Reproducible compound-induced transcriptomics changes in terminally differentiated neurons (NEU), terminally differentiated neurons treated with KCl (NEU.KCL), and induced pluripotent stem cells-derived neural progenitor cells (NPC) were included in the analysis. As a result, we obtained a list of compounds that modulated the expression of transcription factors in one to three cell lines (i.e., transcription factors were within the 100 most upregulated or 100 most downregulated genes by a given compound).

## Results

### TBI-induced gene expression changes after TBI were most prominent in the perilesional cortex and were associated with DNA methylation at the gene promoter region

#### *GSEA analysis of MBD-seq data*

GSEA analysis of the perilesional cortex MBD-seq data suggested that altered DNA methylation in the gene

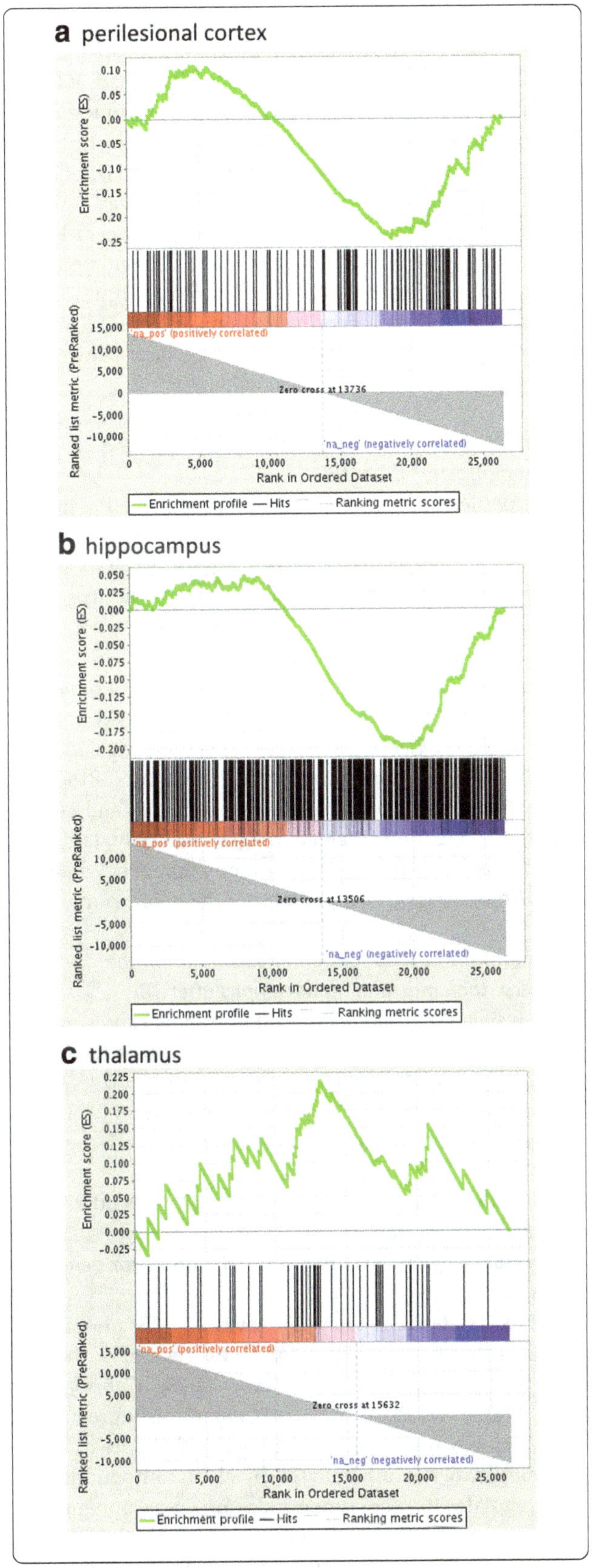


**Fig. 1** Enrichment scores of Gene Set Enrichment Analysis (GSEA) of DNA methylation in gene promoters in the (**a**) perilesional cortex (**b**) ipsilateral hippocampus, and (**c**) ipsilateral thalamus at 3 months after TBI. GSEA indicated significant negative enrichment in the perilesional cortex (FDR q-val. 0.046), but not in the ipsilateral hippocampus (FDR q-val. 0.079) or ipsilateral thalamus (FDR q-val. 0.828)

promoter area was inversely associated with the global gene expression profile (FDR q-val. 0.046) (Fig. 1). Altered DNA methylation in the gene promoter area in the hippocampal (FDR q-val. 0.079) or thalamic samples (FDR q-val. 0.828), however, was not associated with regulated gene expression. Interestingly, changes in DNA methylation in exons were not associated with gene expression in the perilesional cortex (FDR q-val. 0.243), hippocampus (FDR q-val. 0.464), or thalamus (FDR q-val. 0.372). DNA methylation in the gene body area also was not associated with transcriptomics changes in the perilesional cortex (FDR q-val. 0.083), thalamus (FDR q-val. 0.256), or hippocampus (FDR q-val. 0.631).

### *Linear regression analysis of the MBD-seq data*

To find individual genes affected by DNA methylation and TBI from the global DNA methylation profile, we performed a regression analysis to separately assess the TBI effect and methylation effect on gene expression. In the perilesional cortex and ipsilateral thalamus, however, we observed no TBI-induced effect on DNA methylation of individual genes when the gene promoter, exon, or gene body areas were analyzed separately. In contrast, in the hippocampus, TBI affected the DNA methylation of ***Crybg3*** (FDR = 0.0347, estimate = – 1.105 (95% confidence interval [CI]: – 1.2517 to – 0.9598) and ***Mak16*** (FDR = 0.0356, estimate = 4.596, 95% CI: 3.9705 to 5.2219) promoters, which affected their target gene expression. in the hippocampus, no TBI effect on methylation was detected in the exon and gene body regions.

We also used regression analysis to investigate the DNA methylation effect on gene expression. DNA methylation in any of the genomic areas did not appear to affect gene expression in any of the studied brain regions.

### *Methylation of the promoter area*

Analysis of MBD-seq data revealed significantly regulated DNA methylation in the promoter regions of 29 genes (all with increased methylation) in the perilesional cortex (FDR < 0.05). In four of 29 genes (***RGD1566265, Nap1l2, Lrp1b,*** and ***Gpr12***), an increase in promoter methylation was associated with reduced gene expression in the corresponding perilesional cortex (FDR < 0.05). In the hippocampus, none of the 166 methylation changes (97 increased and 69 decreased) in the promoter area were associated with changes in gene expression. In the thalamus, no alterations in promoter methylation were found (FDR < 0.05).

#### *Methylation of exons*

Methylation in exons of 20 genes (15 increased and 5 decreased) was regulated in the hippocampus, but none of the methylation changes were associated with altered expression of the corresponding gene in the RNA-seq data (FDR < 0.05). In the perilesional cortex and thalamus, we observed no changes in exon methylation (FDR < 0.05).

#### *Methylation of gene body areas*

Methylation of the gene body area was not changed in any of the brain areas studied (FDR < 0.05).

### Validation of MBD-seq using pyrosequencing and RNA-seq data using ddPCR failed to confirm a link between promoter methylation and changed gene expression in the perilesional cortex at 3 months after TBI

#### *Validation of gene promoter area methylation and gene expression*

Promoter methylation and expression of ***Lrp1b***, ***Gpr12***, ***Wrd26***, and ***Ppid*** genes in the perilesional cortex were validated with pyrosequencing and ddPCR, respectively, in animals from the same cohort used for the RNA-seq and MBD-seq studies (Table 2). The percentage of methylation per CpG site in the promoter region varied from 49.95 to 87.22%, depending on the gene or the methylation site in each gene (Table 2). Unexpectedly, pyrosequencing indicated that none of the four tested genes in the perilesional cortex had altered methylation in the gene promoter area (Table 2). ddPCR, however, confirmed reduced expression of ***Wrd26*** and ***Ppid*** in the perilesional cortex (Table 2).

### Post-TBI perilesional cortex showed a substantial increase in the expression of four transcription factors

#### *Transcription factors regulating post-TBI gene expression*

As we observed few methylation changes in relation to the large number of transcriptomic changes in the perilesional cortex and ipsilateral thalamus, we next assessed whether chronic post-TBI regulation of gene expression in these brain areas was controlled by transcription factors. To assess whether the transcriptomic changes observed in RNA-seq correspond to alterations in local cell populations we correlated the read counts of transcription factors with the read counts of neuronal, microglial and astroglial markers (Additional files 2 and 3).

#### *Transcription regulatory network of the perilesional cortex*

In the perilesional cortex, integration of SignaLink 2.0 TRN and RNA-seq revealed increased expression in five transcription factors, ***Pax6*** (Fig. 2), ***Tp73*** (Fig. 3), ***Cebpd***, ***Spi1***, and ***Myb***, and decreased expression in ***Etv4*** at 3 months post-TBI (Table 3). ***Pax6*** had 300 targets in the TRN analysis, of which 32 were upregulated and 59 downregulated. ***Tp73*** had 54 targets in the TRN analysis, of which five were upregulated and 11 downregulated. ***Igf1***, the only target of ***Cebpd***, was upregulated in the TRN analysis. ***Spi1*** had three targets in the TRN analysis, of which only ***Lsp1*** was upregulated. According to the TRN analysis, ***Etv4*** had one target, which did not show altered gene expression. In the TRN analysis, ***Myb*** had three targets, none of which showed altered expression in the perilesional cortex.

#### *Validation of transcription factor expression in the perilesional cortex after TBI*

In the perilesional cortex, validation confirmed a significant increase in gene expression of ***Cebpd*** ($p = 0.0003996$), ***Pax6*** ($p = 0.004795$), ***Spi1*** ($p = 0.007592$), and ***Tp73*** ($p = 0.0007992$) (Table 4) at 3 months after TBI.

#### *Transcription regulatory network of the ipsilateral thalamus*

TRN analysis of the ipsilateral thalamus revealed upregulation of ***Pax6***, ***Cebpd***, and ***Spi1***, and downregulation of the ***Etv4*** transcription factor at 3 months post-TBI (Table 3). ***Pax6*** had 19 targets that were upregulated and 14 targets that were downregulated. ***Igf1***, the only target of ***Cebpd***, was upregulated. ***Spi1*** had one upregulated target, ***Lsp1***. ***Etv4*** showed no alteration in gene expression.

#### *Validation of transcription factor expression in the ipsilateral thalamus and hippocampus after TBI*

In the ipsilateral thalamus, validation of gene expression indicated a trend toward increased expression of ***Spi1*** ($p = 0.06633$), but not ***Cebpd*** ($p = 0.2721$), ***Pax6*** ($P = 0.4559$), or ***Tp73*** ($p = 0.3884$) (Table 4) at 3 months after TBI. In the ipsilateral hippocampus, gene expression was unchanged.

### LINCS analysis revealed 118 candidate pharmacotherapies that can regulate transcription factors

#### *Pharmacotherapies regulating transcription factor gene expression*

The LINCS database analysis revealed 118 pharmacotherapies that can modify the gene expression of the top four transcription factors (***Pax6***, ***Tp73***, ***Cebpd***, and ***Spi1***) (Table 5). Expression of ***Cebpd*** was upregulated by 92 compounds and downregulated by two compounds. ***Pax6*** was upregulated by eight compounds and downregulated by six compounds. ***Spi1*** was upregulated by two compounds and downregulated by three compounds. ***Tp73*** was upregulated by five compounds. Interestingly, none of the compounds regulated more than one transcription factor.

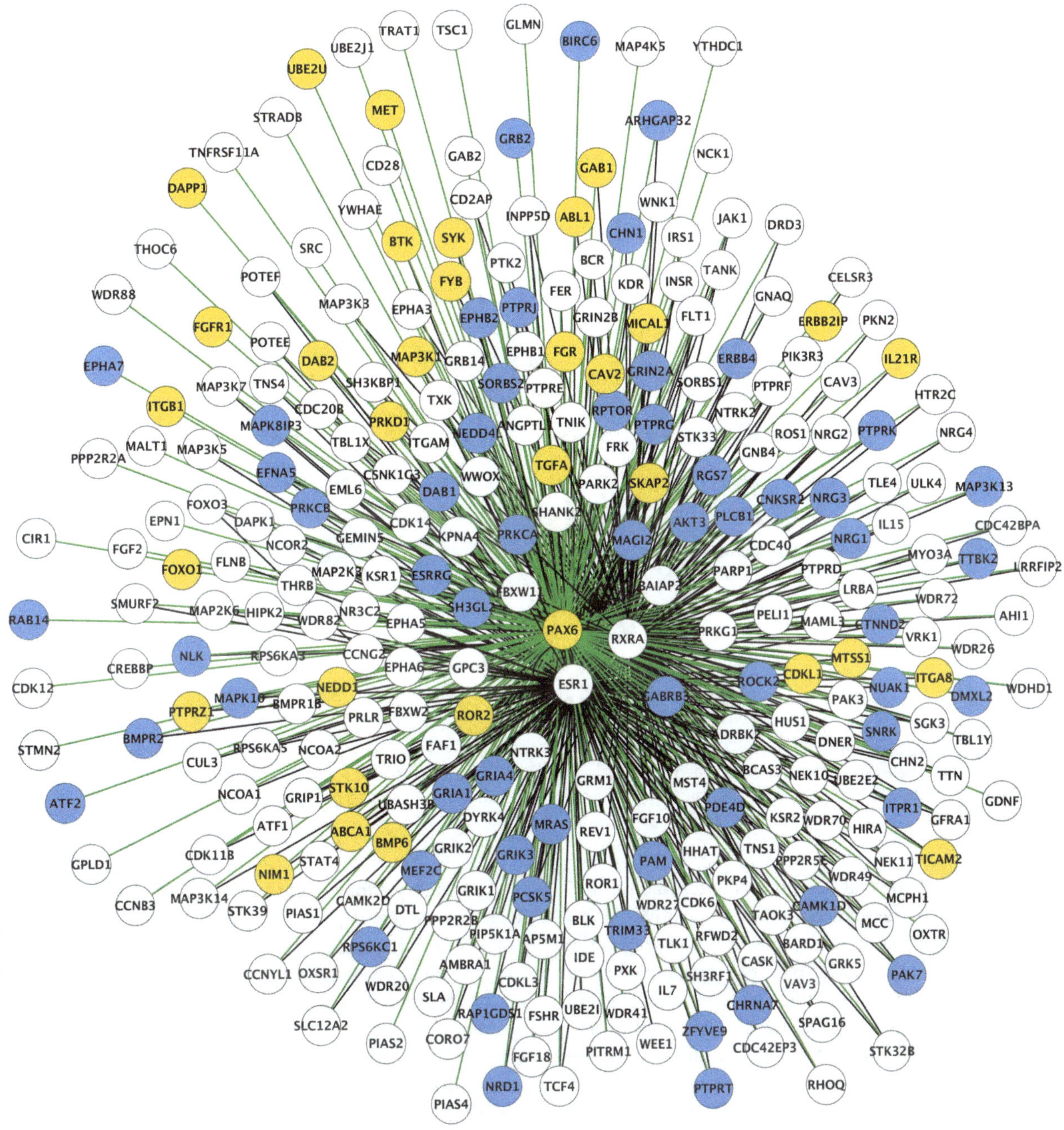


**Fig. 2** SignaLink transcription regulatory network (TRN) of *Pax6* and its targets in the perilesional cortex. SignaLink network analysis revealed 300 targets, of which 36 were upregulated and 59 were downregulated in the perilesional cortex 3 months post-TBI. Color codes: blue circle, downregulation after TBI; yellow circle, upregulation after TBI; white circle, no change in gene expression after TBI; green line, transcriptional interaction with *Pax6*; black line, inter-target interaction

## Discussion

In the present study, we evaluated whether TBI induces long-lasting transcriptomics regulation that is under the control of DNA-methylation. Bioinformatics analysis indicated that transcription factors rather than DNA methylation regulate gene expression at 3 months after TBI. Further, LINCS analysis revealed that several drugs already in clinical use modulate the expression of the identified key regulatory transcription factors ***Cebpd, Pax6, Spi1,*** and ***Tp73***.

### DNA methylation is not a major regulator of chronically altered post-TBI gene expression in our experimental model

Our previous study indicated regulated expression of approximately 5000 genes in the perilesional cortex and

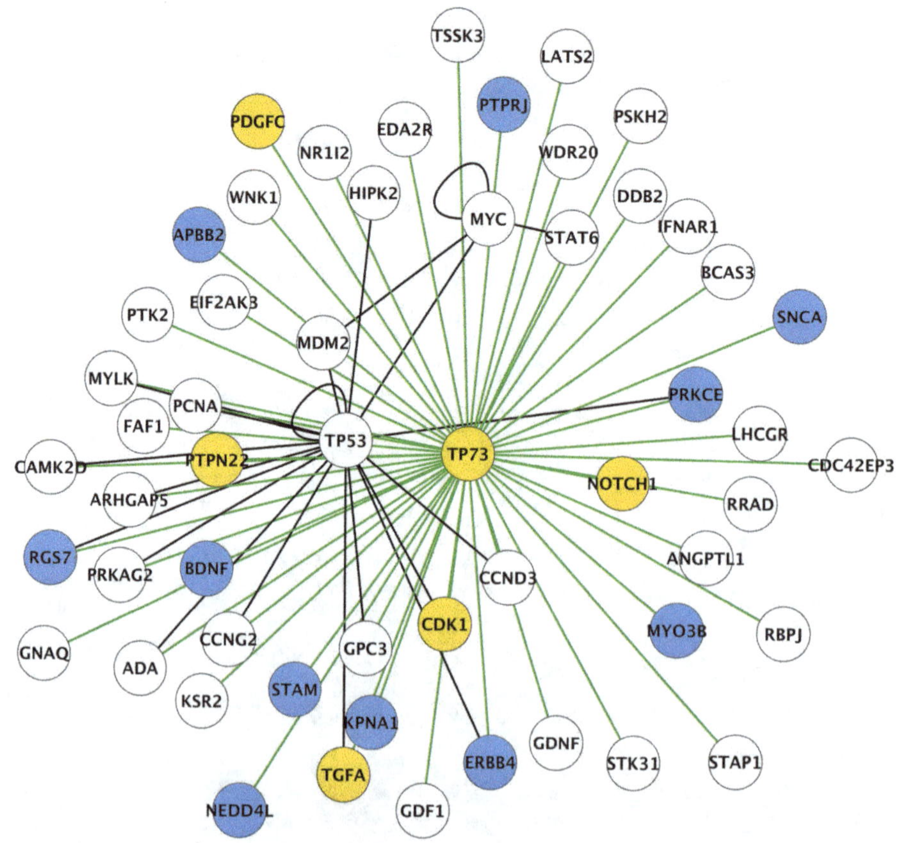


**Fig. 3** SignaLink transcription regulatory network (TRN) of *Tp73* and its targets in the perilesional cortex. SignaLink network analysis revealed 54 targets, of which five were upregulated and 11 were downregulated in the perilesional cortex 3 months post-TBI. Color codes: blue circle, downregulation after TBI; yellow circle, upregulation after TBI; white circle, no change in gene expression after TBI; green line, transcriptional interaction with *Tp73;* black line, inter-target interaction

1900 in the thalamus at 3 months after lateral FPI-induced TBI. in particular, we found a positive enrichment of inflammation-related genes and downregulation of ion channel-related genes [69]. The mechanisms that regulate chronic gene expression, however, remained unclear. Our transcriptomic data suggest that gene expression alterations could not be explained only by changes in the local cell populations [69]. One potential major regulator could be DNA-methylation, which regulates gene expression in several brain diseases, including Alzheimer's' disease [19], Parkinson's disease [51], amyotrophic lateral sclerosis [32], epilepsy [127], and TBI [39, 83, 102, 106]. To explore the significance of DNA methylation as a regulator of chronically detected transcriptomics changes, we carried out genome-wide MBD-seq and RNA-seq from the perilesional cortex, ipsilateral thalamus, and ipsilateral hippocampus at 3 months post-TBI.

Regulated methylation was associated with altered gene expression only in the perilesional cortex. GSEA analysis revealed that the most enriched DNA methylation patterns in the perilesional cortex after TBI were in the gene promoter area. Specifically, MBD-seq indicated altered methylation in promoters of the ***Lrp1b*, *Gpr12*, *Wrd26*,** and ***Ppid*** genes. Pyrosequencing, however, did not confirm the sequencing data. This could relate to a low, although consistent, read count per methylation site in the promoter region (< 200) in the MBD-seq. Our negative findings are in agreement with previous studies in fluid-percussion injury, controlled cortical injury, weight-drop, and blast-induced TBI models, which reported no changes in the promoter methylation of ***Lrp1b*, *Gpr12*, *Wrd26*** and ***Ppid*** genes in cortical, hippocampal, or amygdaloid tissue sampled 3 days to 8 months post-injury [39, 83, 102, 106]. We were not able to reproduce the altered methylation in the rat cortex at 8 months after blast TBI [39], in the rat amygdala at 48 h to 30 d after weight-drop–induced TBI [102], in the rat hippocampus at 3 and 14 d after controlled cortical impact [106], in the rat hippocampus at 7 d after fluid-percussion injury [83], or in the rat hippocampus 3 months after lateral fluid-percussion injury [20]. This is likely related to the different injury types and post-injury delays between the present and previous experimental studies.

**Table 3** SignaLink 2.0 transcription regulatory network (TRN) analysis of differentially expressed transcription factors and their up-regulated and down-regulated target genes in the perilesional cortex and the ipsilateral thalamus at 3 months after traumatic brain injury. The same targets that were up-regulated both in the perilesional cortex and ipsilateral thalamus or down-regulated both in the perilesional cortex and ipsilateral thalamus are bold fonts

| | Perilesional cortex | | | | | Ipsilateral thalamus | | | | |
|---|---|---|---|---|---|---|---|---|---|---|
| TF | Log2FC | FDR | Altered targets/ all targets | Upregulated TF targets | Downregulated TF targets | Log2FC | FDR | Altered targets/ all targets | Upregulated TF targets | Downregulated TF targets |
| *Cebpd* | 1.835 | 3.78E-034 | 1/1 | **IGF1** | – | 1.261 | 7.47E-005 | 1/1 | **IGF1** | – |
| *Etv4* | −1.105 | 2.03E-008 | 0/1 | – | – | −0.697 | 0.00523964 | 0/1 | – | – |
| *Myb* | 1.350 | 0.0042262 | 0/3 | – | – | ns | ns | – | – | – |
| *Pax6* | 1.186 | 5.97E-022 | 91/300 | **ABCA1,** ABL1, BMP6, **BTK,** CAV2, CDKL1, DAB2, **DAPP1, ERBB2IP,** FGFR1, **FGR,** FOXO1, FYB, **GAB1, IL21R,** ITGA8, **ITGB1,** MAP3K1, MET, MICAL1, MTSS1, NEDD1, NIM1, PRKD1, PTPRZ1, ROR2, SKAP2, STK10, SYK, **TGFA,** TICAM2, UBE2U | AKT3, **ARHGAP32,** ATF2, BIRC6, BMPR2, **CAMK1D, CHN1,** CHRNA7, CNKSR2, CTNND2,DAB, DMXL2, EFNA5, EPHA7, EPHB2, ERBB4, ESRRG, GABRB3, GRB2,GRIA1, GRIA4, GRIK3, GRIN2A, ITPR1, MAGI2, MAP3K13, **MAPK10,** MAPK8IP3, MEF2C, MRAS, **NEDD4L,** NLK, NRD1, NRG1, NRG3, NUAK1, PAK7, PAM, PCSK5, PDE4D, PLCB1, PRKCA, **PRKCB,** PTPRG, PTPRJ, PTPRK, PTPRT, RAB14, **RAP1GDS1,** RGS7, ROCK2, RPS6KC1, RPTOR, SH3GL2, SNRK, SORBS2, TRIM33, TTBK2, ZFYVE9 | 0.779 | 8.41E-5 | 33/300 | **ABCA1,** ATF1, **BTK, DAPP1,** EPHB1, **ERBB2IP,** ERBB4, FGF2, **FGR, GAB1,** GRB14, **IL21R,** INPP5D, ITGAM **ITGB1,** PKP4, PRKCA, TCF4, **TGFA** | **ARHGAP32, CAMK1D, CHN1,** DAPK1, GRM1, MAP3K14, **MAPK10, NEDD4L, NRG2, PRKCB, RAP1GDS1,** SRC, STRADB, TRIO |
| *Spi1* | 1.021 | 2.88E-011 | 1/3 | LSP1 | – | 1.310 | 8.57E-006 | 1/3 | **LSP1** | – |
| *Tp73* | 1.328 | 0.01004339 | 15/54 | TGFA, PTPN22, CDK1, PDGFC, NOTCH1 | BDNF, RGS7, **ERBB4,** SNCA, PRKCE, PTPRJ, NEDD4L, KPNA1, APBB2, STAM, MYO3B | ns | ns | 6/55 | MYLK, NEDD4L | RRAD, TGFA, **ERBB4,** PCNA |

*Abbreviations*: *FDR* false discovery rate, *ns* non-significant, *TF* transcription factor

### TRN analysis revealed transcription factors *Cebpd, Pax6, Spi1* and *Tp73* as regulators of chronically altered post-TBI gene expression

To identify the master switch that regulates the massively altered gene expression at 3 months post-TBI, we next investigated the possible contribution of transcription factors by integrating transcriptomics data into the Signalink 2.0 database. Laboratory validation of top hits using ddPCR confirmed the predicted mRNA upregulation of four transcription factors, ***Pax6, Tp73, Cebpd,*** and ***Spi1,*** in the perilesional cortex.

***Pax6*** showed a 6.7-fold upregulation, and almost 30% (91 or 300) of its target genes were regulated in the perilesional cortex. The function of ***Pax6*** in the cerebral cortex is unknown. In the hippocampus, ***Pax6*** controls the differentiation and migration of neuronal progenitor cells (NPC) [37], which show regenerative potential after ischemic injury [88]. Moreover, overexpression of ***Pax6*** improved the cellular viability of SH-SY5Y cells exposed to neurotoxin [119]. These studies suggest that upregulation of ***Pax6*** after TBI could play a reparative role.

***Tp73*** showed a 1.6-fold upregulation, and approximately 30% (15 of 54) of its target genes were regulated in the perilesional cortex after TBI. The Tp73 gene has two promoters, producing two protein isoforms with different functions [86]. The ***ΔNp73*** isoform is anti-apoptotic during development of the mouse superior cervical ganglion neurons [95]. Furthermore, ***ΔNp73*** is vital for long-term

**Table 4** Gene expression validation of genes encoding transcription factors using ddPCR in the rat perilesional cortex, thalamus and hippocampus at three months after TBI

| | *Cebpd* | *Pax6* | *Spi1* | *Tp73* |
|---|---|---|---|---|
| *Perilesional cortex* | | | | |
| Fold change | **2.58** | **1.64** | **1.75** | **6.67** |
| p-value | **0.0003996** | **0.004795** | **0.007592** | **0.0007992** |
| *Thalamus* | | | | |
| Fold change | 1.55 | 1.13 | 1.65 | 0.55 |
| p-value | 0.2721 | 0.4559 | 0.06633 | 0.3884 |
| *Hippocampus* | | | | |
| Fold change | 0.74 | 0.91 | 1.00 | 0.79 |
| p-value | 0.1375 | 0.7308 | 0.6282 | 0.6282 |

***Statistical significances:*** Fold change and corresponding *p*-value (< 0.05) are shown in bolded font

survival of mouse superior cervical ganglion and cortical neurons [66, 94]. The ***TAp73*** isoform, however, induces apoptosis in SAOS-2 and medulloblastoma cell cultures [11, 50]. Further studies are needed to explore the functional consequences of Tp73 upregulation after TBI.

***Cebpd,*** also known as NF-IL6β, regulates immune and inflammatory responses [57, 101]. ***Cebpd*** showed a 2.6-fold upregulation, and its predicted target gene, IGF-1, was also upregulated in the perilesional cortex at 3 months post-TBI. There are some reports of increased expression of ***Cebpd*** in the cortex already at 2 h to 7 d after injury in various experimental models of TBI, including a controlled cortical impact mouse model [48, 105, 128] and a weight-drop rat model [16, 123]. These studies propose a wide time window for the post-injury regulation of ***Cebpd*** and its target IGF-1. It remains a testable hypothesis that chronic upregulation of ***Cebpd*** and *IGF-1* genes relates to the control of chronic inflammation after TBI, as recently suggested in favorable proof-of-concept preclinical studies in injury models [75, 96, 110, 120].

***Spi1*** showed a 1.8-fold upregulation at 3 months post-TBI. ***Spi1*** is expressed in microglia [126], which become activated after TBI [13, 61, 124]. ***Spi1*** encodes PU.1, which appears vital for microglial survival [111]. Our TRN network analysis revealed three gene targets for ***Spi1,*** and of those, ***Lsp1*** was upregulated in the perilesional cortex and ipsilateral thalamus at 3 months post-TBI. ***Lsp1*** was reported to be upregulated in the rat cerebral cortex at 24 h after controlled cortical impact-induced TBI [128]. ***Spi1*** regulates monocyte and macrophage differentiation [100], and has a crucial role in the normal development of T cells, B cells, neutrophils, and macrophages [82], which are important players in the post-TBI systemic inflammatory response [110].

In summary, our findings indicate that four transcription factors, ***Pax6, Tp73, Cepbd,*** and ***Spi1,*** serve as major chronic post-TBI transcriptomics regulators, and are thus potential targets for treatments.

**Table 5** LINCS database analysis identified compounds that up-regulate or down-regulate the gene expression of *Cebpd, Pax6, Spi1* and *Tp73* transcription factors. Identification of compounds regulating the expression of transcription factors were carried out by retrieving compound-induced transcription profiles in terminally differentiated neurons, terminally differentiated neurons treated with KCl, and iPS-derived neural progenitor cells

| TF | Upregulating compounds | Downregulating compounds |
|---|---|---|
| *Cebpd* | aminobenztropine (NEU), BG-1002 (NEU.KCL), BG-1011 (NPC), BIIB021 (NPC), BRD-A06779035 (NPC), BRD-A70591769 (NEU), BRD-A75769921 (NEU.KCL), BRD-A92334183 (NEU), BRD-K01608965 (NPC), BRD-K07381195 (NPC), BRD-K12683703 (NPC), BRD-K15050703 (NPC), BRD-K15935695 (NPC), BRD-K16934333 (NPC), BRD-K20126873 (NPC), BRD-K21374126 (NPC), BRD-K23986500 (NPC), BRD-K24798550 (NPC), BRD-K25164076 (NPC), BRD-K25990552 (NEU), BRD-K28934562 (NPC), BRD-K30229575 (NPC), BRD-K32885145 (NPC), BRD-K36269259 (NEU), BRD-K36313546 (NPC), BRD-K36591038 (NPC), BRD-K36796217 (NPC), BRD-K39597586 (NPC), BRD-K40300908 (NPC), BRD-K41871066 (NPC), BRD-K43631199 (NPC), BRD-K44540157 (NPC), BRD-K49111930 (NPC), BRD-K54331210 (NPC), BRD-K55536701 (NPC), BRD-K57166447 (NPC), BRD-K58808184 (NPC), BRD-K59253994 (NPC), BRD-K62970326 (NPC), BRD-K63494246 (NEU), BRD-K64523453 (NPC), BRD-K65148580 (NPC), BRD-K65657366 (NPC), BRD-K72354054 (NPC), BRD-K73008154 (NPC), BRD-K77888550 (NPC), BRD-K78133682 (NPC), BRD-K79947405 (NPC), BRD-K80062189 (NPC), BRD-K80138901 (NPC), BRD-K80400482 (NEU), BRD-K85133207 (NPC), BRD-K86110682 (NPC), BRD-K91844626 (NEU), BRD-K93158953 (NPC), BRD-K99718824 (NPC), cabergoline (NEU), chlorpromazine (NEU), deoxycholic-acid (NEU), econazole (NPC), farnesylthioacetic-acid (NPC), fluspirilene (NEU), geldanamycin (NPC), GSK-461364 (NPC), GW-3965 (NPC), GW-441756 (NPC), IQ1 (NEU), IQ1 (NPC), isoflupredone (NPC), ITSA-1 (NPC), IWP-2 (NEU), LY-255283 (NPC), LY-294002 (NPC), menadione (NPC), NVP-BEZ235 (NPC), PD-173074 (NPC), PI-828 (NPC), quercetin (NPC), R-96544 (NPC), scoulerine (NPC), serotonin (NPC), spermidine (NEU), SR-142948 (NEU), ST-023431 (NPC), ST-056792 (NPC), suberoyl-bis-hydroxamic-acid (NEU), tamoxifen (NPC), tozasertib (NPC), tranylcypromine (NEU.KCL), triacetylresveratrol (NPC), trichostatin-a (NEU), trifluridine (NPC), vorinostat (NPC) | BRD-K89824424 (NPC), O-1918 (NPC) |
| *Pax6* | acetyl-farnesyl-cysteine (NEU.KCL), BRD-K02409808 (NEU), BRD-K24656059 (NPC), BRD-K45842176 (NPC), clofibric-acid (NPC), rolipram (NPC), SKF-96365 (NPC), thioproperazine (NPC) | apicidin (NEU.KCL), BG-1016 (NPC), BRD-K37650321 (NEU), chrysamine-g (NEU), proadifen (NPC), XMD-1150 (NEU) |
| *Spi1* | BRD-K39172790 (NEU), timosaponin (NEU) | AS-703026 (NPC), genistein (NPC), U-0126 (NPC) |
| *Tp73* | BRD-K16827616 (NPC), BRD-K78133682 (NPC), RG-14620 (NPC), trimipramine (NEU), wortmannin (NEU) | – |

*Abbreviations: NEU* terminally differentiated neurons, *NEU.KCL* terminally differentiated neurons treated with, *NPC* iPS-derived neural progenitor cells, *TF* transcription factor

### LINCS analysis revealed transcription factor-targeting antidepressants and anti-cancer drugs as novel treatment candidates for TBI

Next, we performed a LINCS analysis to identify compounds that modulate the gene expression of ***Pax6, Tp73, Cepbd,*** or ***Spi1***. The largest number of compounds identified targeted ***Cebpd***. Most of the compounds upregulating ***Cebpd*** were bioactive (starting with BRD) without any known therapeutic actions. The analysis, however, also identified antidepressants and anti-cancer drugs that are already used in the clinic. **Tranylcypromine**, an antidepressant and monoamine oxidase inhibitor (MAO-I) [29], is a promising therapy as MAO-Is have neuroprotective effects in mice with TBI [44]. Tranylcypromine also alleviates neurodegeneration and inflammation by inhibiting prostacyclin and arachidonic acid release in calf primary endothelial cells [34, 43]. LINCS analysis also revealed **fluspirilene and chlorpromazine** as upregulators of ***Cepbd.*** Duotherapy with **chlorpromazine** and promethazine was demonstrated to be neuroprotective when assessed at 24 h after brain ischemia in rats [35]. **Chlorpromazine** suppressed neuronal apoptosis in the rat parietal cortex and the CA1 subfield of the hippocampus when assessed at 24 h after ethanol-induced apoptosis [131]. **Chlorpromazine** also reduced the cerebral infarct size when assessed at 24 h post-ischemia in rats [68].

In addition to compounds used in psychiatry, LINCS analysis revealed an anti-cancer drug, **vorinostat**, a histone deacetylase inhibitor (HDAC1–3 and 6) [77] as an upregulator of ***Cepbd***. **Vorinostat** attenuated neurodegeneration and improved neurological outcome when assessed at 24 h after stroke in rats [117]. Interestingly, valproate, another HDAC inhibitor (HDAC1–3 and 8) [6], is neuroprotective and anti-inflammatory in rodent models of TBI and ischemia [18, 55, 132]. **Tamoxifen** was another upregulator of ***Cepbd*** identified by the LINCS analysis. Tamoxifen is a selective estrogen receptor modulator [107] used to treat breast cancer [33]. Tamoxifen reduced the cerebral infarct volume and neuronal apoptosis when assessed at 72 h after fluid-percussion injury in rats [121]. LINCS analysis also revealed two compounds that downregulated ***Cebpd***, O-1918 and BRD-K89824424. Information available from **O-1918** indicates that it is a cannabidiol analog, acting as a selective antagonist of abnormal cannabidiol at the non-$CB_1$/$CB_2$ endothelial receptor [89, 135]. Interestingly, another cannabinoid receptor antagonist, AM630, counteracted the recovery-enhancing effects of leptin [71]. Moreover, SR144528, a cannabinoid receptor antagonist increased TNFα gene expression 24 h after mouse controlled cortical impact (CCI), suggesting that it enhances the inflammatory response [2]. Taken together, these studies suggest that upregulation of ***Cebpd*** favorably modifies the post-TBI outcome.

LINCS analysis revealed **SKF-96365, thioproperazine,** and **rolipram** as upregulators of ***Pax6***. **SKF-96365** is an inhibitor of receptor-mediated calcium entry [84]. In an in vitro model of bovine brain microvessel endothelial cells, SKF-96365 decreased blood-brain barrier permeability [1], a major pathology in TBI. **Thioproperazin** is a neuroleptic that increases dopamine release [12]. Interestingly, dopamine release was decreased at 1 week after TBI in the rat CCI model [109], and an increase in dopamine level by methylphenidate improved spatial memory based on a shorter Morris water-maze latency at 14 d after rat CCI [58]. **Rolipram**, an antidepressant, MAO-I, and phosphodiesterase (PDE) IV inhibitor, also upregulates Pax6 gene expression. It suppresses cytokine production in human and rat T cells [114]. Moreover, **rolipram** inhibits neuronal damage in gerbil CA1 hippocampus 7 d after stroke [53]. **Rolipram** also reduced infarct size, improved neurological outcome, increased anti-inflammatory cytokines, and decreased pro-inflammatory cytokines at 24 h after mouse focal cerebral ischemia [62]. LINCS analysis revealed that ***Pax6*** was downregulated by **proadifen**, a cytochrome P-450 inhibitor [10], and by **apicidin**, a histone deacetylase inhibitor [41]. Interestingly, **apicidin** induced apoptosis in MCF-7 cells through cell cycle regulatory proteins [45] and reversed nitric oxide and inducible nitric oxide synthase expression induced by dexamethasone and RU24858 in a mouse macrophage cell culture [40]. Taken together, upregulation of ***Pax6*** gene expression appears to be a target for favorable modulation of the post-TBI outcome by reversing the reduced dopamine release and reducing neuroinflammation via cytokine release, as suggested by studies of **thioproperazine** and **rolipram**. Moreover, both ***Cepbd*** and ***Pax6*** are upregulated by compounds with an MAO-I mechanism, and are predicted to have favorable effects.

LINCS analysis revealed two compounds that upregulate ***Spi1***. From these, **timosaponin AIII** is a candidate anti-cancer drug [52, 118]. It reverses scopolamine-induced memory impairment in mice [67]. LINCS analysis revealed three compounds that downregulated ***Spi1***. **AS-703026** (also known as pimasertib) and **U0126** are MEK1/2 inhibitors [30, 56]. **U0126** has favorable effects on recovery in various in vivo brain injury models. For example, it reduced infarct size when assessed at 24 h after middle cerebral artery occlusion in rats [27], lesion size when analyzed at 7 d after in mice injured with controlled cortical impact [87], and microglial activation in the ischemia model of spinal cord injury in rats [73]. **Genistein**, a phytoestrogen with a broad spectrum of pharmacological properties, inhibits protein tyrosine kinases and topoisomerase II, and exhibits estrogen-like activity [23, 93]. **Genistein** showed neuroprotective effects when assessed at 48 h after weight-drop–induced TBI [113] and at 24 h after focal cerebral ischemia in rats [4]. Whether downregulators of ***Spi1*** will have favorable effects on more chronic post-TBI outcome remains to be investigated.

LINCS analysis revealed three compounds with some prior information of biological effects, all of which upregulated ***Tp73***. **Wortmannin,** a radiosensitizer, is a phosphoinositide 3-kinase inhibitor [5] that also inhibits mTOR in vitro, a pathway involved in post-TBI recovery and epileptogenesis in several post-injury animal models [8, 92]. **Trimipramine** is a tricyclic antidepressant [103] that reduced interferon-γ production, suppressed T-cell proliferation, and increased interleukin-12 production in concanavalin A-stimulated human whole blood cultures [21]. The effects of **trimipramine** on brain injury, however, are poorly described. **RG-14620** is a protein tyrosine kinase inhibitor with antiproliferative effects [134]. Compounds that upregulate ***Tp73*** expression are interesting candidates for further studies. For example, trimipramine is already used in the clinic and could be repurposed to improve outcome after TBI.

## Conclusions

This is the first analysis of chronic regulation of gene expression after TBI, demonstrating that chronic post-TBI transcriptional regulation is more under the control of transcription factors than DNA methylation. In particular, four upregulated transcription factors ***Pax6, Tp73, Cebpd,*** and ***Spi1,*** appeared as potent regulators of chronic post-TBI gene expression. They regulate the molecular networks contributing to post-injury secondary damage, including apoptosis and inflammation, strengthening the feasibility of therapeutically targeting these molecular networks even after the acute post-TBI period. To complement hypothesis-driven therapeutic approaches, our systems-biology driven unbiased LINCS database analysis revealed several novel treatment candidates. In particular, our data together with a literature search of effects in in vitro and in vivo models of brain injury revealed that antidepressant/neuroleptics such as trimipramine, rolipram, fluspirilene, and chlorpromazine, as well as the anti-cancer therapies pimasertib, tamoxifen, and vorinostat are candidates for further testing to favorably modulate regulated transcriptomics networks and post-TBI outcome.

#### Abbreviations

CCI: Controlled cortical impact; ddPCR: Digital droplet polymerase chain reaction; FDR: False discovery rate; FPI: Fluid-percussion injury; GSEA: Gene Set Enrichment Analysis; HDAC: Histone deacetylase inhibitor; MAO-I: Monoamine oxidase inhibitor; MBD-seq: Methyl-binding domain sequencing; NEU: Terminally differentiated neurons; NEU.KCL: Terminally differentiated neurons treated with KCl; NPC: iPS-derived neural progenitor cells; RIN: RNA integrity number; RNA-seq: RNA-sequencing; STAR: Spliced Transcripts Alignment to a Reference; TBI: Traumatic brain injury; TRN: Transcription regulatory network

#### Acknowledgements

We thank Mr. Jarmo Hartikainen and Mrs. Merja Lukkari for their excellent technical assistance. We are also grateful to Mr. Juha Kekäläinen and Oskari Timonen (MSc) for their excellent help with the bioinformatics analysis.

#### Funding

This study was supported by the Academy of Finland (A.P.), EpiGENet EUROEPINOMICS (A.P.), and FP7-HEALTH project 602102 (EPITARGET)(AP).

#### Authors' contributions

AL and AP wrote the main manuscript text. NP sampled rat brain. AEO, AK, MZ and HKH did NGS sequencing. AL and JP conducted bioinformatics analyses. VN-F and AL made validations. All authors read and approved the final manuscript.

#### Competing interests

The authors declare that they have no competing interests.

#### Author details

[1]Epilepsy Research Laboratory, A. I. Virtanen Institute for Molecular Sciences, University of Eastern Finland, PO Box 1627, FIN-70211 Kuopio, Finland. [2]Epigenetics in Human Health and Disease Laboratory, Central Clinical School, Faculty of Medicine, Monash University, Melbourne, VIC, Australia. [3]Prince of Wales Hospital, The Chinese University of Hong Kong, Sha Tin, Hong Kong SAR. [4]Institute of Biomedicine, University of Eastern Finland, Kuopio, Finland. [5]University of Eastern Finland Bioinformatics Center, University of Eastern Finland, Kuopio, Finland.

#### References

1. Abbruscato TJ, Davis TP (1999) Combination of hypoxia/Aglycemia compromises in vitro blood-brain barrier integrity. J Pharmacol Exp Ther 289:668–678
2. Amenta PS, Jallo JI, Tuma RF, Hooper DC, Elliott MB (2014) Cannabinoid receptor type-2 stimulation, blockade, and deletion alter the vascular inflammatory responses to traumatic brain injury. J Neuroinflammation 11:191
3. Andrews S. FastQC: A quality control tool for high throughput sequence data. 2010. https://www.bioinformatics.babraham.ac.uk/projects/fastqc/. Accessed 25 Nov 2017
4. Aras AB, Guven M, Akman T, Alacam H, Kalkan Y, Silan C et al (2015) Genistein exerts neuroprotective effect on focal cerebral ischemia injury in rats. Inflammation 38:1311–1321
5. Arcaro A, Wymann MP (1993) Wortmannin is a potent phosphatidylinositol 3-kinase inhibitor: the role of phosphatidylinositol 3,4,5-trisphosphate in neutrophil responses. Biochem J 296:279–301.
6. Atmaca A, Al-Batran S-E, Maurer A, Neumann A, Heinzel T, Hentsch B et al (2007) Valproic acid (VPA) in patients with refractory advanced cancer: a dose escalating phase I clinical trial. Br J Cancer 97:177–182
7. Bramlett HM, Dietrich WD, Green EJ, Busto R (1997) Chronic histopathological consequences of fluid-percussion brain injury in rats: effects of post-traumatic hypothermia. Acta Neuropathol 93:190–199
8. Brunn GJ, Williams J, Sabers C, Wiederrecht G, Lawrence JC, Abraham RT et al (1996) Direct inhibition of the signaling functions of the mammalian target of rapamycin by the phosphoinositide 3-kinase inhibitors, wortmannin and LY294002. EMBO J 15:5256–5267
9. Buffo A, Vosko MR, Ertürk D, Hamann GF, Jucker M, Rowitch D et al (2005) Expression pattern of the transcription factor Olig2 in response to brain injuries: implications for neuronal repair. Proc Natl Acad Sci U S A 102: 18183–18188
10. Capdevila J, Gil L, Orellana M, Marnett LJ, Mason JI, Yadagiri P et al (1988) Inhibitors of cytochrome P-450-dependent arachidonic acid metabolism. Arch Biochem Biophys 261:257–263

11. Castellino RC, De Bortoli M, Lin LL, Skapura DG, Rajan JA, Adesina AM et al (2007) Overexpressed TP73 induces apoptosis in medulloblastoma. BMC Cancer 7:127
12. Cheramy A, Besson MJ, Glowinski J (1970) Increased release of dopamine from striatal dopaminergic terminals in the rat after treatment with a neuroleptic: Thioproperazine. Eur J Pharmacol 10:206–214
13. Chiu C-C, Liao Y-E, Yang L-Y, Wang J-Y, Tweedie D, Karnati HK et al (2016) Neuroinflammation in animal models of traumatic brain injury. J Neurosci Methods 272:38–49
14. Colak T, Cine N, Bamac B, Kurtas O, Ozbek A, Bicer U et al (2012) Microarray-based gene expression analysis of an animal model for closed head injury. Injury 43:1264–1270
15. Corrigan JD, Selassie AW, Orman JAL (2010) The epidemiology of traumatic brain injury. J Head Trauma Rehabil 25:72–80
16. Crack PJ, Gould J, Bye N, Ross S, Ali U, Habgood MD et al (2009) The genomic profile of the cerebral cortex after closed head injury in mice: effects of minocycline. J Neural Transm 116:1–12
17. Crawford F, Wood M, Ferguson S, Mathura V, Gupta P, Humphrey J et al (2009) Apolipoprotein E-genotype dependent hippocampal and cortical responses to traumatic brain injury. Neuroscience 159:1349–1362
18. Dash PK, Orsi SA, Zhang M, Grill RJ, Pati S, Zhao J et al (2010) Valproate administered after traumatic brain injury provides neuroprotection and improves cognitive function in rats. PLoS One 5:e11383
19. De Jager PL, Srivastava G, Lunnon K, Burgess J, Schalkwyk LC, Yu L et al (2014) Alzheimer's disease: early alterations in brain DNA methylation at ANK1, BIN1, RHBDF2 and other loci. Nat Neurosci 17:1156–1163
20. Dębski KJ, Pitkanen A, Puhakka N, Bot AM, Khurana I, Harikrishnan KN et al (2016) Etiology matters - genomic DNA methylation patterns in three rat models of acquired epilepsy. Sci Rep 6:25668
21. Diamond M, Kelly JP, Connor TJ (2006) Antidepressants suppress production of the Th1 cytokine interferon-γ, independent of monoamine transporter blockade. Eur Neuropsychopharmacol 16:481–490
22. Diaz-Arrastia R, Kochanek PM, Bergold P, Kenney K, Marx CE, Grimes CJB et al (2014) Pharmacotherapy of traumatic brain injury: state of the science and the road forward: report of the Department of Defense Neurotrauma Pharmacology Workgroup. J Neurotrauma 31:135–158
23. Dixon RA, Ferreira D (2002) Genistein. Phytochemistry 60:205–211
24. Dobin A, Davis CA, Schlesinger F, Drenkow J, Zaleski C, Jha S et al (2013) STAR: ultrafast universal RNA-seq aligner. Bioinformatics 29:15–21
25. Dougall D, Poole N, Agrawal N (2015) Pharmacotherapy for chronic cognitive impairment in traumatic brain injury. Cochrane Database Syst Rev 12:CD009221
26. Edgar R, Domrachev M, Lash AE (2002) Gene expression omnibus: NCBI gene expression and hybridization array data repository. Nucleic Acids Res 30:207–210
27. Farrokhnia N, Ericsson A, Terént A, Lennmyr F (2008) MEK-inhibitor U0126 in hyperglycaemic focal ischaemic brain injury in the rat. Eur J Clin Investig 38:679–685
28. Faul M, Xu L, Wald MM, Coronado VG. Traumatic Brain Injury in the United States: Emergency Department Visits, Hospitalizations and Deaths 2002–2006. Atlanta (GA): Centers for Disease Control and Prevention, National Center for Injury Prevention and Control; 2010. https://www.cdc.gov/traumaticbraininjury/pdf/blue_book.pdf
29. Fava M, Kendler KS (2000) Major depressive disorder. Neuron 28:335–341
30. Favata MF, Horiuchi KY, Manos EJ, Daulerio AJ, Stradley DA, Feeser WS et al (1998) Identification of a novel inhibitor of mitogen-activated protein kinase kinase. J Biol Chem 273:18623–18632
31. Fazekas D, Koltai M, Türei D, Módos D, Pálfy M, Dúl Z et al (2013) SignaLink 2 – a signaling pathway resource with multi-layered regulatory networks. BMC Syst Biol 7:7
32. Figueroa-Romero C, Hur J, Bender DE, Delaney CE, Cataldo MD, Smith AL et al (2012) Identification of epigenetically altered genes in sporadic amyotrophic lateral sclerosis. Idong, editor. PLoS One 7:e52672
33. Fisher B, Costantino JP, Wickerham DL, Redmond CK, Kavanah M, Cronin WM et al (1998) Tamoxifen for prevention of breast cancer: report of the National Surgical Adjuvant Breast and Bowel Project P-1 Study. J Natl Cancer Inst 90:1371–1388
34. Frieling H, Bleich S (2006) Tranylcypromine. Eur Arch Psychiatry Clin Neurosci 256:268–273
35. Geng X, Li F, Yip J, Peng C, Elmadhoun O, Shen J et al (2017) Neuroprotection by chlorpromazine and promethazine in severe transient and permanent ischemic stroke. Mol Neurobiol 54:8140
36. Gentleman SM, Leclercq PD, Moyes L, Graham DI, Smith C, Griffin WST et al (2004) Long-term intracerebral inflammatory response after traumatic brain injury. Forensic Sci Int 146:97–104
37. Glaser T, Jepeal L, Edwards JG, Young SR, Favor J, Maas RL (1994) PAX6 gene dosage effect in a family with congenital cataracts, aniridia, anophthalmia and central nervous system defects. Nat Genet 7:463–471
38. Goodman JC, Cherian L, Robertson CS (2008) Cortical expression of prolactin (PRL), growth hormone (GH) and adrenocorticotrophic hormone (ACTH) is not increased in experimental traumatic brain injury. Acta Neurochir Suppl 102:389–390
39. Haghighi F, Ge Y, Chen S, Xin Y, Umali MU, De Gasperi R et al (2015) Neuronal DNA methylation profiling of blast-related traumatic brain injury. J Neurotrauma 32:1200–1209
40. Hämäläinen M, Lilja R, Kankaanranta H, Moilanen E (2008) Inhibition of iNOS expression and NO production by anti-inflammatory steroids. Pulm Pharmacol Ther 21:331–339
41. Han JW, Ahn SH, Park SH, Wang SY, Bae GU, Seo DW et al (2000) Apicidin, a histone deacetylase inhibitor, inhibits proliferation of tumor cells via induction of p21WAF1/Cip1 and gelsolin. Cancer Res 60:6068–6074
42. Hellmich HL, Rojo DR, Micci M-A, Sell SL, Boone DR, Crookshanks JM et al (2013) Pathway analysis reveals common pro-survival mechanisms of metyrapone and carbenoxolone after traumatic brain injury. PLoS One 8:e53230
43. Hong SL, Carty T, Deykin D (1980) Tranylcypromine and 15-hydroperoxyarachidonate affect arachidonic acid release in addition to inhibition of prostacyclin synthesis in calf aortic endothelial cells. J Biol Chem 255:9538–9540
44. Huang W, Chen Y, Shohami E, Weinstock M (1999) Neuroprotective effect of rasagiline, a selective monoamine oxidase-B inhibitor, against closed head injury in the mouse. Eur J Pharmacol 366:127–135
45. Im JY, Park H, Kang KW, Choi WS, Kim HS (2008) Modulation of cell cycles and apoptosis by apicidin in estrogen receptor (ER)-positive and-negative human breast cancer cells. Chem Biol Interact 172:235–244
46. Immonen RJ, Kharatishvili I, Niskanen JP, Gröhn H, Pitkänen A, Gröhn OHJ (2009) Distinct MRI pattern in lesional and perilesional area after traumatic brain injury in rat - 11 months follow-up. Exp Neurol 215:29–40
47. Ishikawa Y, Uchino H, Morota S, Li C, Takahashi T, Ikeda Y et al (2006) Search for novel gene markers of traumatic brain injury by time differential microarray analysis. Acta Neurochir Suppl 96:163–167
48. Israelsson C, Bengtsson H, Kylberg A, Kullander K, Lewén A, Hillered L et al (2008) Distinct cellular patterns of upregulated chemokine expression supportingok a prominent inflammatory role in traumatic brain injury. J Neurotrauma 25:959–974
49. Johnson V.E., Stewart W., Arena J.D., Smith D.H. (2017) Traumatic Brain Injury as a Trigger of Neurodegeneration. In: Beart P., Robinson M., Rattray M., Maragakis N, editors. Neurodegenerative Diseases. Advances in Neurobiology, vol 15. Springer, Cham. https://link.springer.com/chapter/10.1007/978-3-319-57193-5_15#citeas
50. Jost CA, Marin MC, Kaelin WG (1997) p73 is a human p53-related protein that can induce apoptosis. Nature 389:191–194
51. Jowaed A, Schmitt I, Kaut O, Wullner U (2010) Methylation regulates alpha-Synuclein expression and is decreased in Parkinson's disease patients' brains. J Neurosci 30:6355–6359
52. Kang Y-J, Chung H-J, Nam J-W, Park HJ, Seo EK, Kim YS et al (2011) Cytotoxic and antineoplastic activity of timosaponin A-III for human colon cancer cells. J Nat Prod 74:701–706
53. Kato H, Araki T, Itoyama Y, Kogure K (1995) Rolipram, a cyclic AMP-selective phosphodiesterase inhibitor, reduces neuronal damage following cerebral ischemia in the gerbil. Eur J Pharmacol 272:107–110
54. Kharatishvili I, Nissinen JP, Intosh TKMC, McIntosh TK, Pitkänen A (2006) A model of posttraumatic epilepsy induced by lateral fluid-percussion brain injury in rats. Neuroscience 140:685–697
55. Kim HJ, Rowe M, Ren M, Hong J-S, Chen P-S, Chuang D-M (2007) Histone deacetylase inhibitors exhibit anti-inflammatory and neuroprotective effects in a rat permanent ischemic model of stroke: multiple mechanisms of action. J Pharmacol Exp Ther 321:892–901
56. Kim K, Kong S-Y, Fulciniti M, Li X, Song W, Nahar S et al (2010) Blockade of the MEK/ERK signalling cascade by AS703026, a novel selective MEK1/2 inhibitor, induces pleiotropic anti-myeloma activity in vitro and in vivo. Br J Haematol 149:537–549

57. Kinoshita S, Akira S, Kishimoto T (1992) A member of the C/EBP family, NF-IL6 beta, forms a heterodimer and transcriptionally synergizes with NF-IL6. Proc Natl Acad Sci U S A 89:1473–1476
58. Kline AE, Yan HQ, Bao J, Marion DW, Dixon CE (2000) Chronic methylphenidate treatment enhances water maze performance following traumatic brain injury in rats. Neurosci Lett 280:163–166
59. Kobori N, Clifton GL, Dash P (2002) Altered expression of novel genes in the cerebral cortex following experimental brain injury. Brain Res Mol Brain Res 104:148–158
60. Korcsmáros T, Farkas IJ, Szalay MS, Rovó P, Fazekas D, Spiró Z et al (2010) Uniformly curated signaling pathways reveal tissue-specific cross-talks and support drug target discovery. Bioinformatics 26:2042–2050
61. Koshinaga M, Katayama Y, Fukushima M, Oshima H, Suma T, Takahata T (2000) Rapid and widespread microglial activation induced by traumatic brain injury in rat brain slices. J Neurotrauma 17:185–192
62. Kraft P, Schwarz T, Göb E, Heydenreich N, Brede M, Meuth SG et al (2013) The phosphodiesterase-4 inhibitor rolipram protects from ischemic stroke in mice by reducing blood–brain-barrier damage, inflammation and thrombosis. Exp Neurol 247:80–90
63. Kukacka J, Vajtr D, Huska D, Prusa R, Houstava L, Samal F et al (2006) Blood metallothionein, neuron specific enolase, and protein S100B in patients with traumatic brain injury. Neuro Endocrinol Lett 27(Suppl 2):116–120
64. Laing AJ, Dillon JP, Condon ET, Street JT, Wang JH, McGuinness AJ et al (2007) Mobilization of endothelial precursor cells: systemic vascular response to musculoskeletal trauma. J Orthop Res 25:44–50
65. Langlois JA, Rutland-Brown W, Wald MM (2006) The epidemiology and impact of traumatic brain injury: a brief overview. J Head Trauma Rehabil 21:375–378
66. Lee AF, Ho DK, Zanassi P, Walsh GS, Kaplan DR, Miller FD (2004) Evidence that Np73 promotes neuronal survival by p53-dependent and p53-independent mechanisms. J Neurosci 24:9174–9184
67. Lee B, Jung K, Kim D-H (2009) Timosaponin AIII, a saponin isolated from Anemarrhena asphodeloides, ameliorates learning and memory deficits in mice. Pharmacol Biochem Behav 93:121–127
68. Li H-J, Zhang Y-J, Zhou L, Han F, Wang M-Y, Xue M-Q et al (2014) Chlorpromazine confers neuroprotection against brain ischemia by activating BKCa channel. Eur J Pharmacol 735:38–43
69. Lipponen A, Paananen J, Puhakka N, Pitkänen A (2016) Analysis of post-traumatic brain injury gene expression signature reveals tubulins, Nfe2l2, Nfkb, Cd44, and S100a4 as treatment targets. Sci Rep 6:31570
70. Logan TT, Villapol S, Symes AJ, Kaltschmidt C, Kaltschmidt B (2013) TGF-β superfamily gene expression and induction of the Runx1 transcription factor in adult neurogenic regions after brain injury. Zheng JC, editor. PLoS One 8: e59250
71. Lopez-Rodriguez AB, Mela V, Acaz-Fonseca E, Garcia-Segura LM, Viveros M-P (2016) CB2 cannabinoid receptor is involved in the anti-inflammatory effects of leptin in a model of traumatic brain injury. Exp Neurol 279:274–282
72. Love MI, Huber W, Anders S (2014) Moderated estimation of fold change and dispersion for RNA-seq data with DESeq2. Genome Biol 15:550
73. Lu K, Cho C-L, Liang C-L, Chen S-D, Liliang P-C, Wang S-Y et al (2007) Inhibition of the MEK/ERK pathway reduces microglial activation and interleukin-1-beta expression in spinal cord ischemia/reperfusion injury in rats. J Thorac Cardiovasc Surg 133:934–941
74. Maas AIR, Menon DK, Steyerberg EW, Citerio G, Lecky F, Manley GT et al (2015) Collaborative European NeuroTrauma Effectiveness Research in Traumatic Brain Injury (CENTER-TBI): a prospective longitudinal observational study. Neurosurgery 76:67–80
75. Madathil SK and Saatman KE. IGF-1/IGF-R Signaling in Traumatic Brain Injury. In Kobeissy FH, editor. Brain Neurotrauma: Molecular, Neuropsychological, and Rehabilitation Aspects. Boca Raton (FL); CRC Press/Taylor & Francis; 2015. https://www.ncbi.nlm.nih.gov/books/NBK299190/
76. Marklund N, Bakshi A, Castelbuono DJ, Conte V, McIntosh TK (2006) Evaluation of pharmacological treatment strategies in traumatic brain injury. Curr Pharm Des 12:1645–1680
77. Marks PA, Breslow R (2007) Dimethyl sulfoxide to vorinostat: development of this histone deacetylase inhibitor as an anticancer drug. Nat Biotechnol 25:84–90
78. Matzilevich DA, Rall JM, Moore AN, Grill RJ, Dash PK (2002) High-density microarray analysis of hippocampal gene expression following experimental brain injury. J Neurosci Res 67:646–663
79. McDonald SJ, Sun M, Agoston DV, Shultz SR (2016) The effect of concomitant peripheral injury on traumatic brain injury pathobiology and outcome. J Neuroinflammation 13:90
80. McGinn MJ and Povlishock JT. Cellular and molecular mechanisms of injury and spontaneous recovery. In: Grafman J and Salazar AM, editors. Handbook of Clinical Neurology. Elsevier; 2015. p. 67-87. https://doi.org/10.1016/B978-0-444-52892-6.00005-2
81. McIntosh TK, Vink R, Noble L, Yamakami I, Fernyak S, Soares H et al (1989) Traumatic brain injury in the rat: characterization of a lateral fluid-percussion model. Neuroscience 28:233–244
82. McKercher SR, Torbett BE, Anderson KL, Henkel GW, Vestal DJ, Baribault H et al (1996) Targeted disruption of the PU.1 gene results in multiple hematopoietic abnormalities. EMBO J 15:5647–5658
83. Meng Q, Zhuang Y, Ying Z, Agrawal R, Yang X, Gomez-Pinilla F (2017) Traumatic brain injury induces genome-wide transcriptomic, Methylomic, and network perturbations in brain and blood predicting neurological disorders. EBioMedicine 16:184–194
84. Merritt JE, Armstrong WP, Benham CD, Hallam TJ, Jacob R, Jaxa-Chamiec A et al (1990) SK&F 96365, a novel inhibitor of receptor-mediated calcium entry. Biochem J 271:515–522
85. Michael DB, Byers DM, Irwin LN (2005) Gene expression following traumatic brain injury in humans: analysis by microarray. J Clin Neurosci 12:284–290
86. Moll UM, Erster S, Zaika A (2001) p53, p63 and p73 – solos, alliances and feuds among family members. Biochim Biophys Acta - Rev Cancer 1552:47–59
87. Mori T, Wang X, Aoki T, Lo EH (2002) Downregulation of matrix Metalloproteinase-9 and attenuation of edema via inhibition of ERK mitogen activated protein kinase in traumatic brain injury. J Neurotrauma 19:1411–1419
88. Nakatomi H, Kuriu T, Okabe S, Yamamoto S, Hatano O, Kawahara N et al (2002) Regeneration of hippocampal pyramidal neurons after ischemic brain injury by recruitment of endogenous neural progenitors. Cell 110:429–441
89. Offertáler L, Mo F-M, Bátkai S, Liu J, Begg M, Razdan RK et al. (2003) Selective ligands and cellular effectors of a G protein-coupled endothelial cannabinoid receptor. Mol Pharmacol 63:699–705.
90. Peña-Llopis S, Brugarolas J (2013) Simultaneous isolation of high-quality DNA, RNA, miRNA and proteins from tissues for genomic applications. Nat Protoc 8:2240–2255
91. Pierce JE, Smith DH, Trojanowski JQ, McIntosh TK (1998) Enduring cognitive, neurobehavioral and histopathological changes persist for up to one year following severe experimental brain injury in rats. Neuroscience 87:359–369
92. Pitkänen A, Immonen R (2014) Epilepsy related to traumatic brain injury. Neurotherapeutics 11:286–296
93. Polkowski K, Mazurek AP (2000) Biological properties of genistein. A review of in vitro and in vivo data. Acta Pol Pharm - Drug Res 57:135–155
94. Pozniak CD, Barnabé-Heider F, Rymar VV, Lee AF, Sadikot AF, Miller FD (2002) p73 is required for survival and maintenance of CNS neurons. J Neurosci 22:9800–9809
95. Pozniak CD, Radinovic S, Yang A, McKeon F, Kaplan DR, Miller FD (2000) An anti-apoptotic role for the p53 family member, p73, during developmental neuron death. Science 289:304–306
96. Puche JE, Muñoz Ú, García-Magariño M, Sádaba MC, Castilla-Cortázar I (2016) Partial IGF-1 deficiency induces brain oxidative damage and edema, which are ameliorated by replacement therapy. Biofactors 42:60–79
97. Rall JM, Matzilevich DA, Dash PK (2003) Comparative analysis of mRNA levels in the frontal cortex and the hippocampus in the basal state and in response to experimental brain injury. Neuropathol Appl Neurobiol 29:118–131
98. Ramlackhansingh AF, Brooks DJ, Greenwood RJ, Bose SK, Turkheimer FE, Kinnunen KM et al (2011) Inflammation after trauma: microglial activation and traumatic brain injury. Ann Neurol 70:374–383
99. Risling M, Plantman S, Angeria M, Rostami E, Bellander B-M, Kirkegaard M et al (2011) Mechanisms of blast induced brain injuries, experimental studies in rats. NeuroImage 54(Suppl 1):S89–S97
100. Rosa A, Ballarino M, Sorrentino A, Sthandier O, De Angelis FG, Marchioni M et al (2007) The interplay between the master transcription factor PU.1 and miR-424 regulates human monocyte/macrophage differentiation. Proc Natl Acad Sci U S A 104:19849–19854
101. Roy SK, Wachira SJ, Weihua X, Hu J, Kalvakolanu DV (2000) CCAAT/enhancer-binding protein-beta regulates interferon-induced transcription through a novel element. J Biol Chem 275:12626–12632

102. Sagarkar S, Bhamburkar T, Shelkar G, Choudhary A, Kokare DM, Sakharkar AJ (2017) Minimal traumatic brain injury causes persistent changes in DNA methylation at BDNF gene promoters in rat amygdala: a possible role in anxiety-like behaviors. Neurobiol Dis 106:101–109
103. Salzmann MM (1965) A controlled trial with trimipramine, a new anti-depressant drug. Br J Psychiatry 111:1105–1106
104. Samal BB, Waites CK, Almeida-Suhett C, Li Z, Marini AM, Samal NR et al (2015) Acute response of the hippocampal transcriptome following mild traumatic brain injury after controlled cortical impact in the rat. J Mol Neurosci 57:282–303
105. Sandhir R, Berman NEJ (2010) Age-dependent response of CCAAT/enhancer binding proteins following traumatic brain injury in mice. Neurochem Int 56:188–193
106. Schober ME, Ke X, Xing B, Block BP, Requena DF, McKnight R et al (2012) Traumatic brain injury increased IGF-1B mRNA and altered IGF-1 exon 5 and promoter region epigenetic characteristics in the rat pup hippocampus. J Neurotrauma 29:2075–2085
107. Scholar EM. xPharm: The Comprehensive Pharmacology Reference. Elsevier Inc. 2015. https://doi.org/10.1016/B978-008055232-3.62712-6. https://www.sciencedirect.com/science/article/pii/B9780080552323627126
108. Shannon P, Markiel A, Ozier O, Baliga NS, Wang JT, Ramage D et al (2003) Cytoscape: a software environment for integrated models of biomolecular interaction networks. Genome Res 13:2498–2504
109. Shin SS, Bray ER, Zhang CQ, Dixon CE (2011) Traumatic brain injury reduces striatal tyrosine hydroxylase activity and potassium-evoked dopamine release in rats. Brain Res 1369:208–215
110. Simon DW, McGeachy MJ, Bayır H, Clark RSB, Loane DJ, Kochanek PM (2017) The far-reaching scope of neuroinflammation after traumatic brain injury. Nat Rev Neurol 13:171–191
111. Smith AM, Gibbons HM, Oldfield RL, Bergin PM, Mee EW, Faull RLM et al (2013) The transcription factor PU.1 is critical for viability and function of human brain microglia. Glia 61:929–942
112. Smith DH, Chen XH, Pierce JE, Wolf J a, Trojanowski JQ, Graham DI et al (1997) Progressive atrophy and neuron death for one year following brain trauma in the rat. J Neurotrauma 14:715–727
113. Soltani Z, Khaksari M, Jafari E, Iranpour M, Shahrokhi N (2015) Is genistein neuroprotective in traumatic brain injury? Physiol Behav 152:26–31
114. Sommer N, Löschmann PA, Northoff GH, Weller M, Steinbrecher A, Steinbach JP et al (1995) The antidepressant rolipram suppresses cytokine production and prevents autoimmune encephalomyelitis. Nat Med 1:244–248
115. Statham AL, Strbenac D, Coolen MW, Stirzaker C, Clark SJ, Robinson MD (2010) Repitools: an R package for the analysis of enrichment-based epigenomic data. Bioinformatics 26:1662–1663
116. Subramanian A, Tamayo P, Mootha VK, Mukherjee S, Ebert BL, Gillette MA et al (2005) Gene set enrichment analysis: a knowledge-based approach for interpreting genome-wide expression profiles. Proc Natl Acad Sci U S A 102: 15545–15550
117. Sukumari-Ramesh S, Alleyne CH, Dhandapani KM (2016) The histone deacetylase inhibitor Suberoylanilide Hydroxamic acid (SAHA) confers acute neuroprotection after intracerebral hemorrhage in mice. Transl Stroke Res 7:141–148
118. Sy L-K, Yan S-C, Lok C-N, Man RYK, Che C-M (2008) Timosaponin A-III induces autophagy preceding mitochondria-mediated apoptosis in HeLa cancer cells. Cancer Res 68:10229–10237
119. Thomas MG, Welch C, Stone L, Allan P, Barker RA, White RB (2016) PAX6 expression may be protective against dopaminergic cell loss in Parkinson's disease. CNS Neurol Disord Drug Targets 15:73–79
120. Tien L-T, Lee Y-J, Pang Y, Lu S, Lee JW, Tseng C-H et al (2017) Neuroprotective effects of intranasal IGF-1 against neonatal lipopolysaccharide-induced neurobehavioral deficits and neuronal inflammation in the substantia Nigra and locus Coeruleus of juvenile rats. Dev Neurosci 39:443-459
121. Tsai Y-T, Wang C-C, Leung P-O, Lin K-C, Chio C-C, Hu C-Y et al (2014) Extracellular signal-regulated kinase 1/2 is involved in a tamoxifen neuroprotective effect in a lateral fluid percussion injury rat model. J Surg Res 189:106–116
122. Valiyaveettil M, Alamneh YA, Miller S-A, Hammamieh R, Arun P, Wang Y et al (2013) Modulation of cholinergic pathways and inflammatory mediators in blast-induced traumatic brain injury. Chem Biol Interact 203:371–375
123. von Gertten C, Flores Morales A, Holmin S, Mathiesen T, Nordqvist A-CS (2005) Genomic responses in rat cerebral cortex after traumatic brain injury. BMC Neurosci 6:69
124. von Gertten C, Morales A, Holmin S, Mathiesen T, Nordqvist A-C, Ray S et al (2005) Genomic responses in rat cerebral cortex after traumatic brain injury. BMC Neurosci 6:69
125. Vonder Haar C, Anderson GD, Elmore BE, Moore LH, Wright AM, Kantor ED et al (2014) Comparison of the effect of minocycline and simvastatin on functional recovery and gene expression in a rat traumatic brain injury model. J Neurotrauma 31:961–975
126. Walton MR, Gibbons H, MacGibbon GA, Sirimanne E, Saura J, Gluckman PD et al (2000) PU.1 expression in microglia. J. Neuroimmunol 104:109–115
127. Wang L, Fu X, Peng X, Xiao Z, Li Z, Chen G et al (2016) DNA methylation profiling reveals correlation of differential methylation patterns with gene expression in human epilepsy. J Mol Neurosci 59:68–77
128. White TE, Ford GD, Surles-Zeigler MC, Gates AS, Laplaca MC, Ford BD (2013) Gene expression patterns following unilateral traumatic brain injury reveals a local pro-inflammatory and remote anti-inflammatory response. BMC Genomics 14:282
129. White TE, Surles-Zeigler MC, Ford GD, Gates AS, Davids B, Distel T et al (2016) Bilateral gene interaction hierarchy analysis of the cell death gene response emphasizes the significance of cell cycle genes following unilateral traumatic brain injury. BMC Genomics 17:130
130. Wong Y-H, Wu C-C, Wu JC-C, Lai H-Y, Chen K-Y, Jheng B-R et al. (2016) Temporal genetic modifications after controlled cortical impact-understanding traumatic brain injury through a systematic network approach. Int J Mol Sci 17:216.
131. Wu J, Song R, Song W, Li Y, Zhang Q, Chen Y et al (2011) Chlorpromazine protects against apoptosis induced by exogenous stimuli in the developing rat brain. Burne T, editor. PLoS One 6:e21966
132. Xuan A, Long D, Li J, Ji W, Hong L, Zhang M et al (2012) Neuroprotective effects of valproic acid following transient global ischemia in rats. Life Sci 90:463–468
133. Yang K, Mu XS, Xue JJ, Whitson J, Salminen A, Dixon CE et al (1994) Increased expression of c-fos mRNA and AP-1 transcription factors after cortical impact injury in rats. Brain Res 664:141–147
134. Yoneda T, Lyall RM, Alsina MM, Persons PE, Spada AP, Levitzki A et al. (1991) The Antiproliferative effects of tyrosine kinase inhibitors Tyrphostins on a human squamous cell carcinoma in vitro and in nude mice. Cancer Res 51: 4430–4435.
135. Zakrzeska A, Schlicker E, Baranowska M, Kozłowska H, Kwolek G, Malinowska B (2010) A cannabinoid receptor, sensitive to O-1918, is involved in the delayed hypotension induced by anandamide in anaesthetized rats. Br J Pharmacol 160:574–584
136. Zhang X-Y, Gu C-G, Gu J-W, Zhang J-H, Zhu H, Zhang Y-C et al (2014) Analysis of key genes and modules during the courses of traumatic brain injury with microarray technology. Genet Mol Res Brazil 13:9220–9228

16

# Rapid and ultra-sensitive quantitation of disease-associated α-synuclein seeds in brain and cerebrospinal fluid by αSyn RT-QuIC

Bradley R. Groveman[1†], Christina D. Orrù[1†], Andrew G. Hughson[1], Lynne D. Raymond[1], Gianluigi Zanusso[2], Bernardino Ghetti[3], Katrina J. Campbell[1], Jiri Safar[4], Douglas Galasko[5*] and Byron Caughey[1*]

**Abstract**

The diagnosis and treatment of synucleinopathies such as Parkinson disease and dementia with Lewy bodies would be aided by the availability of assays for the pathogenic disease-associated forms of α-synuclein (αSyn$^D$) that are sufficiently sensitive, specific, and practical for analysis of accessible diagnostic specimens. Two recent αSyn$^D$ seed amplification tests have provided the first prototypes for ultrasensitive and specific detection of αSyn$^D$ in patients' cerebrospinal fluid. These prototypic assays require 5–13 days to perform. Here, we describe an improved α-synuclein real time quaking-induced conversion (αSyn RT-QuIC) assay that has similar sensitivity and specificity to the prior assays, but can be performed in 1–2 days with quantitation. Blinded analysis of cerebrospinal fluid from 29 synucleinopathy cases [12 Parkinson's and 17 dementia with Lewy bodies] and 31 non-synucleinopathy controls, including 16 Alzheimer's cases, yielded 93% diagnostic sensitivity and 100% specificity for this test so far. End-point dilution analyses allowed quantitation of relative amounts of αSyn$^D$ seeding activity in cerebrospinal fluid samples, and detection in as little as 0.2 μL. These results confirm that αSyn$^D$ seeding activity is present in cerebrospinal fluid. We also demonstrate that it can be rapidly detected, and quantitated, even in early symptomatic stages of synucleinopathy.

**Keywords:** Parkinson, Lewy body, Alzheimer, Diagnosis, Synuclein, Amplification, Cerebrospinal fluid, PMCA, RT-QuIC, Prion

## Introduction

Many neurodegenerative diseases are related to the accumulation of specific misfolded proteins. These deposits are identified upon *post-mortem* analysis of brain tissue, allowing definite diagnoses to be made based on specific neuropathological and molecular findings. Less definitive *intra vitam* diagnoses can be proffered based on specific clinical signs, tissue imaging data, pathological examination of peripheral biopsies, and less-than-specific biomarker levels in the CSF. In particular, early diagnosis can be difficult and discrimination between diseases can be complicated by clinical variability and overlaps in clinical features.

Parkinson's disease (PD), multiple system atrophy (MSA), dementia with Lewy bodies (DLB) [or Lewy body dementia] are called α-synucleinopathies due to the abnormal accumulation of aggregates of a protein called α-synuclein (αSyn) in the brain. Although the clinical diagnosis of parkinsonism can be relatively simple, the specific diagnosis of PD, especially at early stages, can be difficult. Adler et al. noted that in patients with possible PD (never treated or not clearly responsive to L-dopa) only 26% had autopsy confirmation as PD, while in probable PD (responsive to medications) the diagnostic accuracy was 82% [1]. In DLB, clinical diagnostic criteria for probable DLB predict αSyn pathology with sensitivity of about 80% [18] but early diagnosis of DLB is less accurate due to the overlapping symptoms with other types of dementia. In addition, in 15–20% of patients with Alzheimer disease (AD) at autopsy,

* Correspondence: dgalasko@ucsd.edu; bcaughey@nih.gov
†Equal contributors
[5]Department of Neurosciences, University of California-San Diego, La Jolla, CA, USA
[1]Laboratory of Persistent Viral Diseases, Rocky Mountain Laboratories, National Institute of Allergy and Infectious Diseases, National Institutes of Health, Hamilton, MT, USA
Full list of author information is available at the end of the article

concomitant DLB pathology can be found, with only a minority of patients having exhibited clear diagnostic features of DLB [20, 34]. However, in patients with AD and diffuse Lewy body pathology, disease duration was shortened [11], indicating that DLB pathology contributes to dementia progression.

Some pertinent tests indirectly measure the effect of α-Syn pathology (e.g., dopamine receptor SPECT or PET scans, and MIBG cardiac scintigraphy), while the sensitivity and specificity of skin, salivary gland and colonic biopsy for PD or DLB has not been established in large scale studies. In these clinical settings of PD and DLB, the presence of a biomarker that indicates that abnormal pathological forms of a αSyn are present would improve diagnostic accuracy not only for prognostic purposes but also for cohort selection in disease-modifying clinical trials for PD. Attempts to determine if cerebrospinal fluid (CSF) levels of total, phosphorylated or oligomeric a-syn are diagnostically useful have been variable and controversial between studies [reviewed in [27]], and the diagnostic utility of immunoassays for these forms of αSyn in CSF remains unclear [21, 31].

However, two recent studies have provided evidence that analysis of a distinct feature of disease-associated forms of αSyn (hereafter abbreviated $\alpha Syn^D$), namely their amyloid seeding activity, may have substantial diagnostic utility for PD and DLB [7, 35]. The rationale for the seeding activity assays is that the $\alpha Syn^D$ deposits contain fibrils, or subfibrillar oligomers, that propagate by a seeded polymerization mechanism in which $\alpha Syn^D$ templates, or seeds, conversion of non-fibrillar αSyn into larger oligomeric or aggregate, fibrillar forms. Mechanistically similar assays called Real-Time Quaking-Induced Conversion (RT-QuIC) have provided ultrasensitive, specific and quantitative diagnostic tests for prion diseases [2, 39]. RT-QuIC assays are multi-well plate-based reactions that can rapidly amplify oligomeric/multimeric prion seeds by as much as a trillion-fold [8, 24, 26, 39]. Prion RT-QuIC assays have been applied successfully to a variety of biological samples including brain [29, 39, 41], cerebrospinal fluid (CSF) [2, 5, 17, 24, 33], whole blood, plasma [26, 38], urine [14], and nasal brushings [23, 40]. They are being widely implemented for the diagnosis of prion diseases in humans and animals. Notably, our recent studies demonstrated provisional 100% diagnostic sensitivity and specificity in diagnosing human sporadic Creutzfeldt-Jakob disease using CSF and/or nasal swabs [4].

Green and colleagues adapted the RT-QuIC approach to synucleinopathies and applied it to a total of 137 PD and DLB cases and controls [7]. Their assay (αSyn RT-QuIC) has given 95 and 92% sensitivity for PD and DLB patients, respectively, with 100% specificity. Soto and colleagues developed a similar assay called αSyn protein misfolding cyclic amplification (αSyn-PMCA) which gave 89% sensitivity for PD and 97% specificity in analyses of 173 total cases and controls [35]. In these assays, 5–40 μl aliquots of CSF are added to reactions containing recombinant αSyn (rαSyn). Any $\alpha Syn^D$ seeds in the sample initiate amyloid fibril formation by the recombinant αSyn which, in turn, enhances the fluorescence of thioflavin T (ThT). The reactions are performed over ~ 5 [7] to 13 days [35]. Sano and colleagues have described an αSyn RT-QuIC assay that detects DLB $\alpha Syn^D$ seeding activity in brain tissue at extreme dilutions in < 4 days [32]. Bernis and colleagues showed that 10% brain homogenate samples from mice inoculated with human MSA or incidental Lewy body disease brain tissue could seed fibrillization of rαSyn in 1–2 days [3]. Here we report that by using a mutant rαSyn substrate and optimized reaction conditions, αSyn RT-QuIC assays on CSF specimens can be completed within 1–2 days with high diagnostic sensitivity and specificity.

## Materials and methods

### Clinical assessment

All subjects provided consent to clinical assessment, including longitudinal follow-up, and to lumbar puncture to obtain CSF, under UCSD IRB-approved protocol #080012. All procedures performed in this study were in accordance with the 1964 Helsinki declaration and its later amendments or comparable ethical standards. Some subjects died during the follow-up period, and had consented to their brains being obtained at autopsy.

All subjects underwent a detailed clinical research assessment, including review of outside medical records, history of cognitive and motor symptoms, mental state examination with the Mini-Mental State Exam or Montreal Cognitive Assessment, and detailed neuropsychological testing, structured physical neurological examination, including the Unified Parkinson's Disease Rating Scale (UPDRS) Part III motor examination. All subjects were enrolled in a research protocol that allowed annual follow-up reassessment and received at least one follow-up assessment after their baseline visit. Neuroimaging (MRI and in some instances FDG PET scan or DaTscan) results were reviewed when available. The research diagnoses were made by consensus of two neurologists who reviewed all of the available clinical information. Research diagnoses followed published criteria: controls had no history of major neurological or psychiatric illness and were normal on cognition and neurological examination; patients with AD met criteria for probable AD (NIA-AA 2011). For PD, criteria proposed by the Movement Disorder Society were used [30], and research guidelines were applied to diagnose PD-MCI [16], PD-dementia and DLB (possible and probable DLB were diagnosed according to McKeith [19]).

### Lumbar puncture and CSF handling

Lumbar punctures (LPs) were performed in the early morning, after a fast of at least 8 h. Subjects were either sitting or lying, and LPs were performed with sterile technique using an atraumatic needle. CSF (15–20 mL) was withdrawn into a polypropylene tube and a sample was sent for analysis of cell count, total protein and glucose to a local laboratory. The remaining CSF was gently mixed, centrifuged at 1500 g for 10 min, then aliquotted in 500 μL fractions into polypropylene cryotubes, flash frozen and stored at − 80 °C.

### Autopsy brain analysis

Procedures at autopsy at the UCSD Alzheimer's Disease Research Center are as follows: the brain is divided sagittally and the left hemibrain is fixed in 10% buffered formalin while the right hemibrain is sectioned coronally and then frozen at − 70 °C in sealed plastic bags. Routinely, tissue blocks from the right hemibrain of the midfrontal, inferior parietal, and superior temporal cortices, primary visual cortex in the occipital cortex, hippocampus, basal ganglia, substantia nigra and cerebellum are removed and placed in 2% paraformaldehyde for subsequent thick sectioning by vibratome. Tissue blocks adjacent to the ones described above are stored at − 70 ° C for subsequent immunoblot analysis for synaptic proteins and Aβ species (soluble and oligomers). Vibratome sections (40 μm thick) are stored in cryoprotective medium at − 20 °C for subsequent immunochemical studies. The formalin-fixed left hemibrain is serially sectioned in 1 cm slices and tissue blocks from the regions described above are processed for histopathological examination by H&E, and Thioflavin-S (Thio-S) to detect tau and β-amyloid deposits. Lewy body pathology is evaluated using phosphorylated α-synuclein immunoreactivity with a mouse monoclonal antibody at 1:20,000 (BioLegend Cat# 825701 RRID:AB 2564891). Pathological diagnoses of AD and DLB are made using National Institute on Aging-Alzheimer's Association (NIA-AA) guidelines [22].

### K23Q rαSyn expression vector preparation

DNA sequences coding for human α-synuclein sequence (Accession No. NM_000345.3) amino acid residues 1–140 (wildtype) were amplified and ligated into the pET24 vector with an N-terminal His-tag (EMD Biosciences) and sequences were confirmed. The α-synuclein K23Q mutation [15] was engineered using Q5 Site-Directed Mutagenesis (NEB) using the primers CCACACCCTGTTGGGTTTTCTCAG and CAGAAGCAGCAGGAAAGAC. The plasmids were transformed into BL21(DE3) *Escherichia coli* (EMD Biosciences).

### *rαSyn protein purification*

Five ml of LB media containing 50 μg/mL kanamycin were inoculated from a glycerol stock of *E. coli* bacteria containing vectors either for wildtype (WT) or K23Q rαSyn protein expression. Following 4–5-h incubation with continuous 225 rpm agitation at 37 °C, 1 L of the autoinduction media [9] also containing 50 μg/mL kanamycin was prepared and the 5 mL starter culture was added. The cells were grown in a shaking incubator at 37 °C, 225 rpm, overnight. The next day cells were harvested by splitting the 1 L culture into four 250 ml conical tubes and centrifuging at 3273×*g*, 4 °C, 10 min.

Cells were lysed using an osmotic shock protocol modified from Paslawski et al. [28]. Using a 25 mL serological pipette, the cell pellets were gently resuspended in 10% volume of room temperature osmotic shock buffer, (25 mL per 250 mL of cell culture before centrifugation) and incubated at room temperature for 10 min. The suspension was centrifuged at 9000×g, 20 °C, 20 min. The supernatant was discarded and the pellet was gently resuspended in 10 mL of ice-cold water per pellet, using a 25 mL serological pipette. The cell suspensions were pooled into two 50 mL tubes to 20 ml each. 20 μL of saturated $MgCl_2$ was added to each 20 mL suspension. The suspension was then mixed and incubated on ice with mild rocking for 3 min. Next, the suspension was centrifuged at 9000×*g*, 4 °C, 30 min. The supernatant was collected in a 100 ml glass beaker that contained a stir bar for rapid continuous mixing while being careful not to incorporate air bubbles. The pH was reduced to pH 3.5 by adding a bolus of ~ 800 μl 1 M HCl followed by additional 25 μl increments as necessary while continuously monitoring the pH. A large amount of white precipitate was generated. The suspension was then incubated with gentle stirring at room temperature for 10 min, avoiding the formation of air bubbles. The tubes were centrifuged at 9000×g, 4 °C, 30 min, and the supernatant was collected in a fresh 100 ml beaker using continuous agitation with a stir bar. The pH was adjusted to 7.5 with an ~ 800 μl bolus of 1 M NaOH followed by 25 μl increments as necessary. The protein extract was then filtered through a 0.45 μm filter. Next, the extract was loaded onto a 5 ml Ni-NTA column (Qiagen) on an Äkta Pure chromatography system (GE) and washed with 20 mM Tris, pH 7.5 at room temperature. The column was further washed with 50 mM imidazole, 20 mM Tris, pH 7.5 which generated a peak that was not collected. A linear gradient up to 500 mM imidazole in 20 mM Tris, pH 7.5, was performed and a peak was collected between 150 and 375 mM imidazole (Additional file 1). This peak was then loaded onto a Q-HP column (GE) and washed with 20 mM Tris, pH 7.5. The column was further washed with 100 mM NaCl, 20 mM Tris, pH 7.5. A linear gradient up to 500 mM NaCl in 20 mM Tris pH 7.5 was performed and a peak was recovered between 300 and 350 mM NaCl. The protein was filtered through a 0.22 μm filter and dialyzed against water overnight at 4 °C using a 3 kDa MWCO dialysis membrane. The next day, the protein was moved into fresh water for another 4 h dialysis. The protein concentration was determined with a UV–VIS spectrophotometer using a theoretical extinction coefficient at 280 nm of 0.36 $(mg/mL)^{-1}$ $cm^{-1}$. The protein was lyophilized in aliquots and stored for a final concentration of ~ 1.0 mg/ml once resuspended in 500 μL of 40 mM phosphate buffer (pH 8.0). These aliquots were stored at − 80 °C until further use.

For comparative studies, human recombinant full-length (1–140 aa) WT αSyn was also purchased from Stratech, (Cambridge, UK).

Endotoxin concentration levels for rαSyn protein purifications was determined using a ToxinSensor Endotoxin Detection kit (GenScript) according to manufacturer's protocol.

## SDS-PAGE analysis

Samples were prepared in 2× sample loading buffer (final concentration: 62.5 mM Tris–HCl, pH 6.8, 5% glycerol, 3 mM EDTA, 5% SDS, 0.02% bromophenol blue, 4 M urea, 4% β-mercaptoethanol) and boiled for 5 min. Proteins were separated by gel electrophoresis using 10% Bis-TrisNuPAGE gels (Invitrogen). For total protein analysis, gels were stained with GelCode Blue Safe Protein Stain (Thermo Scientific, 24,594) according to the manufacture's protocol.

### *Preparation of synthetic wildtype rαSyn fibrils*

A 100 μL solution of 1 mg/ml WT rαSyn in PBS was subjected to continuous 1000 rpm shaking at 37 °C for 3 days in a 1.5 mL tube. The products were ThT-positive, indicating the presence of amyloid, and the $OD_{280}$ and Western blot comparisons of supernatants before and after centrifugation indicated that > 30% of the total rαSyn was insoluble and therefore aggregated.

### *Brain homogenate preparations*

Brain homogenates (BH; 10% *w/v*) were prepared by homogenizing the tissue in PBS using a Bead Beater (Biospec Products; 11079110z) for 1 min at maximum speed. The homogenate was then spun at 2000 xg for 2 min at room temperature and the supernatant was transferred to a new tube and stored at − 80 °C for αSyn RT-QuIC analysis. For αSyn RT-QuIC testing, BHs were serially diluted in PBS.

### *αSyn RT-QuIC protocol*

RT-QuIC reactions were performed in black 96-well plates with a clear bottom (Nalgene Nunc International). We preloaded plates with 6 glass or silica beads (1 mm in diameter, BioSpec Products or 0.8 mm, OPS Diagnostics, respectively) per well. Silica beads were ultimately chosen over the glass beads because of some occasional batch to batch variability that was observed with the glass beads. For brain homogenate seeded reactions, 2 μL of indicated BH dilutions were added to wells containing 98 μL of the reaction mix to give final concentrations of 40 mM phosphate buffer (pH 8.0), 170 mM NaCl, 0.1 mg/ml of the designated rαSyn (filtered through a 100 kD MWCO filter immediately prior to use), and 10 μM ThT. The plate was then sealed with a plate sealer film (Nalgene Nunc International) and incubated at 42 °C in a BMG FLUOstar Omega plate reader with cycles of 1 min shaking (400 rpm double orbital) and 1 min rest throughout the indicated incubation time. ThT fluorescence measurements (450 +/− 10 nm excitation and 480 +/− 10 nm emission; bottom read) were taken every 45 min. After the initial testing (data in Fig. 1) the fluorimeter gain settings were adjusted to maintain the fluorescence response within the readable range.

In the case of CSF seeded reactions, wells pre-loaded with 6 glass or silica beads were given 85 μL of a reaction mix adjusted to give final reaction concentrations of 40 mM phosphate buffer (pH 8.0), 170 mM NaCl, 0.1 mg/ml rαSyn, 10 μM thioflavin T (ThT) and 0.0015% sodium dodecyl sulfate (SDS) and then 15 μL CSF, or dilutions thereof

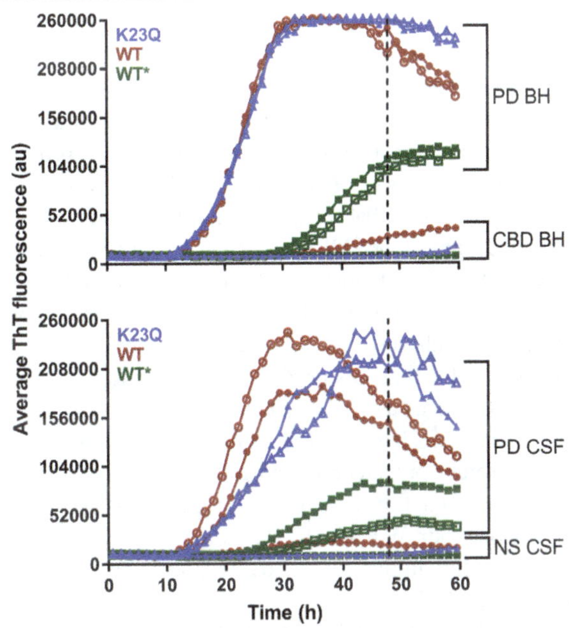


**Fig. 1** Detection of αSyn seeding activity in BH and CSF using K23Q (blue), WT (red) and WT* (green; commercial wild-type rαSyn lacking a 6× histidine tag [7]) substrates. Reactions were seeded in quadruplicate with brain homogenate (BH) (top panel) or CSF (bottom panel) from Parkinson's disease (PD) or non-synucleinopathy (NS) including corticobasal degeneration cases (CBD BH) and healthy donors (NS CSF). For the BH assays, $10^{-3}$ (closed symbols) or $10^{-4}$ (open symbols) brain tissue dilutions from a single PD or NS case were used. For the CSF assays, 15 μl (undiluted) from two PD cases and one NS case was used. Each sample trace represents the average ThT signal of quadruplicate wells. For clarity only every other data point is plotted. The vertical dashed line designates the assay cutoff time used in subsequent analyses

in normal pooled CSF. The reaction plates were subjected to shake-rest cycles as for BH samples above and the reactions classified as RT-QuIC-positive or -negative based on criteria similar to those previously described for RT-QuIC analyses of brain specimens [23, 39]. Briefly, a ThT fluorescence threshold was calculated as the average fluorescence for all samples within the first 10 h of incubation, plus three Standard Deviations (SD). A sample was considered positive overall when at least two of four replicate wells crossed this calculated threshold. When only one of the quadruplicates crossed the threshold, the analysis was repeated.

## Results

### Rapid detection of αSyn$^D$ by αSyn RT-QuIC

In developing our αSyn RT-QuIC, we focused primarily on a recombinant 6× histidine-tagged K23Q mutant of αSyn as a soluble rαSyn substrate for αSyn$^D$-induced fibrillization. Recombinant K23Q αSyn was reported to fibrillize with kinetics similar to wild-type (WT) αSyn when seeded with preformed synthetic WT αSyn fibrils, but was slower to spontaneously fibrillize in the absence of preformed seeds [15]. This latter characteristic, we hypothesized, might improve the sensitivity of an αSyn RT-QuIC assay by enhancing the kinetic distinction between reactions seeded with samples from synucleinopathy cases versus controls. We iteratively optimized the K23Q purification protocol and αSyn RT-QuIC reaction conditions. The best purification protocol to date involves lysis by osmotic shock followed by acid precipitation and sequential metal-ion affinity and ion exchange chromatography steps [28]. No protein impurities were observed by SDS-PAGE analyses of our K23Q mutant rαSyn, our similar preparation of a histidine-tagged WT αSyn, or a commercial wild-type αSyn preparation (without a 6× histidine tag) (WT*) that was used for the previously described αSyn RT-QuIC assay [7] (Additional file 1). However, because lipopolysaccharide (LPS) can contaminate bacterially derived protein preparations and might influence fibrillization, we assayed the three rαSyn preparations and found that whereas our WT and K23Q rαSyn preparations were negative for LPS in this assay (< 0.25 EU/ml), the WT* preparation had ≥ 0.25 EU/ml LPS.

In the αSyn RT-QuIC assay itself, the sample volume, SDS concentration, temperature, bead size and number were particularly influential in improving the speed, sensitivity and specificity of the αSyn RT-QuIC assay for clinical samples (data not shown). Analyses of brain homogenates (BH) and CSF samples from a small initial set of synucleinopathy (PD and DLB) cases and non-synucleinopathy (NS) cases indicated that, whereas the NS brain and CSF specimens gave no positive RT-QuIC reactions above a threshold fluorescence (see Materials and Methods) over the 48-h reaction period, the PD and DLB samples gave positive responses within ~ 18–35 h for BH and ~ 15–24 h for CSF (Figs. 1 and 2; Additional file 2). When prepared in this way, K23Q (Fig. 1, blue traces) and WT rαSyn (red traces) gave similar responses to seeding with PD brain tissue ($10^{-3}$–$10^{-4}$ dilutions; Fig. 1A; Additional file 2) or CSF (15 μl; Fig. 1B; Additional file 2) but the WT rαSyn was more prone to give modest increases in ThT fluorescence in negative control reactions. The WT* rαSyn (green traces), had slower responses and lower maximum ThT fluorescence readings when seeded with PD samples than our WT and K23Q rαSyn substrate preparations. We do not know how the WT* rαSyn was prepared, so either its preparation, its lack of 6× histidine tag, or LPS contamination might be responsible for its weaker responses to seeding compared to our preparations of WT and K23Q rαSyn. With the more rapid PD-seeded reactions with our K23Q or WT rαSyn substrates, we observed decreases in average ThT fluorescence after maximum fluorescence had been achieved. We have observed similar decreases in prion RT-QuIC reactions (e.g. [24]), but their cause has not been determined. Based on these data and the previously published work [15] we have used our K23Q mutant rαSyn preparations in subsequent experiments.

### Blinded analysis of CSF from synucleinopathy cases and controls

We performed blinded analyses of a larger set of CSF specimens obtained *antemortem* from synucleinopathy cases and

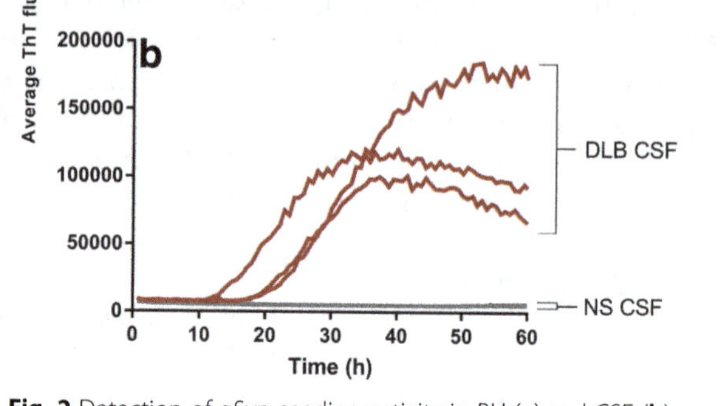


**Fig. 2** Detection of αSyn seeding activity in BH (**a**) and CSF (**b**) from cases with DLB but not non-synucleinopathy cases using K23Q rαSyn. Two μl of $10^{-3}$ dilutions of DLB (red; $n = 3$) or CBD (gray; $n = 3$) BH, or 15 μl (undiluted) CSF from DLB (red; $n = 3$) or healthy donors (NS CSF, gray; $n = 3$) were used per reaction. Each trace represents the average ThT signal of the four replicate wells

controls described in Table 1 and Additional file 3. AD cases ($n = 16$) were included as examples of a neurodegenerative protein misfolding disease that usually, but not always [10], lacks synucleinopathy. As such AD cases were analyzed as a separate category from NS samples. Other types of NS samples, including two progressive supranuclear palsy cases and one corticobasal degeneration case, were also included as controls. For many of the synucleinopathy (PD and DLB) cases, the CSF specimens were collected early in the overall clinical course of disease (Additional file 3). For 8 subjects with PD, the CSF was obtained while motor symptoms and signs were still too mild to warrant treatment with L-dopa or another drug with dopaminergic actions (de novo PD). The consensus diagnosis at follow-up or, if available, the autopsy diagnosis was used as the gold standard diagnosis. Final diagnoses of cases and controls based on 1 year or longer of clinical follow up after the LP, and/or autopsy examination of the brain, was thus used as the final diagnosis (Additional file 3). Two cases (13/020 and 14/045 in Additional file 3) were initially diagnosed with AD but with progression had recurring visual hallucinations that are the most robust of the clinical features that predict DLB. Thus, on follow-up, these cases were given diagnoses of possible DLB.

Almost all of the PD (11/12) and DLB (16/17) CSF samples, including those obtained from the two possible DLB cases, gave positive RT-QuIC responses within 15–35 h (Fig. 3). The average reaction time required to exceed our designated positivity threshold (see Materials and Methods) was similar for the PD and DLB specimens (Fig. 3c). Notably, most of the control cases without any clinical or neuropathological (when available) indication of synucleinopathy were negative in all 4 replicate αSyn RT-QuIC reactions. One case (15/044 in Additional file 3) with a diagnosis of primary progressive aphasia and frontotemporal dementia was positive in 1 of 4 replicate reactions in two independent assays (Fig. 3b; blue "x"). Although it did not meet our criterium of having ≥2 of 4 positive replicate reactions for an overall designation as a positive sample, this case might represent an atypical case of DLB with a clinical diagnosis of primary progressive aphasia [12] with marginally detectable amounts of $\alpha Syn^D$ in the CSF. No $\alpha Syn^D$ was detected by immunostaining in the midfrontal, inferior parietal, and superior temporal cortices, primary visual cortex in the occipital cortex, hippocampus, basal ganglia, substantia nigra and cerebellum; however, this analysis did not include the amygdala, which can be an initial site of $\alpha Syn^D$ accumulation. Thus, while not meeting criteria to be considered positive for $\alpha Syn^D$ seed activity, we cannot rule out the presence of some $\alpha Syn^D$ pathology in this patient at this time.

Overall, the results from this blinded panel indicated diagnostic sensitivities, i.e. the percentage of cases giving positive RT-QuIC responses, of 93% for both PD and DLB. None of the non-synucleinopathy or AD controls met criteria to be considered positive RT-QuIC responses resulting in an apparent specificity of 100%.

### Relative αSyn seeding activities in CSF and brain tissue from PD and DLB cases

To quantify the αSyn RT-QuIC seeding activities in samples from synucleinopathy cases, we performed end-point dilution analyses of frontal cortex brain tissue from representative PD ($n = 1$) and DLB ($n = 3$) cases and CSF samples from 5 DLB cases. All 4 brain samples indicated that positive reactions were obtained out to $10^{-5}$–$10^{-6}$ dilutions of either the PD and DLB tissues (Fig. 4). Positive reactions were obtained from as little as 0.2 μl CSF per reaction well in DLB cases (Fig. 4). Spearman-Kärber analyses [6] provided estimates of the concentrations of seeding activity units giving positive reactions in 50% of replicate reactions, i.e., the 50% "seeding doses" or $SD_{50}$s [39] (Fig. 4). The DLB and PD brain samples contained ~ $10^5$-$10^6$ $SD_{50}$ per mg of tissue while the CSF samples had 4–54 $SD_{50}$s per 15 μl, i.e., our usual sample volume. The latter results indicated that these synucleinopathy CSF specimens had seeding activities that are substantially higher than the minimum detectable level of 1 $SD_{50}$. However, on a per weight basis, seeding activity in brain tissue appeared to be $10^4$–$10^5$-fold higher than the seeding activities measured in PD and DLB CSF specimens (Fig. 4). We note that slightly different conditions were used for the brain homogenate and CSF specimens because neither of the reaction conditions alone was well suited for detecting seeding activity in both types of samples. These

**Table 1** Demographic data and cognitive impairment at the time of lumbar puncture (LP) in studied subjects

| Final diagnosis | n | Age at onset (years) | Age at LP (years) | Mean interval between onset and LP (years) | Sex (M:F) | MMSE[a] |
|---|---|---|---|---|---|---|
| Dementia with Lewy Bodies | 17 | 69.6 ± 7.8 | 73.8 ± 7.8 | 4.2 | 17:2 | 23.0 ± 4.6 |
| Parkinson's Disease | 12 | 63.1 ± 12.0 | 66.0 ± 12.9 | 2.9 | 11:1 | 28.9 ± 1.1 |
| Alzheimer's Disease | 16 | 69.9 ± 9.1 | 73.9 ± 9.1 | 4 | 12:4 | 22.9 ± 3.3 |
| Control[b] | 12 | n/a | 71.3 ± 7.0 | n/a | 4:8 | 28.8 ± 1.2 |
| Other[b] | 3 | 65.7 ± 11.4 | 67.7 ± 10.7 | 2 | 2:1 | 20.5 ± 8.1 |

[a]MMSE: Mini-Mental State Examination, [b]"controls" and "others" were grouped into "non-synucleinopathies" for analysis

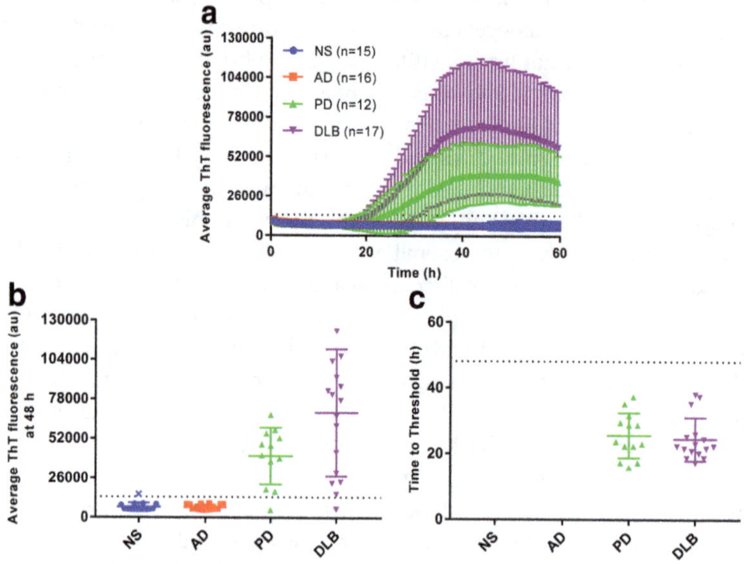


**Fig. 3** Blinded testing of CSF samples by α-synuclein RT-QuIC. Samples from non-synucleinopathy (NS), Alzheimer's disease (AD), dementia with Lewy bodies (DLB) or Parkinson's disease (PD) patients, were tested blinded using the K23Q substrate. Quadruplicate reactions were seeded with 15 μL of CSF. Each sample trace represents the average ThT signal of the four wells. Panel **a** shows the average fluorescence enhancement kinetics for the AD, DLB and PD patients over time along with the associated standard deviation at each time point. Data points in Panel **b** indicate the average fluorescence obtained for each individual case at 48 h. Bars show the average +/− SD for type of case. The dashed line shows the fluorescence threshold for a positive result. Data points in Panel **c** show the hours required for the average fluorescence to exceed the threshold for individual cases. Bars show the average +/− SD for type of case. The dashed line indicates the end of the reaction at 48-h. Blue x symbol indicates sample 15/044 which was tested twice and both times had only one well crossing fluorescence threshold out of the four replicates. This sample was considered negative, as it did not meet our criteria for overall sample positivity (see Materials and Methods)

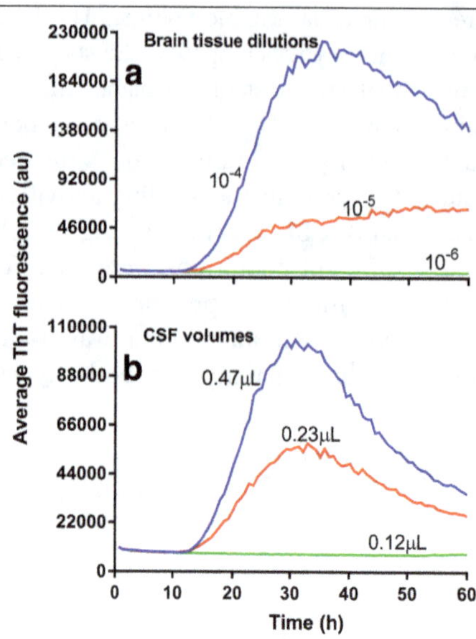


| Disease | Brain sample | $SD_{50}$/mg |
|---|---|---|
| PD | 081017 | $8.89 \times 10^{-4}$ |
| DLB | 2006-005 | $8.89 \times 10^{-5}$ |
| DLB | 2004-016 | $2.81 \times 10^{-6}$ |
| DLB | 2006-020 | $5.00 \times 10^{-6}$ |

| Disease | CSF sample | $SD_{50}$/15μl |
|---|---|---|
| DLB | 10/005 | 54 |
| DLB | 11/037 | 32 |
| DLB | 12/019 | 11 |
| DLB | 12/033 | 5 |
| DLB | 12/046 | 4 |

**Fig. 4** End-point dilutions of synucleinopathy BH (**a**; sample # 081017) or CSF (**b**; sample # 10/005) samples by αSyn RT-QuIC. Each sample trace represents the average ThT signal of quadruplicate wells. Tables to the right of each graph indicate the concentration of $SD_{50}$ units calculated by Spearman-Kärber analysis for these, and additional, cases. End-point dilution experiments used for the additional calculated values shown in the upper and lower panels are provided in Additional files 4 and 5, respectively

different conditions, in addition to differences in absolute seed concentrations, seed characteristics, or sample matrix components, might have affected the relative seeding activities observed in brain and CSF specimens.

### Analytical sensitivity using synthetic αSyn fibrils

Finally, to obtain an indication of the analytical sensitivity of our αSyn RT-QuIC, we prepared synthetic rαSyn fibrils, spiked them into non-synucleinopathy CSF and assayed serial dilutions. As little as 100 ag of the synthetic fibril preparations gave at least 2/4 positive replicate reactions (Fig. 5), which was at least as sensitive analytically as the αSyn PMCA assay [35].

## Discussion

The ability to detect $\alpha Syn^D$ as a causative pathological biomarker for syncleinopathies has important implications in diagnostics, the development of therapeutics, and fundamental studies of $\alpha Syn^D$-based pathogenesis. Recent studies have demonstrated diagnostic utility for αSyn RT-QuIC and closely related αSyn PMCA assays using CSF specimens [7, 35]. Here we present an αSyn RT-QuIC assay with similar diagnostic accuracy but much reduced assay time, i.e. 1–2, rather than 5–13 days. Sano and colleagues detected αSyn seeding activity of DLB brain in 3–4 days [32], but as brain has much higher concentrations of $\alpha Syn^D$ seeding activity than CSF (Fig. 4), it is unclear how well their αSyn RT-QuIC assay would perform with CSF specimens. In any case, our reduced assay time markedly enhances the cost effectiveness and practicality of the αSyn RT-QuIC analyses of CSF. Most of the CSF specimens that we analyzed were collected relatively early in the disease course of the given synucleinopathy. The early detection of $\alpha Syn^D$ is particularly helpful, firstly, because the accuracy of diagnoses based on other clinical indices is poorest in the earlier phases of disease, and, secondly, because the earlier the diagnosis, the earlier that any appropriately targeted therapies can be initiated before further tissue damage is done.

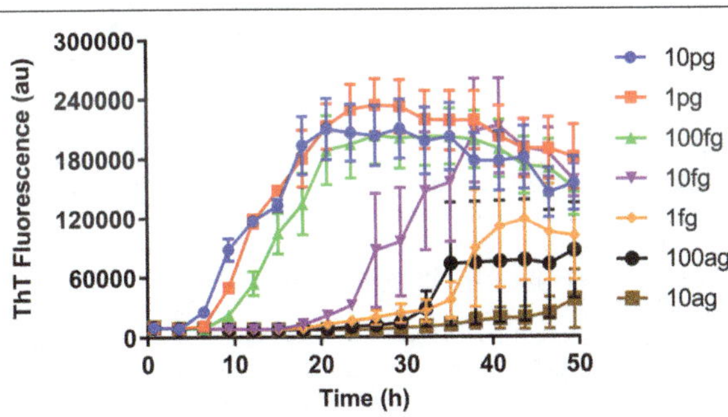


**Fig. 5** End-point dilutions of synthetic seeds spiked into CSF. Synthetic rαSyn fibrils were generated by continuous shaking at 1000 rpm at 37 °C for 3 days in a 1.5 mL tube containing 100 μL of 1 mg/ml WT rαSyn. Samples were monitored by ThT fluorescence. Following fibrilization the samples were spiked into non-synucleinopathy CSF and diluted in 10-fold serial dilutions. Each sample trace represents the average ± SEM ThT signal of quadruplicate wells. For clarity, data points were plotted every fourth point and negative controls, which were all below the positivity threshold, are not displayed

Improvements in the early diagnosis of synucleinopathies should also aid in the selection of suitable patients and controls for therapeutic trials. Furthermore, the ability to serially measure relative levels of $\alpha Syn^D$ in treated and untreated cohorts may provide an alternate means of monitoring the effects of treatments, especially those aimed at reducing the burden of $\alpha Syn^D$ in the brain. Here we have used end-point dilution analysis for quantitation by αSyn RT-QuIC, an approach that has been helpful in many studies using prion RT-QuIC [23, 24, 39]. A potential alternative approach to quantitation from RT-QuIC assays is the comparison of lag phases or times-to-threshold [13, 36] but further studies will be required to document its utility in αSyn RT-QuIC analyses of various specimen types.

Consistent with previous findings for αSyn PMCA [35], αSyn RT-QuIC is capable of detecting subfemtogram amounts of rαSyn fibrils that are orders of magnitude less than those required for more conventional assays such as Western blotting and ELISA, with typical detection limits for total levels of αSyn, in the ng and pg range, respectively. The αSyn RT-QuIC, however, detects only the forms of $\alpha Syn^D$ capable of seeding further αSyn misfolding. How our αSyn RT-QuIC sensitivity for synthetic rαSyn amyloid seeds relates to its absolute sensitivity for any given form of $\alpha Syn^D$ in tissues is difficult to determine accurately because different forms of $\alpha Syn^D$ may have different seeding capacities per unit mass. Nonetheless, based on the average kinetics of seeding using PD or DLB CSF in Fig. 3, one might estimate femtogram levels of seeding capable $\alpha Syn^D$ may exist in the CSF of PD or DLB patient when compared to the synthetic rαSyn amyloid seeding kinetics in Fig. 5. Furthermore, the difference in the average kinetics of seeding using PD or DLB CSF may be indicative of a "strain" difference, similar to what has been observed from CSF samples from different types of CJD cases in prion RT-QuIC reactions [8, 25]. While the difference in the average kinetics is statistically significant (Welch's t-test, $p < 0.02$) between the two seed types, at this point we do not know the basis for this difference, or whether it might be diagnostically useful. It could be due to differences in average seed concentration or seed characteristics, such as potential structural differences between PD and DLB seeds, that contribute to kinetic differences in the αSyn RT-QuIC responses. Testing of much higher numbers of PD and DLB samples is required to discern whether the difference in kinetics is maintained and if it is of diagnostic or mechanistic importance.

As our assay evolved, we saw evidence that several factors, such as sample volume, SDS concentration, temperature, and silica beads, strongly influenced the performance of the assay. However, at present we cannot be sure of the relative importance of these factors individually in allowing the assay to be substantially faster than previously described αSyn RT-QuIC or PMCA assays. Further testing will be necessary to better understand i) the breadth of synucleinopathies that are detected and/or discriminated by αSyn RT-QuIC assays, ii) the diagnostic sensitivities and specificities in clinical settings, iii) the extent to which levels of αSyn seeding activity in CSF or other diagnostic specimens correlates with disease prognosis, and iv) the relevance of $\alpha Syn^D$ seeding activity as a biomarker in therapeutic trials.

## Conclusions

Compared to previously described aSynD seed amplification assays, the use of the raSyn substrate preparation, RT-QuIC reaction conditions, and end-point dilution assays that we describe here allowed for much more rapid detection and quantitation of aSyn seeding activity in CSF of patients with PD and DLB without reductions in diagnostic sensitivity or specificity.

## Additional files

**Additional file 1:** Example of K23Q purification chromatograph, and total protein staining of collected fractions and of the commercial wild-type αSyn (WT*), and our preparation of the WT and K23Q rαSyn substrates. Absorbance spectra (blue) and buffer B gradients (green) for purification of K23Q using a Ni-NTA column (A and B) followed by a Q-HP column (C and D). Arrow in A denotes a peak representing contaminants. Dashed boxes in A and C denote the zoomed regions depicted in B and D. The * in C and D denote contaminants. The red vertical lines in B delineate the peak collected from the Ni-NTA column between 30 and 75% of buffer B1 (containing 100 and 350 mM imidazole, respectively) for further purification on the Q-HP column. The red lines in D indicate the peak collected from the Q-HP column between 30 and 35% of buffer B2 (containing 300 and 350 mM NaCl, respectively) to be used for dialysis and lyophilization. Panels E and F are a total protein Coomassie Blue staining of fractions collected from the Ni-NTA and Q-HP column, respectively. Panel G shows a comparative total protein Coomassie Blue staining of 2 µg of the commercial wild-type αSyn (WT*), and both of our WT and K23Q rαSyn substrate preparations. The staining intensity and apparent molecular weight of the WT* differs from our prepared WT and K23Q due to the lack of a poly-histidine tag [37], therefore a 5-fold higher amount of WT* was run in panel H to investigate for potential contaminants with a higher intensity staining. (TIFF 5283 kb)

**Additional file 2:** Detection of αSyn seeding activity in BH and CSF using K23Q (blue), WT (red) and WT* (green; commercial wild-type rαSyn lacking a 6× histidine tag [7]) substrates as described in Fig. 1 but with standard deviation. For clarity error bars are only displayed in one direction. (TIFF 1254 kb)

**Additional file 3:** Demographic and clinical information for subjects of this study. (XLSX 17 kb)

**Additional file 4:** αSyn RT-QuIC end-point dilution analysis of one Parkinson's (PD; 081017) and three dementia with Lewy bodies (DLB; 2004–16, 2006–005 and 2006–020) brain samples listed in Fig. 4. Reactions were seeded in quadruplicate with two µl of either a $10^{-4}$, $10^{-5}$, $10^{-6}$ or a $10^{-7}$ brain homogenate (BH) dilutions. Each sample trace represents the average ThT signal of quadruplicate wells. (TIFF 852 kb)

**Additional file 5:** End-point dilutions by αSyn RT-QuIC of synucleinopathy CSF samples listed in Fig. 4. Each sample trace represents the average ThT signal of quadruplicate wells. Traces represent 15 (Blue), 7.5 (Red), 3.75 (Green), 1.89 (Purple), 0.94 (Orange), 0.47 (Black), 0.2 (Brown) and 0.1 (Dark Blue) µL of DLBD CSF diluted into normal pooled CSF, when needed, to give overall CSF sample volumes of 15 µL. (TIFF 1383 kb)

**Acknowledgements**

This work was supported in part by the Intramural Research Program of the NIAID, NIH (BC), NIH grant AG05131 (DG), the Parkinson's and Movement Disorder Foundation (BRG), the Shiley-Marcos Alzheimer's Disease Research Center at UCSD (DG), and PHS P30-AG010133 (BG). BRG, CDO, AGH and BC are inventors on a related U.S. Patent pending No. 62/567,079. The authors thank Dr. Daniel Otzen and Cagla Sahin, Aarhus University, Denmark for advice on purification, and Dr. Suzette Priola, Dr. Cathryn Haigh, and Michael Metrick for critical evaluation of this manuscript. We also thank Dr. Christina Sigurdson for establishing contact between BC and DG that made this project possible.

**Authors' contributions**

BC and DG oversaw the project. BRG, CO, LR and AH designed, performed, and helped interpret experiments. DG, GZ and BG provided clinical specimens. BC, BRG, CO, and DG drafted the initial manuscript. All authors read, helped to edit, and approved the final manuscript.

**Competing interests**

BRG, CO, AH, LR and BC are named as inventors on a US provisional patent application related to the technology described herein (see Acknowledgements). The other authors declare that they have no other competing interests.

**Author details**

[1]Laboratory of Persistent Viral Diseases, Rocky Mountain Laboratories, National Institute of Allergy and Infectious Diseases, National Institutes of Health, Hamilton, MT, USA. [2]Department of Neurosciences, Biomedicine and Movement Sciences, University of Verona, Verona, Italy. [3]Indiana University School of Medicine, Indianapolis, IN, USA. [4]Department of Pathology, Case Western Reserve University School of Medicine, Cleveland, OH, USA. [5]Department of Neurosciences, University of California-San Diego, La Jolla, CA, USA.

**References**

1. Adler CH, Beach TG, Hentz JG, Shill HA, Caviness JN, Driver-Dunckley E, Sabbagh MN, Sue LI, Jacobson SA, Belden CM et al (2014) Low clinical diagnostic accuracy of early vs advanced Parkinson disease: clinicopathologic study. Neurology 83:406–412. https://doi.org/10.1212/WNL.0000000000000641
2. Atarashi R, Satoh K, Sano K, Fuse T, Yamaguchi N, Ishibashi D, Matsubara T, Nakagaki T, Yamanaka H, Shirabe S et al (2011) Ultrasensitive human prion detection in cerebrospinal fluid by real-time quaking-induced conversion. Nat Med 17:175–178. https://doi.org/10.1038/nm.2294
3. Bernis ME, Babila JT, Breid S, Wusten KA, Wullner U, Tamguney G (2015) Prion-like propagation of human brain-derived alpha-synuclein in transgenic mice expressing human wild-type alpha-synuclein. Acta Neuropathol Commun 3:75. https://doi.org/10.1186/s40478-015-0254-7
4. Bongianni M, Orrù CD, Groveman BR, Sacchetto L, Fiorini M, Tonoli G, Triva G, Capaldi S, Testi S, Ferrari S et al (2017) Diagnosis of human Prion disease using real-time quaking-induced conversion testing of olfactory mucosa and cerebrospinal fluid samples. JAMA Neurology 74:1–8
5. Cramm M, Schmitz M, Karch A, Zafar S, Varges D, Mitrova E, Schroeder B, Raeber A, Kuhn F, Zerr I (2015) Characteristic CSF prion seeding efficiency in

humans with prion diseases. Mol Neurobiol 51:396–405. https://doi.org/10.1007/s12035-014-8709-6

6. Dougherty RM (1964) Animal virus titration techniques. In: Harris RJC (ed) Techniques in experimental virology. Academic Press, Inc., City, pp 183–186
7. Fairfoul G, McGuire LI, Pal S, Ironside JW, Neumann J, Christie S, Joachim C, Esiri M, Evetts SG, Rolinski M et al (2016) Alpha-synuclein RT-QuIC in the CSF of patients with alpha-synucleinopathies. Ann Clin Transl Neurol 3:812–818. https://doi.org/10.1002/acn3.338
8. Foutz A, Appleby BS, Hamlin C, Liu X, Yang S, Cohen Y, Chen W, Blevins J, Fausett C, Wang H et al (2017) Diagnostic and prognostic value of human prion detection in cerebrospinal fluid. Ann Neurol 81:79–92. https://doi.org/10.1002/ana.24833
9. Fox BG, Blommel PG (2009) Autoinduction of protein expression. Curr Protocols Protein Sci 56:5.23:5.23.1–5.23.18. https://doi.org/10.1002/0471140864.ps0523s56
10. Galvin JE, Lee VM, Trojanowski JQ (2001) Synucleinopathies: clinical and pathological implications. Arch Neurol 58:186–190
11. Graff-Radford J, Aakre J, Savica R, Boeve B, Kremers WK, Ferman TJ, Jones DT, Kantarci K, Knopman DS, Dickson DW et al (2017) Duration and pathologic correlates of Lewy body disease. JAMA Neurol 74:310–315. https://doi.org/10.1001/jamaneurol.2016.4926
12. Grossman M (2010) Primary progressive aphasia: clinicopathological correlations. Nat Rev Neurol 6:88–97. https://doi.org/10.1038/nrneurol.2009.216
13. Henderson DM, Davenport KA, Haley NJ, Denkers ND, Mathiason CK, Hoover EA (2015) Quantitative assessment of prion infectivity in tissues and body fluids by real-time quaking-induced conversion. J Gen Virol 96:210–219. https://doi.org/10.1099/vir.0.069906-0
14. John TR, Schatzl HM, Gilch S (2013) Early detection of chronic wasting disease prions in urine of pre-symptomatic deer by real-time quaking-induced conversion assay. Prion 7:253–258. https://doi.org/10.4161/pri.24430
15. Koo HJ, Lee HJ, Im H (2008) Sequence determinants regulating fibrillation of human alpha-synuclein. Biochem Biophys Res Commun 368:772–778. https://doi.org/10.1016/j.bbrc.2008.01.140
16. Litvan I, Goldman JG, Troster AI, Schmand BA, Weintraub D, Petersen RC, Mollenhauer B, Adler CH, Marder K, Williams-Gray CH et al (2012) Diagnostic criteria for mild cognitive impairment in Parkinson's disease: Movement Disorder Society task force guidelines. Mov Disord 27:349–356. https://doi.org/10.1002/mds.24893
17. McGuire LI, Peden AH, Orru CD, Wilham JM, Appleford NE, Mallinson G, Andrews M, Head MW, Caughey B, Will RG et al (2012) RT-QuIC analysis of cerebrospinal fluid in sporadic Creutzfeldt-Jakob disease. Ann Neurol 72:278–285
18. McKeith IG, Ballard CG, Perry RH, Ince PG, O'Brien JT, Neill D, Lowery K, Jaros E, Barber R, Thompson P et al (2000) Prospective validation of consensus criteria for the diagnosis of dementia with Lewy bodies. Neurology 54:1050–1058
19. McKeith IG, Dickson DW, Lowe J, Emre M, O'Brien JT, Feldman H, Cummings J, Duda JE, Lippa C, Perry EK et al (2005) Diagnosis and management of dementia with Lewy bodies: third report of the DLB consortium. Neurology 65:1863–1872. https://doi.org/10.1212/01.wnl.0000187889.17253.b1
20. Merdes AR, Hansen LA, Jeste DV, Galasko D, Hofstetter CR, Ho GJ, Thal LJ, Corey-Bloom J (2003) Influence of Alzheimer pathology on clinical diagnostic accuracy in dementia with Lewy bodies. Neurology 60:1586–1590
21. Mollenhauer B, Batrla R, El-Agnaf O, Galasko DR, Lashuel HA, Merchant KM, Shaw LM, Selkoe DJ, Umek R, Vanderstichele H et al (2017) A user's guide for alpha-synuclein biomarker studies in biological fluids: Perianalytical considerations. Mov Disord. https://doi.org/10.1002/mds.27090
22. Montine TJ, Phelps CH, Beach TG, Bigio EH, Cairns NJ, Dickson DW, Duyckaerts C, Frosch MP, Masliah E, Mirra SS et al (2012) National Institute on Aging-Alzheimer's Association guidelines for the neuropathologic assessment of Alzheimer's disease: a practical approach. Acta Neuropathol 123:1–11. https://doi.org/10.1007/s00401-011-0910-3
23. Orru CD, Bongianni M, Tonoli G, Ferrari S, Hughson AG, Groveman BR, Fiorini M, Pocchiari M, Monaco S, Caughey B et al (2014) A test for Creutzfeldt-Jakob disease using nasal brushings. New Engl J Med 371:519–529
24. Orru CD, Groveman BR, Hughson AG, Zanusso G, Coulthart MB, Caughey B (2015) Rapid and sensitive RT-QuIC detection of human Creutzfeldt-Jakob disease using cerebrospinal fluid. MBio 6. https://doi.org/10.1128/mBio.02451-14
25. Orru CD, Groveman BR, Raymond LD, Hughson AG, Nonno R, Zou W, Ghetti B, Gambetti P, Caughey B (2015) Bank vole Prion protein as an apparently universal substrate for RT-QuIC-based detection and discrimination of Prion strains. PLoS Path 11:e1004983. https://doi.org/10.1371/journal.ppat.1004983
26. Orru CD, Wilham JM, Raymond LD, Kuhn F, Schroeder B, Raeber AJ, Caughey B (2011) Prion disease blood test using immunoprecipitation and improved quaking-induced conversion. mBio 2: e00078–00011 doi: https://doi.org/10.1128/mBio.00078-11
27. Parnetti L, Castrioto A, Chiasserini D, Persichetti E, Tambasco N, El-Agnaf O, Calabresi P (2013) Cerebrospinal fluid biomarkers in Parkinson disease. Nat Rev Neurol 9:131–140. https://doi.org/10.1038/nrneurol.2013.10
28. Paslawski W, Lorenzen N, Otzen DE (2016) Formation and characterization of alpha-Synuclein Oligomers. Methods Mol Biol 1345:133–150. https://doi.org/10.1007/978-1-4939-2978-8_9
29. Peden AH, McGuire LI, Appleford NE, Mallinson G, Wilham JM, Orru CD, Caughey B, Ironside JW, Knight RS, Will RG et al (2012) Sensitive and specific detection of sporadic Creutzfeldt-Jakob disease brain prion protein using real-time quaking induced conversion. J GenVirol 93:438–449. https://doi.org/10.1099/vir.0.033365-0
30. Postuma RB, Berg D, Stern M, Poewe W, Olanow CW, Oertel W, Obeso J, Marek K, Litvan I, Lang AE et al (2015) MDS clinical diagnostic criteria for Parkinson's disease. Mov Disord 30:1591–1601. https://doi.org/10.1002/mds.26424
31. Sancesario GM, Bernardini S (2015) How many biomarkers to discriminate neurodegenerative dementia? Crit Rev Clin Lab Sci 52:314–326. https://doi.org/10.3109/10408363.2015.1051658
32. Sano K, Atarashi R, Satoh K, Ishibashi D, Nakagaki T, Iwasaki Y, Yoshida M, Murayama S, Mishima K, Nishida N (2017) Prion-like seeding of Misfolded alpha-Synuclein in the brains of dementia with Lewy body patients in RT-QUIC. Mol Neurobiol. https://doi.org/10.1007/s12035-017-0624-1
33. Sano K, Satoh K, Atarashi R, Takashima H, Iwasaki Y, Yoshida M, Sanjo N, Murai H, Mizusawa H, Schmitz M et al (2013) Early detection of abnormal prion protein in genetic human prion diseases now possible using real-time QUIC assay. PLoS One 8:e54915. https://doi.org/10.1371/journal.pone.0054915
34. Schneider JA, Arvanitakis Z, Leurgans SE, Bennett DA (2009) The neuropathology of probable Alzheimer disease and mild cognitive impairment. Ann Neurol 66:200–208. https://doi.org/10.1002/ana.21706
35. Shahnawaz M, Tokuda T, Waragai M, Mendez N, Ishii R, Trenkwalder C, Mollenhauer B, Soto C (2017) Development of a biochemical diagnosis of Parkinson disease by detection of alpha-Synuclein Misfolded aggregates in cerebrospinal fluid. JAMA Neurol 74:163–172. https://doi.org/10.1001/jamaneurol.2016.4547
36. Shi S, Mitteregger-Kretzschmar G, Giese A, Kretzschmar HA (2013) Establishing quantitative real-time quaking-induced conversion (qRT-QuIC) for highly sensitive detection and quantification of PrPSc in prion-infected tissues. Acta Neuropathol Commun 1:44. https://doi.org/10.1186/2051-5960-1-44
37. Tal M, Silberstein A, Nusser E (1985) Why does Coomassie brilliant blue R interact differently with different proteins? A partial answer. J Biol Chem 260:9976–9980
38. Vascellari S, Orru CD, Hughson AG, King D, Barron R, Wilham JM, Baron GS, Race B, Pani A, Caughey B (2012) Prion seeding activities of mouse scrapie strains with divergent PrPSc protease sensitivities and amyloid plaque content using RT-QuIC and eQuIC. PLoS One 7:e48969. https://doi.org/10.1371/journal.pone.0048969
39. Wilham JM, Orrú CD, Bessen RA, Atarashi R, Sano K, Race B, Meade-White KD, Taubner LM, Timmes A, Caughey B (2010) Rapid end-point Quantitation of Prion seeding activity with sensitivity comparable to bioassays. PLoS Path 6:e1001217. https://doi.org/10.1371/journal.ppat.1001217
40. Zanusso G, Bongianni M, Caughey B (2014) A test for Creutzfeldt-Jakob disease using nasal brushings. N Engl J Med 371:1842–1843. https://doi.org/10.1056/NEJMc1410732
41. Zanusso G, Monaco S, Pocchiari M, Caughey B (2016) Advanced tests for early and accurate diagnosis of Creutzfeldt-Jakob disease. Nat Rev Neurol 12:325–333. https://doi.org/10.1038/nrneurol.2016.65

# Permissions

All chapters in this book were first published in ANC, by BioMed Central; hereby published with permission under the Creative Commons Attribution License or equivalent. Every chapter published in this book has been scrutinized by our experts. Their significance has been extensively debated. The topics covered herein carry significant findings which will fuel the growth of the discipline. They may even be implemented as practical applications or may be referred to as a beginning point for another development.

The contributors of this book come from diverse backgrounds, making this book a truly international effort. This book will bring forth new frontiers with its revolutionizing research information and detailed analysis of the nascent developments around the world.

We would like to thank all the contributing authors for lending their expertise to make the book truly unique. They have played a crucial role in the development of this book. Without their invaluable contributions this book wouldn't have been possible. They have made vital efforts to compile up to date information on the varied aspects of this subject to make this book a valuable addition to the collection of many professionals and students.

This book was conceptualized with the vision of imparting up-to-date information and advanced data in this field. To ensure the same, a matchless editorial board was set up. Every individual on the board went through rigorous rounds of assessment to prove their worth. After which they invested a large part of their time researching and compiling the most relevant data for our readers.

The editorial board has been involved in producing this book since its inception. They have spent rigorous hours researching and exploring the diverse topics which have resulted in the successful publishing of this book. They have passed on their knowledge of decades through this book. To expedite this challenging task, the publisher supported the team at every step. A small team of assistant editors was also appointed to further simplify the editing procedure and attain best results for the readers.

Apart from the editorial board, the designing team has also invested a significant amount of their time in understanding the subject and creating the most relevant covers. They scrutinized every image to scout for the most suitable representation of the subject and create an appropriate cover for the book.

The publishing team has been an ardent support to the editorial, designing and production team. Their endless efforts to recruit the best for this project, has resulted in the accomplishment of this book. They are a veteran in the field of academics and their pool of knowledge is as vast as their experience in printing. Their expertise and guidance has proved useful at every step. Their uncompromising quality standards have made this book an exceptional effort. Their encouragement from time to time has been an inspiration for everyone.

The publisher and the editorial board hope that this book will prove to be a valuable piece of knowledge for researchers, students, practitioners and scholars across the globe.

# List of Contributors

**Zsolt Datki, Zita Olah, Lilla Macsai, Amanda Szarvas and Janos Kalman**
Department of Psychiatry, Faculty of Medicine, University of Szeged, Kalvaria sgt. 57, Szeged H-6725, Hungary

**Tibor Hortobagyi**
MTA-DE Cerebrovascular and Neurodegenerative Research Group, Department of Neuropathology, Institute of Pathology, University of Debrecen, Debrecen H-4012, Hungary
Department of Old Age Psychiatry, Institute of Psychiatry Psychology & Neuroscience, King's College London, De Crespigny Park, Denmark Hill, London SE5 8AF, UK

**Katalin Zsuga**
Agrint Kft., Facan sor 56, Godollo H-2100, Hungary

**Livia Fulop and Zsolt Bozso**
Department of Medical Chemistry, Faculty of Medicine, University of Szeged, Semmelweis u. 6, Szeged H-6725, Hungary

**Bence Galik**
Bioinformatics & Scientific Computing, Vienna Biocentre Core Facilities, Dr. Bohr-Gasse 3, 1030 Vienna, Austria

**Eva Acs**
Danube Research Institute, MTA Centre for Ecological Research, Karolina ut 29-31, Budapest H-1113, Hungary

**Angela Foldi**
Sustainable Ecosystems Group, MTA Centre for Ecological Research, Klebelsberg Kuno u. 3, Tihany H-8237, Hungary

**Simon Dujardin, Séverine Bégard, Raphaëlle Caillierez, Cédrick Lachaud, Sébastien Carrier, Sarah Lieger, Vincent Deramecourt, Claude-Alain Maurage, Morvane Colin and Luc Buée**
Univ. Lille, Inserm, CHU-Lille, UMR-S 1172, Alzheimer & Tauopathies, School of Medicine, 1 rue Polonovski, 59045 Lille, France

**Matthew P. Frosch, Simon Dujardin, Jose A. Gonzalez and Bradley T. Hyman**
Department of Neurology, Massachusetts General Hospital, MassGeneral Institute of Neurodegenerative Diseases (MIND), Charlestown, MA, USA
Department of Neurology, Harvard Medical School, Boston, MA, USA

**Nicole Déglon**
Lausanne University Hospital (CHUV), Neuroscience Research Center (CRN), Laboratory of Neurotherapies and Neuromodulation (LNTM), CH-1011 Lausanne, Switzerland

**Christian Klein, Guy Roussel, Susana Brun, Cristina Rusu, Christine Patte-Mensah, Michel Maitre and Ayikoe-Guy Mensah-Nyagan**
Biopathologie de la Myéline, Neuroprotection et Stratégies Thérapeutiques, INSERM U1119, Fédération de Médecine Translationnelle de Strasbourg (FMTS), Université de Strasbourg, Bâtiment 3 de la Faculté de Médecine, Strasbourg, France

**Yuriko Katsumata and David W. Fardo**
Department of Biostatistics, University of Kentucky, 725 Rose Street, Lexington, KY 40536, USA
Sanders-Brown Center on Aging, University of Kentucky, Lexington, KY 40536, USA

**Walter A. Kukull**
National Alzheimer's Coordinating Center, Department of Epidemiology, University of Washington, Seattle, WA 98105, USA

**Peter T. Nelson**
Department of Pathology, Division of Neuropathology, University of Kentucky, Lexington, KY 40536, USA
Sanders-Brown Center on Aging, University of Kentucky, Lexington, KY 40536, USA

**Jun-ichi Kuratsu**
Department of Neurosurgery, Sakurajuji Hospital, Kumamoto, Japan

**Stefanie Beck-Wödl, Marc Sturm, Rebecca Buchert and Olaf Rieß**
Department of Medical Genetics and Applied Genomics, University of Tübingen, Tübingen, Germany

**Klaus Harzer**
Department of Neuropediatrics and Neurometabolic Laboratory, Children's Hospital of the University of Tübingen, Tübingen, Germany

**Elisabeth Latta**
Department of Pediatrics, University Hospital of Marburg, Marburg, Germany

**Hans-Dieter Mennel, Axel Pagenstecher and Ursula Keber**
Department of Neuropathology, Philipps University and University Hospital of Marburg, Baldingerstrasse, 35043 Marburg, Germany

**Christina Moloney, Sruti Rayaprolu, John Howard, Susan Fromholt, Hilda Brown, Matt Collins, Mariela Cabrera, Colin Duffy, Zoe Siemienski and Dave Miller**
Center for Translational Research in Neurodegenerative Disease, University of Florida, Gainesville, Florida, USA
Department of Neuroscience, University of Florida, Gainesville, Florida, USA

**David R. Borchelt and Jada Lewis**
McKnight Brain Institute, Department of Neuroscience, University of Florida, Gainesville, Florida, USA

**Naoki Shinojima, Kenji Fujimoto, Keishi Makino, Kazumichi Yamada, Hideo Nakamura, Shigetoshi Yano and Akitake Mukasa**
Department of Neurosurgery, Kumamoto University Hospital, 1-1-1 Honjo Chuo-ku, Kumamoto 860- 8556, Japan

**Kohei Todaka**
School of Medicine, Kumamoto University, Kumamoto, Japan

**Yoshiki Mikami**
Department of Diagnostic Pathology, Kumamoto University Hospital, Kumamoto, Japan

**Kazutaka Oda, Kazumi Nakamura and Hirofumi Jono**
Department of Pharmacy, Kumamoto University Hospital, Kumamoto, Japan

**Melissa C. Wren and Erik Årstad**
Institute of Nuclear Medicine and Department of Chemistry, University College London, London, UK

**Tammaryn Lashley**
Institute of Neurology, Department of Molecular Neuroscience, Queen Square Brain Bank for Neurological Disorders, University College London, London, UK

**Kerstin Sander**
Radiochemistry, University College London, Kathleen Lonsdale Building, 5 Gower Place,London WC1E 6BS, UK

**Caterina Giacomini, Chuay-Yeng Koo, Ignatius A. Tavares and Jonathan D. H. Morris**
King's College London, School of Cancer and Pharmaceutical Sciences, New Hunt's House, Guy's Campus, London SE11UL, UK

**Natalia Yankova, Wendy Noble and Diane P. Hanger**
King's College London, Department of Basic and Clinical Neuroscience, Maurice Wohl Clinical Neuroscience Institute, Institute of Psychiatry, Psychology & Neuroscience, 5 Cutcombe Road, London SE59RX, UK

**Selina Wray**
UCL Institute of Neurology, Department of Molecular Neuroscience, University College London, 1 Wakefield Street, London WC1N1PJ, UK

**Tamar E. Sztal, Emily A. McKaige, Caitlin Williams and Robert J. Bryson-Richardson**
School of Biological Sciences, Monash University, Melbourne, Australia

**Viola Oorschot**
Monash Ramaciotti Centre for Cryo Electron Microscopy, Monash University, Melbourne, VIC 3800, Australia
Department of Biochemistry and Molecular Biology, Monash University, Melbourne, Australia
Biomedicine Discovery Institute, Monash University, Melbourne, Australia

**Sharon X. Xie**
Perelman School of Medicine (PSOM) at the University of Pennsylvania, Philadelphia, PA, USA

**Gabor G. Kovacs**
Institute of Neurology, Medical University of Vienna, AKH 4J, Währinger Gürtel 18-20, 1097 Vienna, Austria
Center for Neurodegenerative Disease Research (CNDR), Institute on Aging and Department of Pathology & Laboratory Medicine, Perelman School of Medicine (PSOM) at the University of Pennsylvania, HUP Maloney 3rd Floor, 36th and Spruce Street, Philadelphia, PA 19104 - 4283, USA

**John L. Robinson, Edward B. Lee, Theresa Schuck, Virginia M.-Y. Lee and John Q. Trojanowski**
Center for Neurodegenerative Disease Research (CNDR), Institute on Aging and Department of Pathology & Laboratory Medicine, Perelman School of Medicine (PSOM) at the University of Pennsylvania, HUP Maloney 3rd Floor, 36th and Spruce Street, Philadelphia, PA 19104 - 4283, USA

**Douglas H. Smith**
Department of Neurosurgery, Center for Brain Injury and Repair, the Perelman School of Medicine (PSOM) at the University of Pennsylvania, Philadelphia, PA, USA

**P. S. Zeiner**
Edinger Institute (Institute of Neurology), Goethe-University, Heinrich-Hoffmann-Str. 7, D-60528 Frankfurt am Main, Germany
Dr. Senckenberg Institute of Neurooncology, Goethe-University, Frankfurt am Main, Germany

**J. Zinke, S. Bernatz, K. H. Plate and P. N. Harter**
Edinger Institute (Institute of Neurology), Goethe-University, Heinrich-Hoffmann-Str. 7, D-60528 Frankfurt am Main, Germany
German Cancer Research Center DKFZ Heidelberg, Germany and German Cancer Consortium DKTK partner site, Frankfurt/Mainz, Germany

**J. Tichy, M. W. Ronellenfitsch and P. Steinbach**
Dr. Senckenberg Institute of Neurooncology, Goethe-University, Frankfurt am Main, Germany

**S. Stefanović**
Department of Immunology, Institute for Cell Biology, University of Tuebingen, Tuebingen, Germany

**D. J. Kowalewski**
Immatics Biotechnologies GmbH, Tübingen, Germany
Department of Immunology, Institute for Cell Biology, University of Tuebingen, Tuebingen, Germany

**F. Thorsen**
Department of Biomedicine, The Kristian Gerhard Jebsen Brain Tumour Research Center and The Molecular Imaging Center, University of Bergen, Bergen, Norway

**A. Berger**
Institute for Virology Goethe-University, Frankfurt am Main, Germany

**M. T. Forster**
Department of Neurosurgery, Goethe-University, Frankfurt am Main, Germany

**A. Muller**
Department of Oncology, Luxembourg Institute of Health, Luxembourg, Luxembourg

**R. Beschorner**
Department of Pathology and Neuropathology, University of Tuebingen, Tuebingen, Germany

**J. Wischhusen**
Department of Gynecology, University of Wuerzburg, Wuerzburg, Germany

**H. M. Kvasnicka**
Goethe-University, Dr. Senckenberg Institute for Pathology, Frankfurt am Main, Germany

**B. Weide**
Department of Dermatology, University of Tuebingen, Tuebingen, Germany

**William Davidsson, Fausto Chiazza, David Nathanson, Hiranya Pintana, Thomas Nyström, Vladimer Darsalia and Cesare Patrone**
Department of Clinical Science and Education, Södersjukhuset, Internal Medicine, Karolinska Institutet, Stockholm, Sweden

**Josefin Skogsberg**
Boehringer Ingelheim AB, Stockholm, Sweden

**M. Mittelbronn**
Luxembourg Centre of Neuropathology (LCNP), 3555 Dudelange, Luxembourg. Laboratoire National de Santé, Department of Pathology, 3555 Dudelange, Luxembourg
Luxembourg Centre for Systems Biomedicine (LCSB), University of Luxembourg, 4361 Esch-sur-Alzette, Luxembourg
NORLUX Neuro-Oncology Laboratory, Department of Oncology, Luxembourg Institute of Health (L.I.H.), 1526 Luxembourg, Luxembourg

**Claes-Göran Östenson**
Department of Molecular Medicine and Surgery, Karolinska Institutet, Stockholm, Sweden

**Grazyna Lietzau**
Department of Anatomy and Neurobiology, Medical University of Gdansk, Gdansk, Poland
Department of Clinical Science and Education, Södersjukhuset, Internal Medicine, Karolinska Institutet, Stockholm, Sweden

**Thomas Klein**
Boehringer Ingelheim Pharma GmbH & Co. KG, Biberach, Germany

**Juan Carlos Polanco, Chuanzhou Li and Jürgen Götz**
Clem Jones Centre for Ageing Dementia Research (CJCADR), Queensland Brain Institute (QBI), The University of Queensland, Brisbane, QLD 4072, Australia

**Nela Durisic and Robert Sullivan**
Queensland Brain Institute (QBI), The University of Queensland, Brisbane, QLD 4072, Australia

**Anssi Lipponen, Vicente Navarro-Ferrandis, Noora Puhakka and Asla Pitkänen**
Epilepsy Research Laboratory, A. I. Virtanen Institute for Molecular Sciences, University of Eastern Finland, FIN-70211 Kuopio, Finland

**Antony Kaspi, Mark Ziemann, Ishant Khurana and Harikrishnan KN**
Epigenetics in Human Health and Disease Laboratory, Central Clinical School, Faculty of Medicine, Monash University, Melbourne, VIC, Australia

**Assam El-Osta**
Prince of Wales Hospital, The Chinese University of Hong Kong, Sha Tin, Hong Kong SAR

**Jussi Paananen**
Institute of Biomedicine, University of Eastern Finland, Kuopio, Finland
University of Eastern Finland Bioinformatics Center, University of Eastern Finland, Kuopio, Finland

**Bradley R. Groveman, Christina D. Orrù, Andrew G. Hughson, Lynne D. Raymond, Katrina J. Campbell and Byron Caughey**
Laboratory of Persistent Viral Diseases, Rocky Mountain Laboratories, National Institute of Allergy and Infectious Diseases, National Institutes of Health, Hamilton, MT, USA

**Gianluigi Zanusso**
Department of Neurosciences, Biomedicine and Movement Sciences, University of Verona, Verona, Italy

**Bernardino Ghetti**
Indiana University School of Medicine, Indianapolis, IN, USA

**Jiri Safar**
Department of Pathology, Case Western Reserve University School of Medicine, Cleveland, OH, USA

**Douglas Galasko**
Department of Neurosciences, University of California-San Diego, La Jolla, CA, USA

# Index

www.ingramcontent.com/pod-product-compliance
Lightning Source LLC
LaVergne TN
LVHW080712210926
848485LV00003B/452